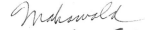

a **LANGE** medical book

Genetics in Primary Care & Clinical Medicine

first edition

Margretta Reed Seashore, MD
Professor of Genetics & Pediatrics
Yale University School of Medicine
New Haven

Rebecca S. Wappner, MD
Professor of Pediatrics & Medical and Molecular Genetics
Indiana University School of Medicine
Indianapolis

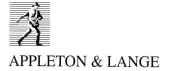

APPLETON & LANGE

Copyright 1996
by Appleton & Lange
A Simon & Schuster Company

96 97 98 99 / 10 9 8 7 6 5 4 3 2 1

Prentice Hall International (UK) Limited, *London*
Prentice Hall of Australia Pty. Limited, *Sydney*
Prentice Hall Canada, Inc., *Toronto*
Prentice Hall Hispanoamericana, S.A., *Mexico*
Prentice Hall of India Private Limited, *New Delhi*
Prentice Hall of Japan, Inc., *Tokyo*
Simon & Schuster Asia Pte. Ltd., *Singapore*
Editora Prentice Hall do Brasil Ltda., *Rio de Janeiro*
Prentice Hall, *Englewood Cliffs, New Jersey*

ISBN: 0-8385-3128-8
ISSN: 1082-9709

Senior Acquisitions Editor: John J. Dolan
Managing Editor: Gregory R. Huth
Production Service: Rainbow Graphics, Inc.
Designer: Libby Schmitz

ISBN 0-8385-3128-8

9 780838 531280

90000

PRINTED IN THE UNITED STATES OF AMERICA

Table of Contents

Preface and Acknowledgments

The authors hope that this book will serve medical students, house staff, and practicing physicians in all branches of medicine by facilitating a review of the principles of modern medical genetics, both basic science and clinical practice. The authors have tried to synthesize their experience and to make the information accessible. The book could not have been written if the authors had not had the benefit of association with many people: those from whom they have learned and those whom they have taught. While too numerous to thank individually, there are some whose support, mentoring, and review have been especially notable.

Yale University and Indiana University students have reviewed much of the material in the courses they have taken at those medical schools; their suggestions have been most helpful.

Several important mentors have shared knowledge, imparted skills, and inspired our efforts: Ira Brandt, MD, W. Roy Breg, MD, Y. Edward Hsia, MD, and Leon E. Rosenberg, MD.

Colleagues have reviewed specific chapters. We have tried to use their advice wisely. Others have assisted us through discussion, book loans, and encouragement: Ray Bahada-Singh, MD, Allen Bale, MD, Nancy Berliner, MD, Bhuwan Garg, MD, Bryan E. Hainline, MD, PhD, Richard Johnston, MD,

Jon Jonsson, MD, PhD, Ora Pescovitz, MD, John Seashore, MD, and David Weaver, MD.

Our families have shaped our lives, provided essential support and patiently endured our preoccupation with this work: Lillie A. and Robert C. Reed; John H., Robert H., Carl J. and Carolyn L. Seashore; C. Diane, Richard D., and Stephen M. Risser; Helen E. Wappner.

The Online Mendelian Inheritance in Man (OMIM), by Victor A. McKusick, MD, with the assistance of Clair Francomano, MD, and Stylios Antonarakis, MD, was an essential source of information without which this book could not have been contemplated, let alone written. The authors recommend that all those delving into medical genetics learn how to use this inestimable resource.

While gratefully acknowledging the help of all the above mentioned individuals, they bear no responsibility for any possible errors, which remains our own.

Margretta Reed Seashore, MD
New Haven, Connecticut

Rebecca S. Wappner, MD
Indianapolis, Indiana

June 1995

SECTION I.
Basic & Clinical Genetics: Bridging the Gap

The Role of Genetics in Medicine

1

Overview

The relevance of human genetic concepts to general medical practice will certainly increase over the coming decades. Genetic advances will have a major effect on all areas of medicine. Genetic factors in cancer, cardiac disease, neurological dysfunction, developmental abnormalities, and psychiatric conditions are becoming increasingly important in the diagnosis and management of these conditions. Advances in clinical genetics have led to the diagnosis of rare inherited disorders such as inborn errors of metabolism, many of which are now screened for in the newborn infant. Screening for the heterozygous states for recessively inherited disorders such as Tay–Sachs disease and sickle cell anemia has created new options for families dealing with the possibility of serious disorders in their children. The lessons learned from these programs will be important when screening for heterozygosity becomes feasible for such common conditions as cystic fibrosis. The use of new techniques based on gene probes, chromosome walking, and recombinant DNA has refined genetic diagnosis in all areas of medicine. Current research to develop practical methods for gene transfer has expanded the possibilities for innovative and even curative gene therapy for certain cancers, infectious diseases, and inherited disorders.

Consider the case of a very ill male infant who nearly dies of a severe infection. Will this outcome happen to another child? Are others in the family at risk? Can X-linked immunodeficiency or an autosomal recessive immune disorder be diagnosed or excluded? If the problem is genetic, is there a possibility for gene therapy to help an affected child in the future? Short-limb syndromes are many and diverse. How can genetic tools help with diagnosis, predicting risk, and prognosis? Coronary artery disease is common. Which families have a defined genetic risk? Can they be identified through genetic screening? Will identifying them make a difference in outcome? These and many similar questions are the province of clinical medicine; they are examples of how the basic and clinical science of genetics will influence the practice of primary care and clinical specialties.

Incidence

The overall incidence of single gene disorders approaches 1 in 100 births (Baird et al, 1988). These conditions, which cross medical specialties, are seen by many different kinds of physicians. The overall incidence of chromosome abnormalities is 1 in 150 at birth, with Down syndrome (trisomy 21) the most common at about 1 in 800. Trisomy 21 remains the most common genetic cause of mental retardation. Both genetic and other factors, presumably environmental, play a role in the development of a large group of common conditions in both children and adults.

McKusick (1992) has compiled a list of medical journal citations referring to published papers about medical conditions that have a genetic component (Figure 1–1). Of some 26,546 papers, 45.7% were published in journals related to nine fields of medical practice, as illustrated in Figure 1–1. The other papers were scattered in various general and scientific journals, such as the *Journal of the American Medical Association, The New England Journal of Medicine, Nature, Science,* and *Lancet.* While genetics, pediatrics, and neurology top the list of specialty journals, the diversity of the other specialties represented is notable. Genetic disorders taken together affect more than 12 million Americans and account for 30% of pediatric hospital admissions and 10% of adult hospital admissions (Hall, 1978). Increasingly, the primary care physician needs to address genetic questions; some are the specific concerns of medical geneticists, but most will involve other physicians as well. The use of genetic tools, which require some understanding of general principles, will form an increasing part of medical practice in the decades to come. The identification of families at risk for genetic disease will come from family history, genetic screening, recognition of risk factors such as maternal and paternal age, and diagnosis of a specific genetic condition in a family member. Some conditions result from single gene mutations (Table 1–1). Others result from undefined genetic and environmental influences (Table 1–2). The physician will need to be aware of the range of gene influence on illness and of the methods for assessing genetic risk. Several cues

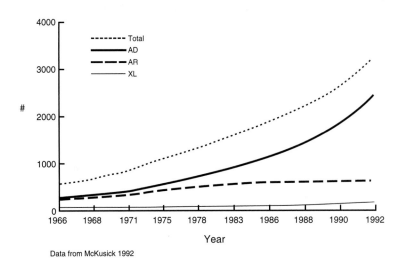

Data from McKusick 1992

Figure 1–1. Medical journal citations that refer to published papers about medical conditions with a genetic component. (Adapted from Burrow GN and Ferris TF (editors), *Medical Complications During Pregnancy*, 4th ed, WB Saunders, 1994.)

Table 1–1. Incidence of some common single gene disorders.

Single Gene Disorder	Incidence
Hypercholesterolemia	1 in 500
Sickle cell anemia	1 in 600 (African ancestry)
Cystic fibrosis	1 in 1600 (European ancestry)
Tay–Sachs disease	1 in 3500 (Ashkenazi Jewish ancestry)
Huntington disease	1 in 5000
Phenylketonuria	1 in 10,000

netic mechanisms provides the key to preventing and treating some inherited conditions.

At some point in considering a genetic condition, the primary care physician or physician specialist will need to consult a clinical geneticist to perform a genetic evaluation or specific tests. In the past, descriptive and inferential approaches played a key role in human genetics. Today modern technology has advanced our understanding of chromosomal abnormalities and of the genes responsible for many Mendelian conditions. The laboratory evaluation of a patient and family often includes the use of molecular tools that vastly increase the power to analyze human genetic pathology. The clinical geneticist should

ought to alert the physician to look for genetic factors (Table 1–3). The need for all physicians to recognize the contribution of genetic factors to the etiology of disease cannot be overemphasized. This is not a capitulation to determinism; an understanding of ge-

Table 1–2. Common conditions that are gene-influenced.

Childhood	Adulthood
Cleft lip and palate	Coronary artery disease
Spina bifida	Diabetes mellitus
Congenital heart disease	Schizophrenia
Juvenile diabetes mellitus	Hypertension
Cancer	Cancer
Pyloric stenosis	Alcoholism

Table 1–3. Features of medical history that raise genetic concerns.

Feature	Risk
Multiple affected family members	Single gene; multifactorial; chromosomal
Family history of known inherited disorder	Risk of being affected with same condition
Maternal age over 35 years at delivery	Chromosome abnormality in baby
Exposure to therapeutic radiation	Gonadal mutation or chromosome rearrangement
Consanguinity (first cousin or closer)	Infant death or malformation; homozygosity for same mutant gene
History of neonatal deaths in the family	Recessive or X-linked disorder; chromosome abnormality

have all these tools at his or her disposal. A physician should expect that the clinical geneticist will

- Obtain a detailed family history
- Construct a pedigree
- Perform a careful examination of the patient and other family members with the purpose of identifying or excluding a genetic cause for the condition
- Perform imaging and laboratory tests to specify the condition more completely
- Assess the prognosis and genetic risk to the individual and family

- Communicate the results of these examinations to the patient and family in a clear, concise way that includes a written report.

The kinds of tests ordered should be directed toward identifying or excluding a recognized particular genetic condition or a recognized genetic mechanism. The possibilities for therapy should be specified; therapeutic options may be undertaken by the clinical geneticist alone or in collaboration with other specialists and the primary physician.

REFERENCES AND SUGGESTED READING

Baird PA et al: Genetic disorders in children and young adults: A population study. Am J Hum Genet 1988;**42:**677.

Buyse ML: *Birth Defects Encyclopedia.* Center for Birth Defects Information Services, Inc., 1990.

Carter CO: Genetics of common single malformations. Br Med Bull 1976;**32:**21.

Hall JG et al: The frequency and financial burden of genetic disease in a pediatric hospital. Am J Med Genet 1978;I:417.

Magnus P, Berg K, Bjerkedal T: Association of parental consanguinity with decreased birth weight and increased rate of early death and congenital malformations. Clin Genet 1985;**28:**335.

Marden PM, Smith DW, McDonald MJ: Congenital anomalies in the newborn infant, including minor variations. J Pediatr 1964;**64:**357.

McKusick VM, Francomano C, Antonarakis S: *Mendelian Inheritance in Man: Catalogs of Autosomal Dominant, Autosomal Recessive, and X-linked Phenotypes,* 10th ed. Johns Hopkins University Press, 1992.

McKusick VM: The morbid anatomy of the human genome: chromosomal location of mutations causing disease. J Med Genet 1993;**30:**1.

Seashore MR: Genetic counseling. In: *Cecil Textbook of Medicine.* Wyngarden JB, Smith LH, Bennett JC (editors). WB Saunders, 1988.

2 Review of Fundamental Genetics

The current study of the human genome has a rich historical background. An historical perspective can put the new developments and advances in the basic science of genetics into focus for clinical medicine. Major historical landmarks are shown in Table 2–1. Genetics had its scientific beginning in 1865 when Gregor Mendel made his now famous observations on the apparent inheritance of certain traits in garden peas. From these observations he developed his principle of the discreet inheritance of traits. Sir Archibald Garrod, physician to the Hospital for Sick Children at Great Ormond Street, observed that some human traits behaved as if they followed the principles set forth by Mendel and developed the notion of "inborn errors of metabolism." Further discoveries identified and clarified the function and structure of DNA culminating with Watson and Crick's discovery, in 1953, that DNA is configured as a double helix. The face of molecular biology changed forever. A few years later, Marshall Nierenberg cracked the genetic code and set the course for modern genetics.

MOLECULAR GENETICS: STRUCTURE AND FUNCTION OF DNA & RNA

DNA (deoxyribonucleic acid), the information-carrying molecule in the cell, directs the synthesis of all proteins. DNA is constructed of the purine and pyrimidine bases adenine, cytosine, guanine, and thymine, each of which is attached to a phosphorylated sugar, deoxyribose. The base attached to the deoxyribose is referred to as a **nucleoside;** with the phosphate added it is a **nucleotide** (Figure 2–1, Figure 2–2). Nucleotides are strung together in a linear order, and the resulting molecule is single-stranded DNA. Two lengths of complementary single-stranded DNA, held together by hydrogen bonding, twist into the double helix recognized as double-stranded DNA (Figure 2–3). The entire complement of DNA is called the **genome.**

RNA, ribonucleic acid, is the molecule that serves as an intermediate between the DNA and the protein whose synthesis it directs. RNA is similar to DNA in structure, except that in RNA the sugar is ribose instead of deoxyribose, and thymine is replaced by a different base, uracil. Also, RNA is usually single-stranded rather than double-stranded like DNA. DNA directs the synthesis of proteins by means of the triplet nucleotide code. Each series of three nucleotides specifies a particular amino acid (Table 2–2). The code is degenerate, which means that some amino acids can be coded for by more than one triplet of nucleotides. The order of triplets that specify amino acids determines the order of the amino acids in the protein. During this process the DNA unwinds, and a single strand is transcribed into RNA, which is then translated into protein on structures known as ribosomes.

The typical gene is a length of DNA which is organized into specialized regions. In humans the structure is not a single continuous gene, as in bacteria, but is made of protein coding sequences called **exons** separated by non-coding intervening sequences called **introns.** On either end of the region containing the introns and exons are the 5′ and 3′ untranslated regions. Ahead of the 5′ untranslated region are the sequences that regulate transcription, including enhancer sequences and other specialized sequences related to transcriptional control and tissue specific expression. At the 3′ end of the gene are specialized sequences relating to termination of transcription.

The sequence of events in the process of converting the information in the gene to a specific protein structure begins with the initiation of RNA transcription. A variety of proteins serve as signals that regulate this process. Further processing of RNA involves splicing out the introns (which are not expressed in the resulting proteins) and rejoining the RNA represented by the exons into the messenger RNA that will be used as the template for translation into protein. The amino acids that make up the protein are ordered when the tRNAs to which they are attached line up along the template. Complex splicing using alternative sites occurs in the production of some proteins and provides variability in the structure of the proteins which can be made from a single gene. Transport to the subcellular organelles for translation into protein occurs, and the newly made protein may then undergo post-translational modification depending on its ultimate destination and function (Figure 2–4).

Types of Molecular Pathology

With increased understanding of the structure and function of human genes has come increased interest

Table 2–1. Historical landmarks in genetics.

Year	Researcher	Development
1866	Mendel	Introduces paper on genetic inheritance in sweet peas: Proceedings of the Brünn Society for Natural History
1902	Boveri Sutton	Discover presence of paired chromosomes in diploid species
1905	Bateson	Names the science of genetics
1908	Hardy Weinberg	Formulate the law that states the behavior of genes in populations
1909	Johannsen	Introduces the word gene
1910	Morgan	Announces chromosomal basis of linkage; sex-linked inheritance *(Nobel Prize 1933)*
1910	Kossel	Discovers nucleic acids adenine and thymine *(Nobel Prize 1910)*
1924	Painter	Announces that males carry both the X and Y chromosome
1941	Beadle Tatum Lederberg	Discover that single enzymes are linked to single genes *(Nobel Prize 1958)*
1945	McClintock	Explains mobile genetic elements *(Nobel Prize 1983)*
1946	Muller	Discovers x-ray mutagenesis
1952	Hershey Chase	Show that genetic material in T_2 phage is DNA *(Nobel Prize 1969)*
1953	Watson Crick	Elucidate double helix structure of DNA *(Nobel Prize 1962)*
1953	Wilkins	Elucidates double helix structure of DNA *(Nobel Prize 1962)*
1956	Tijo Levan	Determine that diploid chromosome number is 46
1958	Meselson Stahl	Elucidate semi-conservative replication
1959	Ochoa Kornberg	Discover RNA polymerase *(Nobel Prize 1959)*
1959	Lejeune	Shows that Down syndrome is trisomy 21
1959	Jacobs Strong	Link Klinefelter syndrome with XXY chromosomes
1959	Ford	Reports Turner syndrome has chromosome constitution of 45, X
1960	Nowell Hungerfold	Report Philadelphia chromosome in chronic myelogenous leukemia (CML)
1960	Patau	Discovers trisomy 13
1960	Edwards	Discovers trisomy 18
1961	Jacob Monod	Offer operon model for regulating gene expression *(Nobel Prize 1965)*
1961	Lyon	Presents hypothesis of X-inactivation
1963	Lejeune	Explains *cri du chat* deletion, mechanism of first deletion syndrome
1965	Holley Khorana Nirenberg	Define nucleotide sequence, alanine tRNA *(Nobel Prize 1968)*
1968	Caspersson	Develops chromosome banding techniques
1969	Delbruck Luria	Develop phage genetics *(Nobel Prize 1969)*
1970	Nathans Smith	Discover restriction endonucleases *(Nobel Prize 1978)*
1972	Berg	Invent in vitro recombinant DNA methods *(Nobel Prize 1980)*
1976	Varmus Bishop	Discover oncogenes *(Nobel Prize 1989)*
1977	Maxam Gilbert Sanger	Invent DNA sequencing methods (Gilbert, Sanger, *Nobel Prize 1980*)
1986	Mullis	Develops polymerase chain reaction (PCR) *(Nobel Prize 1993)*
1989	Tsui Collins	Clone CF gene
1990	Anderson Rosenberg Woo	Develop gene therapy protocols
1990	Friend Fraumeni	Explain role of tumor suppressor gene mutations in inherited cancers
1990	Fearon Vogelstein	Explain role of tumor suppressor gene mutations in acquired cancers

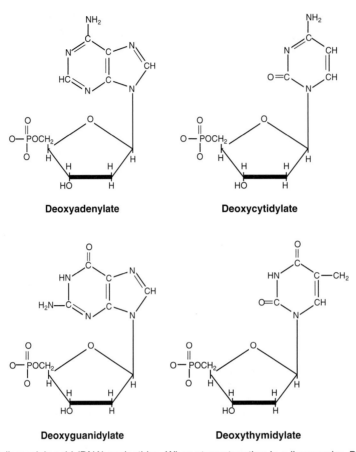

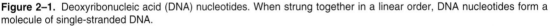

Figure 2–1. Deoxyribonucleic acid (DNA) nucleotides. When strung together in a linear order, DNA nucleotides form a molecule of single-stranded DNA.

in mutations that result in genetic disorders. As human genes are mapped, cloned, and sequenced, the relationship between mutations and changes in structure and function of important proteins has become clearer. This in turn has led to an improved understanding of genetic pathophysiology, ie, the mutations that cause disease.

Specific molecular pathology can be divided into several classes of mutations; the type of mutation influences the expression of the gene and the phenotype. Classes of mutations are shown in Table 2–3. Single base changes can alter the character of proteins. Mutations that affect m-RNA processing can result in the synthesis of abnormal proteins. Deletions and insertions of a single base can change the frame of the triplet code, and deletions and insertions of large pieces of DNA can change the character of the protein. Any of these changes can stop the synthesis of a protein. Abnormal crossover events can result in fusion genes that make non-functional fusion proteins.

Trinucleotide repeats occur in a series within or near by genes. The series usually has a characteristic number of repeats, eg, 30–40 (Figure 2–5). The series can undergo expansion in number during meiosis, and in this way affect the protein that is encoded by a gene. Examples of this kind of change have been seen in a group of disorders affecting the nervous system. This expansion affects phenotype as shown in Table 2–4.

Effects of various changes in genes appear in structural proteins, enzymes, or membrane proteins. General effects of mutations on protein function include the following:

- Loss of protein entirely
- Loss of protein function
- Abnormal protein function
- Quantitative effects
    Subunit imbalance
    Decreased function.

The elucidation of specific mutations has led also to an increase in diagnostic precision. Phenotypically similar conditions can be differentiated through the use of molecular techniques that identify specific ge-

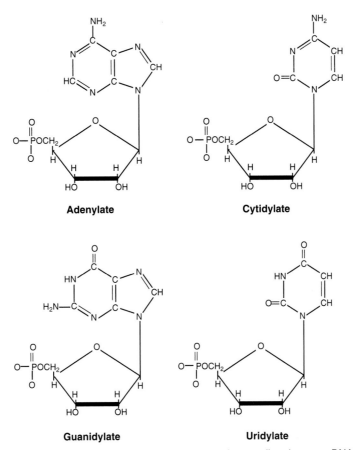

Figure 2–2. Ribonucleic acid (RNA) nucleotides. RNA acts as an intermediate between DNA and the protein whose synthesis it directs.

netic changes. Consequently individuals in families at risk can be tested, and their risks can be clarified.

Mitochondrial Genetics

The vast majority of the genes in the cell reside in the nucleus. Mitochondria, however, have a genome of their own that codes for some of the proteins important in mitochondrial function. The organization of the **mitochondrial genome** is radically different from that of the nuclear genome. The former is circular, as shown in Figure 2–6, and has two DNA strands, light and heavy, each with its own origin of replication. In the mitochondrial genome, bidirectional transcription and translation of mitochondrial DNA (mtDNA) occur; the 16,569 base pairs code for 13 polypeptides (all of which are components of the oxidative phosphorylation pathway), two ribosomal RNAs (rRNAs), and 22 transfer RNAs (tRNAs). The remaining polypeptides that comprise the respiratory chain are encoded by nuclear genes. The mitochondrial genetic code differs from the universal code in the cell's nucleus; for this reason, mitochondrial tRNAs cannot "read" cytoplasmic ribosomes and

vice-versa. Complex processing of the mRNA occurs, but without introns or a 5′ or 3′ untranslated region. Coordinated expression of mitochondrial and nuclear genes for the multienzyme complexes exists, but the mechanism remains unclear. Compactness and efficiency characterize the mitochondrial genome. Transcripts of the mitochondrial genome remain in the mitochondria. The nuclear coded subunits are synthesized in the cytosol and transported into mitochondria, where the complete proteins are assembled.

It is estimated that each human cell has hundreds of thousands of mitochondria and more than 200,000 copies of each mitochondrial gene. If one or several mtDNAs carries a mutation, segregation of that mutation will occur randomly and will follow population distributions—not Mendelian segregation; moreover, distribution will be unequal from one cell to another. More than one type of mtDNA within a cell or tissue is termed **heteroplasmy;** if all the mtDNA are similar, the phenomenon is called **homoplasmy.** Heteroplasmy accounts for some of the variability observed in patients with similar mutations and in tissue types from one patient.

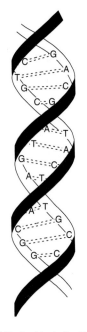

Figure 2–3. DNA double helix. Two lengths of complementary single-stranded DNA, held together by hydrogen bonding, comprise the helical molecule of double-stranded DNA. The entire complement of DNA is called the genome.

First Base (5′)	Second Base				Third Base (3′)
	U	C	A	G	
U	phe	ser	tyr	cys	U
	phe	ser	tyr	cys	C
	leu	ser	Stop	Stop	A
	leu	ser	Stop	trp	G
C	leu	pro	his	arg	U
	leu	pro	his	arg	C
	leu	pro	gln	arg	A
	leu	pro	gln	arg	G
A	ile	thr	asn	ser	U
	ile	thr	asn	ser	C
	ile	thr	lys	arg	A
	met	thr	lys	arg	G
G	val	ala	asp	gly	U
	val	ala	asp	gly	C
	val	ala	glu	gly	A
	val	ala	glu	gly	G

Table 2–2. The genetic code.

A number of mutations in the enzymes of the oxidative phosphorylation pathway have been characterized; these result in abnormal function of the energy cycle and lead to serious disease. Many familial cases of mitochondrial dysfunction that fit autosomal Mendelian patterns have been described; most of the subunits of the multienzyme complexes are encoded by nuclear genes, and this accounts for **autosomal dominant and recessive** patterns. However, a number of pedigrees have shown an odd pattern of vertical inheritance in which affected mothers had substantial numbers of affected offspring of both sexes, but affected fathers had no affected offspring. This pattern has become known as **maternal inheritance.** During oogenesis, the mtDNAs are amplified as much as 200,000 fold; during spermatogenesis, mtDNAs move to the tail and are lost. Maternal mtDNAs are distributed to the daughter cells; no maternal/paternal recombination occurs, however, and segregation at cell division allows different distributions of mutant and normal mtDNAs into each cell. Since that is cytoplasmic inheritance, all offspring would be expected to get only a maternal mitochondrial contribution. Because of the random assortment of the mitochondrial genes after replication, severity is variable, and prediction of the phenotype in different offspring is difficult. Specific disorders of oxidative phosphorylation are discussed in Chapter 16.

Major characteristics of mitochondrial inheritance are shown in Table 2–5.

CYTOGENETICS

The double helical structure of DNA undergoes packaging into the tertiary structure of **chromosomes,** which reside in the nucleus. DNA is associated with two types of proteins: histones, very basic proteins of which there are five classes, and non-histone proteins, which comprise all the other DNA-associated proteins. This combination of DNA, histones, and non-histones is referred to as **chromatin.** The chromatin is further packed into particles called nucleosomes through which the DNA continues and coils around histones. The nucleosomes undergo supercoiling and then packaging into the fiber which is the chromosome (Figure 2–7).

The human genome is organized into a set of 46 chromosomes located in the nucleus of each cell; the genome also includes in the many mitochondrial chromosomes located within each mitochondrion. The smallest human chromosome contains about 50 million base pairs of DNA, while the largest has about 250 million base pairs. Individual chromosomes can be identified during mitosis. Under appropriate staining conditions, their morphology is distinctive, as illustrated in Figure 2–7. The alternating light and dark bands consist of euchromatin (DNA that is transcribed) and heterochromatin (DNA that is transcriptionally silent). The number of bands in each haploid set of chromosomes ranges from 350–1000, depending upon the technique employed. Each band contains a number of genes, depending on their size.

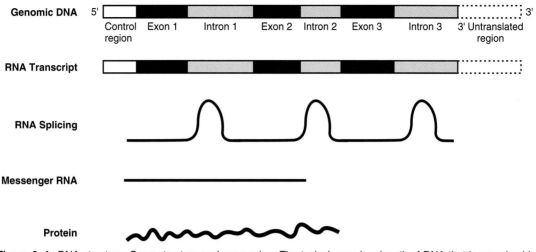

Figure 2–4. DNA structure: Gene structure and expression. The typical gene is a length of DNA that is organized into specialized regions. Human genes are comprised of protein coding sequences called exons, which are separated by non-coding intervening sequences called introns.

The Description of Chromosomes

According to rules established by the Paris convention, for descriptive purposes, the human chromosome complement is arranged according to size and position of the centromere (central constriction) into the **karyotype.** Chromosomes are arranged in pairs from largest to smallest and are numbered as pairs 1 through 22; these are the autosomes that contain most of the genes in the human genome. The twenty-third pair comprises the sex chromosomes. All cells have a pair of sex chromosomes, XX in females and XY in males. The X-chromosome was the first to have specific disease genes mapped to it. To date, at least 50 diseases and 200 genetic markers have been assigned to the X-chromosome. Figure 2–8 is an idiogram of a karyotype according to the Paris convention. Figure 2–9 is a photomicrograph of a karyotype from a normal human cell.

X-inactivation

Beyond the embryonic stage, all somatic cells are hemizygous with respect to the X-chromosome. In each cell in the early embryo (exact stage unknown, perhaps around implantation) either the maternally derived or the paternally derived X-chromosome is inactivated. Only the X-chromosome undergoes inactivation in somatic cells. This inactivation, a form of dosage compensation in females, results in a balance in gene expression between the X-chromosome and autosomal genes, which is necessary because males have only one X-chromosome. In each cell, either the maternally derived or the paternally derived X-chromosome is randomly selected to be inactive; all progeny of that cell inherit the same inactivated X-chromosome. Usually, a structurally abnormal X-chromosome is preferentially inactivated. Exceptions to this rule are provided by X-autosome translo-

Table 2–3. Classes of mutations.

Type of Change	Effect on Genetic Material	Effect on Protein
Single DNA base change	Missense Nonsense Premature stop codon	Abnormal amino acid sequence No protein made No protein made
m-RNA processing	Splice site mutations Cryptic splice site	Abnormal protein Abnormal protein
Deletions, insertions	Frameshift Codon insertions, deletions Gene deletions	Abnormal protein or no protein made Abnormal protein No protein made
Fusion genes	Fusion mRNA	Fusion proteins, abnormal or no function
Triplet repeats	Repeat element insertions, deletions Abnormal methylation	No protein made Transcription termination

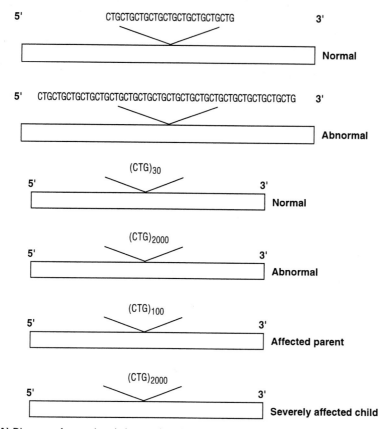

5' CTGCTGCTGCTGCTGCTGCTGCTG 3' Normal

5' CTGCTGCTGCTGCTGCTGCTGCTGCTGCTGCTGCTGCTGCTGCTGCTG 3' Abnormal

$(CTG)_{30}$
5' 3' Normal

$(CTG)_{2000}$
5' 3' Abnormal

$(CTG)_{100}$
5' 3' Affected parent

$(CTG)_{2000}$
5' 3' Severely affected child

Figure 2–5. (A) Diagram of normal and abnormal repeats. **(B)** Relationship between repeat number and phenotype.

cations in which the normal X-chromosome is inactivated, thus preserving the function of the autosome, and by certain X-linked mutations—eg, severe combined immunodeficiency disease (SCID)—where the abnormal X-chromosome is preferentially inactivated in heterozygous females. An important consequence of X-inactivation is somatic cell mosaicism for genes coded for by the X-chromosome. The inactive X-chromosome has the following properties:

1. It is heterochromatic.
2. It replicates late in the cell cycle.

3. Most of its genes undergo inactivation.
4. Once inactivated, the X-chromosome always remains so in somatic cells.
5. An inactivation locus (XIST, Xq13) is expressed by the inactive X-chromosome in all cells.

Some 40 or more genes are known to be inactivated. Some genes on Xp (X_g, MIC2, steroid sulfatase) remain active. A gene on Xq that controls some ovarian functions also remains active. Such active genes are separated by genes that are inactive (Figure 2–10).

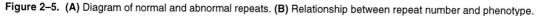

Disorder	Map Location	Repeat	Effect of Expanded Number of Repeats
Myotonic dystrophy	19q13.3	$(CTG)_n$ NI = <30 DM = 50→2000 Premutation = 50–100 Affected = 100–2000	Decreased age of onset and increased severity in general
Huntington disease	4p	$(CAG)_n$ NI = 30–34 Affected = 42–100	Decreased age of onset

Table 2–4. Examples of effects of trinucleotide repeats.

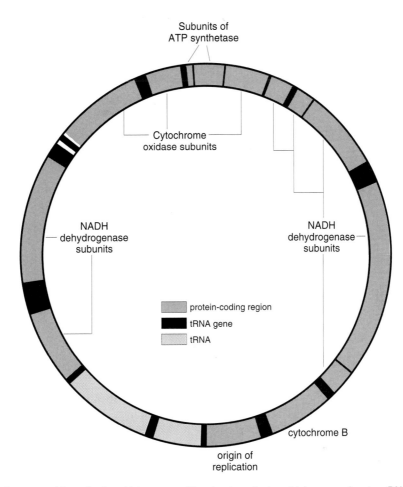

Figure 2–6. Structure of the mitochondrial genome. The circular mitochondrial genome has two DNA strands, light and heavy, each with its own origin of replication. Bidirectional transcription and translation of mitochondrial DNA (mtDNA) is a feature of the mitochondrial genome; the 16,569 base pairs code for 13 polypeptides, two ribosomal RNAs (rRNAs), and 22 transfer RNAs (tRNAs).

Condensed chromatin clumps, which can be seen at the edge of the interphase nucleus, correspond in number to one less than the number of X-chromosomes. Known as Barr bodies, these clumps represent inactive X-chromosomes. At the cellular level, biochemical findings have demonstrated mosaicism for X-linked genes in females who are heterozygous. Glucose-6-phosphate dehydrogenase and ornithine transcarbamylase are examples of proteins for which this kind of cellular mosaicism has been demonstrated. In females heterozygous for an X-linked mutation, two populations of cells—one showing the phenotype of the mutation and one normal with respect to that gene—will be seen. When the female is heterozygous for a pathological mutation, the degree to which she expresses the disorder will depend on the distribution of cells in which the abnormal X-chromosome is active.

Mitosis and Meiosis

With each cell division, it is necessary to replicate the DNA in the cell so that the daughter cells have the same genetic complement as the original cell. This is accomplished faithfully each time a cell divides by the complex mechanisms of mitosis, in somatic cells, and meiosis, in germ cells. In each chromosome, the DNA replicates, the chromosomal

Table 2–5. Characteristics of mitochondrial inheritance.

Characteristic	Description
Inheritance pattern	Maternal
Expression	Variable; Most apparent in energy-demanding tissues
Manifestation	Affects oxidative phosphorylation

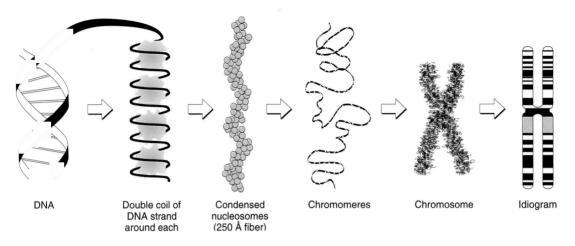

DNA Double coil of Condensed Chromomeres Chromosome Idiogram
DNA strand nucleosomes
around each (250 Å fiber)

Figure 2–7. Tertiary structure of DNA into chromosomes. DNA combines with histones and non-histones to form chromatin. The chromatin is compressed into nucleosomes, which are then supercoiled and packaged to form the chromosome. The smallest human chromosome contains about 50 million base pairs of DNA, while the largest has about 250 million base pairs.

homologs pair, and the pairs separate to provide the normal chromosomal complement in the resulting new cells. Since germ cells are haploid, the first step is replication followed by mitosis; a second division immediately occurs without replication, thus reducing the number of chromosomes to the haploid number again. It is during meiosis that recombination between chromosomes of maternal and paternal origin can occur (Figure 2–11).

The consequences of abnormal mitosis or meiosis are serious. In the germ cell, failure of the chromosomes to separate at the last stages of meiosis results in an unequal number of chromosomes segregating to the daughter cells. This event, called non-disjunction, results in a gamete that has an extra chromosome and one that is deficient. The deficient gamete is not viable. Fertilization of the gamete with an extra chromosome by a normal gamete results in a zygote that is aneuploid. If such a zygote is viable, the child will have trisomy for the chromosome involved, which usually results in an abnormal phenotype (Figure 2–12).

A chromosomal translocation presents a problem for the cell during meiosis, since pairing at reduction division cannot occur normally. Depending on whether the translocation is Robertsonian or reciprocal, the triradial or quadriradial structure that occurs during chromosomal pairing undergoes abnormal segregation. The gamete produced can be normal or aneuploid. It can have a balanced translocation with a normal chromosomal complement, or it can be deficient or duplicated in chromosomal material. Figure 2–13 shows the consequences of each possibility. Because only some possibilities are viable, all are not represented in live offspring. From a practical standpoint, the consequences of translocations to repro-

duction include increased fetal wastage, translocation trisomy, balanced translocation, or normal chromosome complement. Empiric risks to offspring of a balanced translocation carrier depend on the sex of the translocation carrier. Females who carry a 14q21q translocation have about a 10% risk of having an offspring with trisomy 21, while males with the same translocation have less than a 5% risk. Carriers of a 21q21q translocation can have only offspring with trisomy 21. Fortunately this situation is extremely rare.

Sexual Differentiation

In humans, the importance of two normal X-chromosomes for ovarian development—and of a normal X- and Y-chromosome for testicular development—is clear. Studies of structural abnormalities of the X- and Y-chromosomes—and of other exceptional karyotypes—have led to a better understanding of the critical regions or the locations of genes that are responsible for normal gonadal development. For example, deletions and mutations in a gene, Sry, on the Y-chromosome has explained the presence of a male phenotype in individuals with an XX karyotype and a female phenotype in individuals with a 46,XY karyotype. The presence of Y-chromosomal material on one of the X-chromosomes, following exchange between an X-chromosome and a Y-chromosome, explains many of these observations. Sry is on distal Yp between the pseudoautosomal region and the telomere and codes for a regulatory DNA-binding protein.

Chromosomal Abnormalities

The impact of chromosome abnormalities is greatest during fetal life when chromosome abnormalities

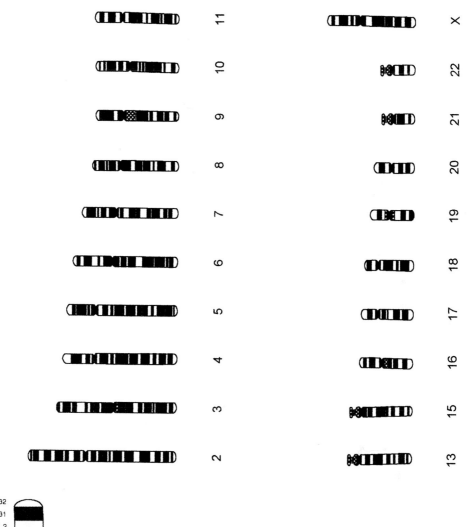

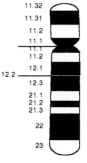

Figure 2–8. **(A)** Idiogram of a typical karyotype, based on rules established by the Paris convention. Chromosomes are ordered according to size. The banding pattern of each chromosome is unique and thus distinguishes that chromosome from all others. **(B)** The banding pattern of chromosome 18 is enlarged to show detail.

have their highest frequency and represent a major cause of fetal loss. Chromosomal abnormalities are found in 7–8% of recognized pregnancies (from about 6 weeks to term). About 50% of abortuses have an abnormal karyotype. Of pregnancies reaching term, about 0.5% have a chromosome disorder. By livebirth the frequency has decreased and, because several of the major autosomal trisomies lead to early death, the frequency in older children and adults is even lower. The frequencies of various

chromosomal abnormalities is quite different in newborns as compared to abortuses, since some aneuploidies are lethal in utero. Abnormalities may be numerical or structural. The syndromes are generally classified according to whether there is extra chromosomal material, deleted chromosomal material, or a normal complement of chromosomal material that has been rearranged. Part or all of a particular chromosome may be missing or may be extra.

Only a few syndromes with trisomy of an auto-

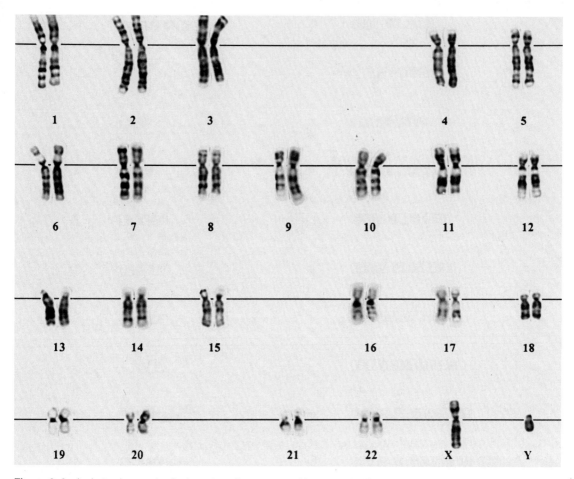

Figure 2–9. A photomicrograph of a karyotype from a normal human cell. (Courtesy of Teresa Yang-Feng PhD, Yale University.)

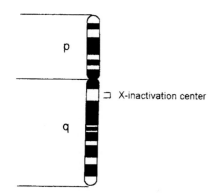

Figure 2–10. X-inactivation. In the human embryo, the maternally derived or the paternally derived X-chromosome in each somatic cell is randomly inactivated. All progeny of the cell inherit the inactivated X-chromosome. Usually, a structurally abnormal X-chromosome is inactivated. Exceptions to the rule include certain X-linked mutations.

some have been described in liveborn individuals; they are trisomies of chromosomes 13, 18, and 21. Occasionally trisomies of other chromosomes—8, 9, or rarely another autosome—have been described in livebirths. Almost always in that case a normal cell line (mosaicism) is also present. In most cases, the mechanism by which the chromosomal abnormality produces the phenotype is not clear. Unlike the single gene traits, these phenotypes result from the effects of more than one gene. The major autosomal abnormalities share a number of phenotypic features that are not distinctive or specific, including mental retardation, cardiac malformations, and growth deficiency. While there is variability within every cytogenetic syndrome, neonatal death and serious congenital malformations are frequent manifestations. Most of the specific cytogenetic syndromes have a constellation of features that distinguish them and allow the clinician to suspect the diagnosis.

Although balanced rearrangements (translocations and inversions) usually do not affect development,

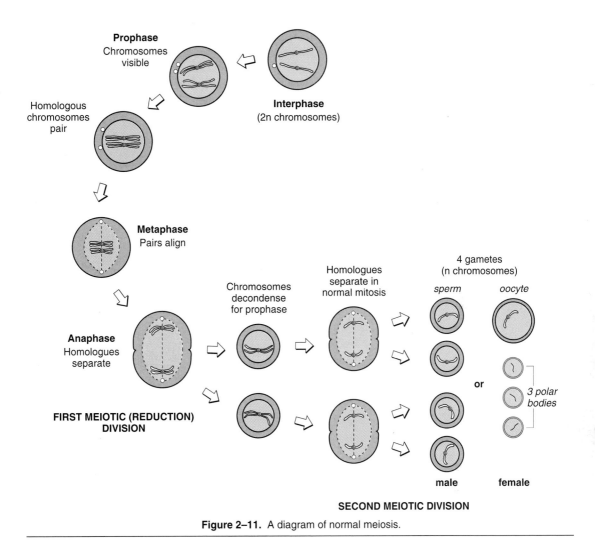

Figure 2–11. A diagram of normal meiosis.

carriers of such abnormalities are at increased risk of having offspring with unbalanced rearranged chromosomes that cause congenital malformations. Microscopically visible as well as submicroscopic deletions that produce recognizable clinical syndromes have been identified. The phenotype in individuals with these deletions seems to result from the loss or interruption of several contiguous genes along the involved chromosome. In such cases, cytogenetic studies can delineate clinical disorders or syndromes, confirm clinical diagnoses, aid in predicting the risk that a chromosome abnormality will recur in a family, and suggest the location of genes responsible for the observed phenotype. Some generalizations about cytogenetic abnormalities can be made:

1. Extra chromosome material (eg, trisomy and duplication) is not as deleterious to development as when the same material is missing (eg, monosomy and deletion).

2. A gain of autosomal material has a greater effect on the phenotype than a gain of sex chromosomes. In the case of the X-chromosome this may be due to inactivation of additional X-chromosomes.

3. Loss of an entire autosome is highly lethal.

4. Lack of one of the sex chromosomes is also deleterious.

5. The lack of an X-chromosome in the presence of a Y-chromosome has never been seen in a liveborn.

6. The vast majority of conceptuses with single X chromosomal constitution fail to survive; the small percentage that do survive have the recognized phenotype of Turner syndrome.

7. Extra sets of chromosomes (triploidy and tetraploidy) have profound effects on development.

8. Haploidy (n = 23) in a conceptus has never been observed.

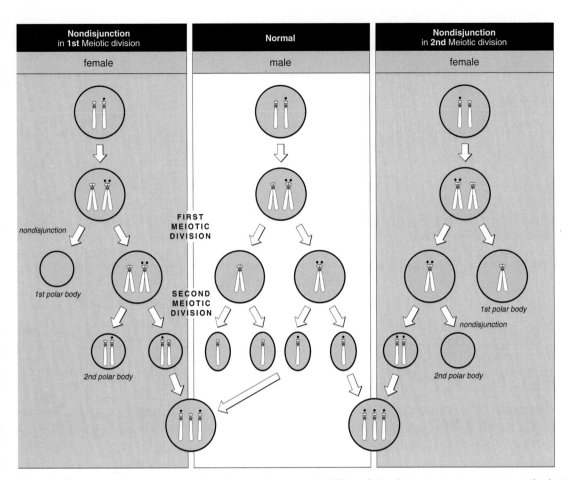

Nondisjunction in **1st** Meiotic division	Normal	Nondisjunction in **2nd** Meiotic division
female	male	female

Figure 2–12. Abnormal meiosis: non-disjunction. In the germ cell, failure of the chromosomes to separate at the last stages of meiosis results in an unequal number of chromosomes segregating to the daughter cells. This event, called non-disjunction, results in a gamete that has an extra chromosome and a deficient gamete that is non-viable. Fertilization of the gamete with an extra chromosome by a normal gamete results in a zygote that is aneuploid. If such a zygote is viable, the child will have trisomy for the involved chromosome, which usually results in an abnormal phenotype.

The types and frequencies of chromosomal abnormalities found in spontaneous abortions are shown in Table 2–6.

Some autosomal deletion syndromes are listed in Table 2–7.

CLINICAL CYTOGENETICS

Major Autosomal Trisomies

Trisomy 21, Down Syndrome (DS): Trisomy 21 (Down syndrome) has been recognized for more than 100 years. Because it is a common and familiar disorder, DS has been studied much more thoroughly than other chromosomal disorders. A number of systems are involved in DS—including the CNS and the skeletal, cardiovascular, and hematopoetic systems—as well as some endocrine glands (Figure 2–14). No

single feature is pathognomonic or diagnostic; an invariable non-specific feature is mental retardation. The Down syndrome phenotype can be produced by duplication of q22.1–q22.2, a small region of chromosome 21 known as the Down syndrome critical region. Whether the activities of a few or many genes within this critical region are responsible for the phenotypic effect remains unknown. Figure 2–15 and Figure 2–16 are karyotypes for chromosome 21 that illustrate trisomy and balanced translocations, respectively.

Common clinical features that help the physician to recognize Down syndrome are listed in Table 2–9.

Recognition of Down syndrome in the neonatal period facilitates prompt diagnosis and management of clinical problems, including congenital heart disease, gastrointestinal malformations, and congenital cataracts. Other clinical issues assume increasing im-

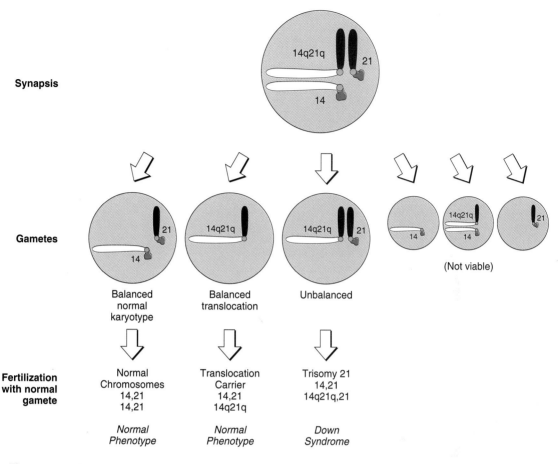

Figure 2–13. Diagram of abnormal segregation of translocation (Robertsonian). If a chromosomal translocation occurs during meiosis, pairing at reduction division cannot occur normally. Depending on whether the translocation is Robertsonian or reciprocal, the triradial or quadriradial structure produced during chromosomal pairing undergoes abnormal segregation. The resulting gamete can be normal or aneuploid; it can have a balanced translocation with a normal chromosomal complement or it can have duplicated chromosomal material.

Table 2–6. Frequency of cytogenic abnormalities in newborns.

Cytogenic abnormality	Rate/1000 newborns[1]
Autosomal abnormalities	
Trisomy 13	0.05–0.27
Trisomy 18	0.10–0.27
Trisomy 21	0.69–1.44
14/21 translocations	0.18–0.27
Sex chromosome abnormalities	
XXY	0.50–1.60
XXX	0.50–1.68
XXY	0.50–1.07

[1] Data from Hassold, Nielson, (1984) and Lubs (1970).

Table 2–7. Chromosome abnormalities in abortuses. (Reproduced, with permission from: Burrow GN and Ferris TF (editors). *Medical Complications During Pregnancy,* 4th ed, WB Saunders, 1994.)

Chromosome Abnormality	Karyotype
Monosomy X	45,X
Monosomy 21	45,XY,–21 or 45,XX,+21
Trisomy	47,+autosome
Double trisomy	48,+2 autosomes
Mosaic trisomy	46/47,+ autosome or 48,+ 2 autosomes
Triploidy	69,XXX, XXY, or XYY
Tetraploidy	92,XXXX or XXYY
Structural abnormalities	Translocations, unbalanced

Table 2–8. Autosomal deletion syndromes. (Reproduced, with permission from: Burrow GN and Ferris TF (editors). *Medical Complications During Pregnancy,* 4th ed, WB Saunders, 1994.)

Syndrome	Region	Critical Chromosomal Location
Greig cephalopolysyndactyly	GCPS	del 7p13
Holoprosencephaly	HOLO	del 7q34
Trichorhinophalangeal/Langer-Gideon syndrome	TRP	del 8q24.1
Wilms tumor, aniridia, genital abnorm, retardation	WAGR	del 11p13
Beckwith-Wiedemann syndrome	BWS	dup 11p15
Retinoblastoma	RB	del 13q14.11
Prader-Willi/Angelman syndrome	PWS/AS	del 15q12
HbH/alpha-thalassemia-mental retardation	ATMR	del 16p13.3
Rubenstein-Taybi syndrome	RTS	del 16p13.3
Miller-Dieker syndrome	MDS	del 17p13
Smith-Magenis syndrome	SMS	del 17p11.2
Charcot-Marie-Tooth disease type 1A	CMT1A	dup 17p11.2–p12
Arteriohepatic dysplasia (Alagille syndrome)	AHD	del 20p11.23–p12.2
DiGeorge/velocardiofacial syndrome	DGS	del 22q11
Cat-eye syndrome	CES	dup 22q11
Duchenne muscular dystrophy/contig genes	DMD	del Xp21
Kallmann syndrome/contig genes	KAL	del Xp22.3
Choroideremia, deafness, clefting, retardation	CDCR	del Xq21

portance in other age groups. These are summarized in Table 2–9. Social support of the family at the time of diagnosis is extremely important; the physician must help them accept the diagnosis and proceed with measures that will help the child to achieve his or her full potential. Children with Down syndrome who receive developmental intervention in early infancy can function at levels previously believed to be impossible (when children with DS were reared in institutions). Social skills often exceed what intelligence measurements would predict. Group living and community-supported work programs help persons with Down syndrome to contribute to their communities and to have productive lives.

Trisomy 13 (Patau syndrome): First described in 1960, trisomy 13 is more lethal and therefore much less common in infants than trisomy 21. The frequency at livebirth for trisomy 13 is about 1 in 12,000. The constellation of malformations seen in this condition makes survival beyond one year of life unusual (Figure 2–17).

Mental retardation as a result of severe brain malformations, frequently holoprosencephaly, is universal in trisomy 13. The phenotype of midline abnormalities that affect face, brain, and heart is often distinctive, but there is variability in the frequency of the associated malformations (Table 2–10). Between 85% and 90% of affected infants die in the first year of life.

Trisomy 18: Trisomy 18 occurs in about 1 in 6000 livebirths. The phenotype of trisomy 18 is not as distinctive as that of the other autosomal trisomies (Figure 2–18). Severe mental retardation is universal. The features which are most recognizable are the prominent occipital shelf, overlapping fingers, and prominent calcaneus (Table 2–10). Long-term survival is uncommon, and about 90% of children with this condition die within the first year of life.

Partial Autosomal Aneuploidy: Though individually rare, partial autosomal aneuploidy as a group is second to trisomy 21 in frequency of chromosomal abnormalities. Reported deletions or duplications have involved almost every chromosome. With better microscopic resolution and new molecular techniques, smaller deletions and duplications continue to be reported. It is believed that excess, loss, or interruption of several contiguous genes along the involved chromosome will explain the phenotypes of these conditions. If more than 1% of the chromosome is involved in a deletion, it is unlikely that the genes are all related to each other. Smaller deletions may contain related genes, as in the globin cluster, or unrelated genes. Since the phenotypes all involve developmental abnormalities, the locations of the deletions may contain important human developmental genes. A few examples of both kinds of deletions illustrate this group of abnormalities (Table 2–8).

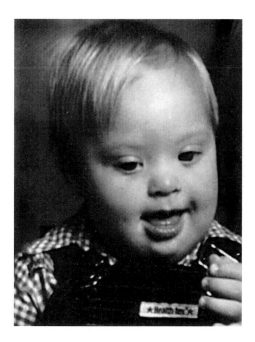

Figure 2–14 Photo of facies; child with Down syndrome. The Down syndrome phenotype can be produced by duplication of q22.1–q22.2, a small region of chromosome 21 known as the Down syndrome critical region. (Reproduced, with permission, from Hathaway WE et al: *Current Pediatric Diagnosis & Treatment,* Appleton & Lange, 1993).

Clinical Consequences of Chromosomal Rearrangements

Rearrangements of chromosomal material can be balanced or unbalanced. If the rearrangement is unbalanced, the phenotype depends upon the genetic material that is added or deleted. One or more genes may be involved. A balanced rearrangement does not result in addition or deletion of genetic material; the phenotype is normal. The rare exception to this rule occurs when the rearrangement is apparently balanced on cytogenetic examination, but there is disruption of a gene or genes—or there is a submicroscopic deletion or addition of genetic material detectable only by molecular means. Rearrangements have major reproductive consequences, however, and these result from the behavior of the rearranged chromosome at meiosis.

How trisomy and other unbalanced chromosome states produce phenotypic abnormalities is unknown. The biologic reasons for non-disjunctional events are also not understood. Advanced maternal age (greater than age 40) clearly has been associated with an increased risk of autosomal trisomy in the fetus. Paternal age has also been examined as a factor in the cause of non-disjunction trisomy 21. Nevertheless, the data show no significant effect of paternal age on non-disjunction.

Sex Chromosome Abnormalities

Abnormalities in number and structure of the sex chromosomes occur among both spontaneous abortuses and liveborns. In contrast to autosomes, sex chromosome abnormalities are associated with less severe phenotypic anomalies. In both males and females, an extra X-chromosome lowers to some extent the intelligence of the individual, thus increasing the frequency of mental retardation (MR) in these individuals. A correlation exists between the number of extra X-chromosomes and the severity of MR and physical abnormalities, so that individuals with three additional X-chromosomes are much more impaired than those with one extra X-chromosome. An extra X-chromosome causes sterility in the male, but not the female. A single extra Y- chromosome has minimal effects; individuals with several extra Y-chromosomes generally have an abnormal phenotype. The clinical features of this group of sex chromosome abnormalities are listed in Table 2–11.

In contrast with the presence of additional sex chromosomes, the presence of only a single sex chromosome has profound effects. A single Y (45,Y) or lack of any X-chromosome is highly lethal, never having been found in recognized pregnancies. Although not always lethal, a single X-chromosome (45,X) usually results in spontaneous abortion of the fetus; a small number of such conceptuses survive to livebirth and have a constellation of anomalies known as Turner syndrome. Clinical features of Turner syndrome are listed in Table 2–11. In these patients, it is important to recognize coarctation of the aorta when it exists; treatment is usually surgical. Administration of growth hormone to improve the short stature associated with Turner syndrome is controversial; while the hormone may increase the growth velocity for a time, ultimate height may not be substantially increased in all affected girls. Replacement therapy with ovarian hormones will result in development of secondary sex characteristics but will not restore fertility. Mental retardation is not a feature of Turner syndrome.

A fragile site at the distal end of the long arm of the X-chromosome is seen in males who have mental retardation and a characteristic facies, along with large testes after puberty. This condition, known as fragile X syndrome, is the most common cause of familial mental retardation. This and other mutations on the X-chromosome account for the excess of mental retardation in males, as compared to females. Although it is inherited as a Mendelian, X-linked condition, fragile X syndrome has a characteristic chromosome marker—the so-called fragile site on the X-chromosome. In addition to this locus, known as FRAXA, two other fragile sites have been identified on Xq27–q28. Termed FRAXE and FRAXF, they are also associated with mental retardation. The molecular pathology is an expansion of trinucleotide repeats, which is discussed in more detail in the gen-

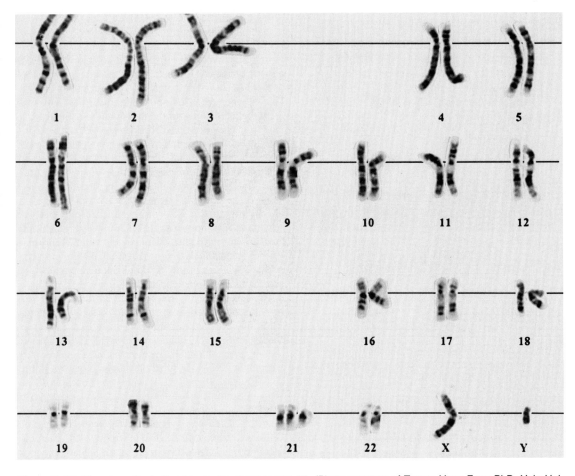

Figure 2–15. Karyotype illustrating trisomy for chromosome 21. (Photo courtesy of Teresa Yang-Feng PhD, Yale University.)

MENDELIAN GENETICS

Conditions that are caused by a mutation at a single gene locus appear in families in a defined pattern, which is referred to as Mendelian. The genetic constitution of the individual, the **genotype,** is not always obvious, and without the molecular genetic tools that are coming into current use, the genotype must be inferred from the pedigree. The **phenotype** can be observed in the individual. In many conditions caused by the same genotype, the phenotype may vary from one individual to another, giving rise to the concept of variable expression. Occasionally the individual carrying an abnormal gene at the locus of interest may have a completely normal phenotype; this phenomenon is known as variable penetrance. These two features lead to difficulties in identifying individuals carrying a mu-

eral section on molecular pathology. The clinical aspects are discussed in Chapter 11.

tant gene, and the tools of modern molecular genetics are brought into play to solve the question.

The three major **Mendelian patterns of inheritance** are autosomal dominant, autosomal recessive, and X-linked. Autosomal refers to the location of the gene on one of the 22 pairs of autosomes; X-linked refers to the location of the gene on the X-chromosome. These patterns are divided into two general types: **dominant,** in which expression of the trait occurs in the presence of only one mutant allele for that trait at the locus, and **recessive,** in which two copies of the mutant allele at the locus are required for obvious expression. Put another way, a mutation is dominant if it is expressed as a definable phenotype when only one copy of the mutation exists at the locus; a mutation is recessive if it is expressed only in individuals with no copy of the normal gene. If the alleles at a particular locus are the same, the individual is said to be **homozygous** for that allele; if they are different, the individual is said to be **heterozygous.** Individuals can be doubly heterozygous for

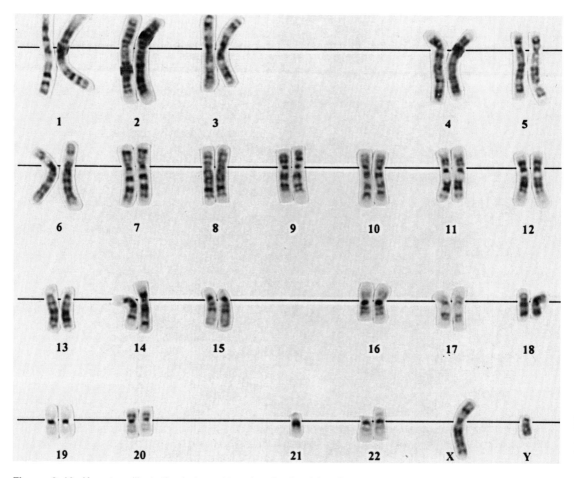

Figure 2–16. Karyotype illustrating balanced translocation involving chromosomes 14, 21 and 45,X,t(14q21q). (Photo courtesy of Teresa Yang-Feng PhD, Yale University.)

Table 2–9. Clinical features of (trisomy 21) Down syndrome.	
Developmental Stage	**Feature**
Neonatal	Hypotonia
	Clinodactyly
	Small ears
	Cataracts
	Transverse palmar crease
	Hearing disability
	Congenital heart disease
	Duodenal atresia
	Typical facies
Infancy, Childhood	Developmental delay
	Ear infections
	Hearing disability
	Atlantoaxial instability
	Seizures
	Visual disability
Childhood into adulthood	Hypothyroidism
	Short stature
	Leukemia
	Mitral valve prolapse
	Intellectual handicap

two different mutant alleles at the locus. **Mendelian principles** can be summarized as follows:

1. Genes are inherited as discreet characters. Acquired characteristics are not inherited.
2. The two alleles at each locus separate during gametogenesis and segregate to different gametes.
3. Loci in the haploid set of genes assort independently to the gametes unless they are tightly linked along the chromosome to each other. This assortment accounts for the Mendelian patterns of inheritance.
4. The major patterns of inheritance that follow Mendelian principles include the following:

Autosomal dominant

- Except for new mutations, every affected person has an affected parent
- Affected persons are usually heterozygous
- Each child of an affected person has a 50% chance of inheriting the abnormal gene
- The two sexes are affected in equal numbers.

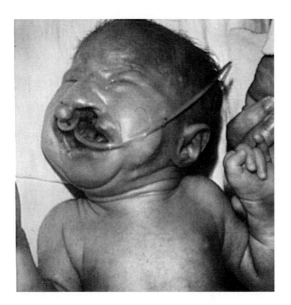

Figure 2–17. Photo of patient with trisomy 13. Frequency at livebirth is about 1 in 12,000. Survival beyond one year of life is unusual. (Reproduced, with permission, from Hathaway WE et al: *Current Pediatrics Diagnosis & Treatment,* Appleton & Lange, 1993.)

Autosomal recessive

- Both parents of an affected person are heterozygous for the mutant gene
- Heterozygotes can sometimes be detected using special tests
- For rare traits there is a high frequency of consanguinity
- Each sibling of an affected person has a 25% chance of being affected
- Each phenotypically normal sibling of an affected person has a 2 in 3 chance of being heterozygous
- The two sexes are affected in equal numbers
- If the recessive genes are allelic, all children of affected parents are affected
- An affected person may have two different mutations at the locus involved.

X-linked recessive

- Males carrying the mutant gene show the trait
- Females carrying the mutant gene generally do not show the trait
- Heterozygous mothers have a 50% chance to transmit the gene to each son or daughter
- Hemizygous affected males transmit the gene to all their daughters **but to none of their sons**
- The gene frequency in females is about twice that in males.

X-linked dominant

- Both males and females carrying the mutant gene show the trait
- Heterozygous mothers have a 50% chance to transmit the gene to each son and daughter
- Hemizygous affected males transmit the gene to all their daughters **but to none of their sons**
- The gene frequency in females is about twice that in males.

Similar phenotypes can be the result of different mutations, whether at the same locus or at a completely separate locus. Recognition of this **genetic heterogeneity** is crucial to accurate genetic diagnosis and thus to accurate counseling and correct medical management of genetic disorders, a need which no medical specialty will escape in the decade to come. Figure 2–19 illustrates a pattern of inheritance that follows Mendelian principles.

NON-MENDELIAN INHERITANCE

Many traits are clearly familial but do not follow Mendelian patterns. Some of these traits are rare conditions; some are very common. Examples include many congenital malformations such as cleft lip and palate, club foot, pyloric stenosis, spina bifida and related neural tube abnormalities—as well as many of the common disorders affecting children and adults such as diabetes, schizophrenia, heart disease, and high blood pressure. Several possible explanations for the increased familial clustering of these conditions can be considered. The two most likely genetic mechanisms are (a) a single locus with several alleles that lead to continuous phenotypes (eg, red cell acid phosphatase activity) and (b) multiple alleles at more than one locus that result in additive effects (eg, height, weight, and skin color). Some effects may represent traits which have important genetic and environmental components.

A number of models have been constructed for continuous and discontinuous traits. The evidence for genetic factors in these traits and conditions is found in family studies, empirical incidence data, and twin studies. Discontinuous traits are those in which a particular phenotype is either displayed or not displayed. Many congenital malformations and common disorders of adults and children fall into this category. For club foot, cleft lip and palate, diabetes, and schizophrenia, eg, the individual either displays the trait or does not. The threshold model is used to explain the genetic role in these conditions. This model states that there is continuous variation of some variable in the population, and above a certain threshold value of that variable, an individual shows the trait of interest. An example might be cleft palate. The variable might

Table 2–10. Common clinical features of trisomy 13 and trisomy 18.

System	Features	
	Trisomy 13	**Trisomy 18**
General	Post-natal growth failure; severe mental retardation; 85% to 90% die before age 1 year	IUGR, post-natal growth failure; severe mental retardation; 90–95% die between six months and 1 year of age; a few long-term survivors
Head, face	Hypertelorism, microphthalmia, malformed ears, microcephaly, cleft lip and palate, epicanthic folds, scalp defect	Microcephaly, pronounced occipital
CNS	Holoprosencephaly, arhinencephaly, seizures	Abnormal small brain, seizures
Cardiac	Congenital malformations, frequent cause of death	Congenital malformations, frequent cause of death
Renal	Malformations, UTI	UTI
Skeleton	Polydactyly	Short sternum, contractures, scoliosis
Genitalia		Hypoplastic labia, cryptorchidism

be time-required-for-movement in the embryo of cells destined to be palate. Above a certain length of time, the trait cleft palate occurs.

Characteristics of Inheritance of Complex Traits

The characteristics of inheritance of complex traits include the following:

- Familial clustering
- No clear Mendelian pattern
- Sex difference in frequency
- No clear biochemical or molecular defect
- Considerable variation in expression within and between families
- Genetic and environmental components are important.

QUANTITATIVE GENETICS

Quantitative genetics is the study of human variation and the principles that govern the role genes play in determining that variation. Toward this end, quantitative genetics examines genes in families and in populations. The frequency of any given gene in a population determines how often the effects of that gene will be seen. The rules of Mendelian inheritance determine the patterns in which the effects of any given gene will be seen within a family. The distribution of genes in populations and in families obeys mathematical rules that allow us to approximate frequencies of genes. As the number of genes under consideration increases, so does the complexity of the related mathematics. When several genes in large families or in large popula-

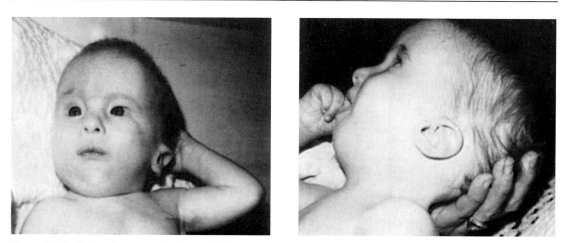

Figure 2–18. Photo of patient with trisomy 18. Long-term survival is uncommon. About 90% of children with trisomy 18 die within the first year of life. (Reproduced, with permission, from Hathaway WE et al: *Current Pediatric Diagnosis & Treatment,* Appleton & Lange, 1993.)

Table 2–11. Features of sex chromosome abnormalities.

Gender	Chromosomes	Phenotype
Female	XO	Turner syndrome
Female	XXX, XXXX	Mental retardation, psychosis; fertile, normal offspring
Male	XYY	Tall stature, learning difficulty
Male	XXY	Klinefelter syndrome
Male	XXYY, XXXYY, XXXXY	Klinefelter syndrome, mental retardation

tions are considered, the mathematical treatment requires sophisticated computer programs. Such programs also help to test models of inheritance for traits whose mode of inheritance has not been determined. Understanding the principles of Mendelian inheritance and the behavior of genes in populations, with particular attention to human disease determining genes, can allow the physician to calculate simple risks for the appearance of genetic traits in families or populations, as the following clinical example suggests.

The family pedigree shown in Figure 2–19 includes a child who has a recessively inherited disorder, eg, cystic fibrosis. This pedigree provides a review of Mendelian principles and allows the estimation of a number of risks of possible interest to the family. These include the risk that another sibling will be born with cystic fibrosis and the risk that a sibling will have an affected child.

According to Mendelian principles, the risk that these parents will have another child with cystic fibrosis is 25%—or 1 in 4—for each future child. These principles alone, however, do not allow clinicians to predict the risk that other family members will have a child with the disorder. For this, princi-

ples of quantitative genetics are needed. For example, what is the risk that a sibling of someone with cystic fibrosis will have a child with the disease? To answer this question two pieces of information are required: the risk that the sibling is heterozygous for the cystic fibrosis gene and the risk that the sibling will marry someone who is heterozygous for the gene. Mendelian principles say that the likelihood that the phenotypically normal sibling of an individual with an autosomal recessive condition is heterozygous for that mutation is 2 in 3. The chance that the sibling will marry a carrier of cystic fibrosis depends on the risk that someone in the general population is such a carrier. This can be calculated as follows:

There are two kinds of genes at the locus in question:

n = normal allele and c = cf allele

If p and q are proportions of each allele, and n is set = p, and c is set = q, then **p + q = 1.**

It is understood that $(p + q)^2$ represents a special case of the binomial theorem $(x + y)^n$ where n = 2, because a person is a random sample of alleles taken

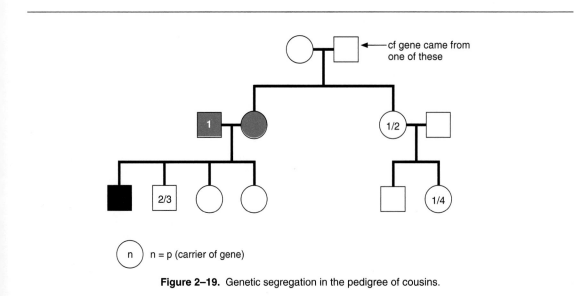

Figure 2–19. Genetic segregation in the pedigree of cousins.

2 at a time. This binomial expression can be expanded to

$$(p + q)^2 = 1 \text{ or}$$

$$p^2 + 2pq + q^2 = 1.$$

The population can thus be described as comprising three kinds of people with respect to the cf gene:

Homozygous normal (p × p) or p²

Homozygous affected (q × q) or q²

Heterozygous (p × q × 2) or 2pq

This is illustrated below in the Punnett square, which is a diagram of matings of heterozygotes:

Parent	N	C
N	NN	NC
C	NC	CC

The relationship among genes and gene frequencies in the population is known as the **Hardy-Weinberg equilibrium.** Note that 2pq can never exceed 0.5, which occurs when the two alleles are equal in frequency. The most useful form of the Hardy-Weinberg relationship is the equation

$$p^2 + 2pq + q^2 = 1.$$

In this case, p and q are allele frequencies, and 2pq is the heterozygote frequency.

The risk to consider is the chance that any member of the general population is a heterozygote for the disorder, cystic fibrosis. In this case, $q^2 = 1$ in 2500, the frequency of the disease in the Caucasian population; assuming that q is small enough so that p approximates 1, the value of 2pq can be calculated as follows:

$$2pq = 2 \times \sim 1 \times 1/50 \approx 2/50 \approx 1/25.$$

Thus, the risk that a sibling of an individual affected with cystic fibrosis will have a child with cystic fibrosis can be calculated in the following equation:

p(sib carries cf gene) × p(passing on gene | carrier) × p(spouse carries gene) × p(passing on gene | carrier)

or

$$2/3 \times 1/2 \times 2/50 \times 1/2 = 1/150.$$

This is 16 times the population risk, which is considerably higher than the general population incidence.

Gene frequencies differ in different ethnic groups. The risks calculated above depend on the frequency of the gene in the population under consideration. If the spouse in the above example were a member of an ethnic group where the disease frequency is only 1 in 10,000 how would that influence q—and thus the risk that the couple will have a child with cystic fibrosis?

Since the disease incidence is q^2, and q^2 is now 1/10,000, the value of 2pq in the equation is:

p(sib carries cf gene) × p(passing on gene | carrier) × p(spouse carries gene) × p(passing on gene | carrier)

or

$$2/3 \times 1/2 \times 2/100 \times 1/2 = 1/300,$$

which is 8 times the risk for the caucasian population.

Is the risk higher if the sibling in question marries someone whose brother or sister has CF? The risk that this couple will have a child with CF is as follows:

p(sib carries cf gene) × p(passing on gene | carrier) × p(spouse carries gene) × p(passing on gene | carrier)

or

$$2/3 \times 1/2 \times 2/3 \times 1/2 = 1/9,$$

which is 277 times the risk for the general population.

The situation becomes much more complex if the sibling marries a first cousin. How does consanguinity affect the probability that these individuals will have a child affected with cystic fibrosis? The genetic risk to individuals who are consanguineous derives from the chance that they each carry deleterious genes that are identical by descent from a common ancestor. The magnitude of this risk depends on the genetic distance that exists between these individuals. The probability that an individual and a first cousin have inherited a gene that is identical (by descent from a common ancestor) is 1 in 8. However, this probability does not apply in this case, since we know that both parents of the affected person and his sibling each carry the mutant/abnormal allele. The equation then becomes:

p(sib carries cf gene) × p(passing on gene | carrier) × p(spouse carries gene) × p(passing on gene | carrier)

or

$$2/3 \times 1/2 \times 1/4 \times 1/2 = 1/24,$$

which is 104 times the risk for the general population.

Figure 2–19 illustrates how the genes of interest segregate in this type of pedigree of cousins.

The reason that consanguinity in a population or a family leads to an increase in the frequency of genetic conditions derives from the fact that consanguineous individuals share genes that have been inherited from a common ancestor. If one gene inherited from a common ancestor carries a mutation, then the related individuals will have a higher risk that each of them carries a copy of the mutant gene. Thus, if two consanguineous persons have a child, that child has an increased chance—compared to a child born to unrelated people—of being homozygous by descent for the mutant gene. If the mutation, when homozygous, causes an abnormal phenotype, the child will be abnormal. The reasons for consanguinity include geographic and ethnic factors. It becomes empirically important when the relationship is that of first cousins, or closer. Under the following conditions, equilibrium is reached and the Hardy-Weinberg proportions apply:

- Random mating
- Large population size
- No selection of the alleles under consideration
- No significant mutation
- No migration.

Obviously no real population meets these constraints precisely, so the use of the Hardy-Weinberg equation is necessarily an approximation. However, very large deviations from the ideal conditions noted above are required to cause major differences in the results of Hardy-Weinberg calculations. In human populations, inbreeding represents one of the most important deviations from Hardy-Weinberg equilibrium. As seen above, blood relatives share genes inherited from a common ancestor. Other deviations from Hardy-Weinberg equilibrium also occur. Stratification of the population alters the observed gene frequency since the sample is not homogeneous. Assortative mating can occur, although the genotype is unknown, because characteristics with a genetic component can sometimes be observable and thus influence choice of mate. Stature and skin color are but two examples. If some gametes do not survive to accomplish fertilization, their genetic contribution will be lost. This unequal viability of gametes can lead to deviations from Hardy-Weinberg equilibrium. **Genetic drift** refers to a perceived unequal distribution of genes in a population because of sampling bias (that is due to a small sample size) or because of chance events in the migration or survival or a population.

Genes from an individual will be lost from the population if that individual does not reproduce. If genotype alters the ability to reproduce, **fitness** decreases. Mutant genes can lead to **selection** in favor of the gene or against the gene, in either the homozygous or heterozygous state. For example, the gene for sickle hemoglobin in the homozygous state leads to sickle cell anemia; in the heterozygous state, the gene

protects against falciparum malaria. This can also alter equilibrium.

Clearly, a better way to estimate whether a person is heterozygous for a particular allele—eg, a way to mark or see the gene of interest—would be of great value to clinicians. The new methods of linkage and molecular analysis provide such a tool.

LINKAGE & MOLECULAR ANALYSIS

Modern molecular genetics has seen the development of tools that have vastly improved the ability to evaluate genetic risks formerly inferred from pedigrees or estimated on the basis of biologic observations far from the site of gene action. Success has depended upon the analysis of human genes, which in turn has relied on the development of various new techniques to analyze and separate proteins, RNA, and DNA. Today, specific molecular pathology is being defined for many human diseases.

In the case of the X-chromosome, location of specific genes has been made by inference from pedigree information; for autosomes, specific genes have been located by linkage to identifiable protein markers, eg, blood groups and HLA antigens. With the development of recombinant DNA technology and the molecular genetic techniques which have followed, the specific chromosomal location of many more genes is known. Polymorphism and non-random assortment of genes due to linkage have allowed the localization of many genes, linkage to specific markers has been established, and many genes of clinical importance have been cloned, sequenced, and molecular pathology defined. It is likely that within the next two decades, the entire human genome will be mapped, and eventually it will be entirely sequenced. The techniques to achieve these goals include somatic cell hybridization, linkage analysis, restriction analysis, DNA fingerprinting, DNA sequencing, and other methods to analyze specific DNA sequences. These approaches have required the ability to detect genes, follow them through families and populations, analyze genetic structure, and correlate structure with function. To identify mutant genes, mutant DNA must be separated from an individual's genome.

Although Mendel's law states that genes assort independently, important exceptions exist, notably, genes that appear to be transmitted together. Such genes must be close together on the same chromosome; for this reason, they are said to be **linked.** Linkage can be useful if one of the genes is easy to detect; the presence of the other gene may then be inferred. The first linkage information was reported in 1911 by E.B. Wilson, who deduced from pedigree information that color blindness is X-linked. Linkage of the Duffy blood group to chromosome 1 was established by observing cosegregation with a heteromorphism on that chromosome. Linkage of myotonic dystrophy to the secretor locus proved useful in some clinical situations.

Somatic cell hybridization between human and mouse cells with observation of cosegregation of expression of known genes with particular human chromosomes has established the chromosomal location of many human genes. New molecular techniques have revolutionized the use of linkage analysis to detect the presence of specific genes. The usefulness of a linkage marker that is easy to measure and is always associated with the presence of the mutant allele can clearly help refine the risk statements for families. Mapping of this kind depends on correlating phenotype (either in the whole individual or in the cell) with the marker. Such markers have been developed; if they are spaced evenly enough along the chromosome, they can be used as landmarks on genetic maps. Three kinds of genetic maps exist:

- Linkage maps
- Cytogenetic maps
- Physical maps.

A linkage map demonstrates that two traits or genes are observed together more often than would occur by chance, thus indicating a deviation from Mendel's law of independent segregation. When a particular allele at a locus (eg, a disease-causing mutation) is associated with an allele at a linked locus—and the association occurs at a greater frequency than is predicted by chance—this deviation is called **linkage disequilibrium.** Today all chromosomes have linkage markers about 10–20 centimorgans (cM) apart. (The cM is a unit of recombination: 10 cM corresponds to 10% recombination, ~ 10^7bp, ~ 1/300 of the genome, or 20–30 functional genetic clusters.)

Cytogenetic maps have been developed through the use of several techniques that have allowed localization of genes to particular chromosomal locations. Such maps require chromosomal banding for fine localization. The technique of somatic cell hybridization with fragmented human chromosomes has been employed. Development of cytogenetic maps has also taken advantage of studies of patients in whom there are single gene disorders segregating with chromosomal deletions or rearrangements. More recently, the technique of in situ hybridization using labelled DNA probes to identify specific chromosomal regions has been used to advantage (Figure 2–20).

Physical maps demonstrate order and spacing of genes. Molecular maps of overlapping clones of DNA, called **contigs,** have been used to establish this order; contigs have led to even finer mapping of genes. A number of methods have been used to detect genes. These include protein sequencing, DNA separation using electrophoretic techniques that detect large and small DNA fragments, DNA sequencing, and cloning techniques that employ plasmids, cosmids, and viruses. Restriction analysis has been very instrumental in establishing linkage and using markers for specific genes. This strategy is particularly useful (if the gene has not been cloned) in establishing the risk that an individual carries the gene of interest. When the gene has been cloned and the molecular pathology has been established, the specific DNA sequence can be used to determine the status of the individual. A short piece of specific DNA—ie, a short string of nucleotides—can be used to identify identical segments of DNA in a tissue sample. Such a piece of DNA is called a **probe.** Probes can be of two kinds:

- **Complementary (c-DNA)** that is reverse-transcribed from mRNA and made double-stranded
- **Genomic DNA**—from small restriction fragments that have been generated from total genomic DNA.

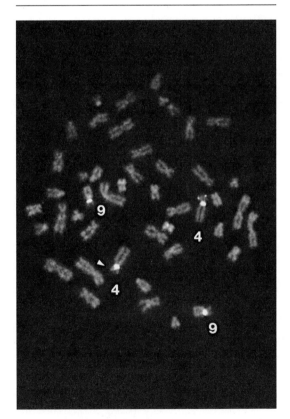

Figure 2–20. Metaphase spreads after fluorescent in situ hybridization (FISH) with probe L6 (D4S166) and a centromere-specific probe for chromosomes 4 and 9. Hybridization signal was detected only on chromosome 4. The arrow indicates chromosome 4, which has a deletion in 4p; the chromosome is lacking the D4S166 sequence. (Courtesy of Theresa Yang-Feng PhD, Yale University.)

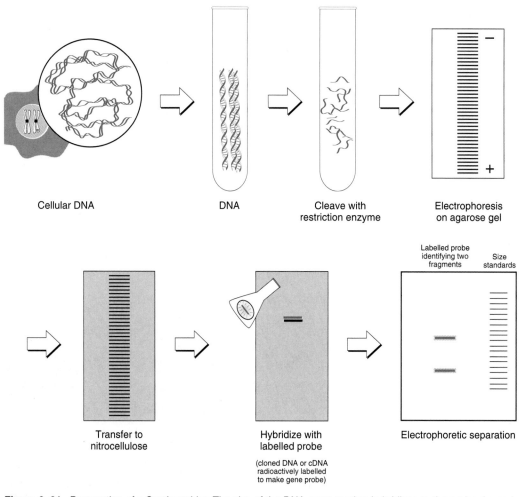

Cellular DNA   DNA   Cleave with   Electrophoresis
                                   restriction enzyme   on agarose gel

Labelled probe
identifying two   Size
fragments   standards

Transfer to   Hybridize with   Electrophoretic separation
nitrocellulose   labelled probe

(cloned DNA or cDNA
radioactively labelled
to make gene probe)

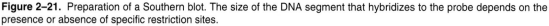

Figure 2–21. Preparation of a Southern blot. The size of the DNA segment that hybridizes to the probe depends on the presence or absence of specific restriction sites.

A probe can be a specific known sequence that is either:

- A synthetic oligonucleotide: A small segment made of a known sequence
- c-DNA that is reverse transcribed from isolated mRNA.

A probe can be an **anonymous sequence** with unknown function and location or an anonymous sequence that is mapped to a specific chromosome; the order of several such segments can be inferred. A DNA probe can be used to detect specific DNA sequences in genomic DNA, eg, a specific oligonucleotide probe to detect a known mutation in genomic DNA (Orkin, β-globin probe).

Restriction analysis uses bacterially derived restriction enzymes that recognize specific DNA sequences. If a mutation changes a restriction site, depending on the location of the site, the size of the fragment that results from the restriction enzyme cleavage varies. Fragments are identified by using a labelled probe as indicator. A radioactive label is often used, but other kinds of labeling can be employed, eg, biotinylation. Polymorphisms in restriction sites (RFLPs) can be used as linkage markers (eg, in cystic fibrosis). By definition, an **RFLP** is a common heritable variation among individuals in DNA nucleotide sequences that results in different DNA fragment lengths, when total genomic DNA is digested by specific bacterial endonucleases—bacterial enzymes that cut DNA reproducibly at specific nucleotide sequences (Botstein, 1980) (Figure 2–21).

In restriction analysis, the locus must be **polymorphic** in order to study it; ie, it must have the following features:

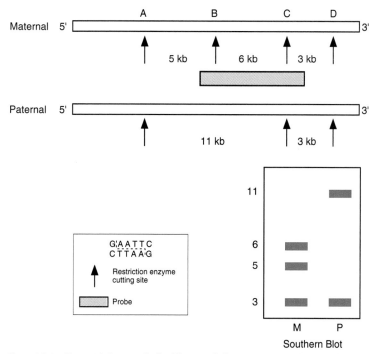

Figure 2–22. A Southern blot with restriction analysis. The restriction enzyme cutting site B is present in the allele of maternal origin but not in the allele of paternal origin, thus enabling the distinction between the two. Cutting by a restriction enzyme will result in different sized fragments from each of those alleles: 5 and 6 kb fragments from the maternal allele and 11 kb fragment from the paternal allele. Both will have a 3 kb allele. A probe spanning sites B and C will identify all the fragments on Southern analysis.

- More than one allele
- The least frequent allele has a frequency of more than 1% (and thus cannot be accounted for by mutation and can be tracked).

Loci are most useful if they are very polymorphic. A diagram of a blot obtained by Southern analysis is shown in Figure 2–22. The sizes of the DNA segments that hybridize to the probe depend on the presence or absence of specific restriction sites.

The method used to obtain these blots is simple in concept. DNA is cleaved by a restriction enzyme into small fragments, then size-fractionated on a gel; the entire electrophoresis is transferred to a nylon membrane and then exposed to a labelled probe, usually P^{32}-labelled DNA. The entire membrane is then placed under unexposed x-ray film, which is exposed only in the location where the radioactive probe has hybridized to its complementary DNA. Specific oligonucleotide probes have been used to hybridize to specific DNA segments in a library.

DNA fingerprinting is based upon the fact that the human genome contains many repetitive sequences. Alu repeats, eg, comprise about 5% of the human genome, and there are a number of other tandem repeats. The numbers of such repeats is unique

to any individual. The method of DNA fingerprinting described by Jeffreys (1985) takes advantage of this fact. Utilizing a single probe and an appropriate restriction enzyme, one can obtain a blot with many bands in a pattern unique to the individual. The likelihood that two individuals will have an identical pattern of DNA fingerprints is extremely small (the precise probability remains controversial); even siblings are not alike in this matter.

The kinds of studies discussed above can be performed on DNA from any tissue source. Blood lymphocytes, skin cells, and fibroblasts are commonly used. In order to amplify amounts of DNA available, the polymerase chain reaction can be used if the DNA sequence of the gene of interest is known. Probes consisting of c-DNA are made from cells actively making m-RNA, and will be representative of the genes being expressed in those cells. Information gained from new techniques of molecular genetic mapping has proven useful in research and clinical applications. In research, eg, the following advances have occurred:

1. Specific molecular pathology has been increasingly identified.
2. Classes of mutations are being delineated.

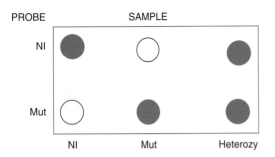

PROBE   SAMPLE

NI

Mut

NI   Mut   Heterozy

Figure 2–23. Dot blot analysis. Blood or other material containing DNA can be analyzed directly for the presence of the mutation when two probes—one complementary to the mutation and one complementary to the normal allele—are used. Homozygous normal, homozygous abnormal, and heterozygous can be distinguished from one another.

3. Size of human genes is being determined.
4. Understanding of gene structure and function is advancing.
5. Human evolution is being clarified.
6. Elucidation of the functional and pathological anatomy of the human genome is occurring.

From the clinical standpoint, linked markers to inherited disease—and the ability to define specific molecular lesions—will be useful for diagnosis, as in the example of cystic fibrosis cited earlier. Better estimation of risk to relatives, better understanding of disease heterogeneity, and improved understanding of multifactorial traits have resulted from increased knowledge of molecular genetics. It is hoped the eventual result will be improved prevention and treatment of inherited diseases.

Consider again the cystic fibrosis example; how have these new techniques been used? Linkage analysis led to localization of the cystic fibrosis gene to chromosome 7. Using chromosome jumping, several groups have succeeded in cloning the gene for cystic fibrosis, a gene that codes for a membrane spanning protein involved in ion transport. Linked DNA markers also have been used for family analysis, carrier detection, and prenatal diagnosis; specific mutation analysis can now be used to establish the presence or absence of the mutations commonly known to result in cystic fibrosis.

While the concepts of linkage analysis are straightforward, the actual analyses often require statistical methods for refinement, particularly when recombination is involved. The landmarks of the map are restriction sites that provide a background upon which mutations have taken place. The usefulness of linked markers depends on their proximity to the gene and the mutation of interest. Because recombination can be a confounding problem, markers to either side of the gene (flanking markers) are useful. If the marker is not the gene itself, the possibility of recombination between the gene and the marker exists. The statistical way to handle that problem is to determine the odds that the association has occurred by chance rather than because of linkage. Because logarithms make this handling simpler, the log of the odds is used; it is called the LOD score. A LOD score of 3 is taken as evidence for linkage. This represents an odds ratio of 1000:1 ($\log_{10}$ of $1000 = 3$).

A disease gene can be linked to a marker locus which can be studied and followed through a family or population. If a large family or a number of families are studied, the case of linkage between two loci, A and B can be considered. Suppose the observation is made that 20% of persons are recombinant, 80%

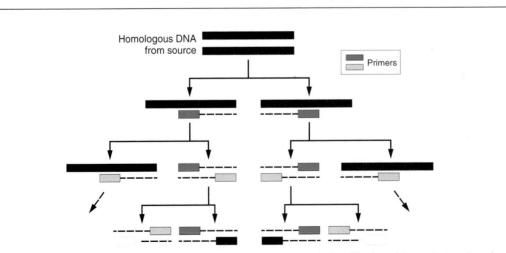

Figure 2–24. Polymerase chain reaction (PCR) (schematic representation). Amplification of the mutant region of a gene with PCR technology is effective in identifying specific mutations.

non-recombinant. Recombination frequency, θ, is thus 20%, and the genes are 20 cM apart. Is this 80:20 significantly different from the null hypothesis, 50:50? The way to determine this is to consider likelihoods of observing the given pedigree at different recombination frequencies testing the likelihoods at each against the 50:50 hypothesis of non-linkage. Calculate likelihood at a given value of θ:

likelihood of the observed data if loci linked at θ

divided by the likelihood of data if loci unlinked

$$\frac{P|\theta_x}{P|\theta = 0.5}$$

This is the **odds ratio,** which is manipulated using the log of odds **(LOD),** or (LOD Score)

$$Z_{\theta x} = \log_{10} \frac{P|\theta_x}{P|\theta = 0.5}$$

The procedure is then to do many families, calculate Z for each family, plot Z for $\theta = 0$ to $\theta = 0.5$, obtain Z for θ_{max}. If Z > 3, this represents 1000:1 odds and is considered significant.

As the specific molecular pathology of various genetic diseases is identified, methodology that detects the presence of mutant genes in individuals who are homozygous or heterozygous for disease genes also becomes more specific. Dot blots that employ DNA probes which are complementary to the specific mutation can be used (Figure 2–23).

Amplification of the mutant region with polymerase chain reaction (PCR) technology is also effective in identifying the presence of specific mutations, when the probes are available.

PCR uses a DNA polymerase from the bacterium *Thermus aquaticus* (Taq polymerase) and small pieces of DNA, about 20 base pairs long, of known sequence, called primers, which flank the region of interest. Under appropriate conditions, the polymerase will use the pieces of DNA as template to synthesize more identical DNA. If the conditions are correct, and the normal and mutant sequences are known and used as primers, DNA that contains the mutation of interest can be distinguished from DNA that does not. If the primers are not more than 1000 base pairs apart, the amplification will be geometric, and at the end of 30 cycles there will be about 1 million copies of the DNA region of interest (Figure 2–24).

These methods can supercede linkage analysis when the appropriate constraints are met. As more of the human genome is mapped, cloned, and sequenced, the means to identify specific mutant genes will become more applicable and more available. A map of the entire human genome consisting of landmarks that include known loci, restriction sites, and the ends of overlapping contiguous clones will soon be available.

REFERENCES AND SUGGESTED READING

Annas GJ: Privacy rules for DNA Databanks: Protecting coded future diaries. JAMA 1993;**270**:2346.

Baird PA, Sadovnick AD: Causes of death to age 30 in Down syndrome. Am J Hum Genet 1988;**43**:239.

Baty BJ, Blackburn BL, Carey JC: Natural History of Trisomy 18 and Trisomy 13: I. Growth, Physical Assessment, Medical Histories, Survival, and Recurrence Risk. Am J Med Genet 1994;**49**:175.

Beighton P (editor): *McKusick's Heritable Disorders of Connective Tissue,* 5th ed. Mosby, 1993.

Bittles AH, Neel JV: The costs of human inbreeding and their implications for variations at the DNA level. Nature Genetics 1994;**8**:117.

Botstein D et al: Construction of a genetic linkage map in man using restriction fragment length polymorphisms. Am J Hum Genet 1980;**32**:314.

Brook JD et al: Molecular basis of myotonic dystrophy: Expansion of a trinucleotide (CTG) repeat at the 3' end of a transcript encoding a protein kinase family member. Cell 1992;**68**:799.

Burrow GN, Ferris TF (editors): *Medical Complications During Pregnancy,* 4th ed, WB Saunders, 1995.

Buxton J, Sherbourne P, Davies J: Detection of an unstable fragment of DNA specific to individuals with myotonic dystrophy. Nature 1992;**355**:547.

Caskey CT: Molecular medicine: A spin-off from the helix. JAMA 1993;**269**:1986.

Caspersson T, Zech L, Johansson C: Differential band of alkylating fluorochromes in human chromosomes. Exp Cell Res 1970;**60**:315.

Childs B et al: Molecular genetics in medicine. Prog Med Genet 1988;7.

Cohen MM, Rosenblum-Vos LS, Prabhakar G: Human cytogenetics: A current overview. Am J Dis Child 1993; **147**:1159.

Collins FC: Cystic fibrosis: Molecular biology and therapeutic implications. Science 1992;**256**:774.

Collins FC: Of needles and haystacks: Finding human disease genes by positional cloning. Clin Res 1991;**39**: 615.

Collins FC et al: The von Recklinghausen neurofibromatosis region on chromosome 17—genetic and physical maps come into focus. (Editorial.) Am J Med Genet 1989;**44**:1.

Cooperative Human Linkage Center: A comprehensive human linkage map with centimorgan density. Science 1994;**265**:2049.

Daniel A, Hook EB, Wulf G: Risks of unbalanced progeny at amniocentesis to carriers of chromosome rearrangements: Data from United States and Canadian laboratories. Am J Med Genet 1989;**31**:14.

Davies KE: *Genome Analysis: A Practical Approach.* IRL Press, 1988.

Day N, Holmes LB: The incidence of genetic disease in a

university hospital population. Am J Hum Genet 1973;**25**:237.

Dietz HC et al: Marfan syndrome caused by a recurrent de novo missense mutation in the fibrillin gene. Nature 1991A;**352**:337.

Dietz HC et al: The Marfan syndrome locus: Confirmation of assignment to chromosome 15 and identification of tightly linked markers at 15q15–q21.3. Genomics 1991B; **9**:355.

Emanuel BS: Molecular cytogenetics: Towards dissection of the contiguous gene syndromes. Am J Hum Genet 1988;**43**:575.

Emery AEH, Rimoin D (editors): *Principles and Practice of Medical Genetics,* 2nd ed, Churchill Livingstone, 1990.

Eunpu DL, McDonald DM, Zackai EH: Trisomy 21: Rate in second-degree relatives. Am J Med Genet 1986;**25**: 361.

Freije D et al: Identification of a second pseudoautosomal region near the Xq and Yq telomeres. Science 1992;**258**: 1784.

Fountain JW et al: Physical mapping of the von Recklinghausen neurofibromatosis region on chromosome 17. Am J Hum Genet 1989;**44**:58.

Fu YH et al: An unstable triplet repeat in a gene related to myotonic muscular dystrophy. Science 1992;**255**: 1253.

Gelehrter TD, Collins FS: *Principles of Medical Genetics.* Williams and Wilkins, 1990.

Greenberg F: Contiguous gene syndromes. Growth, Genetics and Hormones 1993;**9**:5.

Guyer MS, Collins FS: The human genome project and the future of medicine. Am J Dis Child 1993;**147**:1145.

Hall JG: The clinical behavior of hereditary syndromes, with a precis of medical genetics. Pages 1–32 in: *McKusick's Heritable Disorders of Connective Tissue,* 5th ed, Beighton P (editor). Mosby, 1993.

Hassold TJ: A cytogenetic study of repeated spontaneous abortions. Am J Hum Genet 1980;**32**:723.

Hassold TJ, Jacobs PA: Trisomy in man. Annu Rev Genet 1984;**18**:69.

Hawkins JD: *Gene Structure and Expression.* Cambridge University Press, 1991.

Helminen P et al: Application of DNA fingerprints to paternity determinations. Lancet 1988;**1(8585)**:574.

Heitz D et al: Inheritance of the fragile X syndrome: Size of the fragile X premutation is a major determinant of the transition to fill mutation. J Med Genet 1992;**29**: 794.

Hirst MC et al: The identification of a third fragile site, FRAXF, in Xq27–q28 distal to both FRAXA and FRAXE. Human Molecular Genetics 1993;**2**:197.

Hoekelman RA: More and more it seems, "It's all in the genes." Pediatr Ann 1993;**22**:272.

Hook EB, Regal RR: A search for a paternal-age effect upon cases of 47, + 21 in which the extra chromosome is of paternal origin. Am J Hum Genet 1984;**36**:413.

Hook EB, Cross PK, Schreinemachers DM: Chromosomal abnormality rates at amniocentesis and in live-born infants. JAMA 1983;**249**:2034.

Hull C, Hagerman RJ: A study of the physical, behavioral, and medical phenotype, including anthropometric measure, of females with Fragile X syndrome. Am J Dis Child 1993;**147**:1236.

Hunter A et al: The correlation of age on onset with CTG trinucleotide repeat amplification in myotonic dystrophy. J Med Genet 1992;**29**:774.

Inui K et al: Mitochondrial encephalomyopathies with mutation of the mitochondrial tRNALeu (URR) gene. J Pediatr 1992;**120**:62.

ISCN: An International System for Human Cytogenetic Nomenclature-High Resolution Banding. March of Dimes Birth Defects Foundation Birth Defects: Original Article Series 1985;**21(1)**:1.

Jeffreys AJ et al: Amplification of human minisatellites by the polymerase chain reaction: Towards DNA fingerprinting of single cells. Nucleic Acids Research 1988; **16(23)**:10953.

Jeffreys AJ et al: DNA fingerprints and segregation analysis of multiple markers in human pedigrees. Am J Hum Genet 1986;**39(1)**:11.

Jeffreys AJ, Wilson V, Thein SL: Individual-specific fingerprints of human DNA. Nature 1985;**316(6023)**:76.

Jeppesen P, Turner BM: The inactive X chromosome in female mammals is distinguished by a lack of histone H4 acetylaction, a cytogenetic marker for gene expression. Cell 1993;**74**:281.

Kainulainen K et al: Location on chromosome 15 of the gene defect causing the Marfan syndrome. N Engl J Med 1990;**323**:935.

Knight SJL et al: Triplet repeat amplification at the FRAXE locus and X-linked mild mental handicap. Am J Hum Genet 1994;**55**:81.

Knight SJL et al: Trinucleotide repeat amplification and hypermethylation of a CpG island in FRAXE mental retardation. Cell 1993;**74**:127.

Lander ES, Schork NJ: Genetic dissection of complex traits. Science 1994;**265**:2037.

Landgren U et al: DNA diagnostics-molecular techniques and automation. Science 1988;**242**:229.

Loesch DZ, Huggins RM, Chin WF: Effect of Fragile X on physical and intellectual trails estimated by pedigree analysis. Am J Med Genet 1993;**46**:415.

Lyon M: Gene action in the X-chromosome of the mouse (Mus musculus L). Nature 1961;**190**:190.

Mandel JL: Questions of expansion. Nature Genetics 1993; **4**:8.

McConkie-Rosell et al: Evidence that methylation of the FMR-1 locus is responsible for variable phenotypic expression of the fragile X syndrome. Am J Hum Genet 1993;**53**:800.

McKusick V: *Online Mendelian Inheritance in Man.* Johns Hopkins University Press, 1994.

McKusick VM: Medical genetics: A 40-year perspective on the evolution of a medical specialty from a basic science. JAMA 1993;**270**:2351.

Meijers-Heijboer EJ et al: Linkage analysis with chromosome 15q11–13 markers shows genomic imprinting in familial Angelman syndrome. J Med Genet 1992;**29**: 853.

Migeon BR: X-chromosome inactivation: Molecular mechanisms and genetic consequences. Trends in Genetics 1994;**10**:230.

Migeon BR: Role of DNA methylation in X-inactivation and the fragile X syndrome. Am J Med Genet 1993;**47**: 685.

Mikkelsen M et al: Non-disjunction in trisomy 21: Study of chromosomal heteromorphisms in 110 families. Ann Hum Genet 1980;**44**:17.

Mullis K et al: Specific enzymatic amplification of DNA in

vitro: The polymerase chain reaction. Cold Spring Harbor Symp Quant Biol 1986;**51:**263.

Ogata T, Matsuo N: Testis determining gene(s) on the X-chromosome short arm: Chromosomal localisation and possible role in testis determination. J Med Genet 1994;**31:**349.

Redman JB et al: Relationship between parental trinucleotide GCT repeat length and severity of myotonic dystrophy in offspring. JAMA 1993;**269:**1960.

Robinson A, Linden MG: *Clinical Genetics Handbook.* Blackwell Scientific Publications, 1993.

Robinson W et al: Uniparental disomy explains the occurrence of the Angelman or Prader-Willi syndrome in patients with an additional small inv dup(15) chromosome. J Med Genet 1993;**30:**756.

Romeo G, McKusick VM: Phenotypic diversity, allelic series and modifier genes. Nature Genetics 1994;**7:**451.

Root S, Carey JC: Survival in trisomy 18. Am J Med Genet 1994;**49:**170.

Rosenthal N: Molecular medicine: DNA and the genetic code. N Engl J Med. 1994;**331:**39.

Rosenthal N: Molecular medicine: Tools of the trade—recombinant DNA. N Engl J Med 1994;**331:**315.

Rosenthal N: Molecular medicine: Stalking the gene: DNA libraries. N Engl J Med 1994;**331:**599.

Rosenthal N: Molecular medicine: Regulation of gene expression. N Engl J Med. 1994;**331:**931.

Ross DW: *Introduction to Molecular Medicine.* Springer-Verlag, 1992.

Rousseau F et al: A multicenter study on genotype-phenotype correlations in the fragile X syndrome, using direct diagnosis with probe StB12.3: The first 2,253 cases. Am J Hum Genet 1994;**55:**225.

Rousseau F et al: Direct DNA analysis of the fragile X syndrome of mental retardation. N Engl J Med 1991;**24:** 1674.

Royle NJ et al: Clustering of hypervariable minisatellites in the proterminal regions of human autosomes. Genomics 1988(Nov);**3(4):**352.

Sachs ES et al: Chromosome studies of 500 couples with two or more abortions. Obstet Gynecol 1985;**65:**375.

Saitoh S et al: Molecular and clinical study of 61 Angelman syndrome patients. Am J Med Genet 1994;**52:**158.

Schinzel A: Genomic imprinting: Consequences of uniparental disomy for human disease. Am J Med Genet 1993;**46:**683.

Schmickel R: Contiguous gene syndromes: A component of recognizable syndromes. J Pediatr 1986;**109:**231.

Schwartz S, Roulston DR, Cohen MM: Invited editorial: dNORs and meiotic nondisjunction. Am J Hum Genet 1989;**44:**627.

Scriver C: Presidential address: Physiological genetics—who needs it? Am J Hum Genet 1987;**40:**199.

Shapiro LR: The fragile X syndrome. N Engl J Med 1991;**325:**1736.

Shelbourne P et al: Direct diagnosis of myotonic dystrophy with a disease-specific DNA marker. N Engl J Med 1993;**328:**471.

Sherman SJ, Schwartz DB: Eclampsia complicating a pregnancy with neurofibromatosis. J Reprod Med 1992;**37:**469.

Sherman SL, Rogato A, Turner G: Recurrence risks for relatives in families with an isolated case of the fragile X syndrome. Am J Med Genet 1988;**31:**753.

Singer M, Berg P: *Genes and Genomes.* University Science Books, 1991.

Southern EM: Detection of specific sequences among DNA fragments separated by gel electrophoresis. J Mol Biol 1975;**98:**503.

Spence JE et al: Uniparental disomy as a mechanism for human genetic disease. Am J Hum Genet 1988;**42:**217.

Staley LW et al: Molecular-clinical correlations in children and adults with fragile X syndrome. Am J Dis Child 1993;**147:**723.

Sutherland G, Richards RI: DNA repeats—a treasury of human variation. N Engl J Med 1994;**331:**191.

Sutton HE: *An Introduction to Human Genetics.* Harcourt Brace Jovanovich, 1988.

Tamaren J, Spuhler K, Sujanksy E: Risk of Down syndrome among second- and third-degree relatives of a proband with trisomy 21. Am J Med Genet 1983;**15:**393.

Tan AA, Williams EA, Tam PPL: X-chromosome inactivation occurs at different times in different tissues of the post-implantation mouse embryo. Nature Genetics 1993;**3:**170.

Tarleton JC, Saul RA: Molecular genetic advances in fragile X syndrome. J Pediatr 1993;**122:**169.

Taylor AK et al: Molecular predictors of cognitive involvement in female carriers of fragile X syndrome. JAMA 1994;**271:**507.

Therman E, Susman M: *Human Chromosomes: Structure, Behavior, and Effects.* Springer-Verlag, 1993.

Thompson MW, McInnis RR, Willard HF: *Thompson and Thompson Genetics in Medicine.* WB Saunders, 1991.

Tommerup N: Mendelian cytogenetics. Chromosome rearrangements associated with Mendelian disorders. J Med Genet 1993;**30:**713.

Trisomy 21 (Down syndrome): International symposium on trisomy 21. Am J Med Genet Supplement 1990;7.

Turner G et al: Heterozygous expression of X-linked mental retardation and X-chromosome marker fra(X)(q27). N Engl J Med 1980;**303:**662.

Turner G, Turner B: X-linked mental retardation. J Med Genet 1974;**11:**109.

Turner G et al: X-linked mental retardation without physical abnormality (Renpenning's syndrome) in sibs in an institution. J Med Genet 1972;**9:**324.

Warren AC: Evidence for reduced recombination on the nondisjoined chromosomes 21 in Down syndrome. Science 1987;**237:**652.

Warren ST, Nelson DL: Advances in molecular analysis of fragile X syndrome. JAMA 1994;**271:**536.

Watson JD et al: *Recombinant DNA.* Scientific American Books, 1992.

Weatherall DJ: *The New Genetics and Clinical Practice,* 3rd ed. Oxford University Press, 1991.

Wolff DJ, Schwartz S: Characterization of Robertsonian translocations by using fluorescence in situ hybridization. Am J Hum Genet 1992;**50:**174.

Yu S et al: Fragile X genotype characterized by an unstable region of DNA. Science 1991;**252:**1179.

3 Genetic Diagnosis & Gene Therapy

I. GENETIC TESTING, DIAGNOSIS, & COUNSELING

The practicing physician, who will frequently need to consider a genetic diagnosis, must know how to use the genetic tools available and be able to convey the resulting information to a patient and family. Many tests are specialized and their interpretation will require consultation from a clinical geneticist, and the process of genetic diagnosis and counseling may require the skills of the clinical geneticist. Nevertheless, the initial consideration will be in the hands of the primary care physician or medical specialist. The selection of tests will depend on the diagnosis under consideration and the kind of information sought. This chapter will describe the common types of tests in use and the kind of information that they can provide. New tests are being developed and the availability of testing for specific genes or mutations in any given disorder is increasing, but the principles are similar from one disease to another. Testing may determine the specific mutation the patient has or it may only determine the likelihood that the individual carries a mutant gene. The strategy followed may also involve assessing risks to other members of the family. Presymptomatic diagnosis and identification of carriers for recessive or X-linked mutations are possible outcomes. Once specific genetic information has been obtained, the next step is to convey that information to the patient and family. This chapter also will consider the strategies that may facilitate the transfer of this often complex—and alarming—information. Conveying genetic information can have a substantial impact if the news is of previously unforeseen risks to health and reproduction. Questions of privacy and confidentiality will arise within the immediate and extended family. Also, the physician must be prepared to address work-related and school-related issues that may ensue from the results of genetic tests and the identification of family members at risk.

Methods of Genetic Testing

Chromosome Analysis: Any dividing cells can be used for chromosome analysis; common sources of cells include lymphocytes, fibroblasts, and amniocytes. Cells must be in mitosis in order to identify individual chromosomes. Uncultured cells can be used if they are already in mitosis; otherwise, the cells must be placed into culture so that they are dividing. After mitosis is stopped in metaphase, different stains will identify specific features of chromosome morphology and structure. For clinical diagnosis a **karyotype** is prepared after the chromosomes have been stopped in early metaphase. Then a stain, such as Giemsa, is used under appropriate conditions to allow the identification of specific bands, as discussed in Chapter 2. Molecular tools combined with cytogenetic analysis can identify small deletions and rearrangements which cannot be resolved at the level of the light microscope. In the case of the submicroscopic deletions, the use of **fluorescence in situ hybridization (FISH)** may clarify the prognosis by allowing comparison to other patients with the same material deleted. Other molecular strategies may reveal unusual chromosomal mechanisms such as **uniparental disomy.**

Cytogenetic analysis can provide the physician with information which is of diagnostic and prognostic utility. In the patient with multiple congenital malformations, learning disability, or mental retardation, a specific diagnosis may be made. The literature may provide information on outcome in similar cases which may refine the prognosis. The identification of a translocation may explain reproductive loss or a family history of congenital malformations or mental retardation.

Testing for Single Gene Disorders: When the phenotype or the pedigree suggests a single gene disorder, testing aimed at that gene can sometimes provide more specific diagnostic information and risk assessment. The kinds of testing employed depend on how much is known about the gene in question.

Most methods depend on the ability to isolate DNA and identify abnormalities starting with small amounts of material from the patient. Sources are similar to those used for chromosome analysis, but DNA can be isolated from any cell that has a nucleus; cells can be retrieved from hair bulbs, dried blood spots, and solid tissues. Cells do not need to be dividing in order for the DNA to be tested, but sometimes cells such as fibroblasts are placed in culture to increase their numbers.

Some strategies depend on cutting the DNA into pieces which can be separated in an electrophoretic system. This is usually done by employing **restriction enzymes,** enzymes which are isolated from bacteria and cut DNA at specific, predictable sequences called **restriction sites.** When a restriction enzyme is used to cut DNA, the sizes of the pieces depend on the positions of the restriction sites. The restriction sites are inherited within families and are also variable between families just like other single gene traits. This variability, or **polymorphism** leads to variability in size of the pieces of DNA which result from cutting with restriction enzymes, called **restriction fragment length polymorphism (RFLP)** as described in Chapter 2. These RFLPs can be used as **linkage markers** throughout the genome in the same way that polymorphic markers such as HLA types and secretor status have been used.

When the gene has been mapped to a specific chromosome and its location related to molecular markers on that chromosome, **linkage analysis** may provide a way to follow the gene through the family. The basic principles of linkage analysis are discussed in Chapter 2. Although the strategies available depend on the specific gene, the basic procedures do not. In order for linkage analysis to be of clinical use, there must be an identified genetic condition in the proband for which a linkage marker has been identified. In addition, there must be several family members, both affected and unaffected, whose status with respect to the linkage marker is known. The limitation of this test results from the fact that recombination can occur between the homologous chromosomes such that the mutation and the restriction site are no longer linked. The closeness of the linkage marker to the gene of interest determines the likelihood of such recombination between the marker and the gene. Linkage testing will provide a statement of the probability that the individual tested carries the gene of interest, but not usually a definitive statement of the genotype of the individual tested.

When the mutation or mutations causing the disease is known, molecular tests may identify a specific mutation in DNA isolated from the patient. Once molecular testing has determined whether the individual carries the mutation, the information can be used for diagnosis, prognosis, and for determining the status of other members of the family.

Restriction Analysis: Restriction enzymes can be used in linkage analyses to assess genotype within families. RFLPs can be used as linkage markers that allow a gene to be followed through a family. The kinds of answers that result from this kind of study may be either probability statements or definitive statements about genotype. It is important to make this distinction. As shown in Figure 3–1, the usefulness of a linkage marker depends on the proximity to the gene. When the marker and the gene are close, and the recombination frequency is small, the study can provide a meaningful answer for families. The result is usually stated as a probability that depends on the recombination frequency. For example, if the gene and the marker are 5 centimorgans apart (ie, they recombine with a frequency of 5%), the marker and the disease are concordant 95% of the time. That means that an individual in an informative family who carries the linkage marker has a 95% chance of also carrying the disease gene. Similarly, an individual in the family who does not carry the marker has a 95% chance of not carrying the disease gene. It is important to remember that a linkage study requires both affected and unaffected family members, since the marker is only a marker for following that gene within a given family (Figure 3–2).

When the probe used in the restriction study is from the gene which is mutant in the disorder and the restriction site change is within the gene, the result of the test is a statement that the individual does or does not carry the mutation. The study is no longer a linkage study. Clearly this is more specific and thus preferable, but it depends on the gene for the disorder having been cloned. It has limitations when there are many different mutations at a given locus which can cause the disease (Figure 3–3).

Electrophoretic Separations: A variety of methods for electrophoretic separation of DNA is currently in use. Each depends on the differential migration of DNA fragments of varying size on blocks of gel media. Specific kinds of gels, conditions of electrophoresis, types of probes, and other treatments during the process can provide different advantages that allow identification of single base changes, deletions, or insertions in DNA.

A. RNAse Protection Cleavage: RNAse Protection cleavage uses an RNA probe and DNA from a source which hybridize to each other. If the DNA contains a single base change, the hybridization will not be perfect, and there will be a mismatch between the RNA and DNA fragments. The area of mismatch can be cleaved by RNAse, giving two RNA fragments instead of the one which would be produced if there were no mismatch. Using an appropriate probe, these fragments can be detected electrophoretically. The advantage of this technique is that using a normal probe for a known gene, a mutation can be detected without knowing the precise base change in the mutation. Regions of DNA as large as 1000 base pairs can be screened using this method.

B. Denaturing Gel Electrophoresis: Denaturing gel electrophoresis takes advantage of the fact that if there is a single base mismatch between the probe and the DNA from the source, they will separate from each other under denaturing conditions, and two bands will be seen. The denaturing conditions can be temperature changes or changes in concentration of a chemical which denatures DNA, such as urea. Fragments of size up to 1000 base pairs can be analyzed using this method. The benefit of

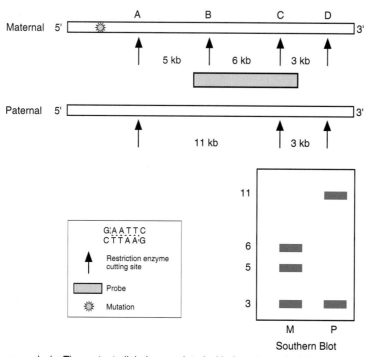

Figure 3–1. Linkage analysis. The mutant allele is associated with the maternal allele and the 5 and 6 kb fragments. It can be followed through the family, as indicated in the following pedigree. The assumption that the presence of the 5 and 6 kb alleles indicates the presence of the mutation is predicated on the lack of recombination between the restriction site and the mutation and on the ability to assign phase to the 5,6 kb fragments.

this method is that if a normal probe is used, the mutation in the DNA from the source need not be known.

C. Pulsed Field Gel Electrophoresis: Pulsed field gel electrophoresis is another electrophoretic technique that employs alternating electric fields in the separation process. The advantage of this technique is that very large pieces of DNA can be separated.

Dot Blots or Slot Blots: Direct mutation analysis can be carried out when probes can be made that recognize the specific mutation. Dot blots (see below) can give direct information about genotype using a probe specific for the mutation, called an **allele specific oligonucleotide (ASO).** These may be done directly without the need for electrophoretic procedures. This method has limitations when there are many different mutations at a given locus which can cause the disease.

Polymerase Chain Reaction (PCR): Polymerase chain reaction (PCR) allows for the amplification of specific segments of DNA containing genes of interest or parts of genes of interest. This development has revolutionized the diagnosis of genetic disorders when the base sequence of the mutation or mutations is known.

PCR amplification using Taq polymerase (discussed in Chapter 2) has several advantages over some of the other techniques in use. To start with,

very small amounts of DNA are required. This makes the procedure suitable for use from sources such as chorionic villus biopsy material, filter paper disks from newborn screening programs, and hair bulbs. In addition, since the reaction can be carried out with multiple primers, several different mutations can be sought at the same time. Because the reaction takes place at a high temperature where few polymerases other than Taq are stable, it is quite specific.

Once DNA has been amplified, it can be used for dot blots or for restriction analysis or directly sequenced. Mutation-specific tests can determine the genotype of the individual accurately. The limitations are that the primers must be specific; if they do not span the mutation in a particular individual, that mutation will not be identified. Examples are in Table 3–1.

THE FAMILY AT GENETIC RISK

There are several ways that a family at risk for a genetic disorder may come to medical attention. Factors that may be helpful in identifying an at-risk family are listed in Table 3–2. Assessment of the genetic risk involves three steps: (1) identifying the nature of the risk, (2) recognizing family members at risk, and (3) helping the family to use the information. The

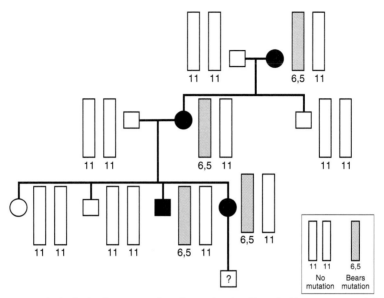

Figure 3–2. Linkage analysis. In the first generation, the mother is affected with an autosomal dominant condition; the mutation resides on her chromosome, which bears the 6,5 kb fragments obtained by restriction enzyme cutting of her DNA. As seen in the previous diagram, she is heterozygous for a restriction site, allowing her two chromosomes to be distinguished from each other. The disease allele can be followed through the family by following the chromosome with the 6,5 kb bands. Diagnosis in the male will depend on the RFLPs of his father, if the patient inherits the 6,5 kb allele from his mother. If he inherits the 11 kb allele, he will be free of the disease within the limits of recombination. If the mutation is on that chromosome but not at the restriction site, the analysis depends upon the absence of recombination between the restriction site marker and the mutation. If the mutation is at the restriction site and the probe recognizes the gene, recombination is not a factor and the analysis is more precise.

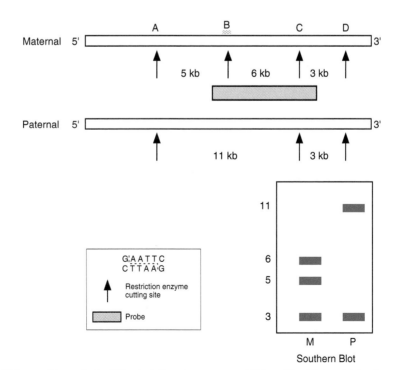

Figure 3–3. Allele-specific analysis. If the mutation changes a restriction site and a probe for the gene is available, direct mutation analysis can be done. A mutation at B is associated with the 5,6 kb fragments and the analysis is not dependent on lack of recombination.

Table 3–1. Examples of specific molecular testing.

Organ System and Disorder	Type of Testing
Endocrine and metabolism	
Congenital adrenal hypoplasia	Specific mutation analysis, linkage analysis
PKU	Specific mutation analysis, linkage analysis
Heart and great vessels	
Marfan syndrome	Fibrillin measurement, specific mutation analysis
Hypertrophic cardiomyopathy	Linkage analysis
Blood	
Thalassemias	Alllele-specific oligonucleotide analysis
Hemophilia A	Specific mutation analysis, linkage analysis
Immune system	
SCID	Adenosine deaminase measurement
Kidney and urinary tract	
Adult polycystic kidney disease	Linkage analysis
Alport syndrome	Mutation, deletion analysis
Skeletal system	
Osteogenesis imperfecta	Collagen secretion, specific mutation analysis
Cancer	
Leukemias	Chromosomal deletions, rearrangements
Nervous system	
Duchenne muscular dystrophy	Deletion analysis, linkage studies, dystrophin analysis
Myotonic dystrophy	Trinucleotide repeat analysis
Fragile-X syndrome	Trinucleotide repeat analysis
Neurofibromatosis	Linkage analysis, specific mutation analysis
Pulmonary	
Cystic fibrosis	Mutation analysis
α-1-antitrypsin deficiency	Mutation analysis

medical consequences of the risk (Table 3–3) and the magnitude of the risk are both important in family decision-making. Similarly, identification of family members at risk will depend upon the genetic mechanism involved. It is essential, therefore, to define the condition in the proband as precisely as possible. It may be helpful to construct a pedigree to diagram the transmission of a gene or a chromosomal translocation through the family (Table 3–4).

Before embarking on an odyssey of this kind, it is important for the patient and family to know what kind of information will be obtained from the testing. Open discussion is valuable as is opportunity for family members to confer privately with the medical professionals involved. Families need to know that such testing may identify others who are at risk for having children with the genetic condition involved or who are at risk for developing the disease itself. They need to be able to explore how they will use this information after it is obtained, what the choices may be, and what other information may be uncovered. The choices may include prenatal diagnosis and pregnancy termination, alternative reproductive technologies, presymtomatic treatment, or even the possibility of presymtomatic diagnosis of a disease for which there is no effective treatment. Molecular genetic studies will show the biologic relationships within the family, and will thus reveal non-paternity

if paternity is not as stated in the pedigree. It is crucial for the family to know about these possible consequences before the testing is done and to discuss any troubling issues with the physician beforehand.

The transfer of genetic information to a family requires good communication skills and a clear understanding of the facts (Table 3–4). There is wide variation in the knowledge with which families come to evaluation. The physician should be selective in con-

Table 3–2. Factors to consider in ascertaining genetic risk.

Ethnic background
Consanguinity
Advanced maternal age

Family history of
  genetic disorder
  mental retardation
  congenital malformations
  early infant deaths
  cancer
  neurologic disease
  renal disease
  skeletal disorders

Table 3–3. Genetic risk associated with ethnic background.

Ethnic Background	Disorder at Higher Risk
Northern European caucasian	Cystic fibrosis PKU
Jewish (Ashkenazi)	Tay-Sachs disease Canavan disease Gaucher disease (non-neuronopathic)
West African	Sickle cell anemia Sickle-C disease
Mediterranean region	β-thalassemia Sickle cell anemia
Asian	α-thalassemia
French-Canadian	Tay-Sachs disease (different mutation from Askenazi mutation) Branched-chain ketoaciduria

veying information that is pertinent to the decisions at hand and not try to deliver a short course in genetics to the family. Nevertheless, the information must be complete and clear. The use of diagrams and photographs of chromosomes or other supporting visual aids will be helpful. While counseling should in general be non-directive, many families will want more than just the facts and will seek guidance about how to use the information provided. It may be helpful to frame the information in terms of choices and the expected outcome of making those choices. This may assist the patient and family to consider what is the best decision for them. It is also possible that not all family members will wish the same information, and each individual's wishes should be honored in the way information is given. The preservation of confidentiality is essential. When the risk to another family member is serious and the proband does not wish these matters discussed with the relevant family member, serious persuasion must be employed. If harm to the other individual is a clear likelihood it may be necessary to breach the confidentiality of the proband.

Once the decision has been made to proceed with genetic evaluation, appropriate testing must be arranged. It is essential for the physician to use a reliable laboratory, since important decisions will result from the answers obtained. Most of the tests involved will require a specialized laboratory.

Results of the evaluation will determine what intervention, if any, should be recommended. Further diagnostic evaluation of individuals carrying a deleterious gene may be warranted, especially if treatment to prevent the onset of symptoms or the development of disease will play a role. Such treatment or prevention options must be thoroughly delineated for the family. If further testing to clarify a chromosomal rearrangement or a mutation or protein deficiency is needed, this should be arranged. There are many disease-specific organizations that provide literature and help to organize support groups that are extremely valuable to patients and families. Introduction to

Table 3–4. Common genetic risk estimates.

Condition in Proband	Genetic Risk of Another Affected	Diagnostic Tools
Chromosome abnormality	1% if parents normal; 3–10% if parents carry a translocation	Cytogenetic analysis; molecular cytogenetic testing
Autosomal recessive disorder	25% if both parents heterozygous; no risk if only one parent heterozygous	Functional tests of protein, enzymology; molecular genetic testing
Autosomal dominant disorder	50% risk if affected parent; no risk if new mutation in proband	Functional tests of protein, enzymology; molecular genetic testing
X-linked disorder	50% risk of affected son or heterozygous daughter if heterozygous mother; no risk to son of affected male; 100% risk of heterozygous daughter of affected male. No risk if proband new deletion or new mutation	Functional tests of protein, enzymology; molecular genetic testing
Multifactorial	Variable; ranges from 2% to 15% depending on condition and number of affected family members	Empirical estimates from literature on similar conditions

Table 3–5. Providing genetic information to patient and family.

Identify genetic disorder in proband

Discuss possible outcomes of further genetic
evaluation

Identify genetic mechanism
    By literature review
    By pedigree analysis
    By specific cytogenic or molecular testing

Discuss results and implications with proband

Draw family pedigree and assess risk to each family
member

Discuss providing information to others in family with
proband

such groups should be provided. The physician may be able to arrange a meeting with another family dealing with the same condition; care must be taken to secure the other family's permission before such an invitation is issued.

There will be times when no specific genetic diagnosis can be made or when no specific genetic hypothesis can be developed. The family may still wish an assessment of the risk to other family members of having the same disorder under consideration. Provision of such information may require empiric data from the literature as well as exclusion of the major genetic mechanisms. Modern cytogenetic techniques can exclude a chromosomal abnormality within the limits of light microscopic resolution and the ability of molecular cytogenetic tools. In the case of a translocation, absence of the balanced translocation in another family member provides assurance of low risk to offspring. Careful biochemical evaluation by a sophisticated laboratory will exclude most recognized biochemical conditions if samples are obtained in an appropriate way. Some biochemical disorders may be difficult to diagnose between episodes of decompensation, and thus the status of the affected individual needs to be considered when the results of such testing are interpreted.

It is difficult to exclude with absolute certainty the presence of a mutant gene of major effect. Present technology does not provide screening testing for such single gene mutations, and so the molecular technology can only confirm a diagnosis suspected on clinical grounds. When more than one family member is affected, a genetic hypothesis can be generated based on the pedigree. When only one individual is affected, knowledge of the literature and a specific diagnosis are needed to assess genetic risk. Often, if a disorder is diagnosed which is known to have a Mendelian mechanism, risk assessment can be offered based on the pedigree and molecular testing offered when available. Gonadal mosaicism can never be excluded and has been reported in some dis-

orders such as osteogenesis imperfecta. When using empiric risks from the literature, it is important to recognize genetic heterogeneity and to be as certain as possible that the risks apply to the disorder in question.

The diagnosis of a genetic disorder can have a major impact on a family beyond the effect on the individual. Asymptomatic individuals may be found to be at risk for developing a serious illness by virtue of their position in the family without their prior knowledge. Relationships may be exposed to be different from family beliefs. Risks of having children with serious disability may be uncovered. Life and health insurance may be jeopardized. Stigmatization and discrimination in the workplace may occur. The physician must try to deal with all these issues in a supportive and sensitive way.

II. GENE THERAPY

The elucidation of molecular mechanisms of disease and the development of recombinant DNA technology has engendered new hope of providing definitive treatment for genetic disorders by replacing defective genes. The hemoglobinopathies were the initial target of gene therapy in the 1980's. Today, human trials in gene therapy are underway for a number of conditions.

Gene therapy aims to transfer new genetic material into cells that bear a mutation, in order to (a) restore normal function to the cell or tissue, (b) repair a genetic defect, or (c) add a new function to the cell. Theoretically, any tissue could be the target of such therapy. Current thinking, however, draws a distinction between therapy for somatic cells and germ cells. Alteration of the genetic material of somatic cells has implications for tissue cells that receive the new gene and for progeny of those cells, if they are capable of mitosis. In contrast, germ cells with altered genetic material allow for transmission of altered genetic material to the offspring of the individual and to future generations. Clearly, this has ethical and biological implications for the evolution of the species—implications that are more far-reaching than those for somatic cell therapy alone. For these reasons, germline gene therapy is not considered suitable at present. All current clinical trials in gene therapy involve somatic cells.

Somatic Cell Gene Therapy

Somatic cell gene therapy may have a role in two different classes of genetic alteration: **constitutional mutations and somatic mutations.** Constitutional mutations, in which every cell of the body bears a

Table 3–6. Steps in development of gene therapy for single gene disorders.

Developmental Step	Key Factors
Understanding of molecular genetics of disease	Gene that is mutant is known Gene is cloned Function and biochemistry of protein is known Tissue-specific expression is achieved
Design of vector	Effectiveness of gene transfer is assured Safety issues are crucial
Strategy to target cell, organ, or tissue	Mitotic or post-mitotic cells are targeted Control of expression is achieved

mutation, are usually represented as *single gene disorders* inherited according to Mendelian principles. In such cases, variability occurs in the expression of most genes from one organ to another. Phenotype depends on (a) the expression of the gene in specific organs and tissues and (b) the effect of the mutation on the structure, metabolism, transport, or other functions of the encoded protein. **With a constitutional mutation,** gene therapy to restore function may be directed to the organs or tissues most affected by the mutation, or therapy may involve the introduction of cells that produce the protein needed. **Somatic mutations** are those in which a somatic cell undergoes a mutation or series of mutations that are passed on to progeny. Cancer represents example of somatic mutations that currently seem most amenable to gene therapy. The aims of gene therapy for cancer include repair of the mutation, restoration of function, or destruction of the malignant cells.

Crucial steps in designing gene therapy for single gene disorders are shown in Table 3–6. Gene therapy for single-gene disorders is based on available knowledge about the molecular pathology of the disorder, including the regulation of expression of the gene, the function and biochemistry of the encoded protein, and the nature of the mutations. Although it may not be essential to define the specific mutation precisely, it is always necessary to identify the mutant gene. The gene, or at the very least the c-DNA for the coding sequence, must be cloned.

Until gene therapy is a well established clinical tool, **designing** a research protocol will be the initial step in any clinical setting. In particular, the design of the vector gene is critical; key concerns include the following:

- Whether expression of the vector gene will be long term or short term
- How such expression will be regulated
- How to achieve sufficient expression in order to restore function
- Identifying the appropriate target cell or organ for the vector gene
- Determining the timing and degree of expression appropriate for the normal function of the organ
- The design of an optimal delivery system—usually a viral vector or a physicochemical vector.

Delivery Systems

Genes can be transferred into cells using viral vectors (transduction) or physicochemical methods (transfection) that include mechanical injection, liposomal transfer, or receptor-mediated transfer. Physical methods of delivery have the advantage of not transferring unwanted viral DNA into the cell; because the transferred genetic material does not usually integrate into a chromosome, however, long term expression does not occur. Short term expression may be effective for cancer cells that are expected to undergo destruction or for cells which undergo rapid turnover, such as respiratory epithelium. However, for treatment of organs such as liver or brain to provide ongoing normal function, long term expression is most desirable.

In the case of a viral vector, the gene to be transferred (the transgene) is inserted into a virus that cannot replicate. Most work in gene therapy has employed viral vectors, in particular, retroviruses that are among the best understood vectors. A good example is the murine-leukemia retrovirus. Adenoviruses, adeno-associated viruses, and herpes viruses are also used as vectors. Even as experience with these vectors increases, efforts to develop improved delivery systems will most likely occur. The targets for gene therapy may include cells that will be implanted and used as protein delivery systems, cells that will be injected to repopulate an organ, or cells within organs or tumors that will be transfected or transduced in vivo.

Constructing a Viral Vector

With transduction, the therapeutic gene must be placed into a virus that can infect the cell of interest and insert the new gene into the cell's genome. The virus must be disabled, however, so that it cannot become an infectious, pathogenic agent. To achieve this goal, the retroviral vector that contains the gene for transduction is modified so that the retrovirus cannot replicate independently. The strategy involves the development of a cell line that contains two retroviral genomes which cannot replicate and become infectious independently and cannot recombine to produce a replication-competent infectious virus.

While the two retroviruses are derived from the same wild type retrovirus, they differ in structure. The retroviral vector contains the gene to be transferred, an internal promotor, the Long Terminal Repeats (LTRs), the packaging signal, and, in research protocols, a selectable marker or reporter gene. In addition, the viral protein genes gag, pol, and env, which have important functions including regulation of viral replication, ability to make the capsid protein, and competence to be infective, are deleted. The second virus does not have a packaging signal; likewise, its LTRs are deleted or modified. Other key DNA sequences are also modified to reduce recombination with the retroviral vector. The second virus contains a polyadenylation signal and viral protein genes that direct the synthesis of proteins which are needed, so that together the two viruses provide the genes needed to reproduce the retroviral vector which contains the gene to be transferred.

Thus, vector design must result in a construct that can infect the cell of interest without allowing recombination which generates a replication-competent virus, since the wild-type viruses that form the basis for the constructs are oncogenic or cytopathic. To prevent this outcome, genes are deleted from viral vectors to make it impossible for the viruses to replicate; but the viruses still have genes that direct the synthesis of viral specific proteins. In vitro, the vector containing the transgene replicates and produces many copies of the vector, which are then used to transduce the target cells to be treated. After the targeted cells receive the vector, it is reverse-transcribed to DNA, which is integrated into the cells' genome that now includes the transduced, therapeutic gene (Figure 3–4).

The production of **adenoviral vectors** follows similar principles, except that the packaging cell line contains a crippled adenovirus into which a *plasmid* containing the gene to be transferred is introduced. Adenoviral vectors are then produced by recombination. Although they can infect non-dividing cells, these vectors do not integrate into the chromosome and thus do not provide long-term expression of the protein.

Current limitations for long-term gene therapy in solid organs include the fact that retroviral vectors that integrate into the genome only do so when they are transferred into dividing cells. In addition, the size of the DNA that can be placed in a viral vector can be a serious limitation, since many clinically important genes are larger than the amount of DNA that viral vectors can accommodate. Ultimately, it would be attractive to target the new gene to the precise site of the mutant gene. Although not yet feasible, ultimately one could replace the mutant gene with a new, normal gene in the correct position and under the appropriate control.

Target Cells in Gene Therapy

Potential targets for gene therapy include circulating cells, cells that comprise solid tissue, cells that can be injected to become protein delivery systems, and bone marrow stem cells. The target tissue determines strategy to some degree, as the following examples illustrate.

Circulating Cells Such as Peripheral Blood Lymphocytes: Circulating cells such as peripheral blood lymphocytes can be removed from the body, transduced with a vector, and returned to the circulation to carry out their restored or new function. This approach has been successful in Phase III human trials involving patients with severe combined immunodeficiency due to adenosine deaminase (ADA) deficiency (Figure 3–5).

Therapy Aimed at Liver Cells: Therapy aimed at liver cells must overcome a significant limitation: the liver has completed its differentiation; thus, hepatocytes are non-dividing. To overcome this limitation, current gene therapy protocols in PKU and hemophilia in animals and hereditary hypercholesteremia in both animal and human trials rely on partial hepatectomy. In vivo transduction of regenerating liver cells with a retroviral vector has resulted in expression of the transduced genes for both phenylalanine hydroxylase and, in other experiments, the gene for the coagulation factor, factor IX. Ex vivo protocols have relied on collagenization of hepatic cells, which are then transduced with the desired vector and returned to the liver by injection into the portal system or the spleen. Partial hepatectomy provides liver cells for the ex vivo transduction;

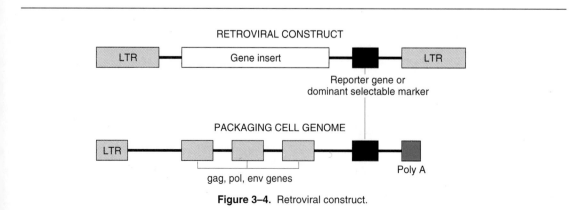

Figure 3–4. Retroviral construct.

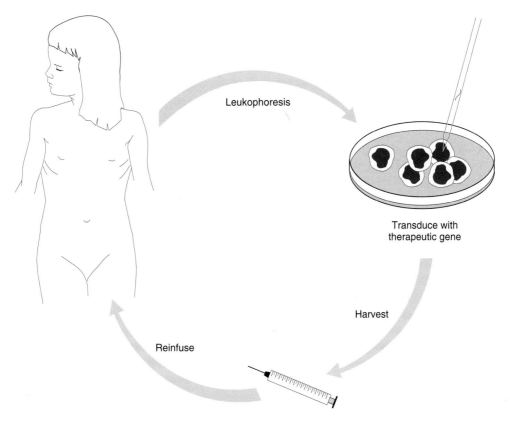

Figure 3–5. Adenosine deaminase (ADA) strategy.

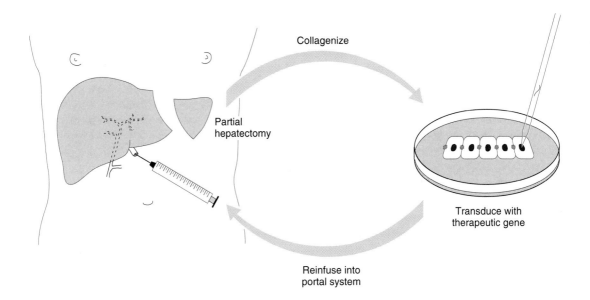

Figure 3–6. Low density lipoprotein (LDL) strategy.

Table 3–7. Gene therapy for cancer.

Cancer Type	Strategy	Mechanism
Brain tumors	TK/gancyclovir	"Suicide" gene
Melanoma	TNF or IL-2	Intracellular cytokine production
Renal cell carcinoma	IL-4	Intracellular cytokine production
Non-small-cell lung cancer	Antisense K-ras	Decrease K-ras protein
Non-small-cell lung cancer	Normal p53	Increase normal p53 protein

subsequent liver regeneration may also play a role in the uptake of the transduced cells. The problem of low level of expression remains to be solved.

Ongoing Human Trials for Familial Hypercholesterolemia: Ongoing human trials for familial hypercholesterolemia employ the low density lipoprotein **(LDL) receptor gene.** The strategy for ex vivo transduction of liver cells is the same as that outlined above. Preliminary results suggest that plasma cholesterol is lowered; expression of the LDL protein itself needs to be proven, and level of expression must be increased (Figure 3–6).

Transduced Keratinocytes, Muscle Cells, Hepatocytes and Fibroblasts: Transduced keratinocytes, muscle cells, hepatocytes and fibroblasts are all being studied for possible application someday in human trials. The use of transduced cells as a protein delivery system is illustrated by animal experiments using keratinocytes transduced with the gene for factor IX, the gene defective in Hemophilia B. Length and level of expression remained to be studied.

The Central Nervous System: The central nervous system is an important potential target for gene therapy. Adenoviral vectors are being studied for this use, as are vectors that can accept larger pieces of DNA than some other vectors and which are derived from viruses that can infect non-dividing neurons, eg, the herpes virus. The safety of the herpes virus remains a major concern, however, since its cytopathic effect is lethal to neurons. This difficulty must be overcome before this form of gene therapy for CNS diseases can progress to human trials.

Airway Epithelium: Airway epithelium is a dividing tissue that is an attractive target for gene therapy for disorders such as cystic fibrosis. Current human trials employ adenoviral and adeno-associated viral vectors transduced with the gene for the protein that is defective in cystic fibrosis, CFTR. The vectors are introduced into the airway directly. The lung mounts an inflammatory response to proteins made by the viral vectors, a problem that requires further engineering of the viral vectors in order to solve.

Hematopoietic Stem Cells: Hematopoietic stem cells are an attractive target for gene therapy because they produce all the cells of the hematopoietic system, and they renew themselves. It is hoped that transducing them with a therapeutic gene will overcome current problems of short term expression and the subsequent need for repeated treatment.

Gene Therapy for Cancer

Gene therapy for cancer is undergoing extensive clinical investigation. Strategies involve genetic manipulation of selected tumor cells inside and outside the body. The basic schemes are shown in Table 3–7. In ex vivo protocols, tumor cells are removed and provided with the desired transgene; the method depends on the particular gene to be inserted. The cells are then returned to a tumor site where, it is hoped, the bioengineered cells will exert their greatest therapeutic effect.

In the in vivo protocols, genes are transferred to the tumor either by physical transfer of DNA or by injecting other cells, such as fibroblasts that have undergone manipulation. A good example is the recent insertion of the thymidine kinase gene from the herpes simplex virus (HSVTK) into brain tumor cells. This experimental approach allows the tumor to metabolize systemically administered ganciclovir to a compound toxic to the tumor cell, while the normal cell is spared. Untransduced tumor cells are also killed, a phenomenon that is incompletely understood.

A second strategy involves utilizing the immune system to destroy tumor cells by inserting a gene into the tumor cells that will make them more immunogenic. Examples include genes for a cytokine such as interleukin-2 (IL-2), tumor necrosis factor, IL-4, or other cytokines. The strategies to accomplish this include: (a) culturing and infecting tumor cells directly or (b) inserting the gene into fibroblasts, mixing these

Table 3–8. Safety concerns in gene therapy.

Risk Category	Safety Concern
Recombination	Recombination to replication-competent pathogenic virus
Toxification	Production of toxic viral protein products

Integration	Integration at a site that disrupts other genes
	  Oncogene disruption causing cancer
	  Tumor suppressor gene disruption causing cancer

Table 3–9. Gene therapy models in animal or human trials.

Disorder	Gene to Replace	Target Cell/Organ	Technique
Familial hypercholesterolemia	LDL receptor	Liver	Ex vivo, viral construct
Severe combined immuno- deficiency disease (SCID)	Adenosine deaminase	T cells	Ex vivo, viral construct, short-term
Hemophilia B	Factor IX	Hepatocytes, keratinocytes, muscle cells	Ex vivo, viral construct
Cystic fibrosis	CFTR	Lung, airway cells	In vivo, viral construct, short term
PKU	Phenylalanine hydroxylase	Liver	Ex vivo, viral construct

with tumor cells that have been removed from the patient, and reinjecting the cells into the tumor. The resulting immunologic response can destroy the tumor. Advantage can also be taken of strategies to correct the genetic defect in the tumor cell that has allowed it to become malignant. Tumors in which the genetic mechanism relies on the dysfunction of a tumor suppressor gene or the activation or overexpression of an oncogene can be attacked by strategies that manipulate those genes. Two examples of this form of gene therapy currently undergoing human trials include the following: (a) the insertion of the normal p53 tumor suppressor gene in tumors that have undergone a mutation in that gene and (b) the use of a gene that transcribes messenger RNA for the oncogene k-ras in the antisense direction to decrease k-ras protein production. Other strategies seek to reverse the resistance of tumor cells to antineoplastic drugs by manipulating the multiple drug resistance genes that confer drug resistance to the tumor cells. Clinical trials using these and similar protocols are underway for melanoma, brain tumors, lung cancer, renal cancers, and ovarian cancers.

The safety of these techniques remains an important concern. Areas of particular uncertainty are listed in Table 3–8. As stated earlier, vector design must result in a construct that can infect the cell of interest without allowing recombination that generates a replication-competent infectious virus, since the wild-type viruses employed in constructing the

vectors are oncogenic or cytopathic. While genes are deleted from viral vectors to make it impossible for the viruses to replicate, they still have genes that direct the synthesis of viral specific proteins. These proteins can stimulate an inflammatory response that leads to destruction of the target cells and thus ends the therapeutic effect of the transgene. Improved understanding the biology of the viruses used for vectors is crucial to design of safe gene therapy.

Another concern is integration of the viral construct into the genome. Integration into the genome is probably necessary for expression to persist, especially in solid organs. Ideally, integration should occur at the site of the mutant allele, so that the normal allele contained in the viral vector would replace the mutant allele and come under its normal control region. Retroviruses appear to integrate into the genome at random; if integration is random, the construct could be integrated in a position that disrupts the gene in that position. Such disruption, if it involved an oncogene or a tumor-suppressor gene, could cause the development of cancer. Thus, learning how to direct the specificity of site selection remains a strategic goal.

Table 3–9 lists representative protocols under investigation to treat various single gene disorders. As with the development of all new therapeutic tools, careful clinical investigation will define the safety, ethical application, and utility of the new techniques in gene therapy.

REFERENCES AND SUGGESTED READING

Anderson WF: Human gene therapy. Science 1992;**256:** 808.

Blaese RM: Development of gene therapy for immunodeficiency: adenosine deaminase deficiency. Pediatric Research 1993;**33:**S49.

Breakefield XO: Gene delivery into the brain using virus vectors. Nature Genetics 1993;**3:**187.

Brown MS, Goldstein JI: Gene therapy for cholesterol. Nature Genetics 1994;**7:**349.

Cournoyer D, Caskey CT: Gene transfer into humans: A first step. N Engl J Med 1990;**323:**601.

Culver K: Clinical applications of gene therapy for cancer. Clin Chem 1994;**40:**510.

Culver KW, Blaese RM: Gene therapy for cancer. Trends in Genetics 1994;**10:**174.

Freeman SM, Zweibel JA: Gene therapy of cancer. Cancer Invest 1993;**11:**676.

Friedmann T: A brief history of gene therapy. Nature Genetics 1992;**2:**93.

Friedmann T: Gene therapy for neurological disorders. Trends in Genetics 1994;**10:**210.

Hershfield MS, Chaffee S, Sorensen RU: Enzyme replacement therapy with polyethylene glycol-adenosine deaminase in adenosine deaminase deficiency: overview and case report of three patients, including two now receiving gene therapy. Pediatric Research 1992;**33:**S42.

Kay MA, Woo SLC: Gene therapy for metabolic disorders. Nature Genetics 1994;**10:**253.

Kay MA, Woo SLC: Gene therapy for metabolic disorders. Trends in Genetics 1994;**11:**300.

Ledley F et al: Development of a clinical protocol for hepatic gene transfer: Lessons learned in preclinical studies. Pediatric Research 1993;**33:**313.

Ledley FD. Designing clinical trials of somatic gene therapy. Ann NY Acad Sci. in press.

Ledley FD: Clinical considerations in the design of protocols for somatic gene therapy. Human Gene Therapy 1991;**2:**77.

Levine F, Friedmann T: Gene therapy. Am J Dis Child 1993;**147:**1167.

Morgan RA, Anderson WF: Human gene therapy. Annu Rev Biochem 1993;**62:**191.

Morsy MA et al: Progress toward human gene therapy. JAMA 1993;**270:**2338.

Mulligan RC: The basic science of gene therapy. Science 1993;**260:**926.

Nabel EG, Plautz G, Nabel GJ: Site-specific gene expression in vivo by direct gene transfer into the arterial wall. Science 1990;**249:**1285.

Ohno T et al: Gene therapy for vascular smooth muscle cell proliferation after arterial injury. Science 1994;**265:**781.

Randall T: Medical news and perspectives: First gene therapy of inherited hypercholesterolemia. A partial success. JAMA 1993;**269:**837.

Rosenberg SA et al: The development of gene therapy for the treatment of cancer. Ann Surg 1993;**218:**455.

Rosenfeld MA et al: Adenovirus-mediated transfer of a recombinant α-antitrypsin gene to the lung epithelium in vivo. Science 1991;**252:**431.

Shapiro LJ: Gene therapy: Possibilities and promise. Pediatric Research 1993;**33:**321.

Tizzano EF, Buchwald M: Cystic fibrosis: Beyond the gene to therapy. J Pediatr 1992;**120:**337.

Wilson JM et al: Ex vivo gene therapy of familial hypercholesterolemia. Hum Gene Therapy 1992;**3:**179.

Immune Function

4

Overview of the Immune System

The immune system is complex and capable of extreme diversity. The development and function of the immune system are under intricate genetic control. This chapter will not focus on the aspects of genetic control of immune function itself. Rather, it will address some major disorders that result from mutations in genes that concern immune function and affect the cellular and protein components of the immune system.

T cells, B cells, macrophages, and granulocytes comprise the cellular component of the immune system and originate from bone marrow stem cells. T cells require a further maturation step in the thymus and macrophages mature from blood monocytes. Cells of the immune system are found in the circulation and in solid organs (Table 4–1). Neutrophils, which are found in the circulation, and monocytes, which are found both in the circulation and in some solid organs, are phagocytic cells.

Plasma cells and B lymphocytes comprise the B cell series. B cells synthesize immunoglobulins; no other cell has this capability. Immunoglobulins synthesized by lymphocytes remain cell-surface immunoglobulins. Those synthesized by plasma cells are secreted into the surrounding tissue. These antibodies bind foreign antigens such as toxic proteins, viruses, and bacteria. They also aid in opsonization of bacteria. T lymphocytes have cell surface receptors that detect foreign substances and bind antigens that have become attached to other host cells. T cells also express other surface proteins that constitute the CD series of proteins, designated by numbers, for example CD3. They can be used as markers to identify T cells. CD8 is associated with cytotoxic ability. T cells expressing this ability are termed cytotoxic T lymphocytes (CTLs) and kill other cells such as tumor cells and cells inhabited by viruses. Helper T cells promote various functions in other cell types.

The protein component includes antibodies, complement, and the cytokines. Cytokines, which are a group of proteins produced by a variety of cell types including lymphocytes, mast cells, macrophages, endothelial cells, fibroblasts, keratinocytes, and other somatic cells, function as secondary signaling proteins. Few mutations in the genes for these proteins are known.

A broad variety of genes control immune function. Mutations in some of these genes derange immune function and cause disease (Table 4–2). In addition, several disorders of immune function appear to have a major genetic component, but no specific mutations have been identified. There are many ways to organize this group of disorders; the organization used here will help to focus them from a genetic standpoint. Granulocytes have a critical role in fighting infection. The genetic disorders that affect granulocyte function result from dysfunction in their phagocytizing and killing functions and are expressed as deficient ability to fight infection. Lymphocytes control biosynthesis of immunoglobulins, provide for diversity in the immune response, and are involved in cytokine synthesis. Disorders that affect lymphocytes disturb a variety of these functions.

Classes of Genetic Disorders of Immune System

Genetic disorders that involve the immune system can be divided into classes that reflect the different components of the system. These classes are:

- Disorders of phagocyte function
- Disorders of B cell function
- Disorders of T cell function
- Combined disorders of T and B cell functions
- Disorders of other proteins relating to immune function
- Complement
- Cytokines.

DISORDERS OF PHAGOCYTE FUNCTION

Chronic Granulomatous Disease (CGD)

Chronic granulomatous disease is the name given to a group of disorders characterized by clinical features listed below:

Table 4–1. Components of the immune system.

Component	Major Function	Origin	Location	Genetic Defects
Phagocytes				
Neutrophils	Phagocytosis, bacterial killing	Bone marrow	Blood	+
Monocytes, macrophages	Phagocytosis, secretory protein production	Bone marrow	All tissues	
Lymphocytes				
B lymphocytes plasma cells	Immunoglobulin production	Bone marrow	Blood, lymph nodes, spleen	+
T lymphocytes, Helper T cells (THs), Cytotoxic T cells (CTLs)	Detect antigens and other foreign material using T cell receptors	Bone marrow; differentiate in thymus	Blood, thymus, lymph nodes, spleen	+
Proteins				
Immunoglobulins	Humoral immunity; antiviral, opsonization, complement activation	B cells, plasma cells	γ-globulin fraction of serum	+
Complement	Opsonization, inflammatory response, release of histamine, cytotoxic to bacteria and tumors	Liver, some macrophages	Plasma	+
Cytokines: interleukins, tumor necrosis factor, interferons	Mediate cell-cell interaction and signalling	Lymphocytes, variety of other cell types	Blood, solid organs	

- Recurrent infections, typically beginning before age 2 years
- Involvement of multiple organ systems
- Formation of granulomas
- Lymphadenitis.

Staphylococcus aureus and other catalase producing organisms are the most common pathogens. Unusual bacteria such as Staphylococcus epidermidis, Pseudomonas, and Serratia marcescens may also cause infection. The disease is caused by the loss of the killing function of phagocytes; bacteria can then grow unchecked. This killing function fails because the respiratory burst does not occur after bacteria are phagocytosed. Normally the reduced nicotinamide adenine dinucleotide phosphate (NADPH) oxidase system converts molecular oxygen to metabolites that kill the phagocytosed bacteria. This complex sys-

Table 4–2. Gene locations for some genes of importance in immunologic disorders.

Gene	Disease	Map Locations
CYBA	Chronic granulomatous disease (recessive)	16q24
CYBB	Chronic granulomatous disease (X-linked)	Xp21
Myeloperoxidase	Myeloperoxidase deficiency	17q21.3–q22
Bruton tyrosine kinase	X-linked Agammaglobulinemia	Xq21.3q22
CD40 ligand	Immunodeficiency with hyper IgM	Xq26.3–27.1
XLP	X-linked lymphoproliferative disease	Xq25–q26
IL2 receptor γ	X-linked SCIDXI*	Xq13.1
Adenosine deaminase	SCID (recessive)	20q12–q13.11
Purine nucleoside phosphorylase	Purine nucleoside phosphorylase deficiency	14q13.1
WAS	Wiscott-Aldrich syndrome	Xp11.3–p11.2
PFC	Properdin factor P deficiency	Xp11.4–p11.2

* SCID = severe combined immunodeficiency disease.

tem has both a cytosolic component and a membrane-associated component that includes ctochrome b. Two subunits, α and β, comprise the cytochrome b component. Several different genes bear mutations that cause CGD. The disorders that result display both autosomal recessive and X-linked inheritance.

Cytochrome b β Chain (CYBB) (MIM 306400): Cytochrome b β chain (CYBB)—the best characterized and most common form of CGD—is X-linked. The 91 KD β-subunit of the cytochrome b component of the NADPH oxidase system is implicated in nearly 60% of cases. The gene, designated CYBB, has been mapped to Xp21 and has been cloned. CYBB is flanked by the genes for Duchenne muscular dystrophy, (DMD) and ornithine transcarbamylase (OTC). Several kinds of mutations, including at least 10 allelic variants, have been described. In at least one of these, no cytochrome b protein is made. The mutations include single base changes, including one that leads to exon-skipping with the resultant deletion of one exon.

Diagnosis is based on absent NBT dye reduction by phagocytes, decreased oxygen uptake during phagocytosis, and abnormal bacterial killing curves. For the X-linked form, diagnostic tests employ linkage analysis using DMD and OTC, genes that flank CYBB, as linkage markers. Molecular testing for the specific mutation can be performed if family studies have identified the specific mutation in that family. Such molecular testing is feasible for prenatal diagnosis.

Prognosis depends on the success of antibacterial treatment since considerable organ damage results from infection. Mortality can be decreased with aggressive antibacterial therapy. Recombinant γ-interferon has been used with some success. The most successful outcomes have been in patients who have undergone successful bone marrow transplantation. An experimental protocol for somatic gene therapy by retroviral transduction of B cells with this gene remains to be proved successful.

Cytochrome b α-Subunit (CYBA) (MIM 233690): Clinically similar to CYBB, this disorder results from mutations in the α-subunit of cytochrome b and shows an autosomal recessive pattern of inheritance. Consanguinity has been reported. Parents of affected individuals sometimes demonstrate intermediate amounts of cytochrome b or NADPH oxidase activity under appropriate stimulation. Complementation by cells from patients with the X-linked form is a feature. The gene, CYBA, has been mapped to chromosome 16q24. The recognized allelic variants include deletions, exon skipping, and single base changes. Compound heterozygosity for two different mutations and homozygosity for the same mutations both result in disease.

Mutations in the two cytosolic components of the NADPH oxidase system can also account autosomal recessive CGD.

G6PD Deficiency (Deficiency of Leukocyte G6PD): The clinical features of G6PD deficiency, the complete deficiency of leukocyte G6PD, are similar to those of CGD. These patients, however, may also have hemolytic anemia. Because of deficient generation of NADPH, leukocytes are unable to kill bacteria. The gene for G6PD is on the X-chromosome and thus the disorder has an X-linked pattern of inheritance. Diagnosis is based on the measurement of leukocyte G6PD and the observation of a deficient bacterial killing curve. The prognosis and treatment are similar to chronic granulomatous disease. Sepsis and extensive organ damage follow the frequent infections, and aggressive antibacterial therapy can lessen these complications and improve prognosis.

Chediak-Higashi Syndrome

The clinical features of Chediak-Higashi syndrome include recurrent bacterial infections, partial albinism with photophobia and nystagmus, an increased incidence of lymphomas, and hepatosplenomegaly. The disorder is quite rare. Pathogenesis involves decreased natural killer (NK) cell activity. Chediak-Higashi syndrome follows an autosomal recessive pattern of inheritance (MIM 214500). The gene or genes responsible have not yet been mapped nor has the protein product been identified. The diagnosis usually rests on finding the characteristic large, eosinophilic, peroxidase-positive inclusions in leukocytes or in other bone marrow derived cells. These granules can also be seen in the lymphocytes of heterozygotes. Prognosis is poor despite aggressive antibacterial measures. Besides the ravages of infection, there is progressive neurologic deterioration and an increased incidence of lymphoma. Patients usually die before 10 years of age.

Job (Hyperimmunoglobulinemia E) Syndrome

A rare condition, Job syndrome is characterized by recurrent abscesses that can be so severe as to require aggressive surgical management. The organism most commonly recovered is *Staphylococcus aureus*. Various abnormalities in granulocyte and lymphocyte function have been reported, but the precise defect is not known. Some patients have an increased serum concentration of IgE. Males and females are affected, and there are reports of affected siblings, suggesting autosomal recessive inheritance (MIM 243700). Autosomal dominant hyper IGE (MIM 147060) is also recognized.

Myeloperoxidase Deficiency

Deficiency of myeloperoxidase (MPO) is common, and very few MPO-deficient individuals have had clinical problems. A predisposition to infection has not been clearly shown. Myeloperoxidase converts hydrogen peroxide to hypochlorous acid, which participates in phagocytic bacterocidal activity. The gene has been mapped to chromosome 17q21.3–q22 and the disorder demonstrates autosomal recessive inheritance (MIM 254600). Some heterozygotes have had half the normal activity of myeloperoxidase. Bacterial killing is delayed but not absent. Peroxidase stain of peripheral blood reveals the absence of the enzyme.

Congenital Neutropenia (Kostmann Syndrome)

Congenital neutropenia results in recurrent bacterial infections that are the major clinical symptom. Only the granulocyte series of white blood cells is affected. The defect is in the receptor (MIM 138971) for granulocyte-stimulating factor (GCSF), a cytokine that directs granulocyte proliferation. One patient responded to treatment with GCSF. Leukocyte adhesion defects are also being defined.

DISORDERS OF B CELL FUNCTION

The disorders of B cell function are disorders of immunoglobulin synthesis and function. The elucidation of the genetic defects has considerably augmented our understanding of this group of disorders.

X-linked Hypoglobulinemia or Agammaglobulinemia (Bruton)

Originally described by Bruton, X-linked hypoglobulinemia or agammaglobulinemia has become better understood since the understanding of B cell function has improved. The most striking clinical feature is recurrent, severe bacterial infections beginning at 5–6 months of age when maternal immunoglobulins have disappeared. Predominant organisms include *Streptococcus pneumoniae* and *Hemophilus influenzae*. Various other gram-positive and gram-negative organisms can also be involved. In contrast to the deficient defense against bacterial infections, affected children usually have a normal immune response to viruses except enteroviruses. Depending on the severity of the immunoglobulin deficiency, presentation can be later and include such protean manifestations as gastrointestinal infections (especially *Giardia lamblia* and *Campylobacter jejuni*), arthritis, and conjunctivitis. The incidence of this rare disorder is about 1 in 100,000.

Pathogenesis involves:

- Deficiency or absence of all five immunoglobulin classes Ig A, M, G, E, D
- Absence of B lymphocytes due to a block in maturation of B lymphocytes from pre-B cells

Genetic evidence suggests that about 50% of patients have a positive family history. The gene locus, designated XLA, (MIM 300300), has been mapped to Xq21.3q22, in keeping with the observation of X-linked inheritance. The protein is a cytoplasmic tyrosine kinase in the src family that has been named Btk (for Bruton tyrosine kinase). Point mutations have been identified in the kinase domain, which is homologous to the Rous sarcoma tyrosine kinase, src, and in the nonkinase SH2 domain; some mutations result in no synthesis of the protein and some mutations produce less than normal amounts of protein or protein with decreased stability. Correlations between genotype and phenotype are now being made. Mutations in the kinase domain affect B cell maturation; nonkinase mutations are less severe and may result in problems in interactions between proteins and in intercellular signaling.

Diagnosis is initially based on deficiency or absence of all five immunoglobulin classes. Absence of B lymphocytes is also a useful diagnostic finding. Linkage analysis using flanking markers is accurate for diagnosis in informative families. In families where the specific mutation in Btk can be identified, specific molecular genetic tools are useful for diagnosis. Treatment includes replacement of immunoglobulin; antibiotics may also be needed. Despite these interventions, long-term prognosis is guarded because of the severity of enteroviral infections later in life. In addition, there may be an increased incidence of leukemia and lymphoma later in life.

Immunodeficiency with Hyper IgM

Immunodeficiency with hyper IgM is marked by recurrent bacterial infections. Pathogenesis involves poor antibody response to bacterial infections, which is a B cell function. In addition, there is some evidence of associated T cell dysfunction. From the genetic standpoint, there are X-linked, autosomal recessive, and autosomal dominant forms. The X-linked form has been well characterized genetically. The gene, designated HIGM1 (MIM 308230) has been mapped to chromosome Xq26.3–27.1. The protein is a membrane glycoprotein called the CD40 ligand (CD40L). This protein is expressed on the surface of T cells and binds CD40, a surface glycoprotein on B cells. The CD40 ligand is found on CD4 and CD8 T cells. This complex controls proliferation and differentiation of B cells and may have a role in immunoglobulin switching. Several types of mutations have been identified, including point mutations, deletions, and nonsense mutations. Diagnosis is made by measuring an increased concentration of IgM (150–1000 mg/dl) along with absent IgA and IgG. Prognosis and treatment are similar to those for Bruton agammaglobulinemia.

IgA Deficiency

The clinical phenotype of IgA deficiency is inconsistent. Most affected individuals are healthy, but an increased frequency of respiratory infections occurs in some persons. In addition, there is a higher frequency of IgA deficiency among patients with several clinical disorders, including cancer, celiac disease, and atopy. Reports of familial incidence of IgA deficiency are incompletely documented, and the mechanism is entirely unclear. In several families the affected individuals have a deletion of an immunoglobulin heavy chain gene on chromosome 14. These patients have deficiency but not total absence of IgA, a secretory immunoglobulin, but most affected persons have no significant clinical symptoms. The plasma cells that make IgA are in lymphoid tissue adjacent to mucous membranes, such as tonsils, adenoids, and gastrointestinal tract. The genes involved are the IgA and IgG heavy chain genes on chromosome 14. Diagnosis depends on measurement of IgA, which is decreased. In some families, it is possible to look for deletions on chromosome 14. In other families, no specific mode of inheritance can be defined. Most likely, IgA deficiency is genetically heterogeneous.

X-linked Lymphoproliferative Syndrome

The clinical features of X-linked lymphoproliferative syndrome are striking. Besides infectious mononucleosis, immunodeficiency, aplastic anemia, and American Burkitt lymphoma, these patients have a very high incidence of fatal EBV infection. Pathogenesis involves severely abnormal B cell function, including no switch from IgM to IgG specific antibody following immunization, no antibody response to EBV following EBV infection, and depressed natural killer cell function. Patients may have variable immunoglobulin abnormalities. Family history in many patients has suggested X-linked inheritance, and the gene, designated XLP (MIM 308240) maps to chromosome Xq25–q26. Diagnostic findings include the observation of abnormal helper/suppressor T cell ratios, abnormal response to mitogens, and lack of antibody to EBV. Prognosis and treatment are not encouraging. Administration of gamma globulin has been used; despite therapy, 60% of patients succumb to fatal EBV infection. Of those who survive, development of American Burkitt lymphoma is not rare.

DISORDERS OF T CELL FUNCTION

DiGeorge Syndrome

DiGeorge syndrome is characterized by clinical features that include:

- Aplasia or hypoplasia of the thymus
- Lymphopenia because of the decreased T cells
- Decreased lymphocytes in lymph nodes

- Dysmorphology including: low-set ears, small jaw, short philtrum, hypertelorism, antimongoloid slant of eyes.

Esophageal atresia may be present. Congenital heart disease is a common feature. The usual cardiac anomalies are truncus arteriosus, anomalous pulmonary drainage, tetralogy of Fallot, and right-sided aortic arch or interrupted aortic arch. Cardiac failure soon after birth is not unusual (Figure 4–1). Hypoparathyroidism with severe hypocalcemia occurs 24–48 hours after birth. The thymus is small or absent, and normal T cell development does not take place. Consequently, chronic infections with viral, bacterial, and fungal pathogens may occur. Incidence, including partial expression, has been estimated at 1 in 4000. DiGeorge syndrome results from abnormal development of the third and fourth pharyngeal arches. The third and fourth pharyngeal arches are the embryologic origin of the thymus and parathyroid glands (Figure 4–2). At about the 12th week of embryologic life, these migrate to their final position. Differentiation of the aortic arch and the philtrum occur at the same time. The abnormal development of these structures in DiGeorge syndrome suggests that a developmental gene or genes may be involved. The observation of deletions or transloca-

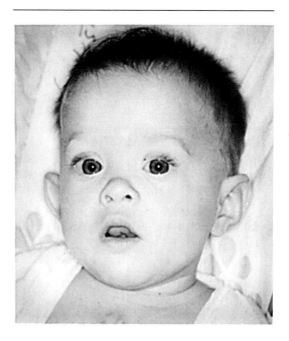

Figure 4–1. Infant with DiGeorge syndrome. Prominent are low-set and malformed ears, hypertelorism, and fish-shaped mouth. Also note the surgical scar from cardiac surgery. (Reproduced, with permission, from Stites DP, Terr AI, and Parslow TG: *Basic & Clinical Immunology.* 8th ed, Appleton & Lange, 1994.)

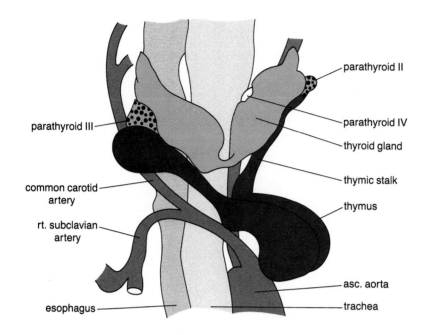

Figure 4–2. Embryologic development of the thymus and parathyroid glands from the third and fourth pharyngeal pouches. (Reproduced, with permission, from Stites DP, Terr AI, and Parslow TG: *Basic & Clinical Immunology.* 8th ed. Appleton & Lange, 1994.)

tions in chromosome 22 involving 22q11 has led to further investigations at that chromosomal location. Submicroscopic deletions have been detected through the use of molecular techniques such as in situ hybridization. Greenberg has estimated that probably as many as 90% of patients with DiGeorge syndrome have a deletion in the critical region at 22q11. Dominant transmission of the syndrome from parent to child has occurred in association with the 22q11 deletion in both parent and offspring. The phenotype of the deletion at 22q11 is now expanding to include some conotruncal cardiac defects without the rest of the DiGeorge syndrome and the velocardiofacial syndrome (MIM 192430). The precise nature of the genetic abnormality remains unknown. Several candidate genes lie in the critical region, including TUPLE1, a developmental gene, and ZNF74, a zinc-finger protein gene. A few patients with the DiGeorge phenotype and other chromosomal abnormalities suggest the presence of other possible loci on chromosome 10p13 and on chromosome 17p13.

Diagnosis is suggested by the characteristic cardiac, facial, and parathyroid abnormalities, along with absence of the thymus. The lymphocyte count is usually but not always low (<1200 μL); numbers of T cells are decreased, and there is poor lymphocyte response to phytohemagglutinin. Maternally derived IgG is present. Some patients appear to have abnormal B cell function. Banded karyotype and molecular

studies directed at 22q11 in situ hybridization techniques should be used to refine the diagnosis postnatally; such studies also can be used for prenatal diagnosis. Both parents should be tested if the child demonstrates a deletion or rearrangement.

Prognosis and treatment depend on the extent of the abnormalities. Cardiac surgery is often needed to correct the cardiac malformation; hypoparathyroidism is treated with calcium and 1,25-cholecalciferol. Any blood for transfusion must be irradiated prior to use in order to prevent graft vs host disease (GVHD). Transplantation with fetal thymus has been successful, providing that the thymus is less than 14 weeks' gestation. Some patients undergo spontaneous remission.

Mucocutaneous Candidiasis

These patients have chronic mucocutaneous candidiasis that responds poorly to treatment. Skin, mucous membrane, and nails are involved. Familial cases and consanguinity have been reported. Recessive inheritance has been assumed (MIM 212050), but the gene has not been mapped or characterized.

Nezelof Syndrome

A rare disorder of T cell function, Nezelof syndrome results in recurrent microbial infections similar to those in other immunodeficiency syndromes. The gene or genes involved have not been identified, but there is evidence for recessive inheritance (MIM 242700). Diagnosis is based on aplasia or dysplasia of the thymus, lymphopenia, and normal immunoglobulins. Delayed hypersensitivity may be abnormal. Because there are so few cases, and the defect has not been defined, it is difficult to be certain about prognosis. However, some patients have died of opportunistic infections.

COMBINED IMMUNODEFICIENCY

Severe Combined Immunodeficiency (SCID)

Severe combined immunodeficiency, formerly called Swiss-type agammaglobulinemia, is characterized by the following clinical features:

- Failure to thrive
- Unrelenting diarrhea
- Recurrent infections within the first 6 months.

The organisms involved include bacterial, viral, and fungal pathogens. Infections are severe and unrelenting: oral candidiasis, pneumonia, chronic otitis media, and sepsis occur. There is absence of lymphoid tissue such as tonsils and lymph nodes. No thymic shadow is present on chest imaging. Affected persons fail to mount an immune response to live virus immunizations or to clinical infection. Systemic, fatal viral infections occur. Patients may develop clinical poliomyelitis, eg, after immunization. Opportunistic infections such as pneumocystis carinii also occur. GVHD also can develop following blood transfusion or engraftment of maternal cells. T and B cell immunity are both lacking. This may result from any of several mechanisms that involve T and B cell maturation, development, and survival.

Diagnosis is initially based on the presence of lymphopenia with absence of both B and T cells, absent thymus, and low concentrations of immunoglobulins in serum. No response of lymphocytes to phytohemagglutinin occurs. Specific, recognized genetic deficits can be sought using appropriate cytogenetic and molecular techniques. Family history may be revealing; an X-linked or autosomal recessive pattern may be helpful. It is useful to recognize that either possibility is compatible with a history of two affected brothers. Prenatal diagnosis has proved successful both by staining for the cell surface markers CD3 and CD11 and by observing the lymphocyte response to mitogens. In addition, X-inactivation patterns have been used to diagnose X-linked SCID prenatally.

Skewed X-inactivation Patterns: The use of skewed X-inactivation patterns for carrier detection of certain X-linked disorders merits more discussion here among the disorders for which it is helpful. As noted in Chapter 2, random inactivation of one X-chromosome occurs in each cell of the body at some time during early development. An exception to this is the **nonrandom X-inactivation pattern** that has been observed in women who are heterozygous for certain X-linked disorders, largely disorders of immune function. This phenomenon has been seen in carriers of SCIDX1; the abnormal X chromosome is preferentially inactivated. It is also seen in carriers of the Wiskott-Aldrich (WAS) gene. The presence of nonrandom X-inactivation can be assayed by examining the methylation patterns that distinguish the active from the inactive X-chromosome, by the study of mouse-human cell hybrids, or by examination of G6PD isozymes. For SCID, this phenomenon is observed in T and B cells. In WAS, it is seen in T cells, B cells, phagocytes and platelets. The skewed pattern is seen in B cells in X-linked agammaglobulinemia. It is **not seen** with X-linked lymphoproliferative syndrome or X-linked hyper-IgM. A test for skewed X-inactivation can also be used for prenatal diagnosis because the question can be asked: Do the affected child and unborn child have same maternal X? This X chromosome presumably carries the mutation.

Prognosis in this group of disorders is poor; the disorder is usually fatal without either restoration of the immune system or complete protection from microbes. No live virus vaccination should ever be given to affected patients. Transfusion with blood-containing lymphocytes is dangerous unless it has first been irradiated to prevent GVHD. Aggressive antimicrobial therapy along with gamma globulin administration may provide some time to prepare for more definitive treatment. Bone marrow transplant has had substantial success, with reports of 50–75% survival rates. For the adenosine deaminase (ADA) deficient form, weekly infusion of a polyethylene glycol complex of adenosine deaminase (PEG-ADA) has been successful in partially restoring ADA activity and immune function. Gene therapy by providing the ADA gene to autologous lymphocytes is currently under investigation; preliminary results are promising (see Chapter 3).

Many genes in the pathway of maturation and proliferation of T and B cells are candidate genes for mutations that result in SCID. Both autosomal recessive and X-linked forms have been recognized; genetic abnormalities have been sought on autosomes and on the X-chromosome. The defined mutations are noted here, but there may be others that are yet to be defined.

SCIDX1 (MIM 300400): SCIDX1, an X-linked form, accounts for 60–80% of cases. The gene product is the B cell surface IL-2 receptor γ (IL-2Rγ). IL-2 is a cytokine that stimulates growth and differentiation of T cells and B cells. To do this, it must interact with its receptor, IL-2R, on the surface of the relevant cells. The gene for the IL-2 receptor was known before it was related to this condition, and thus the gene has a separate designation and MIM number (IL2RG; MIM 308380). The receptor protein has three chains, of which the γ-chain is important for function. This subunit is also shared by two other lymphokine receptors, IL4 and IL7, and perhaps others, accounting for the profound effects of mutations in this subunit. This gene, IL2RG, has been mapped to Xq13.1. Point mutations have been identified in some patients, as have transversion to stop codons, which result in no protein synthesis. Some cases are new mutations, while others are inherited mutations.

SCIDX2 (MIM 312863): SCIDX2, an X-linked condition, is similar to but milder than SCIDX1. It is unclear whether these two are allelic variants.

Adenosine Deaminase (ADA) Deficiency (MIM 102700): Adenosine deaminase (ADA) deficiency is a recessively inherited form of SCID that accounts for about 20% of all cases and about half the recessive ones. The gene for ADA has been mapped to 20q12–q13.11. The deficiency of ADA results in an increased intracellular concentration of deoxy-ATP, which is toxic to T cells but not to B cells. Specific diagnosis can be made by measuring ADA activity and identifying the defect in erythrocytes, leukocytes, cultured fibroblasts, and other tissues. Heterozygotes can also be identified this way. Many allelic variants have been described. Most involve point mutations, but there have been reports of a deletion and of splice site mutations.

Purine Nucleoside Phosphorylase (PNP) Deficiency (MIM 164050): Purine nucleoside phosphorylase (PNP) deficiency has a pathogenesis that is probably similar to ADA deficiency. PNP converts deoxyinosine and deoxyguanosine to their respective purine bases, which are most likely toxic to T cells. PNP maps to 14q13.1. Specific diagnosis can be made by measuring PNP activity and identifying the defect in erythrocytes, leukocytes, cultured fibroblasts, and other tissues. Both homozygotes and heterozygotes can also be identified this way (Figure 4–3).

Bare Lymphocyte Syndrome: The defect in bare lymphocyte syndrome is the lack of production of class I or class II histocompatibility antigens. This provides evidence for the possibility that HLA antigens are important in the differentiation of lymphocytes. Affected siblings have been reported, and autosomal recessive inheritance is considered likely (MIM 209920). Bone marrow transplantation has been successful and prenatal diagnosis has been performed.

Wiscott-Aldrich Syndrome (WAS)

Wiscott-Aldrich syndrome (WAS) is characterized by thrombocytopenia present at birth, recurrent infections usually beginning around 6 months of age, and eczema beginning around age 1 year. The most common organisms are those of the capsular-polysaccharide type, for example, *Streptococcus pneumoniae*,

Hemophilus influenza, and *Neisseria meningitidis.* Incidence is reported to be about 1 in 4 million. The nature of the immune defect is uncertain: B and T cell function are largely normal early, but variable dysfunction appears later.

WAS has long been recognized as an X-linked trait. The locus for WAS has been mapped to Xp11.3–p11.2 (WAS, IMD2) (MIM 301000), proximal to properdin and CYBB. The protein product is unknown, but it may relate to interaction between cell surface proteins. Flanking markers exist, enabling linkage analysis for diagnosis within families with multiple affected members.

Several hematologic laboratory findings are helpful for diagnosis. Platelets are both small in size and decreased in number (platelet count ranges from 5000–100,000/μL). Red cell isohemaglutinins are low or absent. There is no response to immunization with polysaccharide antigens. B and T cell function are largely normal early, but there is depletion of T cells later. Immunoglobulin abnormalities are variable, with decreased IgM and increased IgA and IgE. There is also reduced cell surface CD43, but that is not the primary defect, since the gene for CD43 has been mapped to chromosome 16.

Treatment is directed at bleeding, which can be severe; bloody diarrhea, petechiae, and central nervous system hemorrhage all occur. Attempts to control bleeding with splenectomy have been followed by an increased risk of infection; fatal infections have been reported. Thus, early recognition of infection is critical, and aggressive antibiotic therapy is essential. IV gamma globulin may have a role in treating infection. Bone marrow transplant has been used with some success. An increased risk of lymphoma and leukemia in surviving adults has been reported.

Immunodeficiency Associated with Other Recognized Genetic Disorders

Immunodeficiency can be associated with several recognized genetic disorders including:

- Ataxia-telangiectasia: Selective IgA deficiency is described in about 40% of patients. It may relate to the presumptive defect in DNA repair that is believed to be the basic defect in this disorder.
- Cartilage-hair hypoplasia
- Transcobalamin II deficiency
- Biotinidase deficiency
- 18q-syndrome.

DISORDERS OF COMPLEMENT FUNCTION

Properdin Deficiency

Patients with properdin deficiency present with fulminant meningococcemia, which is often fatal.

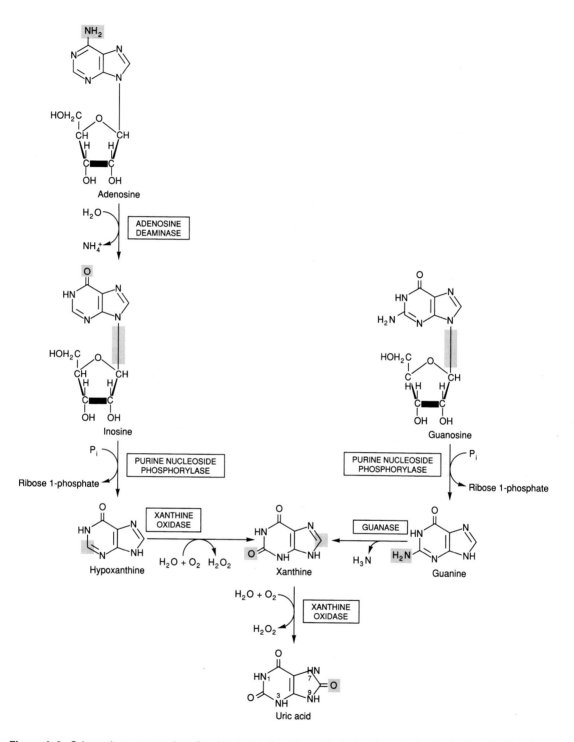

Figure 4–3. Schematic representation of purine metabolic pathway illustrating the critical role of adenosine deaminase and purine nucleoside phosphorylase. (Reproduced, with permission, from Murray RK et al: *Harper's Review of Biochemistry.* 22nd ed. Appleton & Lange, 1990.)

Complement-mediated lysis or phagocytosis occurs weakly in the absence of antibody, since properdin is needed to stabilize C3 convertase in order to maintain the complement cascade. The gene for X-linked properdin factor P (PFC) (MIM 312060) has been mapped to Xp11.4–p11.2 (PFC, PFD) and has been cloned. Flanking markers exist for linkage studies. Mutations are being defined. The deficiency has been reported in several ethnic groups.

Other Immune Function Disorders

Other ill-defined disorders of immune function appear familial. Precise diagnosis and genetic counseling will be more effective when these disorders are genetically defined.

PROSPECTS FOR GENETIC DIAGNOSIS AND THERAPY

With the elucidation of the genetic defects responsible for inherited disorders of immune function comes the promise of improved diagnosis and therapy. The promise of improved diagnosis is already being realized. The number of specific molecular diagnostic tests and linkage studies for disorders that have been mapped but not characterized at the molecular level is increasing rapidly for these immunologic disorders. Gene therapy for ADA deficiency is already in clinical trials. More such protocols will undoubtedly be advanced if gene therapy is shown to be safe and effective.

REFERENCES AND SUGGESTED READING

Aruffo A, Farrington M, Hollenbaugh D: The CD40 ligand gp39 is defective in activated T cells from patients with X- linked hyper-IgM syndrome. Cell 1993;**72:**291.

Berthet F et al: Clinical consequences and treatment of primary immunodeficiency syndromes characterized by functional T and B lymphocyte anomalies (combined immune deficiency). Pediatrics 1994;**93:**265.

Bohler MC et al: A study of 25 patients with chronic granulomatous disease: a new classification by correlating respiratory burst, cytochrome b, and flavoprotein. J Clin Immunology 1986;**6:**136.

Buckley R. Assessing inheritance of agammaglobulinemia: N Engl J Med 1994;**330:**1526.

Chan AC et al: ZAP-70 deficiency in an autosomal recessive form of severe combined immunodeficiency. Science 1994;**264:**1599.

Clark RA: Genetic variation in chronic granulomatous disease. Hosp Prac 1990;(**May):**51.

Cunningham-Rundles: Genetic aspects of immunoglobulin A deficiency. Advances in Human Genetics 1990;**19:** 235.

Densen P et al: Familial properdin deficiency and fatal meningococcemia. N Engl J Med 1987;**316:**922.

Driscoll DA et al: Prevalence of 22q11 microdeletions in DiGeorge and velocardiofacial syndrome: implications for genetic counselling and prenatal diagnosis. J Med Genet 1993;**30:**813.

Elder ME et al: Human severe combined immunodeficiency due to a defect in ZAP-70, a T cell tyrosine kinase. Science 1994;**264:**1596.

Greenberg F: DiGeorge syndrome: an historical review of clinical and cytogenetic features. J Med Genet 1993; **30:**803.

Greer WL et al: X-chromosome inactivation in the Wiskott-Aldrich syndrome: A marker for detection of the carrier state and identification of cell lineages expressing the gene defect. Genomics 1989;**4:**60.

Halford S et al: Low-copy-number repeat sequences flank the DiGeorge/velo-cardio-facial syndroem loci at 22q11. Human Molecular Genetics 1993;**2:**191.

Hall J: CATCH 22. J Med Genet 1993;**30:**801.

Hathaway WE et al: *Current Pediatric Diagnosis and Treatment.* Appleton & Lange, 1991.

Hirschhorn R: Overview of biochemical abnormalities and molecular genetics of adenosine deaminase deficiency. Pediatric Research 1992;**33:**S35.

Hirschhorn R, Hirschhorn K: Immunodeficiency disorders. Pages 1411–1430 in: *Principles and Practice of Medical Genetics,* Emery AEH, Rimoin D (editors), 2nd ed. Churchill Livingstone, 1990.

Horwich AL, Seashore MR, Dwyer JM: Overwhelming sepsis in the adult variant of Wiskott-Aldrich syndrome. Arch Intern Med 1984;**144:**1498.

Hyde RM: *Immunology.* National Medical Series. Williams and Wilkins, 1992.

Johnston RB: The complement system in host defense and inflammation: the cutting edges of a double-edged sword. Pediatr Inf Dis 1993;**12:**933–41.

Korthauer U et al: Defective expression of T-cell CD40 ligand causes X-linked immunodeficiency with hyper IgM. Nature 1993;**361:**539.

Lovering R et al: Genetic linkage analysis indentifies new proximal and distal flanking markers for the X-linked agammaglobulinemia gene locus, refining its localization in Xq22. Human Molecular Genetics 1993;**2:**139.

Lubs HA, Ruddle FH: Chromosomal abnormalities in the human population: estimation of rates based on New Haven Newborn Study. Science 1970;**169:**495–497.

Marsh DG et al: Linkage analysis of IL4 and other chromosome 5q31.1 markers and total serum immunoglobulin E concentrations. Science 1994;**264:**1152.

Miller ME, Hill HR: Disorders of leucocyte function. Pages 1439–1452 in: *Principles and Practice of Medical Genetics,* Emery AEH, Rimoin D (editors), 2nd ed. Churchill Livingstone, 1990.

Nogucki M et al: Interleukin-2 receptor gammachain mutation results in X-linked severe combined immunodeficiency in humans. Cell 1993;**73:**147.

Nunoi H et al: Two forms of autosomal chronic granulomatous disease lack distinct neutrophil cytosol factors. Science 1988;**242:**1298.

Ormerod AD: The Wiskott-Aldrich syndrome. Int J Dermatol 1985;**24:**77.

Puck J: X-linked Immunodeficiency. Advances in Human Genetics 1993;**21:**107.

Puck JM et al: Prenatal test for X-linked severe combined

immunodeficiency by analysis of maternal X-chromosome inactivation and linkage analysis. N Engl J Med 1990;**322:**1063.

Rijkers GT, Sanders LA, Zegers BJ: Anti-capsular polysaccharide antibody deficiency states. Immunodeficiency 1993;**5:**1.

Rosen FS, Alper CA: Complement defects. Pages 1431–1438 in: *Principles and Practice of Medical Genetics,* Emery AEH, Rimoin D (editors), 2nd ed. Churchill Livingstone, 1990.

Saffran DC et al: Brief report: A point mutation in the SH2 domain of Bruton's tyrosine kinase in atypical X-linked agammaglobulinemia. N Engl J Med 1994;**330:**1488.

Schroeder SA et al: *Current Medical Diagnosis and Treatment.* Appleton & Lange, 1992.

Sjoholm AG et al: Dysfunctional properdin in a Dutch family with meningococcal disease. N Engl J Med 1988;**319:**33.

Sprent J, Tough DF: Lymphocyte life-span and memory. Science 1994;**265:**1395.

Standen GR: Wiskott-Aldrich syndrome: new perspective in pathogenesis and management. J R Coll Physicians Lond 1988;**22:**80.

Stites DP, Terr AI, Parslow TG: *Basic and Clinical Immunology.* Appleton & Lange, 1994.

Tsukada S, Saffran DC, Rawlings DJ: Deficient expression of a B cell cytoplasmic tyrosine kinase in human X-linked agammaglobulinemia. Cell 1993;**72:**279.

Volpp BD, Nauseef WM, Clark RA: Two cytosolic neutrophil oxidase components absent in autosomal chronic granulomatous disease. Science 1988;**242:**1295.

White CJ, Gallin JI: Phagocyte defects. Clin Immunol Immunopathol 1986;**40:**50.

Wilson DI et al: DiGeorge syndrome: part of CATCH 22. J Med Genet 1993;**30:**852.

5

Genetics & Cancer

This chapter will focus on four aspects of cancer that are important to the practicing physician:

- Mechanisms of cancer at the cellular level
- Inheritance of cancer as a single gene trait
- The role of chromosomal changes in cancer cells
- Syndromes in which cancer occurs in increased frequency.

The chapter aims to outline the importance of genetic factors in cancer. These factors are of value in arriving at the diagnosis and prognosis for specific cancers. Genetic knowledge and tools can help the physician to identify the presymptomatic patient at risk for developing cancer and to provide genetic counseling for patients and families who have had cancer diagnosed. Chapter 5 will not focus on clinical discussion of individual cancer types or diseases. Discussion of other diagnostic means and treatment options is beyond the scope of this chapter.

CANCER GENETICS AT THE CELLULAR LEVEL

New understanding of the biology of cancer cells is becoming valuable in designing strategies to diagnose and treat cancer effectively. Cancer cells have lost the growth regulation that keeps normal cells in check. By developing characteristics that allow them to avoid the mechanisms that suppress uncontrolled growth, the cells metastasize and grow in new locations. Many proteins are involved in this process:

- Proteins that stimulate cell division
- Receptors that activate the above-mentioned proteins and are in turn activated by other signaling proteins
- Proteins that suppress cell division and growth
- Proteins that control programmed cell death
- Proteins that interact with DNA and control its replication or turn specific genes off or on.

The molecular events that allow cancer to develop involve a broad variety of genes. Mutations, rearrangements, deletions, and amplification in the genes coding for this group of proteins cause the above-stated mechanisms to go awry.

Features that suggest the presence of inherited cancer syndromes are listed in Table 5–1.

Role of Single Genes in Cancer Cells

In 1971 Knudsen proposed a hypothesis for a two-step origin for childhood cancer at the cellular level. The hypothesis was developed on a probabilistic model and arose from considerations of the multiple hit model for colon cancer in adults proposed by Ashley. Retinoblastoma, an eye tumor in children, was observed in some families in an autosomal dominant pattern; in others, it was a sporadic occurrence. Families with dominant inheritance displayed earlier onset and a higher frequency of bilateral tumors. These observations led Knudsen to the idea that cancer might be caused by sequential inactivation of genes important in cell growth, and the proposed mathematical model suggested that two genetic events, "two hits," might be enough (Figure 5–1). In acquired cancer, both hits would be somatic mutations that took place sequentially in a cell which then lost growth control and initiated a malignant tumor. In families in which a dominant inheritance pattern occurred, the first "hit" would be an inherited mutation in one of the genes; the second "hit" would be an acquired mutation in a somatic cell that already had inherited the first hit (Figure 5–2). Such persons would have a greater likelihood of developing cancer than persons without the constitutional mutation, since only one genetic event would be required.

Three critical observations supported this hypothesis over the last two decades. The report in 1976 of retinoblastoma in an individual with a deletion in chromosome 13q was consistent with the inherited first hit of the two hit model; deletion of a normal

Table 5–1. Features that suggest the presence of inherited cancer syndromes.		
Category	**Feature**
Chronological	Early age of onset of cancer
Physical	Multiple primary tumors Congenital malformations in association with cancer
Familial	Affected family members

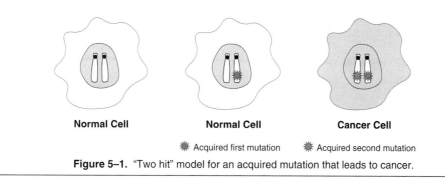

Normal Cell Normal Cell Cancer Cell

☀ Acquired first mutation ☀ Acquired second mutation

Figure 5–1. "Two hit" model for an acquired mutation that leads to cancer.

gene represented the "first hit." The second observation was a family with several members who had the aniridia-Wilms tumor syndrome associated with deletion in chromosome 11p. The third observation was a family with renal cell carcinoma and a translocation between chromosomes 3 and 8.

Clear evidence continues to accumulate that changes in multiple genes are causative in many kinds of cancer. Retinoblastoma provides a prime example of two sequential mutations, one at the RB1 locus on each chromosome 13. Both are needed to cause the cell to become cancerous. In colon cancer, the evidence supports the conclusion that multiple hits at different loci result in the cancer phenotype. The genes involved are now being identified. Examples include proto-oncogenes, oncogenes, and tumor suppressor genes. Many mutations in these genes play a role in the development of cancer.

Cancer can develop after multiple changes in a set of genes. The order in which those changes occur may not be important. Environmental agents may contribute to the accumulation of mutations. Inherited cancer syndromes may result from the inheritance of a mutation that represents the first mutation in the multi-step process. This would decrease the number of mutation events needed to lead to cancerous transformation in a cell, shorten the time span over which tumorigenesis occurs, and lead to an earlier age of onset. It might also make it more likely that more than one kind of cancer would develop in an individual.

Oncogenes

A group of retroviruses called RNA tumor viruses can transform animal cells to tumor cells. The transformation is effected by particular genes known as **viral oncogenes,** which are now known to have arisen from normal gene sequences. All cells contain genes known as **proto-oncogenes** that have homology to these viral oncogenes and probably gave rise to them. The proto-oncogenes code for proteins that affect cell growth and differentiation. By mutation or other alteration, these proto-oncogenes become oncogenes: genes coding for proteins that direct or allow abnormal cell growth. There are several such gene families.

The proto-oncogenes and their derivative oncogenes have distinct mechanisms of action based on the biochemical functions of the oncoproteins whose synthesis they direct. They act as gain-of-function proteins that induce cell division. The biochemical mechanisms through which they act include phosphorylation of proteins (particularly at tyrosine, serine, and threonine residues on the proteins) activation of phospholipid turnover, and interaction with G proteins. These actions are all related to signal transduction within cells and between cells and affect functions within the cells. Currently, there are many

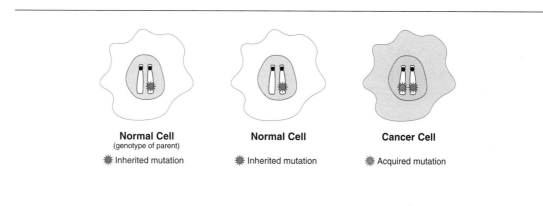

Normal Cell
(genotype of parent)
☀ Inherited mutation

Normal Cell
☀ Inherited mutation

Cancer Cell
☀ Acquired mutation

Table 5–2. Oncogenes related to cancer.

Oncogene	Related Cancer
c-raf	Lung cancer, parotid gland
c-kit	Lung cancer
myc	Small cell lung cancer, colon cancer, lymphoma
N-myc	Neuroblastoma
k-ras	Colon cancer
erbA	Lymphoma, small cell lung cancer
bcr-abl	Chronic myelogenous leukemia
ras	Colon, pancreas, bladder, lung

acquired tumors in which oncogenes are implicated; mutations or overexpression of proto-oncogenes constitute one of the steps in the multistep path to cancer. The ret oncogene, in which a germline mutation occurs in MEN2A and MEN2B, is an example of a single gene disorder involving an oncogene. Examples are provided in Table 5–2, which lists known proto-oncogenes, oncogenes, and tumors in which they are seen.

The identification of oncoproteins or of oncogenes in some tumors may allow for prediction of the severity of the cancer, its response to treatment, its propensity to metastasis. Understanding of the function of these genes may lead to improved therapy by allowing specific sites for development of anticancer drugs, gene therapy approaches, and other targeted approaches.

Tumor Suppressor Genes

The second type of defined gene related to cancer is the **tumor suppressor gene.** The seminal observation was that malignant cells, when fused with normal cells, lost the cancer phenotype; the hybrid cell regained its malignant characteristics after the loss of several chromosomes. These observations suggested that some genes could turn off the malignant transformation. Further investigations led to the identification of a protein called p53, which is mutated in about 50% of human cancers in different tissues; wild type p53 protein can reverse malignant transformation. This is an example of a protein encoded by a tumor suppressor gene. This family of genes encodes proteins that affect cell growth and proliferation; some are DNA binding proteins; others may regulate transcription of other genes in other ways. Several tumor suppressor genes are listed in Table 5–3.

Evidence is accumulating that mutations in RB1 and p53, when present in the same cell, may cooperate in the development of some kinds of tumors, including some sarcomas and carcinoma of lung, breast, cervix, pancreas.

Role of Chromosomal Changes in Cancer Cells

Observations of chromosomal abnormalities in the cells of malignant tumors are as old as the field of cytogenetics. Both constitutional and somatic chromosomal changes are recognized. Individuals with some constitutional chromosomal abnormalities are at increased risk for developing cancer. These chromosomal abnormalities are listed in Table 5–4. Similarly, individuals who have syndromes associated with increased numbers of chromosomal breaks have an increased risk for developing cancer.

Many kinds of cytogenetic abnormalities characterize cancer cells. Loss of chromosomes, addition of chromosomes, and translocations are all seen. These observations have led to the chromosomal localization of some genes that cause cancer. Translocations may disrupt important genes or place two genes in juxtaposition to each other and place genes for growth proteins under new control. Identification of the chromosomal constitution of tumors may provide useful diagnostic and prognostic information. Some are listed in Table 5–5.

Table 5–3. Tumor suppressor genes.

Gene	Protein	Protein Function	Disease	Map Location
p53	p53	DNA binding protein	Sporadic acquired cancer, all kinds; germline mutations, Li-Fraumeni, osteosarcoma	17p13.1
WT1	WT1	Zinc finger DNA binding protein	WAGR, Denys-Drash, Wilms tumor	11p13
WT2	Unknown	Wilms tumor	Wilms tumor	11p13
APC	β-catenin	Cell adhesion molecule	Familial adenomatous polyposis	5q21
NF1	Neurofibromin	G-protein, GTPase activity	Neurofibromatosis 1	17q11
p16	p16	Binds proteins that regulate cell cycle	Familial melanoma	9p21
RB1	RB1	DNA binding	Retinoblastoma, osteosarcoma, other sarcomas	13q14

Table 5–4. Cytogenetic disorders that have an increased risk of cancer.

Cytogenetic Disorder	Cancer Risk
Trisomy 21 (Down syndrome)	Leukemia
del 11p13 (WAGR syndrome)	Wilms tumor
dup 11p15 (Beckwith-Wiedemann syndrome)	Wilms tumor
ring 22	Meningioma
del or translocation, 13q	Retinoblastoma

WAGR = Wilms' tumor, aniridia genital, renal abnormalities.

Table 5–5. Cytogenetic abnormalities recognized in cancers.

Solid Tumors	Cytogenetic Abnormality
Bladder	1, 3, 11, 5q, 9
Testicular	12p
Ewing	t(11:22)(q24;q12)
Chondrosarcoma	t(9:22)(q31;q25)
Neuroblastoma	Double minutes; del(1)(p31–32)
Renal cell carcinoma	del 3p26–p14
Small cell lung	del 3p14–p23
Burkitt lymphoma	Deletions, translocations 2p and 8q
Non-Hodgkin lymphoma	Translocations 2p, 5q, 14q, 11q, 8q
Leukemia	**Cytogenetic Abnormality**
	1p, 3q, 4, 5q, 6q, 11q23, 14, 22q (Philadelphia chromosome; (9,22)(q34;q11) Trisomy 21 in ALL Abnormalities in all chromosomes except Y have been seen in either solid tumors or leukemia

SINGLE GENE DISORDERS THAT PREDISPOSE TO CANCER

A broad variety of single gene disorders are associated with an increased frequency of cancer compared to the general population. Many of these conditions are discussed elsewhere in the appropriate chapter for the system involved. Table 5–6 lists some well recognized associations.

Single Gene Cancer Syndromes

That cancer can run in families has been known for many years. Pedigree analysis has led to the recognition of several family cancer syndromes that are inherited in an autosomal dominant pattern (Figure 5–3). New molecular tools have begun to unravel the genetic basis of these conditions and provide better information for diagnosis, prognosis, and counseling in these families. Several examples are listed in Table 5–7.

Li-Fraumeni Syndrome: Families that have Li-Fraumeni syndrome have multiple members who have cancers characterized by early onset, multiple primaries, and a variety of organs involved. About 50% of people who carry the gene develop cancer by age 30 yrs. These cancers include brain tumors, sarcomas, adrenocortical carcinoma, and leukemia; 50% of women develop breast cancer.

Table 5–6. Inherited syndromes in which development of cancer is a significant risk.

Syndrome	Type of Cancer	Map Location	Gene
Von Hippel Lindau (MIM 193300)	Hemangioblastoma, renal cell carcinoma	3p25	VHL
Tuberous sclerosis (MIM 191100) (MIM 101092)	Renal cell carcinoma, malignant giant cell astrocytomas	9q34; 16p	TSC1 TSC2
Gorlin MIM (109400)	Basal cell carcinoma, fibrosarcoma of jaw cysts, nasopharyngeal carcinomas	9q22	NBCCS
MEN1 (MIM 131100)	Carcinoids, tumor of pancreas, parathyroids, and pituitary	11q13	MEN1
MEN2 (MIM 164761)	Medullary thyroid cancer, malignant pheochromocytoma	10q11.2	RET protooncogene
NF1 (MIM 162200)	Neurofibrosarcoma, malignant schwannoma, rhabdomyosarcoma, glioma	17q11.2	NF1
Peutz-Jegher (MIM 175200)	Gastrointestinal tract, breast, uterus	—	—
Denys-Drash	Wilms tumor, gonadoblastoma	11p13	WT1
Beckwith-Wiedemann (MIM 130650)	Wilms tumor, adrenal carcinoma, hepatoblastoma	11p15	BWS

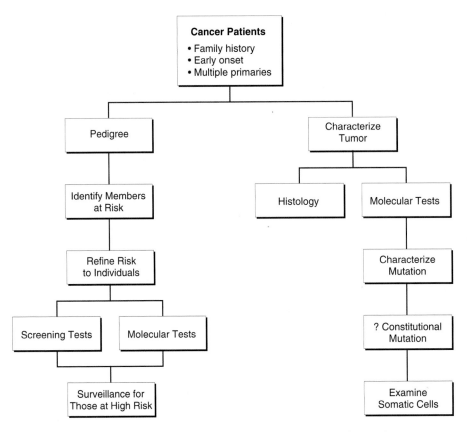

Figure 5–3. Flow chart for screening and testing patients at risk for certain cancers.

The development of cancer follows an autosomal dominant inheritance pattern. Constitutional mutations in the tumor suppressor gene p53 have been identified in these families. Genetic counseling for these families is complex. Members at risk can be offered clinical screening for tumors for which such screening tests are available. Molecular testing is not yet practical, but may become so when there is more information about clinical correlation between the specific mutations and the cancer risk. It is difficult to devise a screening program that will address all the sites at risk. When the mutation(s) better understood, molecular testing may become feasible, but the problems of clinical screening will remain.

Familial Breast Cancer: Familial cancer of the breast comprises about 5% of all breast cancer. The tumors have a variety of types of histology. Early age of onset and the presence of bilateral disease are characteristic. There is clear autosomal dominant inheritance in some families. In 35% of cases, onset is before 35 years of age. This cancer is rare in men, even in these families. A breast cancer susceptibility gene on chromosome 17q21, BRCA1, may account for somewhat less than half of early onset inherited breast cancer. This gene has recently been cloned and

mutations it harbors will soon be correlated with clinical course.

Genetic counseling in affected families is quite challenging. Family history is effective in the identification of women at risk. The use of linkage testing with probes in BRCA1 region is not yet being widely applied. There is more work to do in characterizing the gene and identifying the mutations. Such testing may become valuable in families where autosomal dominant inheritance is clear. Clinical screening strategies may be considered for susceptible women; some women at high risk in families with autosomal dominant inheritance have undergone prophylactic mastectomy. When the pedigree is not definite for autosomal dominant inheritance, the risk of developing breast cancer under the age of 40 years for women whose mother or sister had breast cancer diagnosed under the age of 40 years is 1.5–3 times that for women with an unaffected mother or sister.

Retinoblastoma: Retinoblastoma is an intraocular cancer that develops from a malignant change in retinal cells. It affects 1 in 20,000 children and occurs predominantly in children under four years of age. Most cases are sporadic. However, there is an autosomal dominant form. Mutations in the tumor suppressor gene, RB1, account for the development of this

Table 5–7. Some inherited cancer syndromes with known genes.

Syndrome	Type of Cancer	Map Location	Gene
Li-Fraumeni	Early onset breast cancer, childhood sarcomas osteosarcoma, leukemia, brain tumors, ovarian cancer	17p	p53
Familial melanoma	Melanoma	9p	p16
Familial adenomatous polyposis; Gardner syndrome	Colon cancer, duodenum, gallbladder	5q21	APC
Family cancer syndromes (Lynch)	Colon, breast, uterus, ovary, stomach, pancreas	2p, 3p	MSH2, MLH1
Familial breast cancer	Breast	17q21	BRCA1

cancer in both the sporadic and the inherited form. Bilateral disease is nearly always associated with a constitutional mutation in RB1. Nearly half of all retinoblastomas arise as the result of a constitutional mutation, either inherited from an affected parent or as the result of a new germ-line mutation in the parent. This mutation constitutes a "first hit," and loss of the second RB1 gene results in the development of the tumor. About 10% of persons with this constitutional loss of function of the RB1 gene never develop retinoblastoma. Submicroscopic deletions, deletions, point mutations (missense and nonsense), and splice site mutations are known. Most result in no protein being made.

Genetic counseling in these families begins with the family history. Molecular analysis of the tumor can be used to identify mutations and molecular analysis of the RB1 gene in leukocytes can identify a constitutional mutation in an affected child. Molecular analysis of the RB1 gene in leukocytes of parents, if they are both unaffected, can be used to find out if a parent is heterozygous or the child represents a new mutation. Restriction analysis has been used; specific mutation analysis is more precise when the mutation can be identified. This kind of testing can't exclude germinal mosaicism in a parent (such germinal mosaicism has been described in some autosomal dominant disorders). New mutations in RB1 occur most frequently on the paternal RB1 allele.

Familial Adenomatous Polyps of the Colon (APC): Familial adenomatous polyposis of the colon (APC) has as its hallmark polyps that carpet the colon. In time, these polyps undergo malignant degeneration to colon cancer. This condition is a common cause of inherited cancer, occurring in between 1 in 8000 and 1 in 14,000 people. There is a variable age of onset; the median age for developing malignant degeneration of the polyps is 40 years. Other tumors that occur within the gastrointestinal tract include periampullary carcinoma and cancer of the rectal stump after surgery. Tumors also occur outside the gastrointestinal tract, including thyroid, brain, liver, and desmoid tumors (mesenteric fibromatosis).

A clinically useful ophthalmologic finding is congenital hypertrophy of the retinal pigment epithelium, occurring in about 90% of affected individuals.

The inheritance pattern is autosomal dominant. The gene responsible, APC, is on chromosome 5q21. The protein encoded by this gene is a 95 kD protein called β-catenin, and it is believed to be involved in cell adhesion. Deletions, frameshifts, nonsense mutations are all seen; most result in no protein being made.

In the past, a similar disorder known as Gardner syndrome was considered distinct. Besides colonic polyposis, tumors of the jaw, lipomas, and fibromas are seen. This condition is also the result of mutations in the APC gene.

Genetic counseling can be provided to family members at risk. Molecular techniques provide tools for assessing risk in families where this condition is segregating. Linkage analysis with flanking markers is highly accurate. Direct mutation screening is possible in some families. Currently such testing detects about 98% of affected individuals. When the combination of molecular and clinical testing shows an individual to be unaffected, clinical screening can be less intense. Individuals whose tests indicate that they carry the gene can have more frequent and rigorous clinical screening. Prophylactic colectomy has been chosen by some patients, as virtually 100% of affected persons develop cancer. The risk of the development of other tumors must be kept in mind, but screening for them may be difficult. Since few if any patients develop important symptoms before age 10 years, there is little rationale for screening in that age group. This could change if important presymptomatic therapy is developed. Patients with mental retardation or congenital malformations in addition to adenomatous polyposis coli should have a cytogenetic study to look for a deletion or unbalanced translocation.

Turcot Syndrome: Turcot syndrome is also associated with adenomatous polyps and cancer of the colon. Brain tumors are also frequent. The syndrome is inherited in an autosomal recessive fashion. There is evidence that the gene involved is also on chromosome 5, not far from the APC gene.

Hereditary Non-polyposis Colon Cancer (HNPCC): Hereditary non-polyposis colon cancer should be considered in families in which colon cancer is not associated with segregating adenomatous polyposis. Other cancers in these families include endometrium, stomach, biliary tract, pancreas, and urinary tract. The inheritance pattern is autosomal dominant. At least two different genes are involved in different families, one on chromosome 2p (MSH2) and one on chromosome 3p21 (MLH1). These genes may have to do with mismatch repair or other housekeeping functions. This disorder accounts for 4–13% of colon cancer. Molecular testing will most likely become available when the mutations and their predictive value for the development of disease are better understood. Genes that play a role in colon cancer are listed in Table 5–8.

MENDELIAN DISORDERS OF WHICH CANCER IS A PART

Cancer is part of the clinical picture in several Mendelian disorders. Many of these conditions are discussed elsewhere according to the organ system most consistently involved. However, when a Mendelian condition is diagnosed in an individual, it is important to consider whether cancer is usually associated with that condition. Mendelian disorders in which cancer commonly occurs are listed in Table 5–6.

Leukemia

Several different types of genes have mutations associated with leukemia. Both oncogenes and tumor suppressor genes are involved. These are acquired abnormalities in leukemic cells. The tumor suppressor gene p53 is commonly involved. Acquired chromosomal translocations sometimes result in the juxtaposition of oncogenes with the control regions of other genes. This results in loss of the normal control mechanisms and abnormal expression of these genes. Some translocations involve fusion genes between oncogenes and other genes, eg. c-abl-bcr in chronic myelogenous leukemia associated with the Philadelphia chromosome.

DNA Repair Abnormalities That Predispose to Cancer (Chromosome Breaks)

Xeroderma Pigmentosum (XP) (Several Complementation Groups): The cancers that occur in xeroderma pigmentosum include squamous cell carcinoma, melanomas, adrenal carcinomas, and basal cell cancers. The genetic disorder is autosomal recessive; the most common type maps to chromosome 9q22.

Ataxia-Telangiectasia (AT) (Several Complementation Groups): The cancers that occur in ataxia-telangiectasia include lymphoma, leukemia, lymphoreticular cancers, breast, basal cell carcinoma, and hepatocellular carcinoma. One type maps to chromosome 11q22–q23. There is some evidence that there may be an increased risk of cancer in heterozygous relatives of affected persons, but this is controversial.

Fanconi Anemia: Leukemia and hepatocellular carcinoma occur in Fanconi anemia. The two genetic forms of the anemia are discussed in Chapter 6.

Bloom Syndrome: Patients with Bloom syndrome may develop cancers of the gastrointestinal tract, cervix, and larynx occur. In addition, these patients commonly develop leukemia and lymphoma.

Genetic Implications of Some Common Cancers

Some general principles apply to the consideration of genetic factors in cancer. These include the following:

1. Genes play a major role in the development of cancer.
2. Almost all cancers demonstrate genetic changes at the cellular level.
3. Some persons have constitutional genetic changes that predispose to cancer and are implicated in inherited cancers.
4. Interaction with environmental factors is undoubtedly important but not well understood.

Table 5–8. Genes that play a role in colon cancer.

Gene	Type	Timing	Clinical Observation
k-ras	Oncogene	Acquired	
mye	Oncogene	Acquired	
DCC (18q)	Tumor suppressor	Acquired	Cell adhesion molecule; allelic loss may be useful for prognosis
p53	Tumor suppressor	Acquired	
APC	Tumor suppressor	Both	Constitutional in FAP; acquired in sporadic tumors
MLH1	Mismatch repair gene	Constitutional	Hereditary non-polyposis coli

5. Prevention will require understanding both genetic and environmental factors.
6. Surveillance, early diagnosis, and treatment will have important roles in mitigating the impact of cancer.

Assessing risk within families is an important part of cancer management. Approximately 10% of families with colon cancer are families with a high risk of affected relatives; some of these will represent a recognized dominantly inherited colon cancer syndrome. Other cancers have familial implications as well. Clues to identifying such families include multiple primaries, cancer in other sites in other family members, and early age of onset. For breast cancer, age of onset, affected first degree relatives (sister, mother) and their age of onset and bilaterality are signals of greater risk. First degree relatives of women with bilateral premenopausal breast cancer have the highest risk of developing breast cancer, probably because they are members of families with single gene disease.

The use of molecular knowledge will play an increasingly important role in the assessment of cancer. Molecular technology will be used to perform the following tasks:

- Identify persons at risk
- Clarify diagnosis of specific type of cancers
- Refine prognosis for response to therapy and for metastasis.

This kind of molecular testing is already in use for several kinds of cancer. Familial adenomatous polyposis of the colon is one example. Tumors that demonstrate p53 mutations are another; loss of heterozygosity, amount of accumulation of p53 protein, and identification of recognizable mutations may be useful in predicting survival and aggressiveness of tumors. Therapy that builds on the molecular understanding of cancer is also attractive. Drugs that perform functions of p53 protein or block interaction of p53 and other proteins are under development. Antibodies to p53 protein and drugs that affect action of MDR1 gene (multiple drug resistance gene) may also have a role to play. Gene therapy is not yet a reality but may be on the horizon.

The identification of persons at risk for cancer raises considerable ethical issues. Such identification must be accompanied by a clear plan for action based on the information. When risk assessment is based on family history, the patient is left with a likelihood of developing cancer that frequently approaches 50%. The plan must include methods for clinical screening and careful followup. The physician must have knowledge of the correlations between molecular abnormalities and clinical outcome. Such knowledge is currently in its early stages, but will expand considerably over the next decade. Testing based on molecular analysis must be used carefully; patients and families must be fully informed as to the precision and predictive value of these tests.

REFERENCES AND SUGGESTED READING

Albertsen HM et al: A physical map and candidate genes in the BRCA1 region on chromosome 17q12–21. Nature Genetics 1994;**7:**472.

Albertsen H et al: Genetic mapping of the BRCA2 region on chromosome 17q21. Am J Hum Genet 1994;**54:** 516.

ASHG Ad Hoc Committee on Breast and Ovarian Cancer Screening: Statement of the American Society of Human Genetics on genetic testing for breast and ovarian cancer predisposition. Am J Hum Genet 1994;**55:**i.

Baker E: The politics of breast cancer. Science 1993;**259:** 616.

Baker SJ et al: Suppression of human colorectal carcinoma cell growth by wild-type p53. Science 1990;**249:**912.

Bishop JM: Molecular genetics of cancer. Science 1987; **235:**305.

Budarf M et al: Comparative mapping of the constitutional and tumor-associated 11:22 translocations. Am J Hum Genet 1989;**45:**128.

Burt R: Inherited susceptibility to colorectal cancer. Hosp Prac 1989;(Nov):**43.**

Caldas C et al: Frequent somatic mutations and homozygous deletions of the p16 (MTS1) gene in pancreatic adenocarcinoma. Nature Genetics 1994;**8:**27.

Cance WG et al: Altered expression of the retinoblastoma gene product in human sarcomas. N Engl J Med 1990; **323:**1457.

Carbone DP: Oncogenes and tumor suppressor genes. Hosp Prac (June) 1993;**145.**

Cavenee WK et al: Prediction of familial predisposition to retinoblastoma. N Engl J Med 1986;**314:**1202.

Cho Y et al: Crystal structure of a p53 suppressor-DNA complex: understanding tumorigenic mutations. Science 1994;**265:**346.

Colditz GA et al: Family history, age, and risk of breast cancer. JAMA 1993;**270:**338.

Coppes MJ, Haber DA, Grundy PE: Genetic events in the development of Wilms' tumour. N Engl J Med 1994; **331:**586.

Coppes MJ, Huff V: Denys-Drash syndrome: relating a clinical disorder to genetic alterations in the tumor suppressor gene WT1. J Pediatr 1993;**123:**673.

Cossman J: *Molecular Genetics in Cancer Diagnosis.* Elsevier, 1990.

Danks DM: Colon cancer screening. Science 1994;**264:**13.

Eckert WA, Jung C, Wolff G: Presymptomatic diagnosis in families with adenomatous polyposis using highly polymorphic dinucleotide CA repeat markers flanking the APC gene. J Med Genet 1994;**31:**442.

Emi M et al: A novel metalloprotease/disintegrin-like gene at 17q21 somatically rearranged in two primary breast cancers. Nature Genetics 1993;**5:**151.

Ezzell C: Genomic imprinting and cancer: Mama may have and Papa may have. J NIH Research 1994;**6:**53.

Fearon ER et al: Identification of a chromosome 18q gene that is altered in colorectal cancers. Science 1990;**247:** 49.

Fletcher JA et al: Diagnostic relevance of clonal cytogenetic aberrations in malignant soft-tissue tumors. N Engl J Med 1991;**324:**436.

Futreal D et al: BRCA1 mutations in primary breast and ovarian carcinomas. Science 1994;**266:**120.

Gallie BL: Retinoblastoma gene mutations in human cancer. N Engl J Med 1994;**330:**786.

Goldstein AM et al: Linkage of cutaneous malignant melanoma/dysplastic nevi to chromosome 9p, and evidence for genetic heterogeneity. Am J Hum Genet 1994;**54:**489.

Hall JM et al: Linkage of early-onset familial breast cancer to chromosome 17q21. Science 1990;**250:**1684.

Harris CC: p53: At the crossroads of molecular carcinogenesis and risk assessment. Science 1993;**262:**1980.

Harris CC, Hollstein M: Clinical implications of the p53 tumor-suppressor gene. N Engl J Med 1993;**329:**1318.

Harris H et al: Suppression of malignancy by cell fusion. Nature 1969;**223:**363.

Hodgson SV, Maher ER: *A Practical Guide to Human Cancer Genetics.* Cambridge University Press, 1993.

Hollstein M et al: p53 mutations in human cancer. Science 1991;**253:**49.

Horsthemke B: Detection of submicroscopic deletions and a DNA polymorphism at the retinoblastoma locus. Hum Genet 1987;**76:**257.

Houlston RS et al: Screening and genetic counselling for relatives of patients with breast cancer in a family cancer clinic. J Med Genet 1992;**92:**691.

Hussussian CJ et al: Germline p16 mutations in familial melanoma. Nature Genetics 1994;**8:**15.

Jen J et al: Allelic loss of chromosome 18q and prognosis in colorectal cancer. N Engl J Med 1994;**331:**213.

Juliusson G et al: Prognostic subgroups in B-cell chronic lymphocytic leukemia defined by specific chromosomal abnormalities. N Engl J Med 1990;**323:**720.

Kamb A et al: Analysis of the p16 gene (CDKN2) as a candidate for the chromosome 9p melanoma susceptibility locus. Nature Genetics 1994;**8:**22.

Karp JE, Broder S: Oncology and hematology. JAMA 1994;**271:**1693.

Kern SE et al: Oncogenic forms of p53 inhibit p53-regulated gene expression. Science 1992;**256:**827.

Kinzler KW, Vogelstein B: Clinical implications of basic research: cancer therapy meets p53. N Engl J Med 1994; **331:**49.

Kinzler KW, Vogelstein B: The colorectal cancer gene hunt: current findings. Hosp Prac (Nov) 1992;**51.**

Kinzler KW et al: Identification of a gene located at chromosome 5q21 that is mutated in colorectal cancers. Science 1991;**251:**1366.

Knudsen A: Genetics of cancer: Major developments of the past five years. J NIH Research 1994;**6:**63.

Knudsen A: All in the (cancer) family. Nature Genetics 1993;**5:**103.

Knudsen AG: *Human Cancer Genes.* Raven Press, 1981.

Knudsen AG et al: Chromosomal deletion and retinoblastoma. N Engl J Med 1976;**295:**1120.

Knudsen AG, Hethcote HW, Brown BW: Mutation and childhood cancer: A probabilistic model for the incidence of retinoblastoma. Proc Soc Natl Acad Sci USA 1975;**72:**5116.

Knudsen AG: Mutation and cancer: statistical study of retinoblastoma. Proc Soc Natl Acad Sci USA 1971;**68:** 820.

Lee WH et al: Human retinoblastoma susceptibility gene: cloning, identification, and sequence. Science 1979;**235:** 1394.

Leppert M et al: Genetic analysis of an inherited predisposition to colon cancer in a family with a variable number of adenomatous polyps. N Engl J Med 1990; **322:**904.

Leppert M et al: The gene for familial polyposis coli maps to the long arm of chromosome 5. Science 1987;**238:** 1411.

Levine AJ: The p53 tumor-suppressor gene. N Engl J Med 1992;**326:**1350.

Li FP, Fraumeni JF: Prospective study of a family cancer syndrome. JAMA 1982;**247:**2692.

Lynch HT et al: Familial heterogeneity of colon cancer risk. Cancer 1986;**57:**2089.

Maher ER et al: Evaluation of molecular genetic diagnosis in the management of familial adenomatous polyposis coli: a population based study. J Med Genet 1993;**30:** 675.

Malkin D et al: Germ line p53 mutations in a familial syndrome of breast cancer, sarcoma, and other neoplasms. Science 1990;**250:**1233.

Marx J. Cellular changes on the route to metastasis: Science 1993;**259:**626.

Marx J: Learning how to suppress cancer. Science 1993; **261:**1385.

Mecklin JP: Frequency of hereditary colorectal carcinoma. Gastroenterology 1987;**93:**1021.

Miki Y et al: A strong candidate for the breast and ovarian cancer susceptibility gene BRCA1. Science 1994;**266:** 66.

Moutou C et al: The French Wilms' tumour study: no clear evidence for cancer prone families. J Med Genet 1993; **31:**429.

Mueller RF: The Denys-Drash syndrome. J Med Genet 1994;**31:**471.

Nagase H et al: Correlation between the location of germline mutations in the APC gene and the number of colorectal polyps in familial adenomatous polyposis patients. Cancer Res 1992;**52:**4055.

National Advisory Council for Human Genome Research: Statement on Use of DNA Testing for Presymptomatic Identification of Cancer Risk. JAMA 1994;**271:**785.

Nowak R: Breast cancer gene offers surprises. Science 1994;**265:**1796.

Nystrom-Lahti M et al: Mismatch repair genes on chromosomes 2p and 3p account for a major share of hereditary nonpolyposis colorectal cancer families evaluable by linkage. Am J Hum Genet 1994;**55:**659.

Ogawa O et al: A novel insertional mutation at the third zinc finger coding region of the WT1 gene in Denys-Drash syndrome. Human Molecular Genetics 1993;**2:** 203.

Olson JM, Breslow NE, Barce J: Cancer in twins of Wilms' tumour patients. Am J Med Genet 1993;**47:**91.

Ottman R et al: Practical guide for estimating risk for familial breast cancer. Lancet 1983;**II-1983:**556.

Papadopoulos N et al: Mutation of a mutL homolog in hereditary colon cancer. Science 1994;**263:**1625.

Pelletier J et al: Mutations in the Wilms' tumour suppressor gene are associated with abnormal urogenital development in Denys-Drash syndrome. Cell 1991;**67:**437.

Peltomaki P et al: Genetic mapping of a locus predisposing to human colorectal cancer. Science 1993;**260:**810.

Peng JWP, Kao-Shan CS, Lee EC: Specific chromosome defect associated with small-cell lung cancer: deletion 3p(14–23). Science 1982;**215:**181.

Pierce ER, Weisbord T, McKusick VA: Gardner's syndrome: Formal genetics and statistical analysis of a large Canadian kindred. Clin Genet 1970;**1:**65.

Rowell S et al: Inherited predisposition and breast and ovarian cancer. Am J Hum Genet 1994;**55:**861.

Rowley J: Chromosome abnormalities in cancer. Cancer Genet Cytogenet 1980;**2:**175.

Rowley JD, Aster JC, Sklar J: The clinical applications of new DNA diagnostic technology on the management of cancer patients. JAMA 1993;**270:**2331.

Skolnick MH et al: Inheritance of proliferative breast disease in breast cancer kindreds. Science 1990;**250:**1715.

Slattery ML, Kerber RA: A comprehensive evaluation of family history and breast cancer risk. JAMA 1993;**270:** 1563.

Solomon E, Borrow J, Goddard AD: Chromosome aberrations and cancer. Science 1991;**254:**1153.

Stanbridge EJ: Identifying tumor suppressor genes in human colorectal cancer. Science 1990;**247:**12.

Swift MS et al: Incidence of cancer in 161 families affected by ataxia-telangiectasia. N Engl J Med 1991;**325:**1831.

Tempero M, Anderson J: Progress in colon cancer—do molecular markers matter? N Engl J Med 1994;**331:**267.

Thirman MJ et al: Rearrangement of the MLL gene in acute lymphoblastic and acute myeloid leukemias with 11q23 chromosomal translocations. N Engl J Med 1993;**329:** 909.

Toguchida J et al: Prevalence and spectrum of germline mutations of the p53 gene among patients with sarcoma. N Engl J Med 1992;**326:**1302.

Trent JM, Meltzer PS: The last shall be first. Nature Genetics 1993;**3:**101.

Walker C et al: Predisposition to renal cell carcinoma due to alteration of a cancer susceptibility gene. Science 1992;**255:**1693.

Weinberg RA: Oncogenes and tumor suppressor genes. CA-A Cancer Journal for Clinicians. 1994;**44:**160.

Weinberg R: Tumor suppressor genes. Science 1991;**254:** 1138.

Wiggs J et al: Prediction of the risk of hereditary retinoblastoma using DAN polymorphisms within the retinoblastoma gene. N Engl J Med 1988;**318:**151.

Williams BO et al: Cooperative tumorigenic effects of germline mutations in Rb and p53. Nature Genetics 1994;**7:**480.

Yandell DW et al: Oncogenic point mutations in the human retinoblastoma gene: their application to genetic counseling. N Engl J Med 1989;**321:**1689.

Yunis JJ: The chromosomal basis of human neoplasia. Science 1983;**221:**227.

Blood Disorders

OVERVIEW

Blood disorders are common medical problems and many of them are inherited. The physician should always try to differentiate between acquired and inherited hematologic disorders. Understanding of the genetic mechanisms may lead to more precise diagnosis, clearer prognosis, and better understanding of the risks to other family members. The inherited blood disorders can be categorized as follows:

- Disorders of red blood cells: involve red blood cell production or destruction
- Platelet disorders: involve functional disorders or disorders resulting from decreased platelet production
- White cell disorders: discussed in Chapter 4
- Disorders of coagulation: involve decreased or increased coagulability.

RED CELL DISORDERS

Bone Marrow Dysfunction

Blackfan-Diamond Anemia: (MIM 205900), Autosomal Recessive; (MIM 105650), Autosomal Dominant: Blackfan-Diamond anemia usually presents in the first year of life. In addition to anemia, 25% of affected children also have congenital malformations including thumb abnormalities, hypertelorism, congenital heart disease, and kidney malformations. This is a hypoplastic anemia. Only the red cell series is affected. Apparently there is no maturation of red cells and no reticulocytes are seen. Diagnosis is based on the presence of anemia with normal or increased white cell and platelet count. Red cells may be slightly macrocytic.

Two genetic forms are recognized based on pedigree analysis. In some families, autosomal recessive inheritance is most likely. Vertical transmission in other families suggests autosomal dominant inheritance. The physician must draw on pedigree examination to assign mode of inheritance, since the gene(s) has not been mapped and the molecular pathology is undefined. Treatment with corticosteroid has been the mainstay. In many patients the response to low doses is good. Other patients may re-

quire transfusions. Bone marrow transplant may have a role to play in steroid-unresponsive patients.

Fanconi Anemia (MIM 227650) (MIM 227645): Fanconi anemia presents in early childhood with anemia accompanied by pancytopenia. Congenital malformations (including thumb and renal anomalies, ear malformations, and congenital heart disease) are part of the clinical picture. Microcephaly and mental retardation can also be seen. Some patients have cafe-au-lait spots. Growth failure is common. There is considerable variability both within and between families. An increased frequency of aplastic anemia and AML complicate the second decade of life. Diagnosis is based on the presence of pancytopenia along with the congenital malformations. An increased number of chromosomal breaks is seen on cytogenetic analysis. This is heightened in the presence of diepoxybutane (DEB), a test that is not popular because of the toxicity of DEB.

Autosomal recessive inheritance is the rule. The molecular defect is unknown but it is thought to be related to DNA repair. There are at least two autosomal recessive forms: Fanconi anemia I, which maps to 20q13.2–q13 (MIM 227650), and Fanconi anemia type C, which maps to 9q22.3 (MIM 227645). There are four complementation groups within type C.

Unfortunately, though in most patients the anemia improves after treatment with androgens, this improvement is not lasting. Bone marrow transplant, while successful in some cases, carries the risk of early mortality because other tissues share the DNA repair defect, and this impedes tissue recovery from the toxicity of the preparative regimen for the transplant.

Cofactor Disorders

Disorders in Cobalamin (Vitamin B$_{12}$) Transport: (MIM 275350), Transcobalamin II Deficiency; (MIM193090) Vitamin B$_{12}$-Binding Protein Deficiency; (MIM261100), Enterocyte Cobalamin Malabsorption: Vitamin B$_{12}$ (cobalamin) is converted to two active cofactors, adenosylcobalamin and methylcobalamin. Inherited disorders of their metabolism are discussed in Chapter 13. Inherited disorders in cobalamin transport cause megaloblastic anemia in infancy and childhood. In the adult, cobalamin deficiency is usually due to acquired intrinsic factor deficiency, secondary to an autoimmune syndrome (pernicious anemia). In the first few years of life intrinsic factor deficiency most likely results from an inherited abnormality in intrinsic factor biosynthesis or secretion, unassociated with gastrointestinal pathology. Abnormal transport of cobalamin by the enterocyte causes a clinically similar disorder. Transcobalamin II (TCII), the binding protein that transports the cobalamin-intrinsic factor complex into the portal blood and into cells, can also be deficient on a genetic basis. Deficiency of TCII causes megaloblastic anemia very early in infancy. In contrast to adults with acquired pernicious anemia, children with these inherited disorders of cobalamin transport have diarrhea, vomiting, and failure to thrive in addition to megaloblastic anemia and neurologic dysfunction. Deficiency of TCII is fatal if untreated.

Pathogenesis is based on abnormal transport of cobalamin into cells. Megaloblastic anemia is presumably on the basis of deficient N^5-tetrahydrofolate: homocysteine methyltransferase activity, an enzyme that uses methylcobalamin as a cofactor, but the mechanism is not clear. The pathogenesis of the central nervous system dysfunction is unknown, but is presumably related to deficiency of adenosylcobalamin.

These rare disorders of cobalamin transport are all inherited in an autosomal recessive fashion. The gene for TCII has been mapped to chromosome 22. Inherited deficiency of intrinsic factor (MIM 261000) is recessively inherited; the gene for this protein has been mapped to chromosome 11. The other relevant genes are uncharacterized.

Diagnosis of intrinsic factor deficiency and enterocyte malabsorption can usually be made by finding a low serum cobalamin concentration and an abnormal Schilling test. The diagnosis of TCII deficiency presents more of a challenge because serum cobalamin concentrations can be normal; the major serum binding protein for cobalamin does not facilitate transport into cells, but is normal in TCII deficiency and may result in a normal serum cobalamin concentration. More sophisticated tests of cobalamin binding may be needed to confirm this diagnosis.

The anemia responds to high doses of parenteral vitamin B_{12}. It is not certain whether the neurologic symptoms are reversible.

Hereditary Folate Malabsorption (MIM 229050): Severe megaloblastic anemia beginning in infancy characterizes this rare condition. Neurologic deterioration culminating in mental retardation is a feature, and seizures occur in some affected children. An increased incidence of infections has been reported.

Pathogenesis is based on deficient or absent absorption of oxidized and reduced folate by the gut. Transport of folates into the brain is also abnormal. Folate is essential for DNA synthesis, and deficiency

of it during fetal life may explain both the congenital megaloblastic anemia and the congenital central nervous system abnormalities. The observation of consanguinity and affected sibs suggests autosomal recessive inheritance.

Diagnosis is based on the findings of megaloblastic anemia, formiminoglutamate (FIGLU) in the urine, and decreased folate concentration in serum.

High doses of oral folate or intravenous folate will normalize the serum folate and correct the anemia, but the folate may not reach the central nervous system. Prognosis is uncertain; death has occurred early in some patients, but others have survived with some improvement in central nervous system symptoms. Hemolytic anemia may also be a symptom of inborn errors of folate metabolism (see Chapter 13).

Red Cell Membrane Disorders

The red cell membrane skeleton is responsible for integrity of the cell, its stability during circulation through the spleen, and its shape and deformability. Many proteins, the products of at least eight different genes, comprise the red cell membrane skeleton. Disorders of red cell membrane skeleton proteins result in hemolysis because of abnormal response of the red cell membrane to the stresses of the circulation. Hemolytic anemia and abnormal red cell shape are cardinal features of this group of conditions. There is considerable variability in the clinical syndrome. Disorders of the red cell membrane skeletal structure display at least five clinical phenotypes:

* Hereditary spherocytosis
* Hereditary elliptocytosis
* Hereditary ovalocytosis
* Hereditary acanthocytosis.

Red cell membrane skeletal abnormalities result from mutations in any of the several proteins in the lattice work of proteins that comprise it. The major proteins are:

* α-spectrin
* β-spectrin
* Ankyrin
* Actin
* Protein 4.1
* Band 3.

The last two proteins are numbered by their position during electrophoretic separation. Many mutations in the genes coding for these proteins have been characterized and the correlations between clinical phenotype and molecular genotype are becoming clearer. The disorders are discussed below. Some are listed in Table 6–1.

Spherocytosis: Hemolytic anemia, jaundice, and splenomegaly are major clinical features of spherocytosis. Other features include gallstones, growth re-

Table 6–1. Genetic abnormalities in hereditary red cell skeleton defects.

Clinical Presentation	Molecular Defect	Inheritance	Map Location
Hereditary spherocytosis, classical (MIM 182870)	Deficient spectrin	AD	14q22–q23.2
Hereditary spherocytosis, classical (MIM 182900)	Deficient ankyrin	AD	8p11.2
Hereditary spherocytosis, classical (MIM 109270)	Insertion, band 3 protein	AD	17q21–qter
Hereditary spherocytosis, classical (MIM 182870), (MIM 182900)	Deficient spectrin-protein 4.1 binding	AD	–
Hereditary spherocytosis, severe	Deficient α-spectrin	AR	1q21
Hereditary spherocytosis, severe	Deficient protein 4.1	AR	1p36.2–p34
Hereditary spherocytosis, severe	Deficient β-spectrin	AR	14q22–q23.2
Hereditary elliptocytosis (MIM 182860)	Deficient α-spectrin	AD	1q21
Hereditary elliptocytosis (MIM 182870)	Deletion β-spectrin	AD	14q22–q23.2
Hereditary elliptocytosis (MIM 141700)	Deficient ankyrin	AD	8p11.2
Hereditary elliptocytosis (MIM 130500)	Insertion protein 4.1	AD	1p36–p34
Hereditary elliptocytosis (MIM 130500)	Deficient protein 4.1	AD	1p36–p34
Acanthocytosis, ovalocytosis (MIM 109270)	Deleted protein band 3		
Hereditary elliptocytosis, Melanesian (MIM 109270)	Deleted protein band 3	AD	17q21–q22
Pyropolkilocytosis (MIM 266140)	Several RBC membrane proteins	AR	–
Ovalocytosis (MIM 166900)	Several RBC membrane proteins	AD	–

tardation, and extramedullary hematopoiesis. The diagnosis is suggested by the presence in the blood smear of spherocytes (red cells that are smaller than normal, have less surface area, are spherical in shape without central pallor) in the blood smear. Aplastic crisis may follow parvovirus B_{19} infection. Hemolytic crises can occur after a variety of viral infections and are not usually severe. The balance between red cell production and destruction accounts for some of the clinical heterogeneity. The disease usually presents in childhood, but symptoms in patients with compensated hemolysis are so mild that diagnosis may not be made until later. Some affected children present in the neonatal period with hemolytic jaundice. The anemia is not usually severe, but the jaundice can be severe enough to require treatment. This presentation is usually transitory and does not portend severe ongoing disease. A few patients have severe, transfusion dependent hemolytic anemia. Pregnancy in a woman with spherocytosis who has not had splenectomy may be complicated by hemolytic crisis and persistent anemia. Fetal outcome is usually normal in pregnancies that go to term.

Spherocytosis is the most common cause of hemolytic anemia in those of European Caucasian descent; it affects 1 in 5000 individuals. The disorder appears to be less common in other ethnic groups. Affected red cells are unable to deform during passage through the spleen. They are thus trapped in the spleen and suffer energy depletion, loss of membrane stability and changes in membrane permeability with subsequent disintegration of the membrane. Splenomegaly also ensues. Whether this is the entire explanation for red cell destruction is unclear; the possibility of physical destruction while traversing the small passages in the spleen has not been excluded. Hemolysis is followed by anemia and jaundice.

Both autosomal dominant and autosomal recessive forms of hereditary spherocytosis are known. Many recognized mutations involve spectrin (Table 6–1). Deficiency of spectrin appears to be the most common abnormality. Mutations that cause autosomal dominant spherocytosis include mutations in the β-subunit of spectrin and loss of the ability of spectrin to bind protein 4.1. One family with dominantly inherited spherocytosis had an insertion in the gene for protein band 3, and the protein was not inserted normally into the cell membrane. Deficiency of both spectrin and ankyrin has also been described. The primary defect in this deficiency of both ankyrin and spectrin is probably a deficiency in ankyrin. Spherocytosis accompanied by fatal hydrops fetalis is associated with a deficiency in α-spectrin. In one case, both parents had mild spherocytosis, but the defect was not characterized. Polymorphisms in the α-subunit that do not segregate with the disease have been described.

Spherocytes are seen in the blood smear; anemia, hyperbilirubinemia, and reticulocytosis are other prominent laboratory features of spherocytosis. Osmotic fragility is usually abnormal. Analysis of red cell membrane proteins may clarify the diagnosis.

Choice of treatment depends on the severity of the hemolytic anemia. When the disease is mild, no treatment may be needed. When severe, splenectomy will cure the hemolytic anemia but incurs the increased risk of severe infections associated with splenectomy. Vaccination against pneumococcus and prompt attention to minor bacterial infections may lessen this risk. Antibacterial prophylaxis may be appropriate in some situations. Efforts at repair of the red cell membrane abnormalities have not been reported.

Elliptocytosis: Elliptocytosis is clinically heterogeneous. A mild hemolytic anemia is present in most affected individuals. Occasionally the hemolysis is severe with jaundice. Many patients develop gallstones. In some forms of elliptocytosis the blood group antigens are not appropriately expressed, possibly because the abnormal red cell membrane prevents their association on the cell surface. The condition affects 1 in 2500 persons of Northern European descent.

The defect in the red cell membrane skeleton may prevent the cell from regaining its normal shape after deforming when passing through capillaries, the spleen, and other small spaces in the circulation. Eventually these red cells become subject to hemolysis in the spleen. Red cell life span in vitro is also shortened.

Many mutations in red cell membrane skeletal proteins have been described. They are associated with slightly different phenotypes of elliptocytosis (Table 6–1). Hematologic indices reveal anemia and reticulocytosis. The blood smear shows the elliptical shape of 30–100% of the red cells affected. The severe form may have poikilocytosis, microelliptocytes and red cell fragments. Osmotic fragility may be normal or increased.

Many patients do well without treatment. Some develop gallstones that may need to be removed. When hemolysis is severe, splenectomy may be required. Splenectomy reduces the degree of hemolysis but may not end the hemolysis in all patients. The risk of sepsis that follows splenectomy may be lessened by vaccination against pneumococcus and prompt attention to minor bacterial infections. The use of antibacterial prophylaxis may be wise in some situations.

Ion Transport Abnormalities: Hemolytic anemia apparently due to abnormal permeability of the cell membrane to sodium or to potassium has been described. The abnormalities in ion transport appear to result in a change in water content, either to dehydration or to increased water content. These abnormalities are reflected in red cell appearance. Families with autosomal dominant and autosomal recessive patterns of inheritance exist. The molecular genetics of these disorders is not clear.

Table 6–2 lists some diseases of secondary hemolytic anemia that are associated with genetic disorders.

Table 6–2. Secondary hemolytic anemia associated with genetic disorders.

| Wilson disease |
| Abetalipoproteinemia |
| Congenital erythropoietic porphyria |
| Glycogen storage disease |
| Hemoglobinopathies |

Disorders of Red Cell Metabolism

Red cells depend on glucose for energy metabolism. Since red cells have no mitochondria, the only pathway available for generation of ATP is glycolysis. The cells depend on this pathway for maintenance of ion pumps, to maintain membrane integrity, and to respond to oxidative stress. Inherited deficiencies in the enzymes of glycolysis result in hemolytic anemia because of red cell demise. The more common of these are discussed below (Table 6–3).

Pyruvate Kinase Deficiency (MIM 266200): The clinical features of pyruvate kinase deficiency include hemolytic anemia of varying severity, jaundice, splenomegaly, and gallstones. Heterogeneity in clinical phenotype is characteristic, from presentation in neonatal life to much later onset in adulthood. The neonatal form is more severe, and kernicterus resulting from the severe hyperbilirubinemia has been reported. Affected infants may show growth retardation. Symptoms may improve following splenectomy. Signs of extramedullary hematopoiesis, iron overload, and biliary tract disease occur in many patients. Various stresses—notably viral infection and pregnancy—may lead to worsening of the hemolysis.

Pyruvate kinase (PK) deficiency is one of the more common disorders of red cell metabolism. The incidence appears highest in persons of Northern European ancestry, but all ethnic groups have been reported at risk. A severe form occurs in Amish families.

PK is the rate-limiting enzyme that converts phosphoenolpyruvate to pyruvate. When PK is deficient, the cell cannot make adequate ATP, ion transport is impaired, and the size and shape of the cell become distorted. The cell is then subject to hemolysis.

PK deficiency is inherited in an autosomal recessive fashion. The gene has been mapped to chromosome 15q22–qter. Compound heterozygosity for two different mutations is common. Heterozygotes are usually asymptomatic, but their red cell life span may be decreased. Diagnosis depends on the identification of deficient PK activity in erythrocytes. Most patients have about 5–25% of normal activity.

Table 6–3. Rare disorders of red cell metabolism that cause hemolytic anemia.

Enzyme Deficiency	Clinical Syndrome	Inheritance	Map Location
Hexokinase	Hemolytic anemia (MIM 235700)	AR	10q22
Phosphofructokinase (PFK)	Hemolytic anemia, myopathy, rhabdomyolysis	AR	–
Glucosephosphate	Hemolytic anemia, may require transfusion or splenectomy; hydrops fetalis has been reported	AR	19q31.1
Triosephosphate isomerase (TPI)	Hemolytic anemia, cardiac arrhythmia, neurologic abnormalities; early death	AR	12p13
Phosphoglycerate kinase (PGK)	Severe hemolysis; neurologic abnormalities and myopathy in some; heterozygous females may have hemolytic anemia (MIM 311800)	XL	Xq13
Aldolase	Rare hemolytic anemia; congenital malformations reported in one case	AR	16q22–q24
Glutathione synthetase	Hemolytic anemia (MIM 231900); hemolytic anemia and neurological abnormalities (MIM 266130)	AR	–
γ-glutamylcysteine synthese	Hemolytic anemia; spinocerebellar dysfunction (MIM 230450)	AR	–
Pyruvate kinase (PK)	Hemolytic anemia (MIM 230450)	AR	1q21

Death and kernicterus can occur in the severe neonatal form. Many patients require frequent transfusions. Splenectomy may be lifesaving in patients with severe disease. In others, splenectomy may decrease the need for transfusions but does not relieve the hemolysis.

Abnormal Nucleotide Metabolism

Pyrimidine Nucleotidase Deficiency (MIM 266120): The clinical features of pyrimidine nucleotidase deficiency include hemolytic anemia, hyperbilirubinemia, and splenomegaly. Pathogenesis is based on the accumulation of pyrimidines that cannot leave the cells. The disorder is inherited in an autosomal recessive fashion. It is more common in persons of African, Mediterranean or Jewish descent. Diagnosis is suggested by basophilic stippling of the red cells, the result of degraded ribosomal nucleoprotein. Measurement of decreased pyrimidine nucleotidase activity and of the accumulation of pyrimidine nucleotides confirms the diagnosis. This condition rarely requires transfusions or splenectomy. Gallstones may occur.

Adenosine Deaminase (ADA) Hyperactivity (MIM 102730): Adenosine deaminase (ADA) hyperactivity, a rare disorder, is characterized by hemolytic anemia, reticulocytosis, and mild hyperbilirubinemia. ADA hyperactivity depletes ATP, and the consequences of energy depletion follow. The condition is inherited as an autosomal dominant trait. The gene has been mapped to 20q12–q13.11. Diagnosis is based on the measurement of increased activity of the enzyme. As this is a mild disease, no treatment is usually needed.

Glucose-6 Phosphate Dehydrogenase (G6PD)

Deficiency (MIM 305900): Worldwide, glucose-6 phosphate dehydrogenase (G6PD) deficiency is the most common red cell enzyme defect associated with hemolytic anemia. Episodic hemolysis after exposure to certain drugs or chemicals characterizes this disorder (Table 6–4). Most of the mutations are conditional; they only cause symptoms under certain conditions, usually oxidant stress. A few mutations cause chronic hemolysis. Several clinical syndromes have been described; they include neonatal jaundice, acute hemolytic anemia, and chronic severe hemolytic anemia. Hemolytic anemia may occur in response to drugs, chemicals, or exposure to fava beans (Table 6–5).

An episode of severe hemolytic anemia may be accompanied by hemoglobinuria, renal failure, jaundice, and pallor. G6PD deficiency is common; more than 400,000 people in the world are affected. The population frequency is highest in sub-Saharan Africa, southern Asia, and the Middle East and correlates with the worldwide distribution of malaria.

Table 6–4. Drugs associated with hemolysis in G6PD deficiency.[1]

Acetanilid	Niridazole
Doxorubicin	Nitrofurantoin
Furazolidone	Phenazopyridine
Methylene blue	Primaquine
Nalidixic acid	Sulfamethoxazole

[1] From Beutler E: Glucose-6-phosphate dehydrogenase deficiency. N Engl J Med 1991;**324:**171.

Table 6–5. Factors associated with hemolysis in G6PD deficiency.

Factor	Association With Hemolysis in G6PD Deficiency
Exposure to fava beans	Is most common in Mediterranean countries; amount of bean eaten and season influence severity; specific G6PD mutation may be a factor in severity; interactions of other genes may play a role
Infections	Viral hepatitis, pneumonia, typhoid fever, viral upper respiratory infections, especially in children
Specific mutation	Genetic heterogeneity plays a role in severity and clinical phenotype
Drugs and chemicals	Administration of oxidant drugs may worsen hemolysis
Age of patient	Newborns at higher risk; neonatal jaundice results from combination of hemolysis and immature bilirubin metabolism; genetic and environmental factors influence severity
Age of red cell population	Young cells less susceptible; may be a function of time of previous episode

There is a selective advantage to female heterozygotes because of increased resistance to malaria. Frequency is lowest in Canada, Northern Europe, Russia, and China.

G6PD plays a critical role in red cell energy metabolism. The enzyme is also important in the conversion of hydrogen peroxide to water and thus in the cell's defense against oxidant stress, as suggested in Figure 6–1, which illustrates the G6PD pathway. Hemolysis is related to deficient NADPH production and decreased GSH, but the exact pathophysiology is not clear. Probably integrity of red cell membranes is compromised, but other factors may be important. Hemolysis takes place within and outside the vascular space, and hemoglobinemia occurs.

The X-linked pattern of inheritance has been known for 40 years. Hemizygous males are clearly affected; occasionally heterozygous females have hemolytic episodes. Homozygous affected females have been reported in regions where the gene frequency is high. The gene is mapped to Xq28. It codes for an enzyme that consists of either a dimer or a tetramer of a 515 amino acid protein subunit. More than 300 genetic variants are known; mutations occur throughout the gene; the sites reported to be affected by mutations include the G6P binding site and the NADP binding domain. Efforts at correlating genotype with phenotype correlations are proceeding.

Diagnosis is made by spectrophotometric measurement of G6PD activity. There is increased activity in reticulocytes that may result in falsely high activity after a hemolytic episode when there is reticulocytosis; patients should be re-evaluated after such an episode. A fluorescent spot test is used for screening. Staining with tetrazolium can demonstrate the mosaicism that is characteristic of heterozygotes. Avoidance of precipitating agents is the mainstay of treatment. Transfusion may be needed during an acute crisis.

Hereditary Methemoglobinemia: (MIM 141800), α-Globin; (MIM 141900), (β-Globin Locus): NADH-methemoglobin reductase maintains the iron of hemoglobin in the ferric state. Deficiency of this enzyme results in methemoglobinemia. The major clinical feature is cyanosis without hypoxia. Hereditary methemoglobinemia is inherited in an autosomal recessive fashion.

Hemoglobinopathies

Hemoglobin is made of a protein tetramer that carries four heme groups; each heme group is a protoporphyrin ring containing an iron atom. The molecule's major function is oxygen transport. Hemoglobin tetramers are composed of two α-like subunits and 2 β-like subunits. The specific genes within the α-like clusters and the β-like clusters are expressed sequentially in a developmentally regulated fashion. During late fetal development and early infancy, hemoglobin switches to adult hemoglobin composed of two α-globin subunits and two β-globin subunits. Hemoglobin A, $\alpha_2\beta_2$, is the major component, and hemoglobin A$_2$, $\alpha_2\gamma_2$ is the minor component. During fetal life the g-globin subunit, another subunit in the β-globin gene cluster, replaces the β-globin subunit to form fetal hemoglobin, $\alpha_2\gamma_2$. Earlier in embryonic life, the β-globin chain is replaced by an embryonic β-like chain, e, in Gower

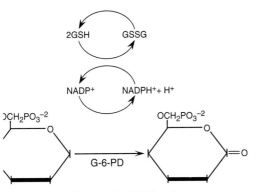

Figure 6–1. G6PD pathway.

Table 6–6. Examples of structural abnormalities of hemoglobin.[1]

Name	Molecular Abnormality	Clinical Feature
Hemoglobin S	β-globin: 6Glu→Val	Sickle cell anemia
Hemoglobin Harlem	β-globin: 6Glu→Val +β-globin; 73Asp→Asn	Sickle cell anemia
Hemoglobin Leiden	β-globin: deletion of codon at position 6 or 7	Unstable hemoglobin
Hemoglobin Gun Hill	β-globin: deletion of 5 codons, positions 91–95	Unstable hemoglobin
Hemoglobin Lepore	γ β-fusion; lost segments of both	Thalassemia-like anemia
Hemoglobin Wayne	α-globin: frame shift from single base deletion	Normal
Hemoglobin Constant Spring	α-globin: base change to termination codon	Thalassemia-like anemia

[1] Data from Phillips, Kagazian.

2 hemoglobin, $\alpha_2\epsilon_2$. Gower 1, another embryonic hemoglobin, has no α-chain and is composed instead of $\zeta_2\epsilon_2$. The genes for the α- and α-like globin chains reside on chromosome 16; the genes for the β- and the β-like globin chains reside on chromosome 11.

Genetic disorders of hemoglobin biosynthesis result from mutations that affect either the α-chain or the β-chain of the hemoglobin molecule (Table 6–6). There are two general classes: deficient protein subunit production and abnormal subunit structure. All have the common feature of anemia, but each has specific features as well. The thalassemias are characterized by quantitative abnormalities in hemoglobin production; they can involve the α- or the β-globin chain. Production of the affected chain can be deficient or absent. Deficient production of one subunit results in imbalance of the two types of subunits; many clinical features of the thalassemias result from this imbalance of globin subunits. Patients with structural variants present with hemolytic anemia and other symptoms and signs, depending on the specific mutation in the affected globin gene.

α-thalassemia (MIM 141800), (α-globin): Since there are two α-globin genes on each chromosome 16, different clinical phenotypes are possible, depending on the number of α-globin genes that are affected. Clinical syndromes have been associated with mutations in or deletions of up to four of the α genes. Furthermore, two mutant or deleted genes can be on the same chromosome 16 (**cis**) or one can be on each chromosome 16 (**trans**). The designations for these situations are:

- (αα/αα), Four normal α-chain genes
- (α-/αα), One abnormal α-chain gene
- (α-/α-), Two abnormal α-genes in *trans*
- (αα/– –/), Two abnormal α-genes in *cis*
- (α-/–/– –), Three abnormal α-genes
- (–/– –/– –/–), No normal α-genes.

The clinical features derive from the genotypes. A mild phenotype results when there are three normal α-chains. Usually these individuals are silent carriers and have no symptoms. The MCV is slightly decreased. Mutations or deletions in two a genes cause a clinical phenotype of mild microcytic anemia, known as α-thalassemia trait. The loss of three α-globin chains gives rise to hemoglobin H disease. Hemoglobin H (β_4) has abnormal oxygen carrying characteristics. These patients have a hypochromic, microcytic anemia. Jaundice and splenomegaly may be part of the picture. There is considerable variation in severity depending on the specific mutations, but in most cases symptoms are mild. When there are no α-globin chains, the patient cannot make any hemoglobin A. These patients make largely hemoglobin Bart's (γ_4), which has very poor oxygen carrying capacity. The clinical phenotype, that of hydrops fetalis, results from severe cardiac failure. The infant dies in utero or shortly after birth.

Worldwide distribution of α-thalassemia is seen, but the group of disorders is most common in Asia, sub-Saharan Africa, the Pacific islands, the Middle East, and the Mediterranean region. In the United States, incidence is higher in persons whose family origins are in those regions. The mutations and deletions in **trans** are more common in Blacks, whereas the mutations and deletions in **cis** are more common in Asians.

Numerous mutations and deletions have been described at the α-globin locus. Deletions are the most common cause of α-thalassemia. The level of expression of α-globin then depends on the molecular anatomy of the rest of the α-globin region. Single base changes also account for some forms of α-thalassemia. These can be nonsense mutations, mutations affecting the initiation codons, and splice site mutations.

Diagnosis is based on hematologic indices and hemoglobin electrophoresis; more specific characterization of the proteins and the genes is more specific, and may be necessary for definitive diagnosis. When the mutation is defined, molecular diagnosis can be used for clinical diagnosis, identification of heterozygotes, and prenatal diagnosis. Population screening for heterozygosity allows individuals to know their risks for having affected children and to use prenatal diagnosis if desired.

Treatment is supportive. In general, α-thalassemia is less severe than β-thalassemia. Since the β_4 tetramer that is produced in α-thalassemia is more soluble than the α_4 tetramer that is produced in β-thalassemia and there is less ineffective erythropoesis. There is no effective treatment for hemoglobin Bart's hydrops fetalis.

β-Thalassemia (MIM 141900), (β-globin locus):

Heterozygotes for β-thalassemia have a mild microcytic anemia (thalassemia trait) and are usually asymptomatic. Thalassemia major presents in the first years of life with a progressively more severe anemia. As extramedullary hematopoiesis occurs in response to the anemia, characteristic bony abnormalities occur, including frontal bossing, protrusion of the cheekbones, and skull abnormalities.

The worldwide distribution of β-thalassemia is similar to that of α-thalassemia. Incidence varies, but the heterozygote frequency is quite high in many parts of the world affected by malaria. The distribution coincides with the distribution of malaria because heterozygotes are resistant to malaria.

Lack of, or decreased production, of β-globin chains results in an imbalance of α- and β-chains, resulting in deficiency of hemoglobin A. The resulting ineffective erythropoesis is an important factor in the development of anemia. The α-chains precipitate and form inclusions that can be seen on electron microscopy and are related to the hemolysis and the ineffective erythropoesis that occur in β-thalassemia. Neonates and infants are protected by the presence of fetal hemoglobin.

Deletions, nonsense mutations, and frameshift mutations are described. Some mutations affect the rate of hemoglobin synthesis. Activation of cryptic splice sites within exons or introns also results in the production of abnormal hemoglobins. There are more than 300 variants. Unequal crossover events lead to the production of fusion hemoglobins with abnormal function. Heterozygosity for β-thalassemia, known as thalassemia minor, can be accompanied by hypochromic anemia. Some mutations result in no synthesis of adult hemoglobin (b^0) and some in decreased production of adult hemoglobin (b^+). Combined heterozygosity for two different thalassemia mutations results in a variable phenotype.

Diagnosis is based on hematologic indices and hemoglobin electrophoresis, which shows increased HbA_2 and HbF. Molecular diagnostic tools are useful if the mutations are defined. They can be employed for clinical diagnosis, heterozygote assignment, and prenatal diagnosis.

Transfusion to control the anemia is the keystone of therapy. The bony abnormalities can be prevented by transfusion to keep the anemia under control. Transfusion, however, results in iron overload with failure of several organs, including liver, lung, heart, pancreas, and endocrine glands. Even without transfusion, hyperabsorption of iron may result in iron overload. Splenectomy may be necessary. Population screening for heterozygosity allows individuals to know their risks for having affected children and to use prenatal diagnosis if desired.

Sickle Cell Anemia (MIM 141900), (β-globin locus):

Anemia that results from hemolysis is the characteristic clinical finding of sickle cell anemia. Infants and young children are at risk for serious infections, especially those caused by *Streptococcus pneumoniae, Hemophilus influenza,* and *Salmonella.* Adults have functional asplenia, and are therefore also at risk for infection. Recurrent episodes of vaso-occlusion that cause abdominal pain, dactylitis, priapism, and renal damage are a major cause of morbidity. Death results from sepsis in the infant or young child and from renal or cardiac failure, stroke, or complications of pregnancy in the adult. The Collaborative Study of Sickle Cell Disease found a median age of death of 48 years in affected females and 42 years in affected males. Sudden death can occur in a vaso-occlusive crisis. Complications of major organ failure play a role in mortality as does toxicity of the narcotics used for pain control. Patients with the SC variant have a longer life span; increased concentrations of fetal hemoglobin are also associated with longer life span.

About 8% of African Americans are heterozygous for the sickle hemoglobin mutation. The birth incidence of sickle cell anemia is 1 in 625. The gene frequency is higher in some areas of sub-Saharan Africa and the Mediterranean regions. In some parts of West Africa, the heterozygote frequency is as high as 25%.

When deoxygenated, sickle hemoglobin takes on an abnormal tertiary structure, causing the cell to assume the sickle shape. The misshapen cells fail to traverse the small capillaries and the spleen, causing obstruction of the small vasculature and leading to hemolysis in the spleen.

The β-globin gene has a single base change (A to T), which results in the substitution of valine for glutamic acid at amino acid position 6 of the protein. Evidence is accumulating that other genes in the β-globin gene cluster influence the clinical expression. Elevated levels of HbF and HbA_2 play a role in reducing severity of symptoms. The presence of α-thalassemia also mitigates severity by decreasing the overall concentrations of HbS.

Diagnosis in both the homozygote and the heterozygote is confirmed by hemoglobin electrophoresis. The sickle hemoglobin is easily identified. Molecular genetic tools are helpful in defining specific diagnosis and in prenatal diagnosis.

Life span is increasing with more aggressive treatment of infection and vaso-occlusive episodes. Newborn screening to identify affected infants and provide them with prophylactic treatment with penicillin has dramatically decreased the mortality rate in the first years of life. Better understanding of the factors associated with longer survival is needed, including improved understanding of the role of other genes in the β-globin cluster. Bone marrow transplant may be a consideration when haplotype analysis within the β-globin cluster suggests the presence of a severe variant. Other structural hemoglobin variants are shown in Table 6–6.

DISORDERS OF PLATELETS

Gulation of blood following injury requires complex interaction between the protein clotting factors and platelets. Disorders of platelet function or secretion are characterized by a bleeding diathesis. Gingival bleeding, mucosal bleeding, menorrhagia, and occasional gastrointestinal bleeding are typical. Several inherited platelet disorders are known.

Glanzmanns Thrombasthenia (MIM 273800): In Glanzmanns thrombasthenia, bleeding begins from birth. The membrane glycoproteins IIb/IIIa are deficient in platelets, which keeps them from forming aggregates in response to stimuli. The disorder is inherited as an autosomal recessive trait. Specific genetic defects have not been identified. Diagnosis is based on the presence of an abnormal bleeding time with normal platelet count and morphology. Laboratory studies to identify the glycoprotein deficiency can be performed if necessary. Outcome is variable, from very mild symptoms to fatal hemorrhage in childhood. Some patients require transfusion.

Bernard-Soulier Syndrome (MIM 231200): The clinical features of Bernard-Soulier syndrome are similar to Glanzmann's thrombasthenia. Deficiency in the platelet membrane glycoprotein complex Ib/IX, which is the von Willebrand factor binding site, is the basis of the condition. The disorder is inherited in an autosomal recessive fashion. A patient with a frameshift mutation in the gene for Ib has been reported, but there may be genetic heterogeneity. Large platelets that fail to aggregate in autologous plasma or ristocetin suggest the diagnosis. The deficiency in membrane glycoprotein Ib/IX can be measured to confirm the diagnosis if necessary. No specific treatment is usually needed, although some patients require transfusion.

X-Linked Thrombocytopenia (MIM 313900): Isolated thrombocytopenia, characterized clinically by easy bruising, has occurred following an X-linked pattern of inheritance. The gene maps to the Wiscott-Aldrich region; the mutation in X-linked thrombcytopenia is probably allelic to that for Wiscott-Aldrich syndrome.

Other Disorders: There are a variety of possible disorders of platelet secretion or storage that are poorly characterized and for which the genetics is not well worked out. Deficiency in α-granules (grey platelet syndrome) has been characterized as a disorder in secretion of platelet proteins.

Coagulopathies

The protein component of the clotting cascade comprises 12 proteins (listed in Table 6–7) and several others. Many inherited abnormalities of the clotting cascade are known. They result from genetic deficiencies of any of the clotting factors I–XIII except for factor XII, prekallikrein, and high molecular weight kininogen. All Mendelian modes of inheritance have been described in this group of bleeding disorders. Often, bleeding or easy bruising begin in infancy and childhood, but the specific diagnosis may not be made until later. Knowing the specific genetic diagnosis can aid in prognosis, genetic risk assessment, and development of a treatment plan.

Factor VIII Deficiency (Classical Hemophilia) (MIM 306700): Classical hemophilia due to factor VIII deficiency is probably the oldest recognized and the best known of the inherited coagulopathies. The disorder occurs in 1 in 10,000 Caucasian males. Bleeding is unusual at birth. However, in severely affected children the disorder may be signaled in the neonatal period by bleeding from the heel prick for newborn screening, from the circumcision site, or from injection sites. Hemoperitoneum and cephalhematoma may also occur. Excessive bruising, bleeding into joints and muscles, and bleeding from sites of injury occur in later childhood and adulthood. Hemarthrosis from recurrent spontaneous bleeding into joints results in serious disability in the older child and adult. Intracranial bleeding in the adult can be acute and fatal. The clinical phenotypes are divided into mild, moderate, and severe.

Factor VIII is a cofactor to factor IX in the activation of factor X. The severity of the clinical syndrome depends on the degree of deficiency of factor VIII. The gene for factor VIII is on chromosome Xq28-qter. The gene has been cloned, and the molecular pathology is being defined. Point mutations, insertions, and deletions are known, and they are all associated with all of the phenotypes. Deletions vary in size up to deletion of the entire gene. All regions of the gene have been involved. In some families, it has been possible to trace the mutation back to a grandmother in whom it appeared de novo. Females may be symptomatic because of unfavorable lyonization. Homozygous affected females do occur; they are usually the offspring of an affected father and a heterozygous mother.

Diagnosis is suggested by a prolonged partial thromboplastin time and is based on measuring factor VIII in blood. In the affected male values may be very low. On average, heterozygous females have 50% of the normal amount. Because of lyonization, this is variable, and biochemical diagnosis of heterozygosity is not always certain. Molecular methods can provide direct analysis of the mutation in some

Table 6–7. Clotting disorders.

Protein Deficiency	Clinical Disorder	Inheritance	Map Location
Vitamin K-dependent proteins			
Prothrombin	Hypoprothrombinemia; dysprothrombinemia; severity of bleeding disorder depends on prothrombin content of blood	AR	11p11–q12
Factor VII	Variable bleeding diathesis; CNS bleeds described	AR	13q34–qter
Factor IX	Christmas disease-hemophilia B; similar to hemophilia A	XL	Xq26–27
Factor X	Variable clinical disorder dependent on specific mutation	AR	13q34–qter
Protein C	Thrombotic disease; homozygous form in newborn with severe thrombosis or purpura fulminans	AD	2q13–q14
Protein S	Thrombosis at young age	AD	3p11.1–q11.2
Fibrinogen	Mild, moderate and severe forms; bleeding diathesis in all; in severe form, neonatal bleeding with intracranial and umbilical cord bleeding; moderate form may have neonatal bleeding and postpartum hemorrhage in mother	AD, AR	4q28 α, β, γ subunits
Factor XIII	Umbilical cord bleeding and intracranial bleeding in neonate; recurrent miscarriage, abnormal wound healing, recurrent bleeding in adult	AR	6p25–p24
Factor VIII	Classical hemophilia	XL	Xq28
Factor V	Bleeding, especially after surgery or injury	AR	1q23
Von Willebrand factor	Mild bleeding especially after surgery or injury; especially mucocutaneous bleeding	AD, AR	12p12–pter
Contact activation of platelets			
Factor XI	Mild bleeding disorder	AR	4q35

families; for others RFLP analysis is needed. In informative families, molecular techniques can be employed for diagnosis of affected males both pre- and postnatally, to establish carrier status in at-risk females, and for prenatal diagnosis.

Replacement of factor VIII is the treatment of choice. Patients with mild disease whose serum factor VIII concentration exceeds 10 u/dl may only need treatment at times of injury or surgery, and may respond to 1-desamino-8-D-arginine vasopressin (DDAVP). Determination of need for treatment depends on the concentration of factor VIII in the blood. In the past, factor VIII has been derived from pooled human blood. Much of the therapeutic advantage of infusion of factor VIII was lost in the last few decades because hepatitis and AIDS have developed in some patients with hemophilia who received many infusions of the factor. Today, heat-treated factor VIII and monoclonal antibody isolated factor VIII are the concentrates employed. Although this obviates the risk of HIV, it does not decrease the transmission of hepatitis B. Immunization against hepatitis B may reduce the chance of that infection. The use of recombinant factor VIII eliminates both risks. Patients who make no factor VIII are at risk for developing antibodies to the factor VIII with which they are treated.

Factor IX Deficiency (Christmas Disease, Hemophilia B) (MIM 306900): The clinical features of hemophilia B are similar to hemophilia A. The incidence is considerably less than hemophilia A; however, approximately 1 in 50,000 males are affected. The disorder exists worldwide and in many ethnic groups. The clotting abnormality is the result of a deficiency in factor IX, a protein that is converted to a serine protease that participates in the activation of factor X.

The disorder is X-linked and has been mapped to Xq26–q27, very near factor VIII. Point mutations and nonsense mutations have been identified and result in a protein with deficient or no clotting activity; mutations have also been described that alter the interaction with other factors in the clotting cascade. Affected females have been reported; unfavorable lyonization is a possible mechanism. Females with X-chromosome abnormalities account for some of these. A deletion at Xq27, and Turner syndrome with only a single X chromosome, have been reported in females affected with hemophilia B. In both of these cases there was a mutation in the factor VIII gene on the remaining cytogenetically normal X. Homozygosity has been seen in a female with an affected father and a heterozygous mother based on consanguinity.

Diagnosis depends on measurement of factor IX in blood; diagnosis of affected males, carrier assignment, and prenatal diagnosis can all be performed using molecular techniques in informative families.

The mild variants may not need any treatment; replacement of factor IX using pooled blood concentrates has had the same success and problems as factor VIII replacement. Use of recombinant factor IX will solve the infection risks. Antibodies to factor IX complicate therapy in about 10% of patients, largely those who make no factor IX as result of gene deletion.

Factor XI Deficiency (Hemophilia C) (MIM 264900): Patients with factor XI deficiency (hemophilia C) usually have a mild bleeding diathesis and usually only have clinically significant bleeding at surgery or after injury. The condition is most common in Jews; incidence in Askenazi Jews in Israel has been reported at 0.1–0.3%. Hemophilia C is seen in many other ethnic groups as well. Deficiency of factor XI (plasma thromboplastin antecedent deficiency) is the basis of the disorder. Factor XI and its activated product bind to platelets during coagulation.

Autosomal recessive inheritance is well documented in this condition. The gene for plasma thromboplastin antecedent is mapped to chromosome 4q35.

Patients have a prolonged activated partial thromboplastin time and a normal prothrombin time. Serious complications are rare; treatment is only needed at the time of surgery or serious injury.

Dysfibrinoginemias: Abnormalities in fibrinogen are rare. The neonatal severe form is characterized by umbilical cord bleeding. Other patients may have a variety of severe kinds of bleeding, including intracranial bleeding. The mortality rate is high in these patients. In the less severe forms, bleeding is less dramatic, but treatment is sometimes needed.

Von Willebrand Disease (MIM 193400): Von Willebrand disease is clinically heterogeneous. Mucocutaneous bleeding is common, but more severe bleeding including postpartum hemorrhage, bleeding with surgery or injury, and bruising often occur. Bleeding into joints and muscles does not usually happen in these patients.

Von Willebrand disease is the most common inherited bleeding disorder. Large studies suggest an incidence of 1–10 in 10,000. An incidence of 1.3% was found in a multiethnic group of children screened for bleeding disorders. The fre-quency is about 5 in one million in some Arab populations.

Von Willebrand factor (vWF) is a multimeric glycoprotein. It is involved in platelet binding to vascular sub-endothelium and in platelet aggregation. vWF also serves as a carrier for factor VIII. Its deficiency is associated with prolonged bleeding. The gene for vWF maps to chromosome 12p12–pter. Many genetic variants have been described (Table 6–7); inheritance is autosomal dominant. Deletions have been associated with the development of an antibody to vWF after treatment with preparations of the factor.

Diagnosis depends on measurement of factor VIII, von Willebrand factor antigen, ristocetin cofactor activity, and ristocetin induced platelet aggregation in platelet rich plasma. Molecular genetic tools can be used if the mutation can be identified or if hybridization studies are informative.

Treatment with preparations of vWF may be needed during surgery or after injury. DDAVP (1-desamino-8-D-arginine vasopressin) mobilizes bound vWF in patients who make some factor and can be used to improve clotting function acutely. Tachyphylaxis to this preparation may occur. Its use is contraindicated in von Willebrand disease type IIb.

Thrombotic Disorders

Antithrombin III Deficiency (MIM 107300): Antithrombin III deficiency is characterized by increased incidence of venous thrombosis, usually in adulthood. Deep vein thrombosis and pulmonary embolus are characteristic, especially during pregnancy or after trauma. The incidence is 1 in 2000 to 1 in 5000. This disorder may account for 2–5% of patients with severe thrombotic disease.

Antithrombin inhibits thrombin, the activated forms of factors XII, XI, IX, X, and kallikrein. The major time of action for antithrombin is during the early stages of activation of the clotting cascade; its deficiency results in a tendency to thrombosis.

The gene for antithrombin maps to chromosome 1q23–q25. The deficiency of antithrombin III is inherited as an autosomal dominant trait. Deletions and nonsense mutations result in deficiency of the protein. Several allelic variants have been described; they involve point mutations in various functional parts of the molecule leading to loss of heparin binding and of inhibition of thrombin. Homozygosity for an antithrombin mutation, a rare occurrence, has been associated with intracardiac thrombosis. Homozygosity for another mutation has been seen in patients with thrombotic disease; heterozygous family members are asymptomatic.

Diagnosis is made by measuring antithrombin in blood; activity is in the range of 25–60% of normal. Prognosis depends on the severity of the thrombotic episodes. Treatment is with anticoagulants. Some patients develop heparin resistance; these patients can be treated with a concentrate of antithrombin III. Prophylactic treatment during pregnancy may be advisable, but warfarin should be avoided since its use is associated with fetal malformations.

Protein C Deficiency (MIM 176860): Protein C deficiency is clinically similar to antithrombin III deficiency, but it may be symptomatic earlier in life. Skin necrosis is sometimes seen after treatment with anticoagulants. Activated protein C is a protease that inactivates factors V and VIII; deficiency thus increases risk of thrombosis. The gene is mapped to chromosome 2. Nonsense mutations result in decreased production in the heterozygous state. Homozygosity has resulted in massive thrombosis in the neonate involving vena cava, and the renal and iliac veins, and pulmonary emboli. Variants with a defective protein are known. Diagnosis is based on finding 40–50% of normal amount or activity of Protein C. Treatment consists of anticoagulation therapy.

Protein S Deficiency (MIM 176880): The clinical features of protein S deficiency are similar to those seen in protein C deficiency. Protein S participates in the inactivation of activated factor V as a cofactor for activated protein C. The disorder is inherited in an autosomal dominant fashion. Treatment consists of anticoagulation.

Activated Protein C Resistance (MIM 227400): A newly recognized disorder, activated protein C resistance is clinically similar to Protein S deficiency, and is due to a mutation in the gene for Factor V. The condition results in resistance of inactivation of Factor V by protein C, and is probably not rare.

REFERENCES & SUGGESTED READING

Agre P: Hereditary spherocytosis. JAMA 1993;**262**:2887.

Agre P, Orringer EP, Bennett V: Deficient red-cell spectrin in severe, recessively inherited spherocytosis. N Engl J Med 1982;**306**:1155.

Antonarakis SE, Kazazian H: The molecular basis of hemophilia in man. Trends in Genetics 1988;**4**:233.

Antonarakis SE et al: Hemophilia A: Detection of molecular defects and of carriers by DNA analysis. N Engl J Med 1985;**313**:842.

Baehner RL, Strauss HS: Hemophilia in the first year of life. N Engl J Med 1966;**275**:524.

Becker PS et al: Beta spectrin kissimmee: a spectrin variant associated with autosomal dominant spherocytosis and defective binding to protein 4.1. J Clin Invest 1993;**92**:612.

Benson RE, Jones DW, Doss WJ: Conformational changes in von Willebrand's factor protein: effects on the binding of factor VIII-coagulant. Am J Hematol 1986;**22**:113.

Bernardi F et al: RFLP analysis in families with sporadic hemophilia A. Hum Genet 1987;**76**:253.

Beutler E: Study of glucose-6-phosphate dehydrogenase: history and molecular biology. Am J Hematol 1993;**42**:53.

Bockenstedt P, Greenberg JM, Handin RI: Structural basis of von Willebrand factor binding to platelet glycoprotein Ib and collagen. J Clin Invest 1986;**77**:743.

Brittenham GM et al: Efficacy of deferoxamine in preventing complications of iron overlead in patients with thalassemia major. N Engl J Med 1994;**331**:567.

Costa FF et al: Linkage of dominant hereditary spherocytosisto, the gene for the erythrocyte membrane-skeleton protein ankyrin. N Engl J Med 1990;**323**:1046.

Donner M et al: Herditary X-linked thrombocytopenia maps to the same chromosomal region as the Wiskott–Aldrich syndrome. Blood 1988;**72**:1849.

Dover GJ, Valle D: Therapy for β-thalassemia–a paradigm for the treatment of genetic disorders. N Engl J Med 1994;**331**:609.

Gallagher PG, Forget BG: Spectrin genes in health and disease. Semin Hematol 1993;**30**:4.

Ginsburg D, Bowie WJ: Molecular genetics of von Willebrand disease. Blood 1992;**79**:2507.

Ginsburg D et al: Human von Willebrand factor (vWF): isolation of complementary DNA (cDNA) clones and chromosomal localization. Science 1985;**228**:1401.

Glader BE: Hereditary red blood cell disorders (excluding haemoglobinopathies and thalasssaemias). Pages 1343–1369 in: *Principles and Practice of Medical Genetics,*

2nd ed. Emery AEH, Rimoin D (editors). Churchill Livingstone, 1990.

Goldsmith MF: Hemophilia, beaten on one front, is beset on others. JAMA 1986;**256**:3200.

Hanspal M et al: Molecular basis of spectrin and ankyrin deficiencies in severe hereditary spherocytosis: evidence implicating a primary defect of ankyrin. Blood 1991;**77**:165.

Hashimi KZ, MacIver JE, Delamore IW: Christmas disease in a female. Lancet 1978;**ii**:965.

Hedner U, Davie EW: Introduction to hemostasis and the vitamin K-dependent coagulation factors. Pages in 2107–2134 in: *The Metabolic Basis of Inherited Disease,* 6th ed. McGraw Hill, 1989.

Higgs DR et al: Negro α-thalassemia is caused by deletion of a single α-globin gene. Lancet 1979;**ii**:272.

Hobbins JC et al: Percutaneous fetal umbilical blood sampling. Am J Obstet Gynecol 1985;**152**:1.

Hurst JA, Baraitser M, Wonke B: Autosomal dominant transmission of congenital erythroid hypoplastic anemia with radial abnormalities. Am J Med Genet 1991;**40**:482.

Iolascon A et al: Ankyrin deficiency in dominant hereditary spherocytosis: report of three cases. Br J Haematol 1991;**78**:551.

Jarolim P et al: Duplication of 10 nucleotides in the erythroid band 3 (AE1) gene in a kindred with hereditary spherocytosis and band 3 protein deficiency (band 3PRAGUE). J Clin Invest 1994;**93**:121.

Lakich D et al: Inversions disrupting the factor VIII gene are a common cause of severe haemophilia A. Nature Genetics 1993;**5**:236.

Ludlam CA. Congenital disorders of haemostasis. Pages 1372–1389 in: *Principles and Practice of Medical Genetics,* 2nd ed. Emery AEH, Rimoin D (editors). Churchill Livingstone, 1990.

Ludomirski A, Weiner S: Percutaneous fetal umbilical blood sampling. Clin Obstet Gynecol 1988;**31**:19.

Lux SE, Becker PS: Disorders of the red cell membrane skeleton: Hereditary spherocytosis and hereditary elliptocytosis. Pages 2281–2339 in: *The Metabolic Basis of Inherited Disease,* 6th ed. Scriver CR et al (editors). McGraw Hill, 1989.

Luzzatto L, Mehta A: Glucose-6-phosphate dehydrogenase deficiency. Pages 2237–2265 in: *The Metabolic Basis of Inherited Disease,* 6th ed. Scriver CR et al (editors). McGraw Hill, 1989.

Macdougall LG et al: Comparative study of Fanconi anemia in children of different ethnic origin in South Africa. Am J Med Genet 1994;**52**:279.

MeEver RP, Majerus PW: Inherited disorders of platelets. Pages 2219–2235 in: *The Metabolic Basis of Inherited Disease,* 6th ed. Scriver CR et al (editors). McGraw Hill, 1989.

Miwa S, Kanno H, Fujii H: Concise review: Pyruvate kinase deficiency: Historical perspective and recent progress of molecular genetics. Am J Hematol 1993;**42:** 31.

Mohandas N, Chasis JA: Red blood cell deformability, membrane material properties and shape: Regulation by transmembrane, skeletal and cytosolic proteins and lipids. Semin Hematol 1993;**30:**171.

Nelson DM, Stempel LE, Brandt JT: Hereditary antithrombin III deficiency and pregnancy: report of two cases and review of the literature. Obstet Gynecol 1985;**65:**848.

Nisen P et al: The molecular basis of severe hemophilia B in a girl. N Engl J Med 1986;**315:**1139.

Oberle I et al: Genetic screening for hemophilia A (classic hemophilia) with a polymorphic DNA probe. N Engl J Med 1985;**312:**682.

Pajor A, Lehoczky D, Szakacs Z: Pregnancy and hereditary spherocytosis: report of 8 patients and a review. Arch Gynecology and Obstetrics 1993;**253:**37.

Palek J: Introduction: red blood cell membrane proteins, their genes and mutations. Semin Hematol 1993;**30:**1.

Palek J, Jarolim P: Clinical expression and laboratory detection of red blood cell membrane material protein mutations. Semin Hematol 1993;**30:**249.

Phillips JA, Kazazian HH: Haemoglobinopathies and thalassaemias. Pages 1315–1342 in: *Principles and Practice of Medical Genetics,* 2nd ed. Emery AEH, Rimoin D (editors). Churchill Livingstone, 1990.

Platt OS et al. Mortality in sickle cell disease: Life expectancy and risk factors for early death. N Engl J Med 1994;**330:**1639.

Powars D, Hiti A: Sickle cell anemia: βS gene cluster haplotypes as genetic markers for severe disease expression. Am J Dis Child 1993;**147:**1197.

Pressley L et al: Genetic basis for hemoglobin-H disease. N Engl J Med 1980;**303:**1383.

Prochownik EV et al: Molecular heterogeneity of hereditary antithrombin III deficiency. N Engl J Med 1983;**308:**1549.

Sadler JE: von Willebrand Disease. Pages 2171–2187 in: *The Metabolic Basis of Inherited Disease,* 6th ed. Scriver CR et al (editors). McGraw Hill, 1989.

Sadler JE et al: Cloning and characterization of two cDNAs coding for human von Willebrand factor. Proc Soc Natl Acad Sci USA 1985;**82:**6394.

Seligsohn U et al: Homozygous protein C deficiency manifested by massive venous thrombosis in the newborn. N Engl J Med 1984;**310:**559.

Simsek S et al: Identification of a homozygous single base pair deletion in the gene coding for the human platelet glycoprotein IB-a causing Bernard–Soulier syndrome. Thromb Haemost 1994;**72:**444.

Tanaka KR, Zerez CR: Red cell enzymopathies of the glycolytic pathway. Semin Hematol 1990;**27:**165.

Valentine WN, Tanaka KR, Paglia DE: Pyruvate kinase and other enzyme deficiency disorders of the erythrocyte. Pages 2341–2365 in: *The Metabolic Basis of Inherited Disease,* 6th ed. Scriver CR et al (editors). McGraw Hill, 1989.

Vehar GA et al: Factor VIII and Factor V: Biochemistry and Pathophysiology. Pages 2155–2170 in: *The Metabolic Basis of Inherited Disease,* 6th ed. Scriver CR et al (editors). McGraw Hill, 1989.

Visochil DH et al: Congenital hypoplastic (Blackfan–Diamond) anemia. Am J Med Genet 1990;**35:**251.

Vulliamy T, Mason P, Luzzatto L: The molecular basis of glucose-6-phosphatase deficiency. Trends in Genetics 1992;**8:**138.

Weatherall DJ et al: The hemoglobinopathies. Pages 2281–2339 in: *The Metabolic Basis of Inherited Disease,* 6th ed. Scriver CR et al (editors). McGraw Hill, 1989.

Werner EJ et al: Prevalence of von Willebrand disease in children: A multiethnic study. J Pediatr 1993;**123:**893.

Wolfe LC et al: A genetic defect in the binding of protein 4.1 to spectrin in a kindred with hereditary spherocytosis. N Engl J Med 1982;**307:**1367.

Reproductive Genetics

7

Background & History

Interest in assessing the well-being of the unborn baby is as old as history itself. Much mythology has surrounded the efforts at predicting fetal sex and normality. Early obstetrical tools were limited to monitoring of variables such as uterine size and maternal weight gain along with auscultation of the fetal heart. By the middle of the twentieth century more invasive tools to assess specific aspects of fetal genetic disease began to be used. Fetal cells obtained from amniotic fluid were first analyzed for the presence of sex-chromatin in the 1950s. The first culture of amniotic cells obtained from amniotic fluid was performed in 1966. The following 30 years have seen an increase in development and more widespread use of amniocentesis and examination of fetal cells. Ultrasound diagnosis of anencephaly was first made in 1972. Advanced ultrasound technology now includes the ability to assess nearly the entire fetal gross anatomy. Fetal blood can be obtained to perform diagnostic studies. In the past decade advances have continued and safety and accuracy of these tools established. New methods and new tools continue to be developed for diagnosis and even therapy for the unborn baby diagnosed with genetic disease. While none of these advances guarantees fetal health, each has vastly improved the odds that families at genetic risk will have a normal baby. The methods will continue to develop and improve.

Interpretation of the results of prenatal diagnostic testing requires knowledge of the types of samples that can be obtained, the techniques in use, the information that can be gained, and the limitations of these tools. The range of samples obtained includes:

- Maternal serum markers of fetal health
- Maternal serum for proteins of fetal origin
- Amniotic fluid for analytes in fluid
- Amniotic fluid for cells of fetal origin
- Chorionic villus for trophoblast cells
- Fetal blood cells of both red cell and white cell series.

The techniques in clinical use to obtain these samples include:

- Amniocentesis to obtain amniotic fluid and fetal cells

- Chorionic villus sampling (CVS) to obtain trophoblast cells
- Cordocentesis to obtain fetal blood cells
- Ultrasound for imaging of fetal anatomy.

Fetal cells are studied using cytogenetic, biochemical, or molecular tools. A variety of analytes that reflect fetal well-being can be measured in amniotic fluid. Several current issues are the subject of continued evaluation and in some cases, controversy. Among these are policy questions surrounding the use of maternal serum screening, the maternal age at which amniocentesis should supersede serum testing, whether all women should be offered amniocentesis, and the cut-off result of serum screening that should trigger amniocentesis for chromosome abnormalities. The safety of invasive tests such as early amniocentesis and chorionic villus sampling continues is still under investigation. New experimental technologies such as pre-implantation diagnosis, using the blastocyst, in association with in vitro fertilization are being investigated. The development of prenatal therapy has focused on early treatment of biochemical disorders and fetal surgery for congenital malformations. There is substantial interest in the primary prevention of birth defects. The observation that maternal intake of appropriate amounts of folic acid prevents neural tube defects has led to its use for prevention of neural tube defects.

TECHNIQUES IN USE FOR DIAGNOSIS

Maternal Serum Screening

The first use of maternal blood to assess fetal health was the measurement of α-fetoprotein (AFP), which was first studied in 1973. Measurement of it in amniotic fluid came into practice in the mid-1980s. AFP is the most prominent protein of fetal origin; it is made in fetal liver. Production peaks between 10 and 13 weeks of gestation and then falls throughout the rest of gestation. The protein can be measured in fetal blood and in amniotic fluid. Excessive amounts of AFP were first observed in amniotic fluid when the fetus had a neural tube defect such as anencephaly or open spina bifida; soon thereafter reports of its measurement in maternal serum appeared. The protein appears in the maternal circulation because of fetal hemorrhage into the maternal circulation at the level of the placenta or diffusion of AFP across the placental membranes. The concentration in maternal serum rises throughout gestation and reaches its highest concentration between 24 and 32 weeks. Excessive concentrations of maternal serum AFP (MSAFP) are associated with a variety of fetal problems. The dependence of the normal range of MSAFP on maternal factors and gestational age is now well recognized; the interpretation of abnormal results as reflecting compromised fetal well-being must take those factors into account.

Abnormally high concentrations of AFP are seen in 80–85% of open neural tube defects. High concentration is also associated with open body wall defects, compromised skin integrity, maternal diabetes, twin pregnancy, impending fetal demise. In about 4% of cases, there is no recognizable abnormality at all; this may reflect a placental abnormality. In 1984 low concentrations of AFP in maternal serum were observed in association with trisomy 21 (Down syndrome) and subsequently with trisomy 18 in the fetus. Because only 30% of fetuses with Down syndrome

are detected this way, other biochemical markers for assessing fetal health have been sought. Three markers are now becoming widely measured in maternal serum to assess the status of the fetus. These are α-fetoprotein (AFP), human chorionic gonadotropin (HCG), and unconjugated estrogen (UE); routine measurement of these may allow detection of 60–70% of fetuses with Down syndrome or trisomy 18 regardless of maternal age. Currently MSAFP screening is recommended for all pregnant women, and screening with the three serum markers is widely used and has become referred to as "triple screening." Follow-up studies when the pregnant patient has an abnormal maternal serum screening test result include the use of detailed ultrasound examination and amniocentesis (Figure 7–1). Elevation of MSAFP demands assessment of fetal anatomy; the frequent abnormalities seen are listed in Table 7–1. Low concentrations of MSAFP and UE along with a high concentration of HCG should alert the physician to the possibility of a trisomy 21; in the case of trisomy 18, all analytes have a low concentration. In this setting, assessment of fetal chromosome constitution is recommended.

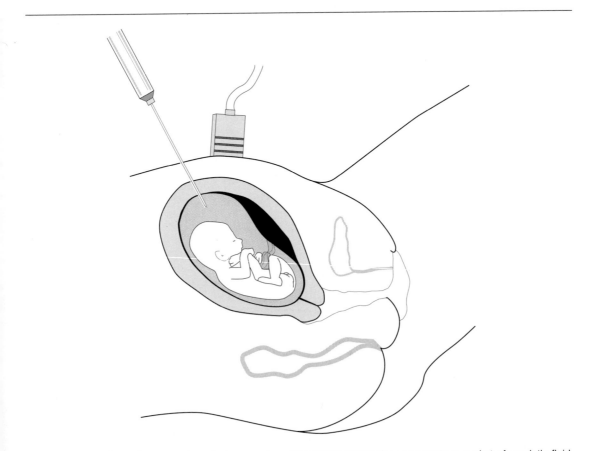

Figure 7–1. An illustration of amniocentesis procedure. Ultrasound guides the operator to a pocket of amniotic fluid, avoiding the placenta.

Table 7–1. Prenatal diagnostic procedures.

Test[1]	Percentage Risk Fetal Loss from Test[†]	Value	Diagnostic Considerations	Further Action
MSAFP	0	↑MSAFP	Open body wall defects, impending fetal demise; congenital nephrosis	Amniocentesis Measure AFP, AChe
Triple screen	0	↓MSAFP ↓UE ↑HCG	Trisomy 21	Amniocentesis; karyotype
Triple screen	0	↓MSAFP ↓UE ↓HCG	Trisomy 18	Amniocentesis; karyotype
Amniocentesis	0.5	Abnormal karyotype	Chromosome abnormality	Review phenotype; counsel about termination or continuing pregnancy
		DNA analysis	Identification of specific mutation; linkage data suggesting disease; eg, cystic fibrosis, muscular dystrophy, hemoglobinopathy	Review phenotype; counsel about termination or continuing pregnancy
		Analyte measurement	Inborn errors of metabolism; endocrinopathies	Review phenotype; counsel about termination or continuing pregnancy; review options for fetal therapy
		Enzyme measurement	Inborn errors of metabolism; specific enzymopathy sought, eg, Tay-Sachs, other leukodystrophies	Review phenotype; counsel about termination or continuing pregnancy; review options for fetal therapy
CVS	0.6	Mosaic chromosomal constitution	Confined placental mosaicism, true fetal mosaicism	Amniotic fluid cell karyotype or fetal blood cell karyotype
		Abnormal karyotype	Chromosome abnormality	Review phenotype; counsel about termination or continuing pregnancy
		DNA analysis	Identification of specific mutation; linkage data suggesting disease; eg, cystic fibrosis, muscular dystrophy, hemoglobinopathy	Review phenotype; counsel about termination or continuing pregnancy
		Enzyme measurement	Inborn errors of metabolism; specific enzymopathy sought, eg, Tay-Sachs, other leukodystrophies	Review phenotype; counsel about termination or continuing pregnancy; review options for fetal therapy

[†] Increase over controls.
[1] MSAFP: maternal serum a-feto protein screening; AChE: acetylcholinesterase; UE: unconjugated estrogen; HCG: human chorionic gonadtropin.

The use of serum triple screening to replace amniocentesis in the assessment of a pregnancy in the mother who is over 35 years of age is under considerable discussion. Historically, maternal age of 35 years or more has been an indication for amniocentesis because of the increase in risk of chromosome abnormalities with advancing maternal age. The use of triple screening to identify the fetus with a chromosome abnormality has been proposed by some as an alternative to amniocentesis in the woman over age 35. There is a drawback to this approach. While amniocentesis, if performed, will identify 100% of such affected fetuses, the maternal serum triple screen will probably only identify 85–90%. Alternatively, some argue that amniocentesis could be avoided in women over age 35 whose screening test results were normal, decreasing the number of amniocenteses performed by 70–75% while picking up 90% of fetuses with Down syndrome. The Clinical Practice Committee of the American College of Medical Genetics currently recommends that maternal age remain an indicator for amniocentesis and not be replaced by serum triple screening at this time. The pregnant woman is faced with a very personal choice to make. She should be carefully counseled about the value of early serum triple screening; the other available options, with their advantages and drawbacks, should be clearly discussed so that she can make an informed decision.

Amniocentesis

Amniocentesis is a widely used technique for prenatal diagnosis. Using this procedure, the physician can obtain amniotic fluid for diagnostic purposes. Fetal cells can be obtained from the fluid and a variety of analytes can be measured. Amniotic fluid volume increases over the course of gestation from about 15 ml to over 350 ml at term. The fetal kidney forms urine and excretes it into the amniotic fluid. Some amniotic fluid is maternal in origin. Analytes measured are of both maternal and fetal origin. Normative data are crucial for interpretation of the results of amniotic fluid analysis, the reference ranges can depend on both maternal and fetal factors. Amniotic fluid is normally sterile and resists infection.

Analytes typical of some biochemical disorders can be measured in amniotic fluid. These analytes include 17-hydroxyprogesterone, which is elevated in congenital adrenal hyperplasia, and some other hormones, amino acids, and organic acids. The use of such measurements in prenatal diagnosis has been supplanted by more direct assessments of enzyme activity or mutation analysis when these are known. The measurement of AFP and acetylcholinesterase (AChE) can be a useful adjunct in the diagnosis of neural tube defects, other open body wall defects, and congenital nephrosis. These measurements should be offered when MSAFP testing reveals an elevated concentration of AFP. Fetal cells obtained from amniotic fluid can be used in the following ways to refine diagnosis in the fetus:

- To measure enzyme activities expressed fibroblast-derived cells
- To use as source of DNA
- To use as a source of cells for chromosome analysis.

Rarely the cells can be used as obtained. For most purposes, it is necessary to culture the fetal cells to obtain numbers large enough for definitive studies. Culture takes 1–2 weeks.

Technical Aspects of Amniocentesis: Midtrimester amniocentesis is usually performed using a transabdominal approach to obtain amniotic fluid from the uterine cavity (Figure 7–1). Approximately 20 ml of amniotic fluid is typically obtained; this represents about 10% of the total amniotic fluid volume and is rapidly replaced. After more than two decades of experience this technique's safety and accuracy have been well established. Ultrasound guidance is used to determine the location of the placenta to help the operator to avoid traversing it, to determine fetal status and location of amniotic fluid, and to look for multiple gestation. Continuous ultrasound surveillance of the needle is usual. The risks of amniocentesis are low in the hands of an experienced operator, and they are almost entirely those of pregnancy loss. In several early collaborative studies the pregnancy loss rate varied from about 1–3.5%. In a large collaborative study supported by the National Institutes of Child Health and Development (NICHD) the percentage of fetal losses did not differ significantly from pregnancies which did not undergo amniocentesis. Most centers now quote a risk of fetal loss of approximately 0.5% above the background rate. Rare instances of needle puncture of the fetus have been reported. Leaking of amniotic fluid is occasionally seen and vaginal bleeding has been reported. Large collaborative studies also found no significant differences in developmental outcome, growth, or congenital malformations between newborns born after amniocentesis and control infants. Some genetic centers are also performing early amniocentesis between 12 and 15 weeks, but the safety of this procedure has not been established. Risks of pregnancy loss after early amniocentesis range from 2–11%.

Chorionic Villus Sampling (CVS)

This procedure is used to obtain trophoblast cells which represent the fetal genetic status early in gestation. Since the cells are rapidly proliferating, they can be used directly without culture for karyotyping, for molecular analysis of their DNA or for measurement of enzyme activities expressed in fibroblast derived cells. In addition, the cells can be cultured to obtain more cells for studies such as enzyme analysis. It takes 1–2 weeks to culture sufficient numbers of cells for further study.

Technical Aspects of CVS: Between weeks 9 and 11 of gestation, under ultrasound guidance, a flexible catheter is introduced into the chorion frondosum and villi are aspirated using negative pressure from a syringe (Figure 7–2). Villi are then dissected under a microscope to obtain cells. If inadequate material is obtained, the procedure can be repeated immediately to obtain an additional sample. The villi in the chorion frondosum are of fetal origin, but they need to be cleaned of decidual tissue to avoid contamination with maternal cells, which would confound the analysis. Since CVS is performed earlier in pregnancy than is amniocentesis it can provide the mother the opportunity to have prenatal diagnostic information before fetal movement is appreciated and before the pregnancy is obvious to others.

Maternal complications from CVS are few; loss of pregnancy is the most significant risk. While this risk is not high, it may be greater than that for amniocentesis. Studies have estimated the fetal loss rate to be higher than the miscarriage rate for amniocentesis when CVS is performed at 9–11 weeks. Fetal loss ranges between 2–13% in published studies; some variation may be related to gestational age, to experience of the operator, or the newness of the technique in early studies. The 1989 NICHD Collaborative Study suggests that following CVS the risk of pregnancy loss is about 1% higher than it is following amniocentesis and is only slightly higher than the background rate of fetal loss of 4% after eight weeks of pregnancy. Of major concern is the small but probably real risk of specific limb deficiency syndromes. This issue remains somewhat controversial. Several studies suggest that oromandibular and limb hypoplasia are more common in infants born after first trimester CVS, particularly when performed prior to seven weeks of gestation. The patient must be provided the most recent information about all of these risks. Current studies suggest that the risk of terminal transverse limb defects may be 3 in 10,000. Some centers no longer perform CVS before 10 weeks of gestational age. Ultrasound examination later in pregnancy can be used to diagnose the presence of such abnormalities following CVS. The use of CVS in multiple gestation is controversial because of the difficulty in being certain that both placentas have been sampled. Amniocentesis may be safer and more reliable.

One technical problem in interpretation is the presence of mosaicism in chorionic villus samples. If mosaicism is found, amniocentesis is usually performed to determine whether or not the observed mosaicism reflects fetal status. Most of the time this mosaicism is not confirmed at amniocentesis or live birth and is apparently confined to the placenta.

Cordocentesis

Cordocentesis provides access to fetal blood when fetal cells obtained by other means are unrevealing or when fetal serum is critical to the diagnostic study. Both cells and serum can be obtained this way. The cells obtained can be used for karyotyping if cells obtained from amniocentesis or CVS suggest mosaicism and confined placental mosaicism cannot be excluded. Results can be obtained in a few days, since the culture of lymphocytes is rapid compared to the culture of amniotic fluid cells. Blood can be used to measure serum proteins. Such proteins include components of the coagulation pathway and measures of immune function such as immunoglobulins. Hemophilia and von Willebrand disease can be diagnosed this way. Platelet function can also be assessed. Critical to this kind of analysis is knowledge of the normal values during fetal life. As the molecular basis for many of the genetic disorders becomes established, direct DNA testing of amniotic fluid cells or chorionic villus cells may supplant the need for cordocentesis in many genetic disorders.

Technical Aspects of Cordocentesis: Using ultrasound for localization, a needle is placed into the

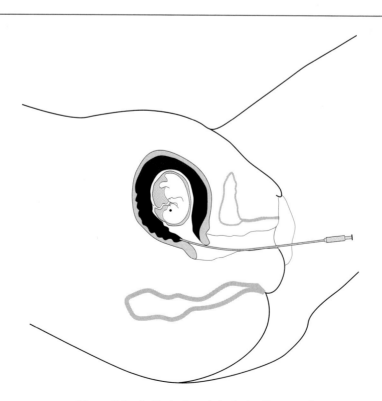

Figure 7–2. An illustration of chorionic villus sampling.

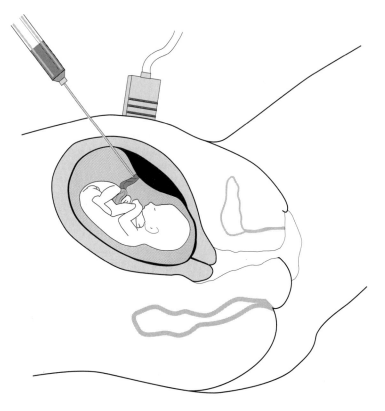

Figure 7–3. An illustration of cordocentesis procedure.

umbilical cord near its insertion into the placenta and fetal blood withdrawn (Figure 7–3). Some studies have reported the use of tocolytic drugs to prevent the onset of labor during cordocentesis and of sedation or neuromuscular blocking agents to decrease fetal movement. Volumes obtained vary from 1–4 ml. Rates of fetal loss range from 0–3%. Unlike amniocentesis and CVS, cordocentesis is performed in only a few specialized centers.

Ultrasound

Ultrasound examination of the fetus provides anatomic and functional information about the unborn baby. It can delineate anatomic structures such as the head, chest, skeleton, and abdominal organs and document fetal growth. Using real time ultrasound both cardiac structure and activity can be assessed. Modern ultrasound can delineate fetal anatomy quite precisely. The four chambers of the fetal heart can be identified; the cerebral ventricles can be assessed as to size and position. Pulmonary and aortic vessels and outflow tracts as well as the cardiac valves can be visualized. Ultrasound examination has revolutionized the diagnosis of congenital malformations and abnormalities in fetal growth.

Technical Aspects of Ultrasound Diagnosis:

Current technology uses non-invasive real-time and static scanners. Transducers produce ultrasound waves that reflect off anatomic structures and are then read as electrical energy. The images created can then be seen on an oscilloscope screen and photographed; real-time images can be videotaped. The several ways to display these images expand the ways they can be used for diagnostic purposes. Examples of congenital malformations which can be diagnosed using ultrasound examination are shown in Table 7–2 and Figure 7–1.

Several retrospective studies of outcome after exposure to diagnostic ultrasound have established the safety of ultrasound at the energy levels used for diagnostic purposes. The energy intensity is not enough to cause thermal damage. Children exposed to intrauterine ultrasound during fetal life show no adverse effects in follow-up as long as 12 years. No damage to maternal structures has ever been reported. The sonologist must be experienced in the diagnosis of congenital malformations. Reference ranges for measurements of such variables as head size, limb length, and body size must be known. Functional correlates with fetal pathology such as filling and emptying of the fetal bladder, right and left ventricular function, and fetal movement must be well understood. The sonologist must also be fa-

Table 7–2. Fetal diagnosis by ultrasound.

Organ Systems	Malformations Identified	Associated Genetic Syndromes and Other Anomalies
Cardiac	Arrhythmias	Maternal autoimmune disease
	Various anatomic	Short-limbed polydactly syndromes; trisomy 13; 9p–13q-
	Valvular anomalies: tetralogy of Fallot, pulmonary and aortic stenosis	Noonan syndrome
	Transposition of great vessels	
	Septal wall defects	Trisomy 21; cardiosplenic defects; Holt-Oram syndrome
	Hypoplastic left heart	
Central nervous system	Spina bifida	Iniencephaly sequence
	Anencephaly	
	Encephalocele	Meckel-Gruber syndrome
	Hydrocephalus	X-linked aqueductal stenosis; Dandy-Walker malformation with or without associated malformations
	Holoprosencephaly	Trisomy 13; Meckel-Gruber syndrome; 18p-syndrome; 13q- syndrome; holoprosencephaly sequence; autosomal dominant holoprosencephaly
	Agenesis of corpus callosum	Trisomy 13; trisomy 18; Aicardi syndrome; Andermann syndrome; FG syndrome
Chest	Diaphragmatic hernia	Tetrasomy 12p (Pallister-Killian syndrome)
	Congenital cysts	
Gastrointestinal	Esophageal atresia	Trisomy 21; other associated anomalies of CNS, urinary tract, heart
	Duodenal atresia	Trisomy 21; other associated anomalies of CNS, urinary tract, heart
	Jejunal-ileal atresia	Cystic fibrosis (rarely)
	Other intestinal atresias	Cystic fibrosis (rarely)
Body wall	Gastroschisis	
	Omphalocele	Trisomy 13, 18; Pentalogy of Cantrell; Beckwith-Wiedemann syndrome; amniotic band sequence
	Cloacal extrophy	Pentalogy of Cantrell
	Bladder extrophy	
Renal	Polycystic disease	Infantile polycystic kidney disease; adult polycystic kidney disease (rarely prenatal); Meckel-Gruber syndrome
		Potter sequence; triploidy
	Obstructive uropathy	"Prune belly" sequence
Skeleton	Osteochondrodysplasia	Jarcho-Levin syndrome; diastropic dysplasia; short-limbed polydactyly syndromes; Camptomelic dysplasia; tetraphocomelia; achondroplasia; thanatophoric dysplasia; asphyxiating thoracic dysplasia (Jeune)
	Fractures	Osteogenesis imperfecta
Head, face, neck	Skull abnormalities	Craniosynostosis syndromes
	Microcephaly	Trisomy 4p; Trisomy 13; Trisomy 18; 4p-; 5p-; 13q-; large number of other genetic syndromes
	Cleft lip, palate	Trisomy 13; some skeletal dysplasias
	Cystic hygroma	Turner syndrome

Table 7–3. Genetic disorders with implications for pregnancy[1]

Disorder	Medical Complications Which Can Occur During and After Pregnancy
Marfan syndrome	Aortic rupture before, during, and **after** labor and delivery
Ehlers-Danlos syndrome	Vascular rupture; uterine rupture
Pseudoxanthoma elasticum	Bleeding, abnormal placentation
Skeletal dysplasias	Respiratory compromise from thoracic dysplasia; pelvic abnormalities requiring operative delivery; decreased mobility of spine, including cervical spine
Cystic fibrosis	Increased fetal wastage, premature labor, pulmonary compromise, cor pulmonale, hypoxia in mother
Myotonic dystrophy	Premature labor; postpartum complications
Neurofibromatosis	Increase in size and number of neurofibromata; eclampsia; thrombocytopenia
Ornithine transcarbamylase deficiency	Acute hyperammonemia and coma at and after delivery
Heterozygosity for disorders of fatty acid metabolism	Jaundice, liver failure
Lysinuric protein intolerance	Thrombocytopenia
Homocystinuria	Thrombophlebitis
Coagulopathies	Post-partum bleeding

[1] Data from Burrow and Ferris.

miliar with the known associations of congenital malformations and genetic syndromes (Table 7–3). Often serial examination must be performed to be certain that a given finding is associated with pathology.

Fetal Diagnostic Methods

Modern prenatal diagnostic techniques can provide a great deal of information about fetal genetic status. Maternal serum screening can identify pregnancies at risk for open body wall defects and chromosome abnormalities and can serve as a screen for fetal well being. Ultrasound when non-focused looks at fetal anatomy in general. Focused ultrasound examination looks at specific anatomical structures. Most other tests are specific to answer a particular question. Cytogenetic studies are done when there is a reason to suspect a chromosomal abnormality because of maternal age, prior chromosomal abnormality or abnormal maternal screening result, or structural abnormality seen at ultrasound examination. Biochemical and molecular studies usually relate to a specific gene, enzyme, metabolite or protein. No test can guarantee that the unborn baby is "normal" or that no genetic problems exist.

The following categories of information can be obtained from available prenatal tests:

- Status of anatomic structures
- Analyte concentration for inborn errors of metabolism
- Chromosomal status

- Specific molecular analysis addressing mutation at risk
- Linkage data to allow calculation of risk in a family at known risk.

Indications for Prenatal Diagnosis

Identification of genetic risk is often based on family history or previous pregnancy outcome. Other factors also indicate that a pregnancy is at increased risk for a genetic disorder. These include:

- Ethnic background with known risk
- Family history of genetic disease
- Paternal or maternal disease
- Adverse outcome in a previous pregnancy
- Maternal age
- Maternal teratogen exposure
- Maternal or paternal exposure to high dose radiation.

Special Considerations in Counseling

The woman and her partner should be part of discussion of options for prenatal diagnosis and for management when abnormalities are identified. The physician who counsels the patient and family in this setting must have expertise regarding the abnormalities that have been diagnosed. The limitations of the diagnostic methods need to be explicitly discussed. Such a discussion will help the couple to make an informed decision about terminating the pregnancy or allowing it to continue.

The decision to terminate a pregnancy is never an easy one. Nevertheless, it is an essential option for a family confronted with the diagnosis in a fetus of a disorder incompatible with life or normal development. For many genetic disorders diagnosed prenatally, particularly chromosome abnormalities and neurologic disorders, no therapy is available, and pregnancy termination is the option favored by most families. If early diagnosis has been made by ultrasound or CVS the woman may decide to terminate the pregnancy at a time when the risks and discomfort for her are lower than they would be with a later termination. The family needs compassionate concern during this decision-making. The woman must have access to appropriate technical expertise. In addition, steps need to be taken to corroborate genetic diagnosis after termination. The physician needs to obtain tissue for cytogenetic, biochemical, or molecular analysis, depending on the nature of the disorder that has been diagnosed prenatally. In the case of a later termination or one in which congenital malformations were identified, a full autopsy on the fetus may be the most suitable procedure. The physician should report results of these corroborative studies to the parents personally. Post-abortion counseling regarding the loss of a baby that was wanted and had serious medical problems is an important adjunct. The family has experienced the loss of a wanted child and is often faced with the risk of recurrence of this unfortunate situation in a subsequent pregnancy.

Planning for an infant with special needs is critical if the decision is to continue the pregnancy. The decision to accept the birth of a child with special needs must be carefully informed. Parents should have an opportunity to talk with parents of children with the same or a similar condition. Discussion with a parent support group may fill this need. The family will need to assess financial, social, and community resources carefully. They must consider the impact on their other children. The consequences of the need for long-term care are important factors when conditions are diagnosed which require multiple medical and surgical interventions or for which no treatment can be offered and chronic custodial care may become necessary. When a congenital malformation such as omphalocele, diaphragmatic hernia, congenital heart malformation, or neural tube defect has been made, delivery should be arranged at a center with the medical and surgical resources needed for optimal care of the child immediately after birth.

PRENATAL THERAPY & OTHER CONSIDERATIONS

Prenatal therapy is still largely an investigative option and has not yet become an available clinical tool. A few examples of effective medical fetal therapy exist for rare inborn errors of intermediary metabolism. Vitamin B_{12}-responsive methylmalonic acidemia has been treated by giving the mother large amounts of vitamin B_{12}; the vitamin crosses the placenta and normalizes the metabolic status of the fetus. Biotin-responsive multiple carboxylase deficiency has been treated by giving biotin to the mother in the same fashion. Fetal surgery is a potentially exciting way to correct fetal congenital malformations early enough to prevent permanent damage. Catheter drainage for bladder obstruction due to posterior urethral valves, hydrocephalus, hydronephrosis, and hydrothorax has been tried with varying success, but outcome has been generally disappointing. There is moratorium on catheter placement for hydrocephalus, but catheter placement for drainage of bladder obstruction and for hydrothorax can be successful in skilled hands. Open fetal surgery in both primate models and humans is being studied. The studies have demonstrated no threat to maternal health or future reproduction related to the fetal surgery. However, premature labor and less than optimal fetal outcome are problems that must be solved if these surgical techniques are to fulfill their promise.

Adoption and Assisted Reproduction

Many families choose to avoid the risk of genetic disease in a child, and instead select adoption or assisted reproduction to avoid these risks. Adoption remains common and popular, but waiting lists are long. Artificial insemination by donor avoids the risks associated with autosomal dominant or autosomal recessive mutations that may be inherited from the father. It also avoids risks resulting from paternal exposure to high dose radiation which may increase the risk of chromosome abnormalities in the offspring. When a family is attempting to avoid a single gene disorder, the donor should be tested for that disorder if possible. In addition, the donor should be tested for any mutations that are common in his ethnic group.

Assisted reproduction employing in vitro fertilization (IVF) using donor egg or sperm is now being used by some families at genetic risk. The selection of the parental gamete depends upon which parent carries a deleterious mutation or chromosomal translocation. IVF using gametes from both members of the couple and subsequent blastocyst diagnosis to address the risk to the fetus is a new tool under investigation. It is costly and time-consuming. The safety of blastocyst development following the diagnostic procedure is unproven. The use of reproductive technology with IVF is expensive; recent estimates range from $44,000 to more than $200,000 per delivery. Such technology also leads to pregnancies with multiple gestation; twins, triplets, and higher order multiple gestations occur considerably more often than in naturally occurring pregnancies.

The ability to diagnose genetic disease and congenital malformations in utero has greatly increased the options for families facing genetic risks and has improved their chances for having healthy children. The importance of identifying those at risk and providing them with appropriate counseling and access to expert diagnostic facilities cannot be overemphasized. The future holds much promise for the improvement of existing diagnostic and therapeutic techniques and for the addition of new ones. Several new diagnostic possibilities are on the horizon. Research is being directed at separation of fetal cells from the maternal circulation, which would allow prenatal diagnosis of some conditions using a sample of maternal blood instead of today's invasive methods. However, enrichment of the sample for fetal cells needs to be improved before such methods can become a clinical reality. Increased molecular understanding of genetic disease will lead to improved assignment of risk for many families. Reproductive technologies would have to be more practical and less costly for the use of pre-implantation diagnosis to become widespread. In addition, the potential risk to the developing embryo must be demonstrated to be small. When prenatal therapy becomes more effective, its use will depend upon safe, accurate prenatal diagnosis.

REFERENCES AND SUGGESTED READING

Ampola MG et al: Prenatal therapy of a patient with vitamin B_{12}-responsive methylmalonic acidemia. N Engl J Med 1975;**293:**313.

Assimakopoulos E, Zheng X, Hobbins JC: The safety of obstetric ultrasonography: concern for the fetus. Obstet Gynecol 1990;**76:**139.

Bahado-Singh RO et al: Invasive techniques for prenatal diagnosis: Current Concepts. In press.

Bell JG, Weiner ST: Cordocentesis. Current Opinion on Obstetrics and Gynecology 1993;**5:**218.

Bergoffen J et al: Diaphragmatic hernia in tetrasomy 12p mosaicism. J Pediatr 1993;**122:**603.

Brambati B, Simoni G: Diagnosis of fetal trisomy 21 in first trimester. Lancet 1983;**i:**586.

Brambati B et al: First trimester fetal diagnosis of genetic disorders: clinical evaluation of 250 cases. J Med Genet 1985;**22:**92.

Brenton DP et al: Pregnancy and homocystinuria. Ann Clin Biochem 1977;**14:**161.

Brodie MJ et al: Pregnancy and the acute porphyrias. Br J Obstet Gynaecol 1977;**84:**726.

Buehler BA et al: Prenatal prediction of risk of the fetal hydantoin syndrome. N Engl J Med 1990;**322:**1567.

Burton BK, Schulz CJ, Burd LI: Limb anomalies associated with chorionic villus sampling. Obstet Gynecol 1992;**79:**726.

Caldwell DC, Williamson RA, Goldsmith JC: Hereditary coagulopathies in pregnancy. Clin Obstet Gynecol 1895;**28:**53.

Canadian Collaborative CVS-Amniocentesis Clinical Trial Group. Multicentre randomised clinical trial of chorionic villus sampling and amniocentesis. Lancet 1989;**1:**1.

Centers for Disease Control. Recommendations for the use of folic acid to reduce the number of cases of spina bifida and other neural tube defects. MMWR 1992;**41:**1.

Chervenak FA, Issacson G, Mahoney MJ: Advances in the diagnosis of fetal defects. N Engl J Med 1986;**315:**305.

Clinton MJ, Niederman MS, Matthay RA: Maternal pulmonary disorders complicating pregnancy. Pages 955–981 in: *Medicine of the Fetus and Mother.* Reece EA et al (editors). Lippincott, 1992.

Collins JC: Reproductive technology: The price of progress. N Engl J Med 1994;**331:**270.

Crandall BF: Alpha fetoprotein. Pages 267–290 in: *Assessment and Care of the Fetus: Physiological, Clinical, and Medicolegal Principles.* Eden RD, Boehm FH (editors). Appleton & Lange, 1990.

Crandall BF et al: ACMG position statement on multiple marker screening in women 35 and older. American College of Medical Genetics Newsletter 1994;**2.**

Cross PK, Hook EB: An analysis of paternal age and 47, +21 in 35,000 new prenatal cytogenetic diagnosis data from the New York State Chromosome Registry: No significant effect. Hum Genet 1987;**77:**307.

Cuckle HS, Wald NJ: Prenatal diagnosis and prognosis. In: *Screening for Down's syndrome.* Lilford RJ (editor). Butterworths, 1992.

Dallaire L, Potier M: Amniotic fluid. Pages 59–122 in: *Genetic Disorders and the Fetus.* Milunsky A (editor). Johns Hopkins Press, 1992.

D'Alton ME, DeCherney AH: Prenatal Diagnosis. N Engl J Med 1993;**328:**114.

de la Cruz F: Report of NICHHD workshop on chorionic villus sampling and limb and other defects, October 20, 1992. Am J Obstet Gynecol 1993;**169:**1.

de la Cruz F: Report of National Institute of Health and Human Development workshop on chorionic villus sampling and limb and other defects, October 20, 1992. Teratology 1993;**48:**7.

Elias S, Simpson JL: Amniocentesis. In: *Genetic Disorders and the Fetus.* Milunsky A (editor). Johns Hopkins Press, 1992.

Ferguson-Smith MA et al: Avoidance of anencephalic and spina bifida births by maternal serum-α-fetoprotein screening. Lancet 1978;**i:**1330.

Fleischer AC, Jeanty P: Obstetric Ultrasonography. Pages 247–258 in: *Assessment and Care of the Fetus: Physiological, Clinical, and Medicolegal Principles.* Eden RD, Boehm FH (editor). Appleton & Lange, 1990.

Gabbe SG, Niebyl JR, Simpson JL: *Obstetrics: Normal and Problem Pregnancies.* Churchill Livingstone, 1991.

Gabrelli S, Pilu G: Prenatal diagnosis of anomalies of the head and neck and central nervous system. Pages 500–524 in: *Medicine of the Fetus and Mother.* Reece EA et al (editors). Lippincott, 1992.

Gabrelli S, Reece EA: Gastrointestinal and genitourinary anomalies. Pages 550–577 in: *Medicine of the Fetus and Mother.* Reece EA et al (editors). Lippincott, 1992.

Golbus MS, Appelman Z: Chorionic villus sampling. Pages 259–265 in: *Assessment and Care of the Fetus: Physio-*

logical, Clinical, and Medicolegal Principles. Eden RD, Boehm FH (editors). Appleton & Lange, 1990.

Golbus MS et al: Prenatal Genetic Diagnosis in 3000 Amniocenteses. N Engl J Med 1979;**300:**157.

Haddow JE et al: Data from an α-fetoprotein pilot screening program in Maine. Obstet Gynecol 1983;**62:**556.

Haddow JE et al: Reducing the need for amniocentesis in women 35 years of age or older with serum markers for screening. N Engl J Med 1994;**330:**1114.

Handyside AH et al: Birth of a normal girl after in vitro fertilization and preimplantation diagnostic testing for cystic fibrosis. N Engl J Med 1992;**327:**905.

Harley HG et al: Detection of linkage disequilibrium between the myotonic dystrophy locus and a new polymorphic DNA marker. Am J Hum Genet 1991;**49:**68.

Harley HG et al: Expansion of an unstable DNA region and phenotypic variation in myotonic dystrophy. Nature 1992;**355:**545.

Hobbins JC et al: Percutaneous fetal umbilical blood sampling. Am J Obstet Gynecol 1985;**152:**1.

Hogge WA, Schonberg SA, Golbus MS: Chorionic villus sampling: Experience of the first 1000 cases. Am J Obstet Gynecol 1986;**154:**1249.

Jackson LG, Zachary JM, Fowler SE: A randomized comparison of transcervical and transabdominal chorionic-villus sampling. N Engl J Med 1992;**327:**594.

Jaffe R, Mock M, Abramowicz J: Myotonic dystrophy and pregnancy: A review. Obstet Gynecol Surv 1986;**31:**272.

Jahoda MGJ et al: Terminal transverse limb defects and early chorionic villus sampling: Evaluation of 4,300 cases with completed follow-up. Am J Med Genet 1993; **46:**483.

Jones KL et al: Pattern of malformations in the children of women treated with carbamazepine during pregnancy. N Engl J Med 1989;**320:**1661.

Kazy Z, Rozovsky IS, Bakharev VA: Chorion biopsy in early pregnancy: a method of early prenatal diagnosis for inherited disorders. Prenat Diagn 1982;**2:**39.

Lockwood CJ, Copel JA, Hobbins JC: Congenital anomalies. Pages 483–557 in: *Assessment and Care of the Fetus: Physiological, Clinical, and Medicolegal Principles.* Eden RD, Boehm FH (editors). Appleton & Lange, 1990.

Longaker MT et al: Maternal outcome after open fetal surgery. JAMA 1991;**265:**737.

Ludomirski A, Weiner S: Percutaneous fetal umbilical blood sampling. Clin Obstet Gynecol 1988;**31:**19.

Macri JN, Haddow JE, Weiss RR: Screening for neural tube defects in the United States. Am J Obstet Gynecol 1979;**133:**119.

Mahoney MJ: Limb abnormalities and chorionic villus sampling. Lancet 1991;**337:**1422.

Manning FA et al: Catheter shunts for fetal hydronephrosis and hydrocephalus. N Engl J Med 1986;**315:**336.

Mastroiacovo P, Botto LD: Chorionic villus sampling and birth defects: A review. Proceedings of the III ASM International Symposium on Birth Defects 1992:149.

Mastroiacovo P et al: Limb anomalies following chorionic villus sampling: A registry based case-control study. Am J Med Genet 1992;**44:**856.

Meizner I, Glezerman MT: Cordocentesis in the evaluation of the growth-retarded fetus. Clin Obstet Gynecol 1992; **35:**126.

Milo R et al: Acute intermittent porphyria in pregnancy. Obstet Gynecol 1989;**73:**450.

Milunsky A: Maternal serum screening for neural tube and other defects. Pages 507–563 in: *Genetic Disorders and the Fetus.* Milunsky A (editor). Johns Hopkins Press, 1992.

Milunsky A: The use of biochemical markers in maternal serum screening for chromosome defects. Pages 565–592 in: *Genetic Disorders and the Fetus.* Milunsky A (editor). Johns Hopkins Press, 1992.

Milunsky A, Alpert E: Results and benefits of a maternal serum α-fetoprotein screening program. JAMA 1984; **252:**1438.

MRS Vitamin Study Research Group. Prevention of neural tube defects: results of the Medical Research Council Vitamin Study. Lancet 1991;**338:**131.

Myring J et al: Specific molecular prenatal diagnosis for the CTG mutation in myotonic dystrophy. J Med Genet 1992;**29:**785.

Neumann PJ, Gharib SD, Weinstein MC: The cost of a successful delivery with in vitro fertilization. N Engl J Med 1994;**331:**239.

NICHD National Registry for Amniocentesis Study Group. Midtrimester amniocentesis for prenatal diagnosis: safety and accuracy. JAMA 1976;**236:**1471.

Nicolaides KH, Thorpe-Beeston, Noble P: Cordocentesis. Pages 291–306 in: *Assessment and Care of the Fetus: Physiological, Clinical, and Medicolegal Principles.* Eden RD, Boehm FH (editor). Appleton & Lange, 1990.

Packman S et al: Prenatal treatment of biotin-responsive multiple carboxylase deficiency. Lancet 1982;**i:**1435.

Palomaki GE, Haddow J: Maternal serum a-fetoprotein, age and Down syndrome risk. Am J Obstet Gynecol 1987;**156:**460.

Pauker SP, Pauker SG: Prenatal diagnosis—why is 35 a magic number? N Engl J Med 1994;**330:**1151.

Pilu G: Prenatal diagnosis of cardiovascular anomalies. Pages 533–549 in: *Medicine of the Fetus and Mother.* Reece EA et al (editors). Lippincott, 1992.

Platt LD et al: Maternal phenylketonuria collaborative study, obstetric aspects and outcome: The first 6 years. Am J Obstet Gynecol 1992;**166:**1150.

Puls LE, Chandler PA: Malignant schwannoma in pregnancy. Acta Obstet Gynecol Scand 1991;**70:**243.

Reece EA: Fetal thoracic malformations. Pages 525–532 in: *Medicine of the Fetus and Mother.* Reece EA et al (editors). Lippincott, 1992.

Reece EA et al: The safety of obstetric ultrasonography: concern for the fetus. Obstet Gynecol 1990;**76:**139.

Reece EA, Copel J: Basic principles of ultrasonography. Pages 489–499 in: *Medicine of the Fetus and Mother.* Reece EA et al (editors). Lippincott, 1992.

Rhoads GG et al: The safety and efficacy of chorionic villus sampling for early prenatal diagnosis of cytogenetic abnormalities. N Engl J Med 1989;**320:**609.

Rodeck CH et al: Long-term in utero drainage of fetal hydrothorax. N Engl J Med 1988;**319:**1135.

Romero R et al: Sonographically monitored amniocentesis to decrease intraoperative complications. Obstet Gynecol 1985;**65:**426.

Romero R, Nores J: Fetal skeletal anomalies. Pages 578–616 in: *Medicine of the Fetus and Mother.* Reece EA et al (editors). Lippincott, 1992.

Rucquoi J: Genetic counselling and prenatal genetic evaluation. Medicine North America 1983;**36:**3359.

Sancho S et al: Analysis of dystrophin expression after activation of myogenesis in amniocytes, chorionic villus cells, and fibroblasts: A new method for diagnosing

Duchenne's muscular dystrophy. N Engl J Med 1993;**329**:915.

Schloo R et al: Distal limb deficiency following chorionic villus sampling? Am J Med Genet 1992;**42**:404.

Seashore MR: Clinical genetics. Pages 218–248 in: *Medical Complications During Pregnancy.* Burrow GN, Ferris TF (editors). WB Saunders, 1994.

Sharma JB, Gulati N, Malik S: Maternal and perinatal complications in neurofibromatosis during pregnancy. Int J Gynaecol Obstet 1991;**34**:221.

Simoni G et al: Efficient direct chromosome analyses and enzyme determinations from chorionic villi samples in the first trimester of pregnancy. Hum Genet 1983;**63**:349.

Simpson JL, Elias S: Isolating fetal cells from maternal blood: Advances in prenatal diagnosis through molecular technology. JAMA 1993;**270**:2357.

Simpson NE et al: Prenatal diagnosis of genetic disease in Canada: Report of a collaborative study. Can Med Assoc J 1976;**115**:739.

Stark CR et al: Short- and long-term risks after exposure to diagnostic ultrasound in utero. Obstet Gynecol 1984;**63**:194.

Steele MW, Breg WR: Chromosome analysis of human amniotic fluid cells. Lancet 1966;**1**:383.

Wald NJ, Cuckle H: Maternal serum-α-fetoprotein measurement in antenatal screening for anencephaly and spina bifida in early pregnancy: Report of U.K. Collaborative Study on α-fetoprotein in Relation to Neural-tube Defects. Lancet 1977;**i**:1323.

Ward H: Review of the development and current status of techniques for monitoring embryonic and fetal development in the first trimester of pregnancy. Am J Med Genet 1990;**35**:157.

Wilson RD, Chitayat D, McGillivray BC: Fetal ultrasound abnormalities: Correlation with fetal karyotype, autopsy findings, and postnatal outcome—five-year prospective study. Am J Med Genet 1992;**44**:586.

Wladimiroff JW et al: Prenatal diagnosis of chromosome abnormalities in the presence of fetal structural defects. Am J Med Genet 1988:289.

Zheng Y, Carter NP, Price CM: Prenatal diagnosis from maternal blood: Simultaneous immunophenotyping and FISH of fetal nucleated erythrocytes isolated by negative magnetic cell sorting. J Med Genet 1993;**30**:1051.

Cardiovascular System

8

STRUCTURAL CARDIAC DEFECTS

The cardiovascular system begins its development during the third week of fetal life. Formation of the heart and major vessels occurs between the third and eighth weeks; cardiac contractions start at 21–22 days. The conduction system, which begins to develop at the fifth week, continues differentiation up to and after birth. The most sensitive time for disturbances in the formation of the cardiovascular system is between the 20th and 50th day of fetal life.

Congenital Structural Cardiac Defects: Congenital structural cardiac defects occur in approximately 8–10 per 1000 births. They are more common in stillbirths (27 per 1000) than live births (4–8 per 1000). The majority of these structural abnormalities occur as isolated cardiac defects. Twenty percent of patients with congenital cardiac defects, however, have more than one cardiac defect, eg, a ventricular septal defect with a patent ductus arteriosus. In addition, approximately 25% (9–45% in various studies) of patients with congenital cardiac defects also have other noncardiac malformations that most commonly involve the musculoskeletal system (9%), central nervous system (8%), urinary tract or kidneys (5%), or gastrointestinal tract (4%); 1.8% have cleft palate. Congenital heart defects account for approximately 25% of all congenital malformations, 50% of deaths from congenital malformations, and 15% of all infant deaths.

Congenital heart defects are usually sporadic, and of multifactorial etiology. About 10% are associated with syndromes, 5–8% result from chromosomal abnormalities, 3–5% are from single gene defects, and 2–3% are related to environmental factors. For isolated defects, the risk of recurrence for an affected sibling ranges from 1–6%. With an affected parent, the risk is as high as 12%; affected mothers are more likely than affected fathers to have affected children. The risk of recurrence doubles with two affected first-degree relatives.

Congenital heart defects that are familial and inherited, either as an isolated defect or as part of a syndrome, have a higher risk of recurrence, depending upon the type of inheritance involved. For example, the risk is 50% for an autosomal dominant trait and 25% for an autosomal recessive trait. For congenital heart disease associated with a teratogen, the risk of recurrence is related to repeat exposure to the agent or maternal disease. For example, each pregnancy of an insulin-dependent diabetic mother carries an 8% chance of congenital heart disease, especially for transposition of the great vessels. And, each pregnancy of a mother with uncontrolled phenylketonuria (PKU) has a 10% risk for major congenital heart disease.

Table 8–1 lists the genetic characteristics of the more common congenital heart defects. The most common, which results in the formation of a bicuspid rather than the normal tricuspid aortic valve, occurs in approximately 1% of the general population. The second most common, ventral septal defect, has an incidence of 1 in 800. Table 8–2 lists common genetic disorders and teratogens, with their associated congenital heart defects. Septal defects are more frequently isolated and sporadic, whereas conotruncal defects (defects in division of the truncus arteriosus, eg, transposition of the great vessels) are more likely to be associated with syndromes and teratogens.

Dextrocardia: Dextrocardia, which occurs in 1 in 10,000 live births, may develop with or without visceral situs inversus. When it occurs without situs inversus, dextrocardia is frequently associated with other major heart defects (MIM 304750). Persons with dextrocardia with situs inversus may also have asplenia-polysplenia syndrome (MIM 208530) or Kartagener syndrome (MIM 244400).

COMMON SYNDROMES WITH CONGENITAL HEART DISEASE AS A MAJOR FINDING

Cornelia de Lange Syndrome (de Lange Syndrome): Cornelia de Lange syndrome (de Lange syndrome) occurs in 1 in 20,000 live births. The major clinical findings include growth deficiency of prenatal onset; microcephaly with severe mental retardation; anomalies of the extremities including micromelia; and a characteristic facies with long eyelashes, bushy eyebrows which meet in the midline (synophrys), anteverted nares, long philtrum, and a characteristic thin downturning upper lip. Twenty-nine percent of patients with Cornelia de Lange syndrome have congenital heart defects, most frequently ventricular septal defects. Although most cases are not inherited, an autosomal dominant pattern of in-

Table 8–1. Congenital heart defects (CHD).

Defect	Incidence in Live Births	Male:Female Ratio	% of CHD	% Associated with Other Birth Defects	Inheritance	Risk for Affected Sibling with Isolated Defect and Negative Family History	Commonly Associated Syndromes; Comments
Ventricular septal defect (VSD)	1 in 800	1:1	24–34.6%	30–40%	Sporadic; AD, AR	3–6%	
Atrial septal defect (ASD)	1 in 2300	1:1.6	5.6–15%	30%	Sporadic, AD	2.5–3%	Holt-Oram, Ellis-van Creveld
Endocardial cushion defect (ECD)	1 in 6500	1:1	2.4–8.6%	75%	Sporadic, AD, AR	1.4–2%	20% of Down have ECD; 30% ECD in Down
Tetralogy of Fallot (ToF)	1 in 2000	1.4:1	3.7–9.2%	30%	Sporadic	2.5%	Goldenhar, DiGeorge
Transposition of the great arteries (TGA)	1 in 3500	2.6:1	2.6–6.0	8%	Sporadic	2%	8% diabetic progeny; maternal collagen vascular disease
Truncus arteriosus communis (TAC)	1 in 30,000	1.6:1	1.1–2.5%	30%	Sporadic	1–6%	
Double outlet right ventricle (DORV)	1 in 30,000		0.6–1%		Sporadic	2%	
Patent ductus arteriosus (PDA)	1 in 1200 term infants	1:1.9	2.6–12.6%		Sporadic, AD, AR	2.5–3%	Fetal rubella exposure
Coarctation of the aorta (AoCo)	1 in 2500	2.3:1	3.4–9.8%	20%	Sporadic, AD	2%	10–15% of Turner.
Aortic stenosis (AoS)	1 in 3000	4:1	3–6%	20%	Sporadic; SVAS, AD	2–3%	Williams (SVAS); 85% have BAV
Bicuspid aortic valve (BAV)	1 in 100	M>F			Sporadic, 17–34% AD	3%	20–40% of Turner
Pulmonary stenosis (PS)	1 in 2000	1:1	10.5%	15%	Sporadic, AD, AR	2–3%	LEOPARD, Noonan, fetal rubella exposure
Pulmonary atresia (PA)	1 in 30,000		1.5%	10%	Sporadic	1%	
Tricuspid atresia (TAt)	1 in 10,000	1:1	1.6%	10%	Sporadic	1%	
Ebstein anomaly (EA)	1 in 30,000		1%	25%	Sporadic	1%	Turner; fetal lithium exposure
Hypoplastic left heart syndrome (HLH)	1 in 12,000	2:1	1–2%	10–37%	Sporadic, AR	1–2%	
Single ventricle (SV)	1 in 30,000		0.9%		Sporadic, AD	2.8%	
Total anomalous pulmonary venous return (TAPVR)	1 in 20,000	4:1	0.6–2.1%	10%	Sporadic, AD	3%	

AD = autosomal dominant, AR = autosomal recessive, SVAS = supravalvular aortic stenosis.

Table 8–2. Genetic disorders and associated congenital heart defects.

Genetic Disorder	VSD	ASD	ECD	CT	PDA	AoCo	AoS	BAV	PS	SV	HLH	TAPVR
Chromosomal												
Trisomy 21	++	+	++	+	+				+	+		
Trisomy 18	++	+		+	++	+		+	+	+	+	
Trisomy 13	++	++		+	+			+	+		+	
Turner Syndrome	+	+				++	+	+			+	+
Triploidy	+	+	+	+	+							
Other	+	+	+	+	+	+	+	+	+	+	+	+
Single Gene Disorders												
Alagille (AD)		+	+	+	+	+			+			
Holt-Oram (AD)	++	++	+	+	+				+		+	+
LEOPARD (AD)							+		++			
Ellis-van Creveld (AR)		++	++							+		
Smith-Lemli-Opitz (AR)		+	+		+	+	+				+	+
Disorders with MCA												
Asplenia-Polysplenia	+	+	+	1	+				+	+	+	+
Beckwith-Wiedemann	+	+		+	+	+					+	
CHARGE association	++	++	+	++	++	+		+				+
Cornelia de Lange	++	+		+		+						
DiGeorge sequence	+			++	+			+	+		+	
Goldenhar s.	+	+		2	+	+						
Noonan s.		+		+	+				++			
Pierre Robin sequence	+	+	+	+	+	+						
Rubenstein-Taybi s.	+			+	+	+			+			
VATER association	++	+		+	+	+					+	
Williams s.	+	+			+		++		+			
Teratogens												
Alcohol	++	++	+	+	+	+			+			
Lithium	+			+	+							
Maternal collagen vascular disease				+	+				+			
Maternal diabetes	+		+	1	+	+			+	+	+	+
Maternal PKU	+	+		2	+	+				+	+	
Phenytoin	+	+		+	++	+	+		+			
Retionic acid	++	+		1,2	+			+	+	+	+	
Rubella	+	+		+	++	+	+		++			+
Trimethadione	+			1,2	+						+	
Valproic acid	++			+	++							

++ = frequently seen; + = may be seen; s = syndrome; AD = autosomal dominant; AR = autosomal recessive; CT = conotruncal defects; MCA = multiple congenital anomalies; 1 = TGA, 2 = ToF; see Table 8–1 for abbreviations for other types of CHD.

heritance has been suggested in some families (MIM 122470). A phenotype similar to de Lange syndrome is seen in patients with duplications of the q25–29 region of chromosome 3.

Ellis-Van Creveld Syndrome: Ellis-van Creveld syndrome, an autosomal recessive chondroectodermal dysplasia (MIM 225500), is frequently seen among the Amish. Affected patients have dispropor-

tionate short stature with short, especially distal, extremities; small thorax; post-axial polydactyly of the fingers; hypoplastic nails and teeth; and a short upper lip bound by a frenula to the alveolar ridge. Approximately one-half of patients with Ellis-van Creveld syndrome have congenital heart defects, most commonly large atrial septal defects.

Goldenhar Syndrome (Oculoauricular Verte-

bral): Goldenhar syndrome (oculoauricular vertebral) is part of the facioauriculovertebral spectrum of defects that occur in 1 in 3000 to 5000 births (MIM 164210, 257700). Abnormal development of the first and second branchial arches results in variable degrees of asymmetric facial hypoplasia, hypoplasia of the external ear (microtia) and middle ear, hearing impairment, preauricular tags and/or pits, and a lateral cleft-like extension of the corner of the mouth. The presence of hemivertebrae or hypoplasia of the vertebral bodies (especially in the cervical area), and ocular epibulbar dermoids (occasionally associated with notches on the upper eyelids) distinguishes Goldenhar syndrome from the less involved **hemifacial microsomia syndrome.** With Goldenhar syndrome, congenital heart disease is common; ventricular septal defects, patent ductus arteriosus, tetralogy of Fallot, and coarctation of the aorta are most frequently noted. Goldenhar syndrome is usually sporadic; familial cases, however, with an autosomal dominant pattern of inheritance have been reported.

Holt-Oram Syndrome (Heart-hand Syndrome: In the Holt-Oram syndrome (heart-hand syndrome, MIM 152900), congenital heart defects are associated with hypoplasia of the upper limb and shoulder girdle. Variable upper limb defects, frequently asymmetric, may include a triphalangeal, finger-like thumb. Atrial septal detects, occasionally with an arrhythmia, and ventricular septal defects are most commonly noted. One-third of affected patients have other cardiac defects, including patent ductus arteriosus and pulmonary stenosis. The disorder is inherited as an autosomal dominant trait that may manifest only as a unilateral thumb abnormality.

Noonan Syndrome: Noonan syndrome, which is of unknown etiology, produces a Turner syndrome-like phenotype, eg, short stature, epicanthal folds and hypertelorism, low posterior hairline with short or webbed neck, shield chest, cubitus valgus, and abnormal ears. In contrast to Turner syndrome, which is associated with an X chromosomal abnormality and seen only in females, Noonan syndrome occurs in both males and females. Fifty percent of patients have short stature; 25% have psychomotor retardation. Affected males may have undescended testes, hypogonadism or small penis. Congenital heart defects are common, including pulmonary valve and supravalvular stenosis, peripheral pulmonary stenosis, septal defects and patent ductus arteriosus. Noonan syndrome is usually sporadic; families with an autosomal dominant pattern of inheritance have been reported, however (MIM 163950).

Williams Syndrome (Idiopathic Hypercalcemia, Supravalvular Aortic Stenosis): Patients with Williams syndrome (idiopathic hypercalcemia, supravalvular aortic stenosis) have a characteristic "elfin" facies with short palpebral fissures, epicanthal folds, periorbital fullness, anteverted nose with long prominent philtrum, micrognathia, and prominent full lips. Short stature, thin build, hoarse voice, brachydactyly, hypoplastic nails and teeth, and bladder diverticulae are frequently noted. Although most patients are moderately mentally handicapped, they have a friendly, loquacious personality. In some patients, especially during infancy, hypercalcemia, hypercalcuria, and nephrocalcinosis may occur. Most patients with Williams syndrome have associated congenital heart disease that may include supravalvular aortic stenosis (SVAS), peripheral pulmonary artery stenosis, pulmonic valvular stenosis, or septal defects. Patients may have other arterial vascular anomalies, including renal artery stenosis and hypoplastic aorta; they are also at increased risk for arterial thromboses and strokes. Williams syndrome is associated with abnormalities in a contiguous gene region at chromosome 7q11.23, which spans and extends beyond the elastin gene locus. Using chromosomal fluorescent in situ hybridization (FISH) studies with probes for the elastin gene, 92–95% of patients with Williams syndrome will have a deletion of one of the elastin genes. Mutations and partial deletions of the elastin gene have also been noted in patients with autosomal dominant isolated SVAS. Williams syndrome is usually sporadic; families with an autosomal dominant pattern of inheritance, however, have been noted (MIM 194050) (Figure 8–1).

Patients with either the **DiGeorge sequence** (MIM 188400) or the **Velocardiofacial syndrome** (MIM 192430), both discussed in detail in the section on immunology, have a high incidence of cardiac malformations. Many of the patients with either of these disorders have a deletion of the q11.2 region of chromosome 22. Because conotruncal defects are common in patients with either the DiGeorge sequence or the VCFS syndrome, and the clinical spectrum of findings in both disorders may be variable, it is recommended that chromosomal FISH studies, employing a probe for chromosome region 22q11.2, be done in all patients with conotrunchal cardiac defects. Congenital heart disease is also common in patients with the **CHARGE** (MIM 214800) and **VATER** (MIM 192350) **associations,** which are discussed in the section on congenital malformations.

Fetal echocardiography and electrocardiography, which have recently become more widely available, are especially helpful during the latter part of pregnancy for prenatal diagnosis of congenital heart defects. Intrauterine arrhythmias can be detected that can often be treated prenatally.

CARDIOMYOPATHIES

Cardiomyopathies are estimated to occur in 1 per 6700 births. Primary cardiomyopathy, which occurs as isolated cardiac disease, is subdivided into hypertrophic, dilated, and restrictive types.

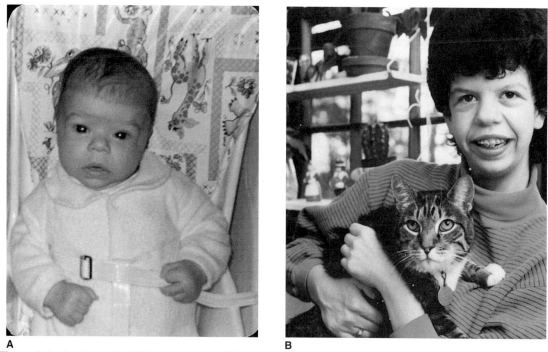

A **B**

Figure 8–1. A patient with Williams syndrome **(A)** at age 4 months and **(B)** at age 14 years. (Courtesy of Barbara Pober, MD, Yale School of Medicine.)

Hypertrophic Cardiomyopathy (HCM): Hypertrophic cardiomyopathy (HCM), which has an incidence of 1 in 30,000, is an important cause of morbidity and mortality in young adults. Massive hypertrophy of the left ventricle, especially of the interventricular septum, occurs with or without obstruction to outflow from the left ventricle. Decreased ventricular filling results from decreased compliance of the thickened ventricular muscles. HCM includes the disorders also known as hereditary ventricular hypertrophy, idiopathic hypertrophic subaortic stenosis (IHSS), and hypertrophic obstructive cardiomyopathy (HOCM). At least 60% of cases are inherited as an autosomal dominant trait with variable expression and incomplete penetrance (MIM 192600). Mutations in the gene responsible for encoding beta-myosin heavy-chains have been found in some patients with HCM. It is postulated that the abnormal myosin may disturb myocardial contractility. Some of the beta-myosin heavy-chain mutations are clinically correlated with more severe disease and a higher incidence of sudden death. In other affected families, linkage studies have mapped HCM to chromosomal locations where genes for troponin I, tropomyosin, and skeletal alpha-actin are located; this suggests that the etiology for HCM may be genetically heterogeneous.

Dilated Cardiomyopathy: Dilated cardiomyopathy, the most common of the cardiomyopathies, is as-

sociated with dilatation of the left ventricular cavity and reduced ejection fractions. Most affected patients also have some degree of left ventricular hypertrophy. The majority of cases of dilated cardiomyopathy are not inherited; only 2% have a positive family history. In some affected families, the disorder is inherited as an autosomal recessive trait (MIM 212110). A mutation in the dystrophin gene, specific for cardiac dystrophin, has been shown in three families with X-linked dilated cardiomyopathy.

Restrictive Cardiomyopathy: Restrictive cardiomyopathy, which results from scarring of the endocardium or myocardium, is associated with impaired diastolic filling of the ventricles. The condition can occur as an isolated, sporadic, disorder; or it can be associated with infiltrative myocardial disorders, many of which are genetic in nature, eg, amyloidosis, hemochromatosis, pseudoxanthoma elasticum, glycogen storage disease, Refsum disease, Fabry disease, and the mucopolysaccharidoses.

Endocardial Fibroelastosis (EFE): Endocardial fibroelastosis (EFE), which occurs in 1 in 4300, may occur as an isolated disorder or be secondary to severe outlet obstruction or to metabolic disorders. Although most cases are sporadic and possibly of viral cause, some are familial with patterns suggestive of autosomal recessive or X-linked inheritance (MIM 305300). EFE also occurs with faciocardiorenal syndrome (MIM 227280).

Cardiomyopathies may also occur with primary carnitine deficiency (carnitine transport defects), fatty acid oxidation defects (secondary carnitine deficiency), mitrochondrial disorders, peroxisomal disorders, Friedreich ataxia, and myotonic and myopathic dystrophies.

CARDIAC CONDUCTION DEFECTS

Congenital Complete Heart Block: Congenital complete heart block, which occurs in 1 in 22,000 live births, is associated with abnormal embryonic development of the AV node and proximal bundle branches. Approximately 25–33% of affected patients have associated congenital heart disease, especially septal defects and transposition of the great vessels. In some affected patients, congenital complete heart block is inherited as an autosomal recessive trait (MIM 234700); in other patients, it is associated with maternal collagen vascular disease.

In adults, conduction defects are most commonly acquired conditions that result from atherosclerosis. Familial cases may be inherited as autosomal dominant or autosomal recessive traits. Patients with inherited metabolic disorders, eg, Fabry disease, hyperoxaluria, and amyloidosis, may also develop cardiac conduction defects.

Wolff-Parkinson-White Syndrome: Wolff-Parkinson-White ventricular pre-excitation syndrome is usually not inherited. Three to four percent of patients with the syndrome will have a positive family history for the disorder; the disorder also may be inherited as an autosomal dominant trait in some families (MIM 194200).

Uhl Anomaly: The Uhl anomaly, an autosomal dominant disorder (MIM 107970), is associated with recurrent ventricular tachycardia, left bundle branch block, and replacement of the right ventricular myocardium with fatty and fibrous tissue (parchment right ventricle). Angiography may be needed to confirm the disorder.

Genetic Syndromes Associated with Cardiac Conduction Defects

Jervell-Lange-Nielsen Syndrome: The Jervell-Lange-Nielsen syndrome, an autosomal recessive disorder (MIM 220400), is associated with severe congenital deafness, prolonged QT and large T waves, syncope, and sudden death.

Romano-Ward Syndrome: The Romano-Ward syndrome, an autosomal dominant trait, has clinically findings similar to those of the Jervell-Lange-Nielsen syndrome except that hearing impairment does not occur.

LEOPARD Syndrome: The LEOPARD syndrome, also autosomal dominant in inheritance pattern (MIM 151100), is characterized by cutaneous lentigenes (dark pigmented macules), EKG abnormalities, ocular hypertelorism, subpulmonic stenosis, genital anomalies, growth retardation, and deafness. Some patients with LEOPARD syndrome also have a hypertrophic cardiomyopathy. The cardiac conduction disturbance is characterized by a prolonged PR interval, widened QRS complex, left anterior hemiblock, or complete heart block.

Cardiac conduction defects may also be seen with inherited neurologic disorders, eg, Friedreich ataxia, and myotonic and muscular dystrophies.

DYSLIPOPROTEINEMIAS

In the United States, one-half of all deaths result from atherosclerosis and coronary artery disease. Many genetic dyslipoproteinemias are associated with abnormalities in the metabolism of plasma lipoproteins and their associated apolipoproteins, which, in turn, significantly increase the risk for atherosclerosis. Because dyslipoproteinemias involve both elevations and reductions in lipoproteins and apoproteins, as well as deficiencies of enzymes and cofactors, the current descriptive name, dyslipoproteinemias, is preferred over the prior term, hyperlipoproteinemias.

Plasma Lipoproteins: Plasma lipoproteins are composed of varying amounts of free and esterified cholesterol, triglycerides, phospholipids, and proteins termed apolipoproteins. The lipoproteins can be separated on the basis of their density, charge, or size. By ultracentrafugation, plasma lipoproteins can be classified in order of increasing density, as follows: chylomicrons (the least dense), very low density lipoproteins (VLDL), low density lipoproteins (LDL), intermediate density lipoproteins (IDL), and high density lipoproteins (HDL) (the most dense).

Chylomicrons, the largest particles, formed in the small intestine, are considered exogenous lipoproteins, whereas VLDL, the next largest, formed in the liver, are considered endogenous lipoproteins. Both chylomicrons and VLDL are highest in lipid content and the major carriers of triglycerides. Low-density lipoproteins (LDL) are smaller lipoproteins, rich in cholesterol and cholesterol esters. Elevated levels of LDL are positively correlated with an increased risk for atherosclerosis and coronary artery disease. LDL and IDL are of intermediate size and are formed during the metabolism of VLDL. Elevated IDL is usually only seen in pathologic states. High density lipoproteins (HDL), the smallest particles, highest in protein content, are negatively correlated with the risk for atherosclerosis. While higher levels of HDL may lessen the risk of atherosclerosis and coronary artery disease, lowered levels of HDL increase the risk.

Lipoproteins can also be separated by electrophoresis, in order of increasing mobility and charge, into chylomicrons, beta-lipoproteins (LDL), pre-beta-lipoproteins (VLDL), and alpha-lipoproteins (HDL). The Fredrickson classification of hyperlipoproteinemias is based on the electrophoretic findings (Table 8–3).

Apolipoproteins (apo): Apolipoproteins (apo) are the lipid-free proteins of lipoproteins that (a) bind and transport lipids and (b) function as cofactors for many of the enzymes involved in lipoprotein metabolism. They are synthesized as pre-apoproteins which undergo post-translational processing to apolipoproteins. Table 8–4 lists the apolipoproteins, their chromosomal gene locations, associated lipoproteins, and functions. ApoA-I and apoC-I are activators of lecithin-cholesterol acyltransferase (LCAT). LCAT catalyzes the transfer of a fatty acid from lecithin to cholesterol creating cholesterol esters. ApoB-100 and apoE are recognition molecules for the LDL receptor. ApoB-48 enhances binding of apoE to LDL receptors. ApoC-II is an activator of lipoprotein lipase. Lipoprotein lipase hydrolyzes triglycerides of circulating chylomicrons, VLDL, and IDL into free fatty acids and glycerols. The genes for the major peripheral apoproteins are members of a common ancestral sequence. One gene cluster, which includes apoE–apoC-I–apoC-II, is located on chromosome 19; another gene cluster involves apoA-I–apoC-III–apoA-IV on chromosome 11.

Disorders of Apolipoproteins
Disorders of Apolipoprotein A:
A. Familial apoA-I Deficiency: Familial apoA-I deficiency (MIM 107660) may occur alone or in association with apoC-III deficiency (MIM 234550). Both deficiencies are rare autosomal recessive disorders associated with markedly reduced plasma HDL, severe coronary atherosclerosis, corneal clouding, and cutaneous and tendonous xanthomas. Mutations in the apoA-I gene and inversions of the apoA-I–apoC-III locus have been noted in some of the patients with this condition. A structural variant of apoA-I, ApoA-I Milano, is associated with abnormal electrophoretic mobility of HDL and lowered plasma HDL levels. This mutation, however, does not appear to increase cardiovascular risk.

B. Tangier Disease: Tangier disease (MIM 205400) is a rare, autosomal recessive disorder associated with the accumulation of cholesterol esters in the reticuloendothelial system and other tissues. Enlarged, orange-yellow tonsils and adenoids, splenomegaly, and peripheral neuropathies occur. Affected homozygotes have markedly decreased levels of apoA-I, apoA-II, HDL, and total cholesterol. Variable degrees of hypertriglyceridemia may occur. Heterozygous carriers have HDL and apoA-I levels that are approximately one-half normal. About one-fourth of carriers and nearly one-half of affecteds over the age of 35 show signs of atherosclerosis. The basis for the disorder is unknown; altered synthesis of HDL and accelerated

catabolism of apo A-I and/or apo A-II may be involved.

Disorders of Apolipoprotein B: ApoB-100 and apoB-48 are products of the same gene locus. ApoB-100, formed in the liver, is a full-length translation product of the gene. ApoB-100 is the major apolipoprotein of VLDL and LDL. ApoB-48, in contrast, is a shorter gene product that contains only 2152 of the 4563 amino acid residues of apoB-100. ApoB-48, formed in the intestine, is the major apolipoprotein of chylomicrons.

A. Abetalipoproteinemia: Abetalipoproteinemia (MIM 200100), an autosomal recessive disorder, is associated with functional absence of both apoB-100 and apoB-48. The exact molecular defect is unknown; defective post-translational processing or incorporation of apoB into lipoproteins may be involved. Plasma post-prandial chylomicrons, VLDL, and LDL are absent. Clinical manifestations include severe fat malabsorption, acanthocytosis of erythrocytes, spinocerebellar ataxia, peripheral neuropathy, ceroid myopathy, and pigmentary retinopathy. The neurologic findings result from the associated defect in intestinal absorption and transport of tocopherol (vitamin E).

B. Hypobetalipoproteinemia: Hypobetalipoproteinemia (MIM 145950), an autosomal dominant disorder, is associated with decreased production of mRNA for apoB-100 and apoB-48. Patients with the homozygous affected form of hypobetalipoproteinemia have clinical findings similar to those seen with abetalipoproteinemia. Heterozygotes for hypobetalipoproteinemia have partial reduction in apoB-100 and apoB-48 levels. Although heterozygotes usually have minimal clinical symptoms, they may show neurological findings.

C. Normotriglyeridemic Abetalipoprotinemia: Normotriglyeridemic abetalipoprotinemia (MIM 107730) is characterized by the production of truncated forms of apoB-100. Acanthocytosis and ataxia occur.

D. Chylomicron Retention Disease: Chylomicron retention disease, an autosomal recessive disorder, results from the absence of apoB-48. Affected patients display fat malabsorption, ataxia, and neuropathy.

Disorders of Apolipoprotein C:
A. Lipoprotein Lipase (LPL) Deficiency: Lipoprotein lipase hydrolyzes triglycerides in chylomicrons and VLDL in extrahepatic tissues. Patients with lipoprotein lipase (LPL) deficiency (MIM 238600), an autosomal recessive disorder, present with eruptive xanthomas, hepatosplenomegaly, and repeated attacks of abdominal pain and pancreatitis. Fasting chylomicrons are markedly elevated. HDL as well as LDL plasma levels are lowered. The condition, however, does not appear to increase the risk for atherosclerosis.

B. Deficiency of apoC-II: Deficiency of apoC-II (MIM 207750), an activator for LPL, produces

Table 8–3. Classification of hyperlipoproteinemias.

Electrophoretic Phenotype	Increased Lipoproteins	Plasma Elevations	Atherosclerotic Risk	Incidence	Associated Defect	Associated Genetic Disorders
Ia	Chylomicrons	Triglyceride	Not increased	Rare	LPL deficiency; LPL inhibitor	LPL deficiency
Ib	Chylomicrons	Triglyceride	Not increased	Rare	ApoC-II deficiency	ApoC-II deficiency
IIa	LDL	Cholesterol	High	1 in 500 (FH) 5 in 100 (PH)	LDL receptor, apoB-100 binding site defects (FH); Multifactoral (PH)	Familial hypercholesterolemia (FH); Polygenic hypercholesterolemia (PH); Familial combined hyperlipoproteinemia
IIb	LDL + VLDL or IDL	Cholesterol and triglycerides	High	1 in 100	Elevated apoB levels	Familial combined hyperlipoproteinemia
III	beta-VLDL	Cholesterol and triglycerides	High	1 in 100	ApoE2/E2 genotype; remnant removal disease	Familial dysbetalipoproteinemia
IV	VLDL	Triglycerides	May be increased	Genetic uncommon, secondary common	Overproduction and decreased clearance of VLDL	Familial hypertriglyceridemia (mild forms); Familial combined hyperlipoproteinemia
V	Chylomicrons + VLDL	Triglycerides	May be increased	Uncommon	Apo E4/E4 genotype	Familial hypertriglyceridemia (severe forms); Familial combined hyperlipoproteinemia

Apo = apoprotein; IDL = intermediate-density lipoprotein; LDL = low-density lipoprotein; LPL = lipoprotein lipase; VLDL = very-low-density lipoprotein.

Table 8–4. Apolipoproteins.

Apolipoprotein (apo)	Chromosomal Gene Location	Associated Lipoproteins	Function
A-I	11q23–24	Chylomicrons, HDL	Cofactor for LCAT
A-II	1p23–21	Chylomicrons, HDL	Transport of HDL
A-IV	11q23–24	Chylomicrons, HDL	Unknown
B-100	2p24–23	Chylomicrons and chylomicron remnants, VLDL, IDL, LDL	Ligand for LDL receptor, transport of VLDL, IDL, LDL
B-48	2p24–23	Chylomicrons and chylomicron remnants, VLDL, IDL	Chylomicron transport
C-I	19q13.1	Chylomicrons, VLDL, IDL, HDL	Cofactor for LCAT
C-II	19q13.1	Chylomicrons, VLDL, IDL, HDL	Cofactor for LPL
C-III	11q24–23	Chylomicrons, VLDL, IDL, HDL	Unknown
D	3p14.2	HDL	Unknown, possibly transport of cholesterol esters between lipoproteins
E	19q13.1	Chylomicrons and chylomicron remnants, VLDL, IDL, HDL	Ligand for remnant receptor and LDL receptor
F		HDL	Possibly involved in cholesterol transport or esterification
G		VLDL	Unknown
H	17	Chylomicrons, VLDL, HDL	Beta-2-glycoprotein I
Lp(a)	6q	LDL, HDL	(Abnormal apo)

p = short arm of chromosome, q = long arm of chromosome; HDL = high-density lipoprotein; IDL = intermediate-density lipoprotein; LCAT = lecithin-cholesterol acyltransferase; LDL = low-density lipoprotein; LPL = lipoprotein lipase; VLDL = very-low-density lipoprotein.

a clinical picture similar to LPL deficiency, except that affected patients do not have xanthomas or hepatomegaly. Changes in plasma lipoproteins are not as dramatic as that seen with LPL deficiency.

C. Familial Inhibitor to LPL: The presence of a familial inhibitor to LPL, possibly an autosomal dominant trait (MIM 118830), is associated with fasting hyperchylomicronemia, pancreatitis, and eruptive xanthomas during childhood. All three disorders of apolipoprotein C metabolism are associated with a type I hyperlipoproteinemia phenotype.

Apolipoprotein E: ApoE is necessary for the binding of chylomicron remnants and large triglyceride-rich VLDL to the LDL receptor. ApoE has three major isoforms—apoE2, apoE3 and apoE4—which are determined by 3 different alleles at the same genetic locus. The isoforms differ in binding affinity to the LDL receptor; apoE3 has the most affinity, apoE4 has less; and apo E2 has the least. The normal homozygous apoE3/E3 genotype is seen in 60% of the population. Approximately 18% of the population are compound heterozygotes for apoE3/E2 and apoE3/E4.

A. ApoE2/E2: The homozygous genotype apoE2/E2, a latent defect seen in 1% of the population, may lead to type III hyperlipoproteinemia (primary dysbetalipoproteinemia, MIM 144500) if other factors associated with the development of hyperlipo-

proteinemia are present, eg, diabetes, obesity, or hypothyroidism. Type III hyperlipoproteinemia is characterized by increased plasma cholesterol and triglycerides. Accumulation of cholesterol-rich remnant lipoproteins that are derived from partial degradation of chylomicrons and VLDL also occurs. Lipoprotein electrophoresis shows a characteristic abnormal "broad beta" band due to the presence of "beta"-VLDL. Affected patients have premature atherosclerosis that affects the carotid and coronary arteries and the abdominal aorta. A distinctive xanthoma stiata palmaris is present in 50% of patients; tuberoeruptive and periosteal xanthomas may also occur.

B. ApoE4/E4: The homozygous genotype apoE4/E4 may result in Type V hyperlipoproteinemia (MIM 238400), a severe form of familial hypertriglyceridemia.

Apolipoprotein (a) [Lp(a)]: Lp(a) is a variant of LDL that consists of an LDL-like molecule that has one or two copies of a glycoprotein termed Lp(a) [apo(a)] attached to its apoB-100 by a disulfide bond. Lp(a) is highly homologous to plasminogen and closely linked to the plasminogen gene on chromosome 6. At least 20 common alleles have been identified at the Lp(a) locus; multiple isoforms exist. Approximately 20% of the population have high levels of Lp(a) that are associated with a doubling of the risk for atherosclerosis (MIM 152200). With elevation of both LDL and Lp(a), the risk is about 5 times higher. The exact mechanism for the increased risk is unclear. It is thought, however, that after arterial wall endothelial damage, Lp(a), which is present in atherosclerotic plaques along with fibrinogen and fibrin, may adhere to fibrin forming a complex that sticks to arterial walls. Alternatively, Lp(a) may inhibit the activation of plasminogen and the dissolution of fibrin clots.

LDL Receptor

Cholesterol is needed for the synthesis of cell membranes, steroid hormones, and bile acids. Cells can synthesize cholesterol de novo. By means of the LDL receptor and receptor-mediated endocytosis, cells are also able to internalize circulating exogenous cholesterol from cholesterol-rich LDL, IDL, or chylomicron remnants. The gene for the LDL receptor is on the short arm of chromosome 19 (19p13.2–13.1); the cDNA has been sequenced. Multiple allelic mutations in the LDL receptor locus are associated with type IIa hyperlipoproteinemia. The defects have included: (a) faulty synthesis of receptors, which is the most common form of abnormality, (b) synthesis of the receptors but failure of post-translational processing or localization of the receptor at the cell surface, (c) defects in LDL-receptor binding or recycling, or (d) defects with proper binding but failure of the receptors to internalize LDL.

Hyperlipoproteinemias

Familial Hypercholesterolemia (Type IIa Hyperlipoproteinemia): Familial hypercholesterolemia (type IIa hyperlipoproteinemia, MIM 143890), an autosomal dominant disorder, is associated with elevation of plasma total cholesterol and LDL. Deposition of LDL-derived cholesterol in issues leads to severe premature atherosclerosis. Reduced clearance of plasma LDL and IDL results from defective LDL receptors.

A. Heterozygous Form: Approximately 1 in 500 persons is a heterozygote for familial hypercholesterolemia. These heterozygotes have approximately one-half of the normal number of functioning LDL receptors. Their mean plasma LDL is 2 to 3 times that of the normal population. Total cholesterol levels average 350 mg/dl, with a range of 270 to 550 mg/dl. VLDL and triglycerides are usually normal but may be elevated. Elevated plasma cholesterol is present from birth. Clinical manifestations, however, are usually not noted until after the age of 20. Xanthomas may occur in the Achilles tendons and in extensor tendons of the fingers. Tuberous and subperiosteal xanthomas may be noted over the elbows and knees. Arcus cornea and palpebral xanthomas are found in about 50% of heterozygotes over the age of 30. Fifty percent of heterozygotes develop coronary artery disease, which usually occurs by age 50 in males and by age 60 in females. The incidence of coronary artery disease is 3 to 6 times that found in the general population. In heterozygotes, the incidence of cerebral vascular accidents is even higher, at 20 times the general population rate.

B. Homozygous Form: A more severe, homozygous form of the disorder occurs in approximately 1 in 1 million. Affected patients have virtually no LDL receptor activity. Plasma LDL levels are 4–6 times normal; total cholesterol levels range between 600 and 1200 mg/dl. Generalized atherosclerosis with symptomatic coronary artery disease and cardiac valvular involvement, xanthomas, and arcus cornea are usually present by mid-childhood. Most patients with homozygous familial hypercholesterolemia do not survive past age 30; deaths have occurred as early as age 18 months. Figure 8–2 shows cutaneous xanthomas in homozygous familial hypercholesterolemia. Prenatal diagnosis has been accomplished by measuring LDL receptor activity in cultured amniocytes.

Genetic mutations in the apoB-100 locus at the binding site domain have a similar clinical picture to that of familial hypercholesterolemia. This disorder also occurs in 1 in 500 persons and is inherited as an autosomal dominant trait.

Polygenic Hypercholesterolemia: Polygenic hypercholesterolemia, which occurs in 5% of the adult population, is noted in 85–90% of patients with moderate elevation cholesterol and LDL. The disorder is of multifactorial etiology. Increased synthesis of apoB or cholesterol, or increased susceptibility to dietary cholesterol may be involved. Environmental factors may also contribute to the development of atherosclerosis in these individuals, eg, high-fat or high-cholesterol diets, obesity, diabetes mellitus, smoking, or lack of exercise. Patients usually have a type IIa electrophoretic phenotype; occasionally a type IIb phenotype is noted. First degree relatives have a 2–6% risk for coronary artery disease.

Familial Combined Hyperlipoproteinemia: Familial combined hyperlipoproteinemia (MIM 144250) is the most common genetic disorder associated with premature atherosclerosis. It occurs in 1% of the population and is inherited as an autosomal dominant disorder with high penetrance. About one-third of patients have elevated plasma cholesterol; one-third have elevated plasma triglycerides; and, one-third have elevation of both cholesterol and triglycerides. Elevated plasma lipid levels are usually lower than those noted with familial hypercholesterolemia or familial hypertriglyceridemia. Types IIa, IIb, IV, or occasionally V lipoprotein electrophoretic patterns may be noted. The electrophoretic pattern may vary among members of the same family. Children with the disorder usually only have hypertriglyceridemia; hypercholesterolemia may later develop. Xanthomas do not usually occur. Patients with markedly elevated

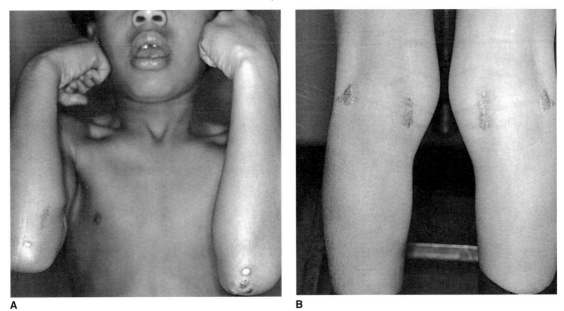

A   **B**

Figure 8–2. Homozygous hypercholesterolemia in a 7-year-old boy. Cutaneous xanthomas had been present since the age of 4 years. **(A)** Elbows; **(B)** popliteal fossa. (Reproduced, with permission from Oski FA, et al (editors): *Principles and Practice of Pediatrics,* 2nd ed, JB Lippincott, 1994.)

plasma triglycerides may develop pancreatitis. Approximately 10% of patients develop coronary artery disease before the age of 60 years. The exact defect is unknown; the moderately elevated apoB levels noted in affected patients may result from increased apoB synthesis. The diagnosis is established by excluding other types of hyperlipoproteinemias on the basis of clinical and laboratory findings. Evaluation of family members may also be required to establish the diagnosis.

Familial Hypertriglyceridemia: Familial hypertriglyceridemia (MIM 145750), an autosomal dominant disorder, occurs in 0.2–0.3% of the population. Moderate elevation of plasma triglycerides (250-500 mg/dl) and VLDL occur. Type IV, or rarely type V electrophoretic phenotypes are noted. Cholesterol is not elevated. The disorder is usually not expressed in childhood. Expression in adults may be enhanced by environmental factors which also contribute to hypertriglyceridemia, eg, diabetes mellitus, obesity, alcoholism, and estrogen therapy. The defect is unknown; overproduction of endogenous triglyceride or delayed catabolism of VLDL may be involved. As with familial combined hyperlipoproteinemia, the diagnosis is established by family studies and exclusion of other types of hyperlipoproteinemias.

Severe Form of Familial Hypertriglyceridemia: A more severe form of familial hypertriglyceridemia (MIM 144650) is associated with a type V electrophoretic pattern, elevated triglycerides in the 600 to 3000 mg/dl range, and the presence of fasting chylomicronemia. Eruptive xanthoma, recurrent ab-

dominal pain, and pancreatitis are noted in affected adults. Other environmental factors and disorders that predispose to hypertriglyceridemia, eg, diabetes mellitus, are frequently present in symptomatic patients.

Other Disorders of Lipoprotein Metabolism

LCAT Deficiency: Lecithin-cholesterol acyltransferase (LCAT) exists in two species in plasma, one with specific activity for HDL, and the other with activity towards VLDL and LDL. Deficiency of both species, termed LCAT deficiency (MIM 245900), is associated with corneal opacities, anemia, target cells and proteinuria, which may progress to renal failure. Unesterified cholesterol and phospholipids are deposited in tissues. Fish eye disease (MIM 136120) results from deficiency of LCAT specific for HDL. Affected patients present with corneal opacities as young adults. Both disorders of LCAT, inherited as autosomal recessive traits, are associated with an increased risk for atherosclerosis.

Deficiency of HTGL: Hepatic triglyceride lipase (HTGL) hydrolyzes HDL triglycerides and surface phospholipids. Deficiency of HTGL is associated with eruptive and plantar xanthomas and early atherosclerosis. Plasma triglycerides, cholesterol, and HDL are moderately elevated. HDL has greatly increased triglyceride content.

Deficiency of Cholesterol Ester Transport Protein: Cholesterol ester transport protein (CETP) facilitates the exchange of HDL cholesterol esters between HDL and VLDL, IDL and LDL. Deficiency of CETP (MIM 118470) results in elevated levels of HDL; affected patients are clinically asymptomatic.

Other Disorders of Lipid and Cholesterol Metabolism

Cerebrotendinous Xanthomatosis: Cerebrotendinous xanthomatosis (MIM 213700), a rare autosomal recessive disorder, is associated with deficient activity of hepatic mitochondrial 26-hydroxylase. Affected patients have deficient biosynthesis of bile salts, especially cholic acid and chenodeoxycholic acid. Increased levels of intermediates in bile salt biosynthesis accumulate in most tissues and are excreted in bile, feces, and urine. Clinical manifestations include progressive dementia, cerebellar ataxia, spinal cord paresis, tuberous and tendonous xanthomas, cataracts, and early atherosclerosis of variable age of onset. Affected patients frequently respond to treatment with chenodeoxycholic acid.

Phytosterolemia (Beta-sitosterolemia): Phytosterolemia (beta-sitosterolemia, MIM 210250) is characterized by subcutaneous and tendonous xanthomas and premature atherosclerosis. Elevated plasma and tissue levels of sitosterol and other plant, and often shellfish, sterols are noted. The defect is unknown; increased absorption or decreased biliary and fecal excretion of these compounds may occur. Treatment includes dietary avoidance of the compounds.

Certain other genetic disorders also are associated with an increased risk for myocardial infarction and atherosclerosis. Included are metabolic disorders, eg, homocystinuria, Fabry disease, lysosomal acid lipase deficiency, and the mucopolysaccharidosis; disorders of connective tissue, eg, Marfan syndrome and pseudoxanthoma elasticum; and sickle cell anemia.

OTHER GENETIC DISEASES WITH MAJOR CARDIAC INVOLVEMENT

Mitral Valve Prolapse: Mitral valve prolapse (MVP, MIM 157700) is the most common genetic cardiac disorder. It is inherited as an autosomal dominant trait with variable expression. Expression is age-dependent. An incidence of 6% in neonates, 1% in children and adolescents, and 4–8% in adults has been reported. Under 50 years of age, females are more likely to be affected than males. Equal sex expression is seen in older persons. Many affected patients have a thin, tall body build. Abnormalities of the thoracic skeleton, eg, pectus excavatum, scoliosis, "straight back syndrome," and narrow AP chest diameter are frequently noted. Although MVP usu-

ally occurs as an isolated, inherited disorder, it may also occur in patients with congenital heart defects, especially ASD, and with disorders associated with abnormalities of connective tissue, eg, Marfan syndrome, Ehlers-Danlos syndrome, fragile X syndrome, Klinefelter syndrome, osteogenesis imperfecta, or Stickler syndrome. MVP may also result from myocardial involvement in the myotonic and muscular dystrophies.

Marfan Syndrome: Marfan syndrome (MIM 154700), a disorder of connective tissue, occurs in 1 in 10,000 persons. Marfan syndrome results from a defect in fibrillin, a microfibrillar protein found in connective tissue, often associated with elastin. The fibrillin gene, which has been isolated, is located on the long arm of chromosome 15. The disorder is inherited as an autosomal dominant trait. As many as 30% of cases are not inherited and result from new mutations in the fibrillin gene; advanced paternal age is often noted. The major clinical findings involve the skeletal, ocular, and cardiac systems. Clinical manifestations have a wide variability. Cardiac complications, however, may show a familial pattern. The skeletal findings include tall stature, long and thin extremities (dolichostenomelia), thin hands and feet with long fingers and toes (especially of the great toe) (arachnodactyly), pectus carinatum or excavatum, scoliosis (60% of patients), kyphosis (30–60%), joint hypermobility, and flat feet. The ocular findings include dislocated lens with often upward and outward displacement of the lens (50–80%), myopia, and retinal detachment. The cardiac manifestations include mitral valve prolapse, mitral regurgitation, aortic regurgitation, dilatation of the aortic root, and dissecting aortic aneurysm. Occasionally pulmonary artery root dilatation is seen. The aortic disease results from a defect in the tunica media of the ascending aorta, which is associated with degeneration of the elastic lamellae. Affected patients are usually thin; decreased subcutaneous tissue occurs. A relatively smaller muscle mass than average and hypotonia may be noted. Hernias, cutaneous striae, spontaneous pneumothorax, apical lung blebs, asymptomatic dural ectasia, and a high, narrow arched palate may occur. Table 8–5 lists the clinical manifestations and diagnostic criteria for Marfan syndrome.

Although clinical signs may be present from infancy, the diagnosis of Marfan syndrome is usually made during or after childhood. A severe infantile or neonatal form of the disorder also occurs that may or may not be a distinct disorder. Clinical findings that may be helpful in distinguishing Marfan syndrome characteristics include a reduced upper to lower body segment ratio. The lower body segment is obtained by measuring from the top of the pubic symphysis to the floor; the upper body segment is determined by subtracting the lower body segment from the total height. The upper to lower body segment ratio aver-

Table 8–5. Manifestations of Marfan syndrome.

Diagnostic requirements:
1. In the absence of an affected first-degree relative: involvement of the skeleton and at least two other systems; at least one major manifestation. (25–30% of cases are sporadic, paternal age effect)
2. With an affected first-degree relative: involvement of two or more systems; at least one major manifestation preferred, but this will depend somewhat on the family's phenotype (autosomal dominant inheritance)
3. Negative amino acid testing for homocystinuria while not taking pyridoxine supplements

Skeletal	**Cardiovascular**
Anterior chest deformity: especially asymmetric pectus excavatum or carinatum	Aorta: dilatation of ascending aorta,* aortic dissection,* aortic regurgitation
Dolichostenomelia, not due to scoliosis (long extremities; lowered upper to lower segment ratio)	Mitral value: mitral regurgitation, mitral valve prolapse, calcification of mitral annulus
Arachnodactyly (long, thin fingers and toes; excessive length of great toe)	Abdominal aortic aneurysm
Vertebral column deformities: scoliosis, thoracic lordosis or reduced thoracic kyphosis	Arrhythmia
Tall stature, compared to unaffected family members	Endocarditis
High, narrow arched palate and dental crowding	**Pulmonary**
Acetabular protrusion	Spontaneous pneumothorax
Abnormal appendicular joint mobility: hypermobility, congenital flexion contractures	Apical bleb
Ocular	**Skin and integument**
Ectopia lentis*	Striae distensae
Flat cornea	Hernias: inguinal, umbilical, diaphragmatic, or incisional
Elongated globe	**Central nervous system**
Retinal detachment	Caudal dural ectasia (radiographic or imaging finding)*
Myopia	Intrapelvic meningocele
	Dilated cisterna magna
	Learning disability
	Hyperactivity

* = major manifestation. Adapted from Beighton, P, editor: *McKusick's Heritable Disorders of Connective Tissue,* 5th ed, Mosby-Year Book, 1993, and Beighton P et al: International nosology of heritable disorders of connective tissue. Amer J Med Gen 1988;29:581.

ages 0.93 in normal Caucasian adults. It is different in African Americans; the ratio is also somewhat higher during puberty. Adult Marfan individuals have a lower ratio that is approximately 0.85. With Marfan syndrome there is an increased arm span to height ratio. The arm span, measured from fingertip to fingertip, is usually equal to or less than the height. The Steinberg "thumb sign" is positive when the thumb extends beyond the ulnar surface of the hand when the thumb is held closely against the palm, under the fingers, in a fist. The Walker-Murdock "wrist sign" is positive when the first and fifth fingers overlap when they are placed around the opposite wrist. These two "signs" reflect the long, thin extremities and digits seen in persons with Marfan syndrome and other forms of arachnodactyly. The ratios and "signs" should not be used as diagnostic tools for Marfan syndrome. They may be helpful, however, when considering the disorder.

Over 90% of deaths in patients with Marfan syndrome occur as a result of cardiac involvement from their disease. Deaths in patients younger than 4 years of age are usually associated with MVP. Deaths in adult Marfan patients usually occur from aortic complications. The average age of death is 40 in males and 50 in females. Between 66–75% of Marfan patients die from severe aortic and/or mitral regurgitation, or aortic root dissection. Sixty-nine percent of Marfan patients develop aortic root dilatation. As many as 21% have aortic root dissection. Beta-blockers may reduce the incidence of aortic dissection. Combined aortic valve and aortic arch replacement has been beneficial in these patients.

Because of clinical similarities, all persons suspected of having the Marfan syndrome should have amino acid testing to exclude homocystinuria. The differential diagnosis also includes Klinefelter syndrome, Stickler syndrome, marfanoid hypermobility syndrome, and congenital contractural arachnodactyly.

Suggested Reading

Cheitlin MD, Sokolow M, McIlroy MB, editors. Pages 359–571, 585–637 in: *Clinical Cardiology,* 6th ed, Appleton & Lange, 1993.

Devereaux RB, Brown WT: Structural heart disease. Pages 192–221 in: *The Genetic Basis of Common Diseases,* King RA, Rotter JI, Motulsky AG, editors, Oxford University Press, 1992.

Emmanuel R, Withers R: The cardiomyopathies. Pages 1263–1272 in: *Principles and Practice of Medical Genetics,* 2nd ed, Emery AEH, Rimoin DL, editors, Churchill Livingstone, 1990.

Frias JL: Genetic Issues of Congenital Heart Defects. Pages 237–243 in: *Pediatric Cardiology,* Gessner IH, Victoria BE, editors, WB Saunders, 1993.

Godfrey M: The Marfan syndrome. Pages 51–123 in: *McKusick's Heritable Disorders of Connective Tissue,* 5th ed, Beighton P, editor, Mosby-Year Book, 1993.

Gotto AM: Etiology, diagnosis and treatment of the lipid transport disorders. Pages 23–49 in: *Progress in Cardiology,* Yu PN, Goodwin JF, editors, Lea & Febiger, 1988.

Hoffman JI, Congenital Heart Disease, Ped Clin N Amer 1990; **37**;1:25.

Jones KL, *Smith's Recognizable Patterns of Human Malformation,* 4th ed, WB Saunders, 1988.

Kelley DP, Strauss AW, Mechanisms of Disease: Inherited cardiomyopathies. New Eng J Med 1994;**330:**913.

Kreisberg RA, Segrest JP, editors. *Plasma Lipoproteins and Coronary Artery Disease,* Blackwell Scientific, 1992.

Marinetti GV, *Disorders of lipid metabolism,* Plenum Press, 1990.

Michels VV, Riccardi VM: Congenital heart defects. Pages 1207–1238 in: *Principles and Practice of Medical Genetics,* 2nd ed, Emery AEH, Rimoin DL, editors, Churchill Livingstone, 1990,

Motulsky AG, Brunzell JD: The Genetics of Coronary Atherosclerosis. In: *The Genetic Basis of Common Diseases,* King RA, Rotter JI, Motulsky AG, editors, Oxford University Press, 1992.

Park MK: *The Pediatric Cardiology Handbook,* Mosby-Year Book, 1991.

Pierpont MEM, Moller JH, editors: *Genetics of cardiovascular disease,* Martinus Nijhoff, 1987.

Riopel DA: The heart. Pages 237–253 in: *Human Malformations and Related Anomalies,* Steven RE, Hall JG, Goodman RM, eds, Oxford University Press, 1993.

Robinson A, Linden MG: *Clinical Genetics Handbook,* 2nd ed, Blackwell Scientific, 1993.

Scriver CR, Beaudet AL, Sly WS, Valle D, editors: Lipoprotein and lipid metabolism disorders. Pages 1127–1302 in: *The Metabolic Basis of Inherited Disease,* 6th ed, Part 7.

Utermann G: Coronary heart disease. Pages 1239–1262 in: *Principles and Practice of Medical Genetics,* Emery AE, Rimoin DL, editors, 2nd ed, Churchill Livingstone, 1990.

Whittemore R, Wells JA, Castellsague X: A second-generation study of 427 probands with congenital heart defects and their 837 children. JACC 1994;**23:**1459.

Kidney & Urinary Tract

9

ROLE OF GENETICS IN RENAL DISEASE

Genetic factors play an important role in the development of renal disease. The variety of kidney diseases that results from genetic mutations is diverse. Single gene disorders can involve only the kidney, or they may affect multiple systems. For some disorders, recognition of the pattern of inheritance is all the genetic information we have. In other disorders, elucidation of the genes that relate to renal disease provides an important key to our understanding of pathogenesis. Specification of the genetic abnormality can clarify prognosis by allowing clinicians to compare the affected individual with others who have the same molecular pathology. Molecular analysis and definition of the mutations involved can also allow the physician to assess risk to other family members with more precision than pedigree analysis or the usual diagnostic tools can achieve.

General Approach to Renal Disease and Genetics

Inherited renal disease can be divided into three categories:

- Major inherited disorders of renal structure or function
- Recognized genetic disorders in which renal manifestations are a significant or usual feature
- Other associations in which renal disease may be a frequent or occasional feature.

In this chapter, single gene disorders that have renal disease as a major manifestation are discussed. In some single gene disorders, renal manifestations are a major part of the syndrome, but other features are clinically distinguishing. In other genetic disorders and dysmorphic syndromes, renal manifestations are reported occasionally. In the tables included in this chapter, genetic disorders are categorized according to the type of renal manifestation they commonly display. The tables also list some rare conditions that have renal manifestations but are not recognized as chromosomal or single gene disorders.

When renal disease is found in association with other findings, a thorough physical examination, patient history, and family history must be comple-

mented by a review of the literature. This approach will help to ensure the diagnosis and to assess the possible or likely role of genes in the pathogenesis.

Tumors

Tumors of the kidney are an important type of cancer in which genetic factors play a role. These tumors are discussed in Chapter 5.

Disorders of the Kidney

Disorders that affect the kidney may involve the entire renal parenchyma or only the glomerulus or tubules. Genetic disorders may be expressed at the gross anatomical level as cystic disease, dysplasia, or even complete agenesis of the kidney. In addition to dysplasia and agenesis of the kidney, other malformations of the urinary tract may occur, either alone or in association with other abnormalities. Such developmental defects and malformations of the urinary tract may have a genetic component. In some conditions, a decrease in glomerular function results in varying degrees of renal failure, including end-stage renal disease. In other conditions, the renal tubular transport mechanism is the site of clinically important mutations. Toxic metabolites resulting from inborn errors of metabolism can damage the kidney. Examples are listed in Table 9–1.

Some metabolic disorders that involve the kidney are discussed in detail in the chapters on intermediary metabolism.

Disease that Primarily Affects the Glomerulus

Many disorders that affect connective tissue have glomerular disease as a manifestation.

Hereditary nephritis takes many forms. In addition to the primary inherited forms, nephritis can be associated with other genetic disorders. Inherited conditions that primarily affect glomerular function have been distinguished on the basis of clinical features, anatomic pathology, and pattern of inheritance. Accumulating knowledge of molecular pathology is clarifying this group of disorders and providing diagnostic tools.

Alport Syndrome: The best understood of the disorders that primarily affect glomerular function is Alport syndrome. The condition is characterized clin-

Table 9–1. Disorders of intermediary or cellular metabolism associated with renal manifestations.

Renal Manifestation	Disorder and MIM Number
Interstitial nephritis	MMA
Hemolytic-uremic syndrome	MMA (cblC)
Secondary renal tubular disease	
Renal Fanconi syndrome	Cystinosis Galactosemia Hereditary fructose intolerance Wilson disease Tyrosinemia
Aminoaciduria	Hartnup syndrome
Renal stones	Primary hyperoxaluria Hypercalciuria Uric acid
Renal tubular acidosis	Osteopetrosis Glycogen storage disease Carnitine palmitoyl transferase deficiency Kearns-Sayres syndrome
Cysts	Zellweger syndrome Glutaricaciduria IIA (231680)

ically by hematuria, proteinuria, progressive renal failure, eye abnormalities, and deafness. Hematuria and proteinuria reflect the glomerulopathy. Ocular findings include keratoconus and myopia, which frequently cause visual symptoms. Sensorineural hearing loss is the result of cochlear malfunction. Hypertension is a frequent feature of Alport syndrome.

Glomerular damage is characterized by ultrastructural abnormalities of the glomerular basement membrane (Figure 9–1). Progressive damage to the basement membrane results in loss of glomerular filtration and hence renal failure. Genetic heterogeneity within Alport syndrome has been recognized for many years. Considerable debate about possible autosomal or X-linked inheritance has occurred in the literature. Pedigrees that are consistent with X-linked, autosomal recessive, and autosomal dominant inheritance have all been observed. The X-linked form comprises about 85% of all cases, but typically shows severe expression in the affected male. The heterozygous female rarely progresses to renal failure, but she may have hematuria. Considerable clinical heterogeneity has been reported. Some pedigrees have shown typical renal disease, but deafness has been absent. Age of onset for end-stage renal disease defines a juvenile and an adult form of the syndrome.

The molecular identification and characterization of genes and their mutations associated with Alport syndrome has clarified the diagnosis and management of patients with the condition. In families in which Alport syndrome is segregating, all of the mutations found to date occur in one of the subunits of the α-chain of type IV collagen. A major component of basement membranes, type IV collagen is ex-

pressed in the glomerulus, the cornea, and the cochlea, and is consistent with findings of nephritis, keratoconus, and sensorineural hearing loss. Type IV collagen is composed of 6 subunits, 4 of which map to autosomes. Two subunits, α5 and α6, map to the same location on the X-chromosome as that for the X-linked form of Alport syndrome. The mutation in type IV collagen compromises the integrity of the basement membranes in the glomerulus, the cochlea, and the cornea, and leads to the clinical abnormalities mentioned above.

The X-linked and most common form of Alport syndrome (MIM 301050) maps to Xq22. Mutations in the gene for the α5 subunit of type 4 collagen, COL4A5, account for the majority of cases of this form of Alport syndrome. Deletions, point mutations, exon skipping, and nonsense mutations that result in no protein synthesis have all been observed. A considerably rarer form of the X-linked variant is Alport syndrome associated with diffuse esophageal leiomyomatosis (MIM 308940). This condition has been shown to have a contiguous deletion of portions of the genes for subunit α5 and α6.

The autosomal recessive form (MIM 203780) is clinically similar to the X-linked form, and has been associated with mutations in the α3 and in the α4 subunits, both of which map to chromosome 2q35–37. The autosomal dominant form (MIM 104200), which tends to have a later age of onset than the other forms, has not yet been mapped; neither have molecular defects been recognized for this form. Subunits α1 and α2 of type IV collagen map to chromosome 13q33–34; no forms of Alport syndrome are as yet associated with them.

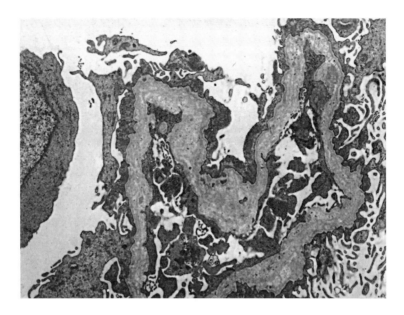

Figure 9–1. Electron micrograph of glomerular basement membrane of a patient with Alport syndrome. There is irregular thickening of the basement membrane with typical laminations and loss of the normal trilaminar structure. Magnification 5750x. (Courtesy of Michael Kashgarian, MD, Yale University School of Medicine.)

The diagnosis of Alport syndrome is suspected on clinical grounds, is corroborated at renal biopsy by glomerular findings on light microscopy, and is confirmed by identification of classical basement membrane ultrastructural abnormalities on electron microscopy. In many families, molecular studies can confirm the presence of a mutation or deletion. Although the correlation of mutation and clinical course is not yet completely specific, the molecular analysis is of some prognostic value and may help to differentiate between autosomal and X-linked Alport syndrome when pedigree information fails to do so. In addition, awareness of the molecular pathology allows clinicians to provide more accurate risk assessment to the family.

The juvenile form of Alport syndrome results in end-stage renal disease by age 30; the adult onset form may not demonstrate renal failure until the fifth decade of life. Female heterozygotes for the X-linked form rarely have significant renal damage. While medical management of hypertension and renal failure can suffice temporarily, most patients eventually require dialysis. In many of these cases, renal transplant has been the ultimate renal replacement therapy.

Other Familial Types of Nephritis: A number of familial nephropathies affect glomerular basement membranes. These are listed in Table 9–2. No molecular defects have been clearly demonstrated in these disorders (Figure 9–2). It is interesting to speculate whether any are allelic to one of the forms of Alport syndrome, but the evidence to resolve this question

does not exist yet. Several inherited disorders affecting the components of complement are sometimes associated with nephritis. Other disorders of hematologic and immune function can also occasionally affect the kidney.

Hereditary Nephrosis

Nephrosis or nephrotic syndrome consists of proteinuria, hypoproteinemia, edema, and hyperlipidemia. The condition can result from various kinds of glomerular injury. Nephrosis can occur as part of various inherited syndromes or as isolated hereditary nephrosis.

Congenital Nephrosis (Finnish Type) (256300): Congenital nephrosis is characterized by a clinical picture of nephrotic syndrome that is evident at birth. Infants have proteinuria, hypoproteinemia, and hyperlipidemia. Edema increasing to the point of anasarca, delayed ossification, low birth weight, and progressive renal failure complete the clinical picture. The disorder is most widely recognized in Finland, where it affects 1 in 8000 infants. However, congenital nephrosis occurs worldwide.

The pathogenesis remains uncertain. In affected fetuses, abnormal foot processes in capillary walls of the glomerulus and accumulation of basement membrane-like material can be seen by electron microscopy. In affected infants, dilated tubules, tubular atrophy, glomerular sclerosis, and fibrosis are seen, but the process by which these abnormalities develop is unknown. Autosomal recessive inheritance is well

Table 9–2. Renal manifestations associated with genetic conditions: nephritis.

Malformation	Genetic Condition	Inheritance	Map Location	Gene
Nephritis				
	Nail-patella syndrome 161200	AD	—	—
	Alport syndrome 104200	AD	—	—
	Familial nephritis, without deafness or ocular defect 161900	AD	—	—
	Benign familial hematuria (thin-basement-membrane nephropathy) 141200	AD	—	—
	Macrothromobcytopathy, nephritis, and deafness (153650)	AD	—	—
	Macrothromobcytopathy, nephritis, deafness, and leukocyte inclusions (153640)	AD	—	—
	Alport syndrome (203780)	AR	2q35–37	COL4A3 COL4A4
	Schminke immunoosseous dysplasia (242900)	AR	—	
	Thoracic asphyxiating dystrophy	AR	—	
	Alport syndrome (301050)	XLR	Xq22	COL4A5

established. The gene has been mapped to chromosome 19q12–13.1 in Finnish families. Although a number of candidate genes have been excluded, the mutant gene in this disorder has not been established. No other loci have been implicated in congenital nephrosis, but genetic heterogeneity has not been excluded.

Diagnosis depends on clinical features, as well as histologic and ultrastructural abnormalities in the glomerulus. The diagnosis can be suspected prenatally when high α-fetoprotein in the amniotic fluid accompanies normal maternal serum α-fetoprotein. This finding is not exclusive to congenital nephrosis, but is diagnostic in families known to be at risk because of a previously affected child. Molecular diagnosis may become possible once linkage markers

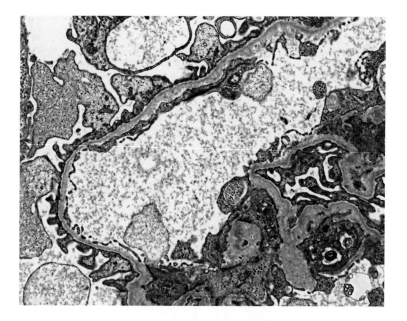

Figure 9–2. Electron micrograph of glomerulus from a patient with thin basement membrane disease. There is marked attenuation of the basement membrane to less than one half the normal thickness for an age-matched control. Magnification 6600x. (Courtesy of Michael Kashgarian, MD, Yale University School of Medicine.)

near the locus or the gene itself are identified. The disorder progresses during the first two years of life and is usually fatal. Patients die of infection or of renal failure. Dialysis or renal transplant are the only effective treatments.

Other Disorders Associated with Nephrosis: Several dysmorphic syndromes have been associated with nephrosis. Their pathogenesis is uncertain. Microcephaly hiatus hernia nephrotic syndrome (MIM 251300) is a recessively inherited disorder. Immunoosseous dysplasia (MIM 242900) is accompanied by nephrosis and spondyloepiphyseal dysplasia. A syndrome of concomitant microcephaly and nephrosis has been reported in consanguineous families. Immune factors may play an important role in the development of nephrosis. While the existence of many HLA associations with nephrosis suggests an inherited immunologic mechanism for the disorder, a link between specific immunologic abnormalities and nephrosis remains unproven (Table 9–3).

Diseases Affecting the Renal Tubules

A broad variety of inherited disorders affect tubular structure and function. A molecular abnormality may affect the tubule alone or it may affect many different kinds of cells. Abnormalities that affect the renal tubule can lead to a deficiency in the transport function of the tubule or result in anatomic disruption.

Primary Renal Tubular Disease: Cystinuria, an autosomal recessive disorder of transport that results in renal stones, is discussed in Chapter 19. Other disorders associated with renal stones are also discussed in that chapter. An X-linked syndrome that includes nephrolithiasis with renal wasting of potassium, phosphate, uric acid, and calcium has not been well defined. Also discussed in Chapter 13 are iminoglycinuria and Lowe syndrome, an autosomal recessive disorder associated with ocular, central nervous system, and amino acid transport abnormalities.

Renal Tubular Acidosis: Renal tubular acidosis is usually characterized by acidosis and an alkaline urine. Several forms exist, and all three Mendelian modes of inheritance have been described. Renal tubular acidosis associated with osteopetrosis and carbonic anhydrase deficiency is discussed in Chapter 13.

Autosomal Dominant Renal Tubular Acidosis (RTA I) (179800): Autosomal dominant renal tubular acidosis is characterized clinically by acidosis and nephrocalcinosis. The pathogenesis involves abnormal distal tubular function, specifically the transport of hydrogen ion. Bicarbonate wasting, hypercalciuria, and hypokalemia are biochemical features. Growth retardation is a common clinical feature. Therapy consists of administration of bicarbonate to normalize the acidosis. Many pedigrees in the literature are consistent with autosomal dominant inheritance. The gene has not been mapped or cloned.

Autosomal Recessive Renal Tubular Acidosis (RTA III) (267200): Autosomal recessive renal tubular acidosis is associated with bicarbonate wasting in the proximal renal tubule. Infants present with failure to thrive, acidosis, and hypokalemia. Occasionally, nephrocalcinosis is seen. Alkali therapy is the mainstay of treatment. Autosomal recessive inheritance has been established, but the gene has not been mapped.

Autosomal Recessive Renal Tubular Acidosis with Deafness (267300): Renal tubular acidosis with deafness is distinct from RTA III. These patients have progressive sensorineural deafness. Two forms with distinct ages of onset have been distinguished. Usually onset is in infancy, with failure to thrive and acidosis. Sensorineural hearing loss is usually severe. When onset occurs during adolescence, the phenotype is milder, and growth and development are normal. Some patients have renal calculi. Treatment with alkali improves growth but has no effect on accompanying deafness. Pathogenesis remains uncertain. Reported pedigrees show affected siblings with normal parents and consanguinity, which suggests autosomal recessive inheritance. The condition has not been characterized at the molecular level, and the gene has not been mapped.

X-Linked Recessive Renal Tubular Acidosis Type II (312400): Males with X-linked recessive renal tubular acidosis type II have bicarbonate wasting,

Table 9–3. Renal manifestations associated with genetic conditions: nephrosis.

Malformation	Genetic Condition	Inheritance	Map Location	Gene
Nephrosis				
	Nail-patella syndrome (161200)	AD		
	Hereditary persistence of α-fetoprotein (104150)	AD		
	Microcephaly, hiatal hernia, nephrotic syndrome (251300)	AR		
	Congenital nephrosis (256300)	AR		
	Familial Mediterranean fever (249100)	AR		
	Sialic acid (N-acetylneuraminic acid) storage disease (269920)	AR		

acidosis, and sometimes growth and mental retardation. The presence of congenital cataracts, hypotonia, and cognitive dysfunction helps to differentiate this condition from Lowe syndrome. Pedigree evidence points to X-linked inheritance; clinical symptoms have not been reported in heterozygous females. The gene has not been mapped, and the molecular pathology remains uncertain.

Renal Fanconi Syndrome: The renal Fanconi syndrome is characterized by aminoaciduria, phosphaturia, glucosuria, and sometimes renal tubular acidosis, with resulting hypophosphatemia, hypokalemia, and rickets or osteomalacia. The best understood cause of Fanconi syndrome is cystinosis, which is discussed in Chapter 13. The renal tubular dysfunction that characterizes this syndrome is seen also in various genetic conditions that damage the renal tubules. Disorders associated with renal tubular damage are listed in Table 9–1.

Idiopathic Adult Fanconi Syndrome (134600): Cases have been reported of isolated familial Fanconi syndrome without cystinosis or other recognized genetic disorders associated with renal tubular damage. A number of families demonstrate multiple affected generations, with pedigrees that support autosomal dominant inheritance. Considerable variability in clinical features exists both within and between families. The symptoms that first garner clinical attention may result from osteomalacia and may include pain in weight-bearing joints, back pain, and abnormal gait. Some patients present initially with renal failure. Hypertension is not a regular feature. Proteinuria may be a sign in the asymptomatic patient who undergoes a routine urinalysis. Presentation during adult life is usual, but affected children sometimes are identified during a family evaluation. Rarely, a child may be diagnosed because of the development of rickets. Skeletal abnormalities improve after treatment with phosphate and vitamin D. Patients who progress to renal failure may require dialysis or transplantation.

CYSTIC DISEASE

Multiple cysts of the kidney are the defining feature of several single gene conditions that are thought to account for at least 10% of cases of end-stage renal disease. These conditions, Table 9–4 which share many pathologic and clinical features, are distinguished by differences in clinical presentation and pathology and by different modes of inheritance. Increasing elucidation of molecular genetic abnormalities that lead to cystic diseases of the kidney is improving the clinical understanding of these disorders and providing tools for more precise diagnosis in individuals and families. The involvement of other organs, in addition to the kidney, provides a valuable clue to the diagnosis, as does a carefully obtained family history. In addition, awareness of the nature of the involvement in other organs should help to clarify prognosis for genetic syndromes that include cystic kidneys, and should improve the ability to provide accurate genetic counseling.

Polycystic Kidney Disease

Adult (Autosomal Dominant) Polycystic Kidney Disease (APKD) (MIM 173900): In the majority of cases, APKD is characterized by the presence of numerous cysts of the kidney (Fig. 9–3). Other organs including liver, spleen, pancreas, testis, and ovary can also be involved. Most patients are asymptomatic for the first three or four decades of life. After that, abdominal pain, back pain, hypertension, and renal failure ensue. Renal concentrating ability is impaired, renal stones can occur, and hematuria can be significant. Between 5% and 10% of affected individuals have cerebral aneurysms that can result in vascular accidents. Abnormalities of the mitral, tricuspid, and aortic valves also occur. A small but intriguing percentage of patients have onset early in infancy or childhood, some with evidence of prenatal onset. Most commonly, these children are the offspring of a mother with later onset APKD. The mechanism for this early onset is not yet clear, but it seems to be correlated with more rapidly progressive disease. This is reminiscent of the anticipation that accompanied early research into disorders characterized by trinucleotide repeats; final elucidation of the mechanisms in APKD awaits molecular characterization of the gene. APKD with onset in infancy has been accompanied by skeletal malformations including polydactyly, tibial agenesis, and syndactyly in the child of an affected mother. The association is unexplained.

In the United states, APKD affects between 1 in 400 and 1 in 1000 people and accounts for 6–8% of end-stage renal disease. While all ethnic groups are affected, the disorder appears to be less frequent in those of African origin. Large numbers of fluid-filled cysts cover the surface and fill the parenchyma of the kidney, greatly enlarging its size. These cysts, highly variable in size, begin in Bowman's capsule and ultimately destroy the entire renal parenchyma. The resulting distortion of the renal microvascular system may contribute to the pathogenesis of hypertension.

Linkage studies have shown that at least two genetic loci account for APKD. One was mapped to chromosome 16p nearly a decade ago and has now been localized more finely to chromosome 16p13.3. This locus on chromosome 16, PKD1, accounts for about 85% of cases in families of European origin. The specificity in other ethnic groups remains to be clarified. A region isolated on chromosome 16 contains the most likely candidate gene. Its transcript, PBP, has not been fully characterized, and its function remains unknown. Thus, the manner in which mutations in PBP may lead to renal cystic disease is

Table 9–4 Renal manifestations associated with genetic conditions: cysts, dysplasia.

Malformation	Genetic Condition	Inheritance	Map Location	Gene
Cysts, Dysplasia				
	Adult polycystic kidney disease PKD1 (173900)	AD	16p13	
	Adult polycystic kidney disease PKD2 (173910)	AD	4q	
	Medullary cystic kidney disease (174000)	AD		
	Tuberous sclerosis (191100)	AD	9q33–q34	
	von Hippel Lindau syndrome (193300)	AD	3p25–p26	
	Ehlers-Danlos syndrome	AD		
	Apert syndrome (101200)	AD		
	EEC syndrome (129300)	AD		
	Bilateral renal agenesis (191830)	AD		
	Laurence-Moon-Biedl-Bardet (245800)	AR		
	Zellweger syndrome (214100)	AR	7q11	
	Majewski Short-Rib polydactyly (263520)	AR		
	Fryns syndrome (229850)	AR		
	Medullary cystic disease (NPH1) (256100)	AR	12p23–cen	
	Ivemark syndrome (263200)			
	Ectromelia-icthyosis syndrome	AR		
	Infantile polycystic disease ARPKD, (263200)	AR	6p21–cens	
	Roberts syndrome (268300)	AR		
	Goldston syndrome (267010)	AR		
	Finnish nephrosis (256300)	AR		
	Meckel-Gruber syndrome (249000)	AR		
	Renal dysplasia and retinal aplasia (266900)	AR		
	Asphyxiating thoracic dystrophy (208500)	AR		
	Radial aplasia syndrome (208500)	AR		
	Lowe syndrome (309000)	XLR	Xq24–26	
	Oral-facial-digital syndrome I (311200)	XLR		

unclear. Haplotype analysis in the region suggests heterogeneity and, as in many other genetic disorders, more than one mutation in this gene may be responsible for APKD. A second locus, PKD2, has been mapped to chromosome 4q. Some data suggest that onset may occur later in families whose mutation resides in this locus, and that when this occurs, APKD may be somewhat milder. Other loci related to APKD may also exist. Additional molecular studies are needed to resolve this question.

Ultrasound examination to identify renal cysts is widely performed for diagnosis in families at risk. The likelihood of identifying affected individuals through the use of renal ultrasound is greater than 80% in patients above the age of 30 years and approaches 100% in patients age 40 or above. Ultrasound is less definitive in younger persons.

Molecular studies can complement ultrasound examination for diagnosis and can refine the risk estimates in individuals and families. Since the specific molecular lesions in the putative gene, PBP, have not

been elucidated, linkage studies using markers that flank the gene on chromosome 16 are the mainstay of molecular diagnosis. Thus, an informative family is critical to the analysis. For the 10–15% of families who do not have the mutation on chromosome 16, other avenues must be pursued. Linkage analysis using markers close to the locus on chromosome 4q can be used in families with an established linkage to chromosome 4. In families for whom the molecular studies are not informative, ultrasound examination of kidneys and liver is the major safe and secure method of diagnosis.

Presymptomatic diagnosis may help to identify affected individuals for whom early management of hypertension and incipient renal failure may improve prognosis. Such early diagnosis can also play a role in identifying unaffected family members who are suitable as donors for renal transplant. Prenatal diagnosis using linkage analysis has been successful in identifying affected fetuses who carry the gene. Occasionally fetuses with the early onset form and the

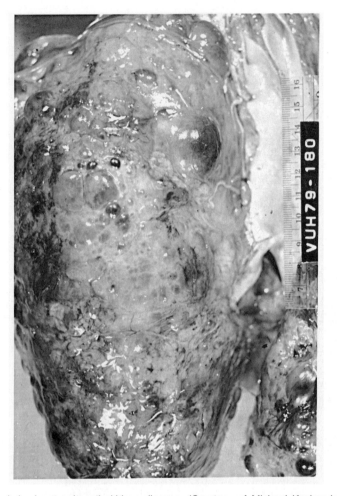

Figure 9–3. Autosomal dominant polycystic kidney disease. (Courtesy of Michael Kashgarian, MD, Yale University School of Medicine.)

variant associated with skeletal malformations have been diagnosed by ultrasonography.

Many persons with APKD survive to the sixth or seventh decade of life with minimal or no symptoms. Estimates suggest that about 50% of individuals who carry the gene will be symptomatic by age 58 years. The factors that lead to variability in survival are not certain. Prognosis seems to depend somewhat on age of onset. The associated hypertension, a major factor in prognosis, must be aggressively treated. Pain is a significant symptom that requires ongoing management. Cysts may become infected, and this represents a life-threatening situation. Many patients go on to renal failure and require dialysis and renal transplant. Pretransplant removal of the enlarged native kidneys is controversial. A small group of patients will have very early onset in infancy or childhood. Their prognosis for renal failure is much higher, but they can survive.

Infantile Polycystic Kidney Disease (Autosomal Recessive Polycystic Kidney Disease—ARPKD) (263200): In distinction to autosomal dominant polycystic kidney disease, the recessive form —autosomal recessive polycystic kidney disease or ARPKD—appears in childhood, usually in early infancy. The large, polycystic kidneys are often appreciated prenatally, and they may be large enough to cause difficulty at delivery (Figure 9–4). Pulmonary hypoplasia may result from oligohydramnios or from physical compression of the fetal lungs by the enlarged kidneys. Complete renal failure may be present, or it may develop over the first months. When prenatal renal failure with oligohydramnios has occurred, typical Potter's facies may be present: flat nose, epicanthal folds, and the appearance of having been "flattened". The mortality rate in the neonatal period is about 50%, and death usually results from pulmonary insufficiency. The liver lesions that are al-

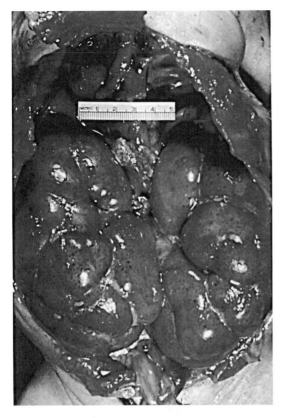

Figure 9–4. Gross appearance of kidneys *in situ* in autosomal recessive, infantile onset polycystic kidney disease. (Photo courtesy of Dr. Michael Kashgarian, Yale School of Medicine).

ways a part of this disorder include proliferation and ectasia of bile ducts, development of cysts, and periportal fibrosis that may result in esophageal varices. Hypertension is common in these patients.

Autosomal recessive polycystic kidney disease is the most common cystic disease of the kidneys in childhood. Its incidence has been estimated at 1 in 10,000 to 1 in 40,000. The cysts appear to arise within tubules, rather than in the glomerulus. The mechanism by which the cysts develop remains uncertain. Autosomal recessive inheritance has been recognized for decades. Linkage studies have shown that the recessive disorder is not linked to the gene on chromosome 4q, which is involved in one of the forms of the autosomal dominant polycystic kidney disease, PKD2. Recently, a gene for ARPKD has been mapped to chromosome 6p21–cen. It is unclear whether this represents the only locus, and no candidate genes have been uncovered. The nature of the mutation or mutations also remains unknown. In mice, an autosomal recessive polycystic kidney disease has been mapped to a region that is homologous to a locus on human chromosome 13. It is unclear whether this locus is related to human ARPKD.

Diagnosis of ARPKD can be confirmed by ultrasound examination that reveals large kidneys with dilated tubules and multiple cysts. Hepatic cysts and hepatic fibrosis are also seen. Prenatal ultrasound examination can identify some affected fetuses, but the kidneys may appear normal in early fetal life, and the abnormalities may not be apparent until as late as 30 weeks of gestation. Linkage studies using markers near the gene on chromosome 6 may help to ensure the diagnosis in informative families. Nearly half of the affected patients die in the first months of life. Death in the immediate neonatal period usually results from pulmonary insufficiency. With ventilatory support, approximately 50% of affected patients who survive the first year may be alive by age 10. Their renal function may be only moderately impaired, or progressive loss of renal parenchyma may lead to renal failure. Aggressive medical management, including bilateral nephrectomy and peritoneal dialysis, has contributed to a longer lifespan and allowed some children to survive to receive a renal transplant. Hepatic fibrosis and hepatic cysts are common in these patients but do not appear to compromise liver function early in life. Portal hypertension, however, may occur in patients who survive early infancy and childhood.

Medullary Cystic Disease

Autosomal Dominant Medullary Cystic Disease (174000):
Autosomal dominant medullary cystic disease has an earlier age of onset than PKD1 and PKD2. Clinical features include the loss of urinary concentrating ability and the presence of small kidneys with multiple cysts. Tubular dysfunction, including salt and potassium wasting, occurs. In contrast to PKD1, hypertension and pain are usually absent. The pathology consists of medullary cysts that involve the collecting ducts. The disorder is inherited in an autosomal dominant fashion, but the gene has not been mapped, and the molecular pathology is unknown. Diagnosis relies on ultrasound examination. Renal failure progressing to death is common. Dialysis and renal transplant are the only therapeutic options.

Autosomal Recessive Medullary Cystic Disease (Familial Juvenile Nephronophthisis, NPH1) (256100):
Autosomal recessive medullary cystic disease usually manifests in early childhood and is a frequent cause of childhood renal failure that requires renal transplantation. The clinical features include loss of renal concentrating ability with polyuria and polydipsia, anemia, growth failure, and salt wasting. Hypertension and pain are not features. The pathology is similar to adult onset medullary cystic disease. Many pedigrees provide evidence of autosomal recessive inheritance. The locus has been mapped to chromosome 2p24.1. The molecular pathology remains uncertain, however. Linkage studies can contribute to diagnosis in informative families. Genetic

heterogeneity has not been excluded, so more than one locus may exist. Ultrasound examination provides diagnostic information. The disorder typically progresses to renal failure and death, and dialysis and renal transplant are the only therapeutic hope.

Oral-Facial-Digital Syndrome Type I

An X-linked disorder, oral-facial-digital syndrome Type I includes, in addition to cystic kidneys, characteristic facies with cleft jaw and tongue, clinodactyly, syndactyly, and central nervous system abnormalities, including mental retardation. Though it is usually lethal in males, the syndrome has been reported in one live-born male. Affected females can develop renal failure.

Other Inherited Disorders That Include Cystic Renal Disease

Many disparate genetic disorders have cystic renal disease as a major characteristic. These disorders are distinguished by the presence of other features that can involve many systems. Examples include multiple congenital malformations, urinary obstruction, retinitis pigmentosa, or a specific constellation of clinical, biochemical, or ana- tomical abnormalities that constitute a syndrome. The presence of other findings, in addition to cystic renal disease, should alert the physician to one of these disorders. For some of these conditions, diagnosis must be based on clinical examination, imaging studies, and examination of microscopic anatomy. For other conditions that have cystic renal disease as a feature, molecular diagnostic tools will prove useful.

Renal Vascular Disease

Renal artery stenosis can be associated with recognized genetic disorders, in particular, neurofibromatosis and Williams syndrome. It is well known that hypertension, especially that of early onset, runs in families. The increased frequency in African Americans is also well recognized. While the specific genetic factors have not yet been elucidated, attention is being directed to the genes that control angiotensin metabolism.

DEVELOPMENTAL DEFECTS & MALFORMATIONS OF THE URINARY TRACT

Renal Agenesis, Dysgenesis, & Dysplasia

Complete agenesis of the kidney is a dramatic and lethal condition that occurs in 1 in 3000–4000 births. Infants are stillborn or die soon after birth. Potter's facies, a constellation of facial deformations, results from deformation in a uterus that contains too little amniotic fluid (Figure 9–5 and Tables 9–5, 9–6 and 9–7). Potter's facies is not specific for renal

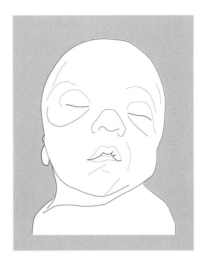

Figure 9–5. Typical facies as described by Potter of stillborn with absent kidneys. Note the pressed-in nose, exaggerated folds under the eyelids, and mishapen face.

agenesis; this disorder can be seen in other conditions with reduced amniotic fluid volume. Bilateral renal agenesis is usually a sporadic event. Nevertheless, bilateral re-nal agenesis can show familial aggregation, alone or in association with recognized genetic conditions.

The presence of other malformations provides important information for assessing the role of genetic factors. If a specific syndrome is identified, the genetic risks are those associated with the syndrome. Isolated renal agenesis has recurred in families with and without parental consanguinity. Both concordant and discordant identical twins have been reported, and new dominant mutations may play a role in this phenomenon. McKusick has listed bilateral renal agenesis in the dominant catalog (MIM 191830). The gene involved is unknown. For couples who have

Table 9–5. Renal manifestations associated with genetic conditions: Phenotypic features of the infant with renal agenesis.

Feature	Manifestation
Potter's facies	Flattened nose Prominent inner canthal fold sweeping below the eyes Recessed chin Enlarged ears
Pulmonary hypoplasia	Pulmonary failure
Talipes equinovarus	
Large, oval adrenals (may be mistaken for kidneys)	

Table 9–6. Renal manifestations associated with genetic conditions: Conditions associated with Potter facies.[1]

Bilateral renal agenesis
Oligohydramnios of any etiology
Severe hypoplasia or dysplasia of kidneys
Intrauterine urinary obstruction
Prune belly syndrome
Infantile polycystic kidney disease (MIM 263200)
Other cystic dysplasias of kidney
Branchiootorenal dysplasia (MIM 113650)
Multiple congenital anomalies associated with renal malformations

[1] See Curry (1984); Pramanik (1977); Fantel (1975).

had one affected child, the risk of having a second affected child is 1–4%. This is higher than the risk for the general population, but lower than the risk for a second affected child in the case of single gene disorders. The risk that a parent or sibling of child with renal agenesis will have a non-lethal renal malformation (8–9%) is also higher than the risk for the general population. Ultrasound examination will identify most cases of renal agenesis. Prenatal ultrasound examination can identify the disorder in a fetus at risk, although the precision of prenatal diagnosis remains uncertain.

Branchiootorenal Dysplasia (BOR) (MIM 113650)

An autosomal dominant condition, branchiootorenal dysplasia (BOR) is characterized by preauricular ear pits, a cochlear malformation with hearing loss, branchial clefts, dysplastic cup-shaped ears, and renal dysgenesis. Variability among family members occurs; a parent with renal dysgenesis can have a child with unilateral renal agenesis or bilateral renal agenesis and Potter's facies. BOR has been mapped to chromosome 8q, but the gene has not been identified.

Urinary Tract Obstruction

Urinary tract obstruction can occur at the level of the ureteropelvic junction (UPJ), the entrance to the bladder, or within the urethra itself. Hydronephrosis is associated with a large number of genetic syndromes (Table 9–8). UPJ obstruction and posterior urethral valves can lead to severe urinary tract obstruction, hydronephrosis, and secondary renal abnormalities. Association with the Prune belly syn-

Table 9–7. Renal abnormalities associated with genetic conditions: renal agenesis.

Malformation	Genetic Condition	Inheritance	Map Location	Gene
Renal Agenesis				
	Triploidy	Chromosomal		
	4p, 18q, trisomy 21	Chromosomal		
	Trisomy 22(pter→q11)	Chromosomal		
	Cat-eye syndrome (trisomy or tetrasomy 22pter–q11)	Chromosomal		
	Branchio-oto-renal dysplasia (113650)	AD	8q	
	Klippel-Feil syndrome (148900)	AD		
	Multiple lentigenes syndrome	AD		
	Bilateral renal agenesis (191830)	AD		
	Glycerol kinase deficiency (191830)	AD		
	Branchiootorenal dysplasia (113650)	AD		
	Opitz-G syndrome (145410)	AD		
	Roberts syndrome (268300)	AR		
	Thrombocytopenia–absent radius syndrome (274000)	AR		
	Multiple pterygium syndrome (265000)	AR		
	Renal-retinal syndrome (Senior-Loken) (266900)	AR		
	Rokitansky syndrome (congenital absence of vagina) (277000)	AR		
	Lenz dysplasia (with microphthalmia) (309800)	XLR		
	Kallmann syndrome (308700)	XLR	Xp22.3	KAL

Table 9–8 Renal manifestations associated with genetic conditions: hydronephrosis, duplications.

Malformation	Genetic Condition	Inheritance	Map Location	Gene
Hydronephrosis, Duplications				
	Apert syndrome (101200)	AD	10q26	FGFR2
	EEC syndrome (129900)	AD	7q21.3–q11.2	
	Multiple lentigenes syndrome	AD	—	—
	Thanatophoric dysplasia (187600)	AD	—	—
	Congenital nephrogenic diabetes insipidus, Type II (125800)	AD	—	—
	Presacral teratoma with sacral dysgenesis (176450)	AD	—	—
	Hydronephrosis with UPJ obstruction (143400)	AD		
	Pallister-hall syndrome (146510)	AD	2q32–q31	HOXD10
	Diabetes mellitus and insipidus with optic atrophy and deafness (222300)	AR	4p	—
	Johanson-Blizzard syndrome (243800)	AR		
	Laurence-Moon-Biedl syndrome (209900)	AR	16q21	
	Congenital lipodystrophy (269700)	AR	—	
	Schinzel-Giedion syndrome (269150)	AR	—	—
	Roberts syndrome (268300)	AR	—	—
	Megacystis-microcolon-intestinal hypoperistalis syndrome (249210)	AR	—	
	Urofacial syndrome (236730)	AR	—	—
	Meckel-Gruber syndrome (249000)	AR	—	—
	Dyssegmental dwarfism (224400)	AR	—	
	Perlman syndrome (267000)	AR	—	
	Smith-Lemli Opitz syndrome (270400)	AR	7q34–qter	
	Xanthinuria (278300)	AR	2	
	Holoprosencephaly, familial alobar (236100)	AR	18pter–q11	
	Coffin-Lowry syndrome (303600)	XLR	Xp22.2–p22.1	
	Otopalatodigital syndrome, Type II (304120)	XLR	—	
	α-thalassemia/mental retardation syndrome (301040)	XLR	Xq21.1–q12	—
	Nephrogenic diabetes insipidus, Type I (304800)	XLR	Xq28	AVPR2

drome is now well known. This constellation of sequelae to urinary tract obstruction includes deficiency of abdominal wall musculature, undescended testes, and renal abnormalities. Prognosis depends upon severity of the renal abnormalities. If renal function is severely compromised during intrauterine life, the consequences of oligohydramnios, including Potter's facies and pulmonary hypoplasia, may occur, and death from pulmonary insufficiency may supervene. Attempts at prenatal urinary drainage have had some success when the urinary obstruction is diagnosed early in prenatal life (see Chapter 7). Exstrophy of the bladder is a severe developmental abnormality in which the bladder is exteriorized and urinary drainage is external. Genetic etiologic factors have not been identified.

Several groups of malformation sequences have associated urinary tract abnormalities. The urorectal septum malformation sequence is associated with renal agenesis, bladder dilatation, hydronephrosis, and urethral absence. Urinary tract abnormalities are part of the VATER sequence (vertebral abnormalities, anal malformations, tracheoesophageal fistula, radial dysplasia, renal abnormalities). The MURCS association includes Mullerian duct aplasia, renal aplasia, and perithoracic somite dysplasia. No genetic factors for these conditions are known. Congenital absence of the vagina (Rokitansky-Mayer-Kunstler syndrome) (MIM 277000) is associated with renal agenesis, solitary kidney, and abnormalities of the renal pelvis. Some evidence exists for autosomal recessive inheritance in this syndrome.

Hypospadias is a common developmental abnormality; the incidence is estimated to be 1 in 300 to 1 in 1000 males. The condition results from incomplete fusion of the urethral folds during development. Etiologic factors include male pseudohermaphroditism and congenital adrenal hyperplasia (see Chapter 12). Sex chromosome mosaicism, XO/XY and XX/XY, may also result in hypospadias (see Chapter 2). Genetic studies in isolated hypospadias have not identified Mendelian segregation. Empiric recurrence risk in brothers has been put at 10–17%. Risk to sons of affected men is not well established; in a small number of families, autosomal dominant inheritance may operate. Hypospadias is a feature of a large number of syndromes (Table 9–8). The association between renal dysplasia and middle ear anomalies is recognized, but genetic factors have not been clarified.

Genetic factors play an important role in the etiology of abnormal structure and function of the kidney and urinary tract. Chromosomal abnormalities, single gene mutations, and interactions between genes and environmental factors may all be implicated. A careful family history is important in the attempt to establish genetic risks. Establishing the extent to which other organ systems are involved may help to diagnose a genetic syndrome. Particular attention should be paid to the eye, ear, heart, and central nervous system when looking for other abnormalities. The confirmation of a genetic condition will help establish prognosis, identify other problems needing attention, and provide risk assessment for family members.

REFERENCES AND SUGGESTED READING

Antignac C et al: Deletions in the COL4A5 collagen gene in X-linked Alport syndrome. J Clin Invest 1994;**93:**1195.

Auchterlonie IA, White WP: Recurrence of the VATER association within a sibship. Clin Genet 1982;**21:**122.

Aula P et al: Prenatal diagnosis of congenital nephrosis in 23 high-risk families. Am J Dis Child 1978;**132:**984.

Bankier A et al: A pedigree study of perinatally lethal renal disease. J Med Genet 1985;**22:**104.

Barker DF et al. Identification of mutations in the COL4A5 collagen gene in Alport syndrome. Science 1990;**248:**1224.

Bear JC et al: Autosomal dominant polycystic kidney disease: New information for genetic counselling. Am J Med Genet 1992;**43:**548.

Blyth H, Ockenden BG: Polycystic disease of kidneys and liver presenting in childhood. J Med Genet 1971;**8:**257.

Bodziak KA, Hammond WS, Molitoris BA: Inherited diseases of the glomerular basement membrane. Am J Kidney Dis 1994;**23:**605.

Brenton DP et al: Adult presenting idiopathic Fanconi syndrome. J Inherited Metab Dis 1981;**4:**211.

Brown MT et al: Progressive sensorineural hearing loss in association with distal renal tubular acidosis. Arch Otolaryngol 1993;**119:**458.

Brown R et al: Molecular cloning of the human Goodpasture antigen demonstrates it to be the α-3 chain of type IV collagen. J Clin Invest 1992;**89:**592.

Cain DR et al: Familial renal agenesis and total dysplasia. Am J Dis Child 1974;**128:**377.

Carlisle EJ, Donnelly SM, Halperin ML: Renal tubular acidosis (RTA): Recognize the ammonium defect and pHorget the urine pH. Pediatr Nephrol 0199;**5:**242.

Carter CO, Evans K, Pescia G: A family study of renal agenesis. J Med Genet 1979;**16:**176.

Chapman AB et al: Intracranial aneurysms in autosomal dominant polycystic kidney disease. N Engl J Med 1992;**327:**916.

Chen YC, Woolley P: Genetic studies on hypospadias in males. J Med Genet 1971;**8:**153.

Curry CJR et al: The Potter sequence: A clinical analysis of 80 cases. Am J Med Genet 1984;**19:**679.

Davison JM, Lindheimer MD: Renal disorders. Page 828 in: *Maternal-Fetal Medicine: Principles and Practice,* 2nd ed. Creasy K, Risnik R (editors). WB Saunders, 1989.

Duncan PA et al: The MURCS association: Mullerian duct aplasia, renal aplasia, and cerviothoracic somite dysplasia. (Abstract) Orthop Trans 1979;**3:**120.

Ehruch JHH et al: Association of spondylo-epiphyseal dysplasia with nephrotic syndrome. Pediatr Nephrol 1990;**4:**117.

Escobar LF et al: Urorectal septum malformation sequence. Am J Dis Child 1987;**141:**1021.

European Polycystic Kidney Disease Consortium. The polycystic kidney disease gene encodes a 14kb transcript and lies within a duplicated region on chromosome 16. Cell 1994;**77:**881.

Fick GM, Gabow PA: Natural history of autosomal dominant polycystic kidney disease. Ann Rev Med 1994;**45:**23.

Friedman AL, Trygstad CW, Chesney RW: Autosomal dominant Fanconi syndrome with early renal failure. Am J Med Genet 1978;**2:**225.

Frymoyer PA et al: X-linked recessive nephrolithiasis with renal failure. N Engl J Med 1991;**325:**681.

Gabow P: Autosomal dominant polycystic kidney disease. N Engl J Med 1993;**329:**332.

Gabow P, Bennett WM: Renal manifestations: Complication management and long-term outcome of autosomal dominant polycystic kidney disease. Semin Nephrol 1991;**11:**643.

Garty BZ et al: Microcephaly and congenital nephrotic syndrome owing to diffuse mesangial sclerosis: An autosomal recessive syndrome. J Med Genet 1994;**31:**121.

Germino G et al: The gene for autosomal dominant polycystic kidney disease lies in a 750-kb CpG-rick region. Genomics 1992;**13:**144.

Gillerot Y et al: Oral-facial-digital syndrome Type I in a newborn male. Am J Med Genet 1993;**46:**335.

Gillespie GAJ et al: CpG island in the region of an autosomal dominant polycystic kidney disease locus defines the 5′ end of a gene encoding a putative proton channel. Proc Soc Natl Acad Sci USA 1991;**88:**4289.

Gillessen-Kaesbach G et al: New autosomal recessive lethal disorder with polycystic kidneys type Potter I, characteristic face, microcephaly, brachymelia, and congenital heart defects. Am J Med Genet 1993;**45:**511.

Grantham J: Polycystic kidney disease: Hereditary and acquired. Adv Intern Med 1993;**38**:409.

Hack M et al: Familial aggregation in bilateral renal agenesis. Clin Genetics 1974;**5**:173.

Hannig VL et al: Presymptomatic testing for adult onset polycystic kidney disease in at-risk kidney transplant donors. Am J Med Genet 1991;**40**:425.

Hasstedt SJ, Atkin CL: X-linked inheritance of Alport syndrome: Family P revisited. Am J Hum Genet 1983;**35**:1241.

Hasstedt SJ, Atkin CL, San Juan AC: Genetic heterogeneity among kindreds with Alport syndrome. Am J Hum Genet 1985;**38**:940.

Hayslett JP: Pregnancy complicated by renal disorders. Pages 1086–1096 in: *Medicine of the Fetus and Mother.* Reece EA et al (editors). Lippincott, 1992.

Heimler A, Lieber E: Branchio-oto-renal syndrome. Am J Med Genet 1986;**25**:15.

Hossack KF et al: Echocardiographic findings in autosomal dominant polycystic kidney disease. N Engl J Med 1988;**319**:907.

Igarashi T et al: Persistent isolated renal tubular acidosis–A systemic disease with a distinct clinical entity. Pediatr Nephrol 1994;**8**:70.

Ives E, Coffey R, Carter CO: A family study of bladder extrophy. J Med Genet 1980;**17**:139.

Kestila M et al: Congenital nephrotic syndrome of the Finnish type maps to the long arm of chromosome 19. Am J Hum Genet 1994;**54**:757.

Kimberling WJ, Pieke-Dahl S, Kumar S: The genetics of cystic diseases of the kidney. Semin Nephrol 1991;**11**:596.

Lemmink HH et al: Aberrant splicing of the COL4A5 gene in patients with Alport syndrome. Human Molecular Genetics 1994;**3**:317.

Lewis SME et al: Joubert syndrome with congenital hepatic fibrosis: Entity in the spectrum of oculo-hepato-renal disorders. Am J Med Genet 1994;**52**:419.

Long WS et al: Idiopathic Fanconi syndrome with progressive renal failure: A case report and discussion. Yale J Biol Med 1990;**63**:15.

McDonald RA, Avner ED: Inherited polycystic kidney disease in children. Semin Nephrol 1991;**11**:632.

Moerman P et al: Pathogenesis of the Prune-belly syndrome: A functional urethral obstruction caused by prostatic hypoplasia. Pediatrics 1984;**73**:470.

Moyer JH et al: Candidate gene associated with a mutation causing recessive polycystic kidney disease in mice. Science 1994;**264**:1329.

Myers JC et al: Molecular cloning of α5(IV) collagen and assignment of the gene to the region of the X chromosome containing the Alport syndrome locus. Am J Hum Genet 1990;**46**:1024.

Neinstein LS, Castle G: Congenital absence of the vagina. Am J Dis Child 1983;**137**:669.

Ni L et al: Refined localization of the Branchiootorenal syndrome gene by linkage and haplotype analysis. Am J Med Genet 1994;**51**:176.

Parfrey PS et al: The diagnosis and prognosis of autosomal dominant polycystic kidney disease. N Engl J Med 1990;**323**:1085.

Peral B et al: Evidence of linkage disequilibrium in the Spanish polycystic kidney disease I population. Am J Hum Genet 1994;**54**:899.

Pramanik AK et al: Prune-Belly syndrome associated with Potter (renal nonfunction) syndrome. Am J Dis Child 1977;**131**:672.

Reeders ST: Multilocus polycystic disease. Nature Genetics 1992;**1**:235.

Reeders ST, Breuning MH, Davies A: Highly polymorphic DNA marker linked to adult polycystic kidney disease on chromosome 16. Nature 1985;**317**:542.

Renieri A et al: Single base apir deletions in exons 39 and 42 of the COL4A5 gene in Alport syndrome. Human Molecular Genetics 1994;**3**:201.

Roodhooft AM, Birnholz J, Holmes I: Familial nature of congenital absence and severe dysgenesis of both kidneys. N Engl J Med 1984;**310**:1341.

Saito A et al: A deletion mutation in the 3′ end of the αr(IV) collagen gene in juvenile-onset Alport syndrome. J Am Soc Nephrol 1994;**4**:1649.

Schinzel A, Homberger C, Sigrist T: Case report: Bilateral renal agenesis in male sibs born to consanguineous parents. J Med Genet 1978;**15**:314.

Shokeir MHK: Expression of "adult" polycystic renal disease in the fetus and newborn. Clin Genet 1978;**14**:61.

Steenman MJC et al: Loss of imprinting of IGF2 is linked to reduced expression and abnormal methylation of H19 in Wilms' tumor. Nature Genetics 1994;**7**:433.

Sujansky E et al: Attitudes of at-risk and affected individuals regarding presymptomatic testing for autosomal dominant polycystic kidney disease. Am J Med Genet 1990;**35**:510.

Sumfest JM, Burns MW, Mitchell ME: Aggressive surgical and medical management of autosomal recessive polycystic kidney disease. Urology 1993;**42**:309.

Svensson J: Male hypospadias, 625 cases, associated malformations and possible etiological factors. Acta Paediatr Scand 1979;**68**:587.

Turco AE et al: Molecular genetic diagnosis of autosomal dominant polycystic kidney disease in a newborn with bilateral cystic kidneys detected prenatally and multiple skeletal malformations. J Med Genet 1993;**30**:419.

Urioste M, Arroyo A, Martinez-Frias ML: Campomelia, polycystic dysplasia, and cervical lymphocele in two sibs. Am J Med Genet 1991;**41**:475.

van Lieburg AF et al: Patients with autosomal nephrogenic diabetes insipidus homozygous for mutations in the aquaporin 2 water-channel gene. Am J Hum Genet 1994;**55**:648.

Warkany J: The kidney. Pages 1037–1040 in: *Congenital Malformations.* Warkany J (editor). Year Book Medical Publications, 1971.

Yoshikawa N et al: Non-familial hematuria associated with glomerular basement membrane alterations characteristic of hereditary nephritis: comparison with hereditary nephritis. J Pediatr 1987;**111**:519.

Zerres K et al: Mapping the gene for autosomal recessive polycystic kidney disease (ARPKD) to chromosome 6p21–cen. Nature Genetics 1994;**7**:429.

Zerres K, Mucher G, Rudnik-Schoneborn. Autosomal recessive polycystic kidney disease does not map to the second gene locus for autosomal dominant polycystic kidney disease on chromosome 4. Hum Genet 1994;**93**:697.

Zonana J, DiLiberti JH: Congenital and herediary urinary tract disorders. Pages 1273–1289 in: *Principles and Practice of Medical Genetics,* 2nd ed. Emery AEH, Rimoin D (editors). Churchill Livingstone, 1990.

Digestive & Pulmonary Systems

10

A number of diverse genetic conditions affect the digestive tract. In some, the digestive tract is the major site of involvement. In others, it is only one of many organs altered by the genetically determined dysfunction. This chapter will describe some of the more common and well defined genetic conditions in which gastrointestinal signs and symptoms are prominent. Two disorders are discussed here which might also be discussed as pulmonary disorders: cystic fibrosis and α-1-antitrypsin deficiency. They are placed here for convenience. Cancers of the digestive tract are considered in Chapter 5.

CONGENITAL ABNORMALITIES WITH A GENETIC COMPONENT

Pyloric Stenosis

Non-bilious vomiting commencing between the first and the fourth weeks of life is the most characteristic clinical feature of pyloric stenosis. If the diagnosis is not made promptly, failure to thrive, dehydration, and hypochloremic alkalosis eventually occur. In contrast to disorders accompanied by nausea or pain, babies with pyloric stenosis appear hungry and feed vigorously, only to vomit in a projectile fashion shortly after nursing. The incidence of pyloric stenosis varies among differing ethnic groups. Representative frequencies include: 1.5–3 in 1000 in Caucasians, 1 in 10,000 in Asians, and 0.5 in 1000 in persons of African origin. Familial incidence is well known, but no Mendelian pattern has been recognized. Several studies provide empiric risk figures to use in genetic counseling. Recurrence risk in a family with one affected child depends on the sex of the index case and may be related to birth order. First-born sons of affected mothers have the highest frequency (Table 10–1).

Diagnosis is made by palpation of the classical "olive" in the right upper quadrant of the abdomen or by ultrasound imaging of the hypertrophic and elongated pyloric muscle. Treatment consists of surgical repair by pyloromyotomy. Prognosis is excellent for complete recovery. Care must be taken to achieve fluid and electrolyte balance prior to surgery, if diagnosis has not occurred early enough to avoid dehydration and hypochloremic alkalosis. Genetic dis-

orders associated with vomiting are listed in Table 10–2.

Hirschsprung Disease

Hirschsprung disease is most commonly diagnosed in infancy. The average age at diagnosis has decreased over the past several decades. The neonate most commonly presents with complete intestinal obstruction or partial obstruction with alternating constipation and diarrhea, vomiting, and distention. Enterocolitis is common and is the major cause of mortality in these patients. Morbidity and mortality associated with enterocolitis are greater in infants diagnosed after the first month of life and in infants with longer aganglionic segments. In the older infant, chronic constipation is the most prominent finding, along with failure to thrive and abdominal distention. In this age group, the diagnosis can be delayed owing to diagnostic odysseys.

Incidence is about 1 in 5000 newborns. There is a preponderance of males, with a ratio of male to females of 3.75:1. The pathogenesis of Hirschsprung disease is based on the absence of ganglion cells in the myenteric and submucosal plexus in the large bowel. Ganglion cells are of neural crest origin and normally migrate to the intestine between 8–12 weeks of gestational age. Either this fails to occur in Hirschsprung disease or the ganglion cells are destroyed. Aganglionosis of the colon is associated with spasm in the affected segment of colon and compromise of peristaltic function. Constipation then occurs with subsequent diarrhea due to the obstruction. Length of the affected segment varies between and within families: 8% involve the entire

Table 10–1. Recurrence risks in pyloric stenosis.		
Percentage Affected Female	Percentage Affected Male	Risk to Relative
18.9	5.5	Son
7.0	2.4	Daughter
10.8	6.6	Brother
3.8	2.8	Sister

Table 10–2. Genetic disorders associated with vomiting.

Condition	Genetic Mechanism
Pyloric stenosis	Multifactorial
Intestinal atresia	
Duodenal atresia	Down syndrome; trisomy 21
Multiple atresia	Recessive (MIM 243150)
Apple peel atresia	Recessive (MIM 243600)
Meconium ileus	Cystic fibrosis; autosomal recessive
Central nervous system disorders	
Hydrocephalus	X-linked aqueductal stenosis
Metabolic	
Adrenal insufficiency	Autosomal recessive
Renal tubular acidosis	Autosomal recessive, autosomal dominant, x-linked recessive
Disorders of carbohydrate metabolism (see chapter inborn errors)	
Galactosemia	Autosomal recessive
Hereditary fructose intolerance	Autosomal recessive
Disorders of organic acid metabolism	Autosomal recessive
Methylmalonic, propionic acidemia	Autosomal recessive
Disorders of ammonia metabolism	
Various urea cycle abnormalities	Autosomal recessive
OTC deficiency	X-linked
Disorders of amino acid metabolism	
Tyrosinemia	Autosomal recessive
Branched chain aminoaciduria (MSUD)	Autosomal recessive

colon, 30% the rectum alone, and 40% the recto-sigmoid.

Familial incidence without any Mendelian pattern has long been recognized. Several studies have attempted to establish an empirical risk for occurrence of Hirschsprung disease in first degree relatives of affected individuals, in order to provide genetic counseling for families with an affected child or parent. These data have been somewhat complex. Recurrence risk within families ranges in various studies from 1.8–8.2% and depends on the sex of the affected index patient and the length of the aganglionic segment (Table 10–3). None of these studies has shown risks of the magnitude seen in simple Mendelian disorders. The exception to this generalization is the observation of a number of families showing a pattern of dominant inheritance for long segment aganglionosis. Consequently this long segment form of Hirschsprung disease has been listed in the autosomal dominant section of the McKusick catalog (MIM 142623).

Recently molecular analysis has shed new light on this disorder. In some affected families, the presence of Hirschsprung disease segregated with markers located at a region on chromosome 10q. These observations directed attention to genes in the region of 10q. Mutations and deletions in the RET oncogene mapped to 10q11.2 were observed in patients with Hirschsprung disease. The same gene is involved in multiple endocrine neoplasia, MEN2B, (see Chapter 13) but the mutations in Hirschsprung disease are different from those in MEN2B. Missense and frameshift mutations as well as deletions affect the tyrosine kinase domain of the protein. Mutations have largely been identified in single cases, but in some families the same mutation has been seen in more than one affected family member. All the mutations that have been identified are in the RET oncogene. The RET oncogene plays a role in Drosophila development and is expressed in the developing nervous system of the mouse, so a relationship to Hirschsprung disease is plausible. The patients reported to have microscopic deletions in 10q have had

Table 10–3. Recurrence risks and sex incidence in Hirschsprung disease.

Source	Percentage Recurrence in Sibs	Percentage Recurrence in Other Relatives	Percentage Male/Female Incidence (Long Segment)	Percentage Male/Female Incidence (Short Segment)
Bodian and Carter	5.9	7.9	1.5	3.6
Madsen	4.6	4.6	2.2	2.9
Passarge	4.8	6.4	2.0	6.9
Garver	3.7	8.2	1.4	3.6

dysmorphic facies as well, suggesting the disruption of contiguous genes. Aganglionosis has been reported in a variety of other conditions, some of which can be viewed as possible neurocristopathies.

Diagnosis is currently confirmed by observing the lack of ganglion cells in rectal biopsy material. As the role of the described mutations becomes clearer, there may be a place for molecular diagnosis. Attempts at prenatal diagnosis by measuring amniotic fluid disaccharidases have failed. Surgical resection of the affected segment is the definitive treatment. Care must be taken to see that the resection includes the entire aganglionic segment and that ganglion cells exist in the remaining proximal colon. If enterocolitis supervenes, it must be promptly recognized and treated.

Anorectal Malformations

Developmental abnormalities of the anus are diverse, ranging from covered anus to complete rectal and anal agenesis. There may be other associated malformations, particularly involving the genitourinary tract. The incidence of this group of anomalies has been estimated to be 1 in 3000–4000 births. Familial recurrence has been reported. There are families with affected sibs of both sexes and families in which the pattern of inheritance is compatible with X-linkage. Anorectal malformations may be seen in association with some recognized dysmorphic syndromes. For the most part, however, incidence is sporadic. Treatment consists of surgical repair. Very high defects may require more than one procedure to achieve correction. Continence may be compromised.

Intestinal Atresias

Intestinal atresias can involve any part of the intestine from the duodenum to the rectum. Familial incidence has varied with the location and distribution of the atretic segment or segments. Atresia of multiple segments of intestine associated with imperforate anus is considered to be recessively inherited. Duodenal atresia occurs in 20–30% of children who have Down syndrome.

Apple-peel jejunal atresia takes its name from the appearance of the small bowel, which twists around the marginal artery. Because the mesentery is absent, the resulting appearance resembles the continuous peel of an apple that has been pared. Several families in the literature have multiple affected siblings. The disorder has been classified as autosomal recessive (MIM 243600). No candidate gene has been identified, and the disorder has not been mapped. Treatment of all intestinal atresias is surgical. Prognosis depends on the extent of the atresias and on the presence of associated anomalies.

Abdominal Wall Defects

Omphalocele and gastroschisis are the two common forms of abdominal wall defects seen in infants. Since they are very different conditions, they will be considered separately.

Omphalocele: The term omphalocele refers to the herniation of abdominal contents in the umbilical stalk. Occasionally the sac ruptures, but usually there is a covering. Omphalocele occurs in about 1 in 2000 births. During fetal life, the midgut migrates to the umbilical stalk and then returns. Omphalocele represents a failure of the midgut to return or a failure of the abdominal wall to close after the return of the gut. Abdominal contents remain in the umbilical stalk, forming the omphalocele sac. This can include only intestine or it may also contain liver, spleen, and/or stomach. In contrast to gastroschisis, the umbilical cord inserts into the sac. (Figure 10–1) Omphalocele may be an isolated abnormality or it may be one feature of a syndrome or chromosome abnormality. More than 50% of patients with omphalocele have associated abnormalities, often the result of chromosome abnormalities. Several syndromes that include omphalocele are thought to represent single gene defects. Of particular interest is Beckwith-Wiedemann syndrome (MIM 130650). In addition to omphalocele, the clinical features of Beckwith-Wiedemann syndrome are macroglossia and somatic overgrowth that may include hemihypertrophy. Hypertrophy of pancreatic islets with resultant hyperinsulinism causes severe hypoglycemia in affected infants dur-

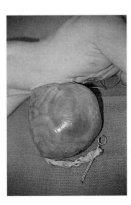

Figure 10–1. An infant with omphalocele. Note that the intestine is covered by a sac. (Courtesy of John H. Seashore, MD, Yale University School of Medicine.)

ing the neonatal period. The central nervous system impairment in some affected infants may be the result of unrecognized and untreated hypoglycemia. Several tumors have an increased frequency in patients with Beckwith-Wiedemann syndrome. These include Wilms tumor, adrenal carcinoma, rhabdomyosarcoma, neuroblastoma, and hepatoblastoma. Considerable variability in the clinical findings exists among patients.

The observation of vertical transmission of Beckwith-Wiedemann syndrome through two and sometimes three generations in many families supports the possibility of single gene inheritance. Affected siblings and cousins have been reported in other families, as have concordant monozygotic twins. Molecular analysis has played a role in explaining some of these observations. There are several reports of disruption of a region of the short arm of chromosome 11. Duplications involving 11p13–pter have been seen, both as part of various rearrangements and as isolated duplications. Several genes of potential interest map to this location, including IGF2 (insulin-like growth factor). The genetic mechanism involved in familial Beckwith-Wiedemann syndrome is unclear; imprinting, single gene mutations, or contiguous gene duplications involving 11p15 have all been proposed.

In addition to these observations, there are reports of familial incidence of isolated omphalocele in which both autosomal dominant and autosomal recessive mechanisms have been proposed. Aside from the recognized Mendelian syndromes of which omphalocele is a feature, familial omphalocele is usually an isolated anomaly. Diagnostic studies in a patient with omphalocele should include a search for other associated congenital malformations by physical examination or appropriate imaging studies, a standard karyotype, and an examination using microscopic or molecular methods to identify duplications or rearrangements involving 11p.

Repair of omphalocele is surgical and may involve staged repair if the liver or a large amount of bowel is within the omphalocele and the abdominal cavity is decreased in size. Overall prognosis depends on whether there are associated malformations or a recognized chromosomal abnormality. Hypoglycemia should be anticipated and aggressively treated in Beckwith-Wiedemann syndrome. Vigilance in identifying Wilms tumor early is important and should include periodic renal ultrasound examination.

Gastroschisis: Gastroschisis is characterized by a defect in the abdominal wall, usually to the right of the umbilicus (and not involving it) (Figure 10–2). The umbilical cord is normally inserted, and the intestine herniates through the defect in the abdominal wall. The intestine is not covered by a membrane but suffers from its exteriorization during fetal life and is often ischemic and thickened.

The incidence has been estimated at 2 in 10,000. The ratio of males to females is 1.5:1. Pathogenesis is un-

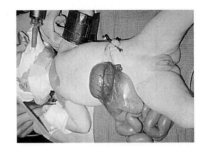

Figure 10–2. An infant with gastroschisis. (Courtesy of John H. Seashore, MD, Yale University School of Medicine.)

known, but gastroschisis is considered by some to involve an undefined ischemic event that compromises the abdominal wall. Familial incidence has been reported, but it is uncommon. Sibling recurrence has been estimated at 3.5%. Gastroschisis has been reported in identical twins. One report describes a family that had one child with gastroschisis and a second child with omphalocele. Treatment is surgical; the repair may need to be done in stages. Prognosis is usually good, and associated abnormalities are rare. Associated anomalies in abdominal wall defects are listed in Table 10–4.

Diaphragmatic Hernia: A few familial recurrences have been reported, but there is no clear evidence for major genetic factors.

Tracheoesophageal Fistula: Familial occurrence of tracheoesophageal fistula, including recurrence in siblings, has been reported. In addition, several families seem to demonstrate vertical inheritance, including one family in which an unaffected father had two affected children born of different mothers. Empiric information suggests a risk of 3–4% that an affected parent will have an affected child, 0.5–2% for recurrence in a sibship that includes one affected child, and 20% for recurrence if two siblings are affected. Table 10–5 lists some gastrointestinal abnormalities associated with genetic disorders.

Disorders of Intestinal Transport
Lactase Deficiency (MIM 223100 Adult Lactase Deficiency); (MIM 223000 Congenital Lactase Deficiency): Inability to digest lactose is com-

Table 10–4. Associated anomalies in abdominal wall defects.

Defect	Associated Anomalies
Gastroschisis	Malrotation Intestinal atresia More than one anomaly rare
Omphalocele	Malrotation Intestinal atresia Cardiac malformations Genitourinary More than one anomaly frequent

Table 10–5. Gastrointestinal abnormalities in recognized genetic syndromes.

Abnormality	Genetic Condition Sometimes Associated	Genetic Mechanism or Map Location
Intestinal atresia Duodenal atresia Multiple atresia Apple peel atresia	Down syndrome (MIM 223400) (MIM 243150) (MIM 243600)	Trisomy 21 Possibly recessive Possibly recessive Recessive
Gastroschisis	(MIM 230750)	Reported in siblings; possibly recessive

Omphalocele	Beckwith-Wiedemann syndrome (MIM 130650)
	Omphalocele-cleft palate syndrome, lethal
	(MIM 258320)
	Isolated familial omphalocele (MIM 164750)
	Trisomy 13
	Trisomy 18
	Shprintzen syndrome (MIM 182210)
	    Learning disability, dysmorphic facies, and
	    scoliosis; pharynx and larynx hypoplasia with
	    omphalocele
	OEIS Complex (MIM 258040)
	    (Omphalocele-exstrophy-imperforate anus-
	    spina defects)
	Otopalatodigital syndrome, Type II
	(MIM 304120)
		Dominant inheritance; imprinting or duplica-
		tion at 11p13–15
		Possibly recessive
		Unknown; possibly dominant
		Trisomy 13
		Trisomy 18
		
		?Autosomal dominant
		
		?Autosomal recessive
		
		?X-linked

Annular pancreas	Down syndrome; trisomy 21	Trisomy 21
Pancreatitis	(MIM 167800)	Dominant families

Anorectal malformations	VATER and VACTERYL complex
	(MIM 192350)
	Some affected sibs, (MIM 207500)
	Townes-Brock syndrome
	Cat-eye syndrome
	Most not genetic
	OEIS Complex (MIM 258040)
	    (Omphalocele-exstrophy-imperforate anus-
	    spina defects)
		
		?Autosomal recessive
		
		Chromosome 22 deletion
		
		?Autosomal recessive

Achalasia	(MIM 200400)	Some sib recurrences; possibly recessive
Hirschsprung disease (aganglionosis of colon)	(MIM 142623) Down syndrome Deletion chromosome 13 Neuroblastoma NF1 MEN2 Pheochromocytoma Congenital central hypoventilation Waardenburg syndrome Cartilage hair dysplasia Shprintzen syndrome	Mutations in RET oncogene (10q11.2) in some Trisomy 21

mon in adults. Deficiency of lactase in the mucosa of the small bowel is responsible for this condition. Symptoms vary with age and lactose exposure. Diarrhea is a particularly prominent symptom and may be severe after a large lactose load. Presentation in infancy is uncommon and is marked by both diarrhea and vomiting that may result in malnutrition. The frequency of this condition varies considerably among differing ethnic groups. Incidence is high in those of African descent, as well as in Asians and people from the Mediterranean regions. As many as 70% of African Americans suffer from lactase deficiency. The difference in frequency between onset in infancy and onset in later childhood and adulthood is best explained on a genetic basis. Both the adult onset form

and the congenital form are inherited in an autosomal recessive fashion. Clearly, however, genetic heterogeneity exists in the lactases. The genes involved have not been mapped.

Diagnosis is based on the presence of reducing substances in the stool. The history of the relationship to lactose ingestion may be strong enough to suggest the diagnosis without any need for diagnostic testing. The gastrointestinal symptoms respond to elimination of lactose from the diet. Careful reading of food labels is important since milk solids containing lactose are a common constituent of prepared foods. The use of milk that is specially treated to remove lactose may be helpful.

Sucrase-isomaltase Deficiency (MIM 222900): Osmotic diarrhea, abdominal distention, and failure to

Table 10–6. Genetic disorders associated with peptic ulcer.

Disorder	Inheritance	Molecular Pathology
MEN1 (includes inherited Zollinger-Ellison)	Autosomal dominant (MIM 131100)	11q13
Familial giant hypertrophic gastritis (Menetrier disease)	Autosomal dominant (MIM 137280)	Not mapped
ABO blood type (association with blood group O)	Autosomal dominant	9q34
Hyperpepsinoginemia (duodenal ulcer)	Autosomal dominant (MIM 126850)	Not mapped
Gastrocutaneous syndrome (peptic ulcer-hiatal hernia, multiple lentigines, cafe-au-lait spots, hypertelorism, and myopia	Probably autosomal dominant (MIM 137270)	Not mapped
Tremor-nystagmus-duodenal ulcer syndrome	Probably autosomal dominant (MIM 190310)	Not mapped

thrive characterize this disorder of carbohydrate absorption in infants and children. The condition may continue to produce symptoms into adulthood. While this condition is rare in North Americans, the incidence is as high as 10% in Alaskan natives. The inheritance pattern is autosomal recessive. The gene for lactase-phlorizin hydrolase, the protein that is abnormal in this condition, maps to chromosome 2q21. Diagnosis is based on measurement of sucrose in the stool. Treatment with a diet deficient in sucrose is successful.

Glucose-galactose Malabsorption: More than 20 years ago, Elsas described this rare condition characterized by severe unrelenting diarrhea in an infant. The clinical presentation of glucose-galactose malabsorption has not changed. Watery diarrhea occurs on an osmotic basis; the stool is characterized by a low pH and the presence of both glucose and galactose. Life-threatening dehydration may occur and can proceed to death unless treated.

Glucose-galactose malabsorption is inherited as an autosomal recessive condition. The deficient protein is a sodium/glucose cotransporter that resides in the membrane of intestinal mucosa. This transporter also functions in the renal tubule, which explains the aminoaciduria sometimes seen in these children. This protein is encoded by the SGLT1 gene that maps to chromosome 22q13.1. Several different point mutations have been described. Treatment with a diet restricted in both glucose and galactose is essential for survival in infancy. Fructose is well tolerated. The glucose and galactose intolerance may improve with age.

Gluten Enteropathy: Gluten enteropathy can occur in more than one member of a family. However, none of the evidence points to a single gene mechanism. A role for the immune system has been proposed.

Inflammatory Bowel Disease

Crohn Disease: Familial incidence has been reported in Crohn disease, but the frequency does not support a Mendelian mechanism. Concordance has been reported in monozygotic twins and discordance in dizygotic twins.

Ulcerative Colitis: In ulcerative colitis, familial aggregation without a clear genetic mechanism oc-

curs. The empiric risk to first degree relatives of an affected individual is 4–16%. A susceptibility gene has been proposed, as has the possibility that there may be a dominant form with earlier onset and more severe disease. Table 10–6 lists some genetic disorders associated with peptic ulcer.

LIVER DISORDERS

Biliary Atresia

Several inherited conditions associated with biliary atresia are listed in Table 10–7.

Bilirubin Metabolism

Bilirubin is a metabolite of the porphyrin moiety of the heme molecule. Its synthesis takes place in the spleen, where senescent red blood cells are broken down. Bilirubin is bound to albumin and transported in the blood to the liver, where it is conjugated with glucuronide by the enzyme UDP-glucuronyl transferase and excreted in the bile. There are several inherited disorders of bilirubin metabolism. The severity of their clinical manifestations is related to the presence of unconjugated bilirubin and its toxicity.

Unconjugated Bilirubin

Crigler-Najjar Syndrome: The two forms of Crigler-Najjar syndrome, type I and type II, are rare.

Table 10–7. Inherited disorders associated with biliary atresia.

Inherited Disorder	Inheritance
Extrahepatic biliary atresia	MIM (210500) Autosomal recessive
Lambert syndrome (branchial dysplasia, clubfoot, inguinal hernia, and biliary atresia)	MIM (245550) Autosomal recessive
Alagille syndrome	MIM (118450) Autosomal dominant
Meckel syndrome	MIM (249000) Autosomal recessive

Patients with type I (MIM 218800) present with severe, non-hemolytic jaundice in the neonatal period. Their serum concentration of unconjugated bilirubin is high (25–50 mg/dl). Affected infants have a high risk for developing kernicterus. There is complete absence of UDP-glucuronyl transferase in the liver.

Diagnosis is based on the high concentration of unconjugated bilirubin in the blood without evidence of either hemolysis or hepatic parenchymal disease. Neurologic damage is severe; most affected infants do not survive despite phototherapy and plasmapheresis to relieve the hyperbilirubinemia. Occasional patients have survived infancy, and some of those have developed late kernicterus. The explanation for this heterogeneity is unknown. Phenobarbital, which induces UDP-glucuronyl transferase, has no effect. Liver transplant has improved outcome in a few patients. The possibility for gene therapy is an attractive one. Type II (MIM 143500) Crigler-Najjar syndrome is a milder disorder with serum bilirubin concentrations ranging from 8–20 mg/dl. Although some mild CNS damage has been reported, the disorder usually has a more benign course than the neonatal form. UDP-glucuronyl transferase deficiency.

The gene UGT, which maps to chromosome 2, is involved in both forms of Crigler-Najjar syndrome, as well as Gilbert's syndrome. The molecular pathology of its described mutations is intriguing. Normal transcription of the gene results in several different forms of the enzyme because of overlapping transcriptional units.

A. Type I: Patients with type I Crigler-Najjar syndrome have had deletions as well as nonsense mutations that result in no synthesis of protein. The inheritance pattern for type I is autosomal recessive; the patients who have been studied appear to have two copies of the mutant gene.

B. Type II: In contrast, type II Crigler-Najjar syndrome shows an autosomal dominant inheritance pattern. One patient with type II was heterozygous for a missense mutation in this gene. It would appear that some mutations are expressed in the heterozygous state as mild disease and others are expressed in the homozygous state as severe disease.

Gilbert Syndrome: Gilbert syndrome (MIM 143500) is a common condition characterized by mild unconjugated hyperbilirubinemia that is worsened by fasting or intercurrent illness. Bilirubin concentration rarely exceeds 3mg/dl. Patients are usually asymptomatic, but some may complain of fatigue. Jaundice is visible on physical examination. The disorder is associated with reduced UDP-glycuronyl transferase activity in the liver. The inheritance of this condition is considered autosomal dominant, since many families fit this pattern of inheritance. However, the genetic mechanism is unknown. No adverse outcome is associated with this condition. Gilbert syndrome maps to the same location as Crigler-Najjar syndrome and is allelic with that group of syndromes.

Conjugated Bilirubin

Dubin-Johnson Syndrome (MIM 237500): Dubin-Johnson syndrome is an autosomal recessive condition characterized by isolated conjugated hyperbilirubinemia. Patients are usually asymptomatic except for the obvious jaundice. The serum bilirubin concentration can range from 2–25 mg/dl, but it is predominantly the conjugated form. Excretion of conjugated bilirubin from hepatocytes is abnormal. The liver is deeply pigmented. This condition is not rare. The gene, designated DJS, has been mapped to chromosome 13q34, but the molecular pathology is unknown. No adverse outcome is associated with this condition.

Rotor Syndrome (MIM 237450): This common benign condition is clinically similar to Dubin-Johnson but lacks the deep pigmentation of the liver. Excretion of conjugated bilirubin from hepatocytes is abnormal. The inheritance pattern is autosomal recessive; several consanguineous families have been described. The gene has not been mapped.

Alagille Syndrome (MIM 118450): Arteriohepatic dysplasia is a dominantly inherited condition first described by Alagille. This condition is characterized by pulmonary artery dysplasia, liver disease, and distinctive dysmorphic facies. Other features include posterior embryotoxon, a pigmentary retinopathy, and a paucity of intrahepatic bile ducts. The gene is mapped to chromosome 20p11.2, but the molecular pathology is unknown.

α-1-Antitrypsin Deficiency (MIM 107400)

The phenotype of α-1-antitrypsin deficiency in infancy and childhood differs strikingly from that in adult life. In childhood, infants can present with cholestatic jaundice that can progress to cirrhosis, liver failure, and death. Young adults suffer the early onset of emphysema that advances rapidly and results in serious deterioration of pulmonary function. The manifestations of the disorder stem from a mutation in the gene for α-1-antitrypsin. It may be helpful here to note the terminology used for α-1-antitrypsin. The gene is termed PI, for protein inhibitor, and the protein itself is called Pi. The variant proteins were originally described according to their electrophoretic mobility. ZZ refers to homozygosity for the common mutation, MM to homozygosity for the common normal allele, and MZ for the heterozygote. Thus, the description Pi ZZ denotes homozygosity for the common mutation; such an individual is affected with α-1-antitrypsin deficiency. The hepatic manifestations in Pi ZZ individuals result from the inability of the liver cell to secrete the abnormal α-1-antitrypsin, which remains in the hepatocyte and impairs its function. Infants who develop cirrhosis from α-1-antitrypsin deficiency are homozygous for the mutant protease inhibitor.

When α-1-antitrypsin cannot perform its function as an inhibitor of the protease neutrophil elastase, this elastase can destroy the proteins in the extracellular matrix of the alveolar walls of the lung parenchyma, as well as the proteins of basement membranes. This process also destroys the integrity of the lung and results in emphysema. Adults who develop this phenotype are also homozygous for a mutant α-1-antitrypsin allele or doubly heterozygous for two deficiency alleles. However, heterozygous individuals may have an increased frequency of emphysema and increased susceptibility to environmental lung damage. Occasionally, liver disease beginning in the fifth decade of life has been reported.

The gene for α-1-antitrypsin (PI) has been mapped to chromosome 14q32.1 and has been cloned. More than 75 specific mutations have been identified, including nucleic acid substitutions, nonsense mutations, and deletions. The mutations result in decrease or loss (null alleles) in α-1-antitrypsin activity. The PI Z mutation is an amino acid substitution that changes the charge, thus accounting for the differing electrophoretic mobility and altering the tertiary structure of the molecule (Figure 10–3).

The gene is a frequent one in the Caucasian population; 5% of Caucasians in the United States are MZ heterozygotes; the frequency is similar in Europe. This may represent a founder effect. The Z allele is rarely found in African Americans or Asians.

Diagnosis is usually based on the measurement of α-1-antitrypsin in serum. Individuals of the PI ZZ phenotype have very low serum concentrations; those with null mutations make no α-1-antitrypsin. The use of molecular tools to specify the mutation and to perform family studies is becoming more widespread. For the infantile presentation, prognosis for longevity is poor, and treatment is directed toward the hepatic failure. Liver transplantation may prove to be a successful treatment. Affected adults are at risk for pulmonary emphysema and should avoid environmental lung toxins, particularly cigarette smoke. The use of intravenous infusions of α-1-antitrypsin has been associated with a halt in the development of emphysema. Protocols for gene therapy using aerosolized vectors supplied with a transgene are under investigation (see Chapter 3).

Cystic Fibrosis (CF) (MIM 219700)

The clinical manifestations of cystic fibrosis (CF) involve several organs, in particular, the pancreas,

lungs, and intestinal tract. About 85% of patients with CF have pancreatic insufficiency, which can lead to malabsorption, failure to thrive, and malnutrition. Meconium ileus occurs in about 10% of neonates with CF. Lung disease occurs in most patients; it is usually milder in individuals without pancreatic insufficiency. Liver disease—most commonly biliary cirrhosis that may be localized—occurs in about 5% of affected patients who typically have pancreatic insufficiency; in a small percentage of these individuals, portal hypertension and gastrointestinal bleeding develop. Males usually have abnormal development of the vas deferens, which leads to infertility in about 95%.

The incidence of CF among Caucasians is 1 in 2500. The frequency is lower in other ethnic groups. Pathogenesis involves abnormal chloride transport across the membranes of secretory epithelia in the lungs, pancreas, small intestine, and sweat glands. This abnormal chloride transport leads to abnormal water transport, which in the lung results in thick inspissated mucous that damages the respiratory tract, leads to obstruction, and provides ideal conditions for bacterial growth that results in fibrosis. In these patients, *Pseudomonas aeruginosa, Staphlococcus aureus,* and *Hemophilus influenzae* are common offending organisms. In the pancreas, a similar process results in thick inspissated mucous that damages pancreatic ducts and leads to pancreatic insufficiency.

Autosomal recessive inheritance has been recognized for more than 40 years. The recent elucidation of the molecular pathology provides an understanding of the pathophysiology. The gene for the protein that is abnormal in CF, CFTR (cystic fibrosis transmembrane regulator), has been mapped to 7q31.1 through the use of positional cloning techniques. The large gene (27 exons) directs the synthesis of a 1480-amino acid transmembrane protein that regulates chloride transport (Figure 10–4).

Two hydrophobic transmembrane domains, two nucleotide binding sites, and a highly charged regulatory domain are important for the physiologic activity of CFTR. The protein, which functions as a chloride channel, plays a key role in chloride conductance in a variety of tissues—most notably, sweat glands, intestinal mucosa, airway cells, and pancreatic ducts. Phosphorylation of the channel allows it to respond to cAMP, and in turn allows chloride to pass

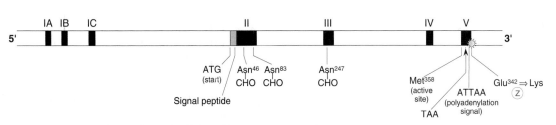

Figure 10–3. Mutations in the gene for α-1-antitrypsin. (Redrawn from Garver, RI)

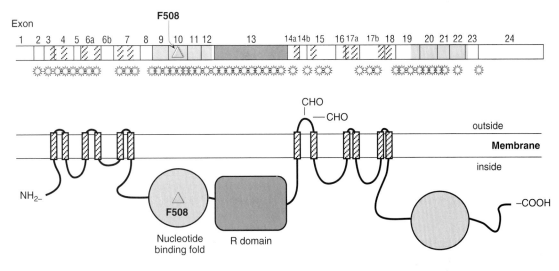

Figure 10–4. Representation of the gene for CFTR and the protein, with some mutations indicated (redrawn after Tsui).

through; but the mechanism of action is not yet clear. Many mutations have been identified in the CFTR gene. The most common is a deletion of an entire triplet codon in exon 10 at position 508 of the protein (DF508), which removes a phenylalanine from the protein at its nucleotide binding fold.

In the DF508 mutation, CFTR is not properly processed and fails to localize in the membranes of epithelial cells. This mutation accounts for about 70% of cases in Caucasians. Many of the more than 240 other mutations also involve the nucleotide binding site; mutations also occur in the membrane spanning portion of the molecule. Single base substitutions and nonsense mutations are known, as are splice site mutations and deletions, which result in a frame shift. This leaves open the possibility that an abnormal protein will be synthesized or that no protein will be made (Table 10–8).

In some milder mutations, the protein appears to be localized correctly but does not function normally. The mildest mutations are expressed as isolated in-

fertility in males, with little or no evidence of pancreatic or lung disease.

Traditionally, diagnosis depends on measurement of a sweat chloride concentration >70mm/L. Measurement of trypsin in the stool may be helpful. Experience is developing with newborn screening for CF through the measurement of immunoreactive trypsinogen in dried blood spots. It is believed that early diagnosis should be beneficial, but this has not been proven conclusively yet. Molecular analysis of DNA for specific mutations can play a role in diagnosis. The correlation between clinical findings and specific mutations is not clear. Homozygosity for the DF508 deletion is usually associated with the severe form of the disease, including pancreatic insufficiency and pulmonary disease. Substantial variability occurs between patients, and some individuals with that genotype have less severe disease. In general, some alleles are more frequently associated with mild disease and some with severe disease (Table 10–9).

The clinical phenotype in persons heterozygous for

Table 10–8. Examples of some CF mutations.

Mutation	Phenotype	Ethnic Group
DF508	Severe	American Caucasians, French, Celtic populations
R553X	Less severe	English/Welsh
W1282X; DF508; G542X; N1303K; splice site 1717	Severe	Ashkenazi Jews, Israel
G542X; R553X; Splice site 1717	Severe	Netherlands
A455E	Less severe	Netherlands

Table 10–9. Cystic fibrosis: clinical correlations with mutations.

Severe pulmonary disease; pancreatic insufficiency, meconium ileus	ΔF508/ΔF508; ΔF508/"severe allele"; ΔF508/nonsense mutation; nonsense mutation/nonsense mutation
Mild pulmonary disease, pancreatic sufficiency; later diagnosis	uncharacterized allele/"mild allele"; "mild allele"/"mild allele"

DF508 and another mutation depends to a large degree on the other mutation. Nonsense mutations leading to a stop codon at the other allele tend to be associated with severe disease, whether present in the homozygous state or as combined heterozygotes with the DF508 mutation or another severe mutation. Some of the characterized mutations are associated with milder disease. While these correlations can be very helpful, the lack of ability to predict the phenotype perfectly—based on the genotype—has created a challenge for genetic counseling. Programs performing heterozygote screening and prenatal diagnosis must prepare patients and families for the fact that identification of some genotypes will lead to uncertainty. Furthermore, although it is theoretically possible to identify nearly 90% of heterozygotes, most programs cannot screen for all possible genotypes and therefore must focus on the common ones. This can be quite precise when the population consists of an ethnic group in which the correlations are well known. It is considerably more complex when the population to be screened is diverse. For these reasons, interpreting the results of molecular testing can be complicated.

Aggressive pulmonary therapy seems to improve outcome; pancreatic enzyme replacement has improved prognosis. The use of DNAse to clear the respiratory tract of bacterial and leukocyte debris is investigational but promising, as is the use of antiproteases and corticosteroids to reduce damage from inflammatory cells and their proteolytic enzymes. Substantial hope exists for gene therapy that replaces the CFTR gene in the respiratory tract through the use of a genetically modified viral vector (see Chapter 3). Efforts are underway to determine whether measurements of immunoreactive trypsinogen in dried blood spots can improve newborn screening for cystic fibrosis. Since malnutrition occurs in the first year of life in infants with pancreatic insufficiency, early diagnosis and treatment may improve outcome by preventing or reducing the degree of malnutrition. In addition, early diagnosis will facilitate the recognition and prompt treatment of pulmonary infection. The availability of additional modes of treatment, including gene therapy, would strengthen the argument for newborn screening.

REFERENCES AND SUGGESTED READING

Anderson MP et al: Demonstration that CFTR is a chloride channel by alteration of its anion selectivity. Science 1991;**253:**202.

Bealer JF et al: Nitric oxide synthase is deficient in the aganglionic colon of patients with Hirschsprung's disease. Pediatrics 1994;**93:**647.

Bodian M, Carter CO: A family study of Hirschsprung disease's. Ann Hum Genet 1963;**26:**261.

Bosher LP, Shaw A: Achalasia in siblings. Am J Dis Child 1981;**135:**709.

Bosma PJ et al. Sequence of exons and the flanking regions of human bilirubin UDP-glucuronosyl-transferase complex and indentification of a genetic mutation in a patient with Crigler-Najjar Type I. Hepatology 1992;**15:**941.

Bronstein MN et al: Pancreatic insufficiency, growth, and nutrition in infants identified by newborn screening as having cystic fibrosis. J Pediatr 1992;**120:**533.

Bugge M, Petersen MB, Christensen MF: Monozygotic twins discordant for gastroschisis. Am J Med Genet 1994;**52:**223.

Buist AS: α-1-antitrypsin deficiency in lung and liver disease. Hosp Pract 1989;**(May):**5.

Campbell PW et al: Cystic fibrosis: Relationship between clinical status and F508 deletion. J Pediatr 1991;**118:**239.

Carter CO, Evans KA: Inheritance of congenital pyloric stenosis. J Med Genet 1969;**6:**233.

Cheadle J et al: Mild pulmonary disease in a cystic fibrosis child homozygous for R553X. J Med Genet 1992;**29:** 597.

Chevalier-Porst F et al: Mutation analysis in 600 French cystic fibrosis patients. J Med Genet 1994;**31:**541.

Chowdhury JR, Lahiri P, Chowdhury NR: Hereditary jaundice and disorders of bilirubin metabolism. Pages 1367–1409 in: *The Metabolic Basis of Inherited Disease,* 6th ed. Scriver CR et al (editors). McGraw Hill, 1989.

Chowdhury JR, Lahiri P, Chowdhury NR: Inherited disorders of bilirubin metabolism. Pages 1135–1164 in: *Principles and Practice of Medical Genetics,* 2nd ed. Emery AEH, Rimoin D (editors). Churchill Livingstone; 1990.

Collins FS: Cystic fibrosis: Molecular biology and therapeutic implications. Science 1992;**256:**774.

Crystal RG: The α-1-Antitrypsin gene and its deficiency state. Trends in Genetics 1989;**5:**411.

The Cystic Fibrosis Consortium. Correlation between genotype and phenotype in patients with cystic fibrosis. N Engl J Med 1993;**329:**1308.

Denayer L et al: Reproductive decision making of aunts and uncles of a child with cystic fibrosis: Genetic risk perception and attitudes toward carrier identification and prenatal diagnosis. Am J Med Genet 1992;**44:**104.

Dhorne-Pollet S et al: Segregation analysis of Alagille syndrome. J Med Genet 1994;**31:**453.

Edery P et al: Mutation of the RET protooncogene in Hirschsprung's disease. Nature 1994;**367**:378.

Eriksson S: α-1-Antitrypsin deficiency: Lessons learned from the bedside to the gene and back again. Chest 1989; **95**:181.

Farag TI et al: Second family with "apple-peel" syndrome affecting four siblings: Autosomal recessive inheritance confirmed. Am J Med Genet 1993;**47**:119.

Fewtrell MS et al: Hirschsprung's disease associated with a deletion of chromosome 10 (q11.2q21.2): A further link with the neurocristopathies? J Med Genet 1994;**31**:325.

Freud E et al: Familial chronic recurrent pancreatitis in identical twins. Arch Surg 1992;**127**:1125.

Gan KH, Heijerman HGM, Bakker W: Correlation between genotype and phenotype in patients with cystic fibrosis. N Engl J Med 1994;**330**:865.

Garver KL, Law JC, Garver B: Hirschsprung disease: A genetic study. Clin Genet 1985;**28**:503.

Garver RI et al: α-1-Antitrypsin deficiency and emphysema caused by homozygous inheritance of non-expressing α-1-Antitrypsin genes. N Engl J Med 1986;**314**:762.

Gasparini P et al: Nine cytic fibrosis patients homozygous for the CFTR nonsense mutation R1162X have mild or moderate lung disease. J Med Genet 1992;**29**:558.

Gasparini P et al: Screening of 62 mutations in a cohort of cystic fibrosis patients from North Eastern Italy: Their incidence and clinical features of defined genotypes. Hum Mutation 1993;**2**:389.

Hammond KB et al: Efficacy of statewide neonatal screening for cystic fibrosis by assay of trypsinogen concentrations. N Engl J Med 1991;**325**:769.

Hershey DW et al: Familial abdominal wall defects. Am J Med Genet 1989;**34**:174.

Highsmith WE et al: A novel mutation in the cystic fibrosis gene in patients with pulmonary disease but normal sweat chloride concentrations. N Engl J Med 1994;**331**: 974.

Jarmas AL et al: Hirschsprung Disease: Etiologic implications of unsuccessful prenatal diagnosis. Am J Med Genet 1983;**16**:163.

Jordan SC, Kangarloo H. Renal cystic diseases. Pages 1291–1303 in: *Principles and Practice of Medical Genetics,* 2nd ed. Emery AEH, Rimoin D (editors). Churchill Livingstone, 1990.

Kartner N et al: Mislocation of delta F508 CFTR in cystic fibrosis sweat gland. Nature Genetics 1992;**1**:321.

Kerem E et al: The relation between genotype and phenotype in cystic fibrosis-analysis of the most common mutation (delF508). N Engl J Med 1990;**323**:1517.

Klein MD, Hertzler JH: Congenital defects of the abdominal wall. Surgery 1981;**152**:805.

Klein MD, Kosloske AM, Hertzler JH: Congenital defects of the abdominal wall. JAMA 1981;**245**:1643.

Kleinhaus S et al: Hirschsprung's disease: A survey of the members of the Surgical Section of the American Academy of Pediatrics. J Pediatr Surg 1979;**14**:588.

Lewis MPN, Gazet JC: Hereditary calcific pancreatitis in an English family. Br J Surg 1993;**80**:487.

Miedzybrodzka ZH et al: Evaluation of laboratory methods for cystic fibrosis carrier screening: Reliability, sensitivity, specificity, and costs. J Med Genet 1994;**31**:545.

Okayama H et al: Characterization of the molecular basis of the α-1-Antitrypsin F allele. Am J Hum Genet 1991; **48**:1154.

Omenn GS, McKusick VM: The association of Waarden-berg syndrome and Hirschsprung megacolon. Am J Med Genet 1979;**3**:217.

Pachnis V, Mankoo B, Constantini F: Expression of the c-ret proto-oncogene during mouse embryogenesis. Development 1993;**119**:1005.

Passarge E: Genetic heterogeneity and recurrence risk of congenital intestinal aganglionosis. Birth Defects: Original Article Series 1972;**8**:63.

Passarge E: Developmental defects of the gastrointestinal tract. Pages 1117–1124 in: *Principles and Practice of Medical Genetics,* 2nd ed. Emery AEH, Rimoin D (editors). Churchill Livingstone, 1990.

Passarge E: The genetics of Hirschsprung's disease. N Engl J Med 1967;**276**:138.

Pletcher BA et al: Familial occurrence of esophageal atresia with and without tracheoesophageal fistula: Report of two unusual kindreds. Am J Med Genet 1991;**39**:330.

Riordan JR et al: Identification of the cystic fibrosis gene: Cloning and characterization of complementary DNA. Science 1989;**245**:1066.

Ritter JK, Crawford JM, Owens IS: Cloning of two human liver bilirubin UDP-glucuronosyl-transferase cDNAs with expression in COS-1 cells. J Biol Chem 1991;**266**:1043.

Ritter JK et al: Identification of a genetic alteration in the code for bilirubin UDP-glucuronosyl-transferase in the UGT1 gene complex of a Crigler-Najjar Type I patient. J Clin Invest 1992;**90**:150.

Romeo G et al: Point metations affecting the tyrosine kinase domain of the RET proto-oncogene in Hirschsprung's disease. Nature 1994;**367**:377.

Rommens JM et al: Identification of the cystic fibrosis gene: Chromosome walking and jumping. Science 1989; **245**:1059.

Sato T, Saitoh Y: Familial chronic pancreatitis associated with pancreatic lithiasis. Am J Surg 1974;**127**:511.

Seashore JH. Congenital abdominal wall defects. Clinics in Perinatology 1978;**5**:61.

Seashore JH et al: Familial apple peel jejunal atresia: Surgical, genetic, and radiographic aspects. Pediatrics 1987; **80**:540.

Shen-Schwarz S, Fitko R: Multiple gastrointestinal atresias with imperforate anus: Pathology and pathogenesis. Am J Med Genet 1990;**36**:451.

Shoshani T et al: Association of a nonsense mutation (W1282X), the most common mutation in the Ashkenazi Jewish cystic fibrosis patients in Israel, with presentation of severe disease. Am J Hum Genet 1992;**50**:222.

Tizzano EF, Buchwald M: Recent advances in cystic fibrosis research. J Pediatr 1993;**122**:985.

Tsui LC, Buchwald M: Biochemical and molecular genetics of cystic fibrosis. Adv Hum Genet 1991;**20**:153.

Warren J, Evans K, Carter CO: Offspring of patients with tracheo-oesophageal fistula. J Med Genet 1979;**16**:338.

Waters DL et al: Pancreatic function in infants identified as having cystic fibrosis in a neonatal screening program. N Engl J Med 1990;**322**:303.

Weinberg SE: Recent advances in pulmonary medicine. N Engl J Med 1993;**328**:1389.

Weterman IT, Pena AS: Familial incidence of Crohn's disease in the Netherlands and a review of the literature. Gastroenterology 1984;**86**:449.

Wilfond BS, Fost M: The cystic fibrosis gene: Medical and social implications for heterozygote detection. JAMA 1990;**263**:2777.

11

Brain & Nervous System

STRUCTURAL BIRTH DEFECTS

Congenital malformations of the nervous system are common birth defects that result in significant morbidity and mortality. They may occur as isolated defects or in association with malformation syndromes.

Defects Associated With Hypoplasia, Hyperplasia, and Abnormal Segmentation

Congenital Microcephaly: Congenital microcephaly reflects an undersized or underdeveloped brain. Microcephaly commonly occurs in association with genetic syndromes, congenital infections, and fetal teratogens. It may also occur as a primary, isolated condition that may be associated with polygenic or multifactorial inheritance, or be inherited as an autosomal dominant (MIM 156580), autosomal recessive (MIM 257200), or X-linked recessive (MIM 309590) trait. Affected individuals have varying degrees of mental handicaps and neurologic abnormalities.

Macrocephaly: Macrocephaly may reflect true megalencephaly, or a hyperplastic brain. It may also be associated with conditions that result in increased cranial size, eg, hydrocephalus, storage disorders, or bone dysplasias. True megalencephaly is a benign, autosomal dominant trait with male predominance (MIM 153470). Isolated unilateral megalencephaly, or hemimegalencephaly, is uncommon and associated with seizures and mental retardation.

Aprosencephaly: Aprosencephaly, a rare condition, is characterized by abnormal development of structures derived from the diencephalon and the facial components of early prechordal mesoderm. Marked craniofacial disproportion with extreme microcephaly, an intact skull, sloping forehead, and prominent supraorbital ridges are noted. The facies may resemble holoprosencephaly. The hypothalamus and posterior pituitary are hypoplastic or absent. Aprosencephaly may occur as an isolated defect or as part of a syndrome.

Holoprosencephaly: Holoprosencephaly results from failure of separation of the embryonic forebrain (prosencephalon) into two symmetric cerebral hemispheres. The defect may be complete (alobar); affected patients have a single ventricle and severe malformations of midline facial structures. Midline facial anomalies range from cyclopia (single eye) without a nasal structure to a small forehead with hypotelorism. Midline clefts of the palate are common. Severe neurologic impairment and neuroendocrine deficiencies are noted. Less severe forms (semilobar and lobar) are known. Holoprosencephaly may occur as a sporadic condition; very rarely is it inherited as an autosomal dominant (MIM 157170) or autosomal recessive (MIM 236100) trait. One-half of cases are associated with trisomy 13 or 18, or with other chromosomal abnormalities. Environmental etiologies include congenital infections, maternal diabetes, and fetal alcohol syndrome.

Defects Associated With Faulty Proliferation and Migration of Neurons

Lissencephaly: Lissencephaly (MIM 247200) consists of a smooth cerebral cortex with absent or decreased gyral formation that results from abnormal neuronal migration during early fetal life. Areas of pachygyria (thick, broad gyri) may also occur. Affected neonates have severe neurological impairment, hypotonia, and seizures. Most die by 2 years of age. Lissencephaly is frequently seen with Neu-Loxova syndrome (MIM 256520), an autosomal recessive disorder, and with the Miller-Dieker syndrome (MIM 247200), which is associated with a deletion at chromosome 17p13.3. Lissencephaly may result from cytomegalovirus congenital infection, or maternal use of alcohol, valproic acid, or retinoic acid.

Agenesis of the Corpus Callosum: Although agenesis of the corpus callosum (MIM 217990) may be seen in normal persons, it is frequently associated with other central nervous system malformations and syndromes.

Hydrocephalus

Hydrocephalus: Hydrocephalus (MIM 236600) is defined as a relative increase in the intracranial volume of cerebrospinal fluid compared to the size of the brain. Hydrocephalus may be associated with primary atrophy of cerebral parenchyma as is seen in **hydrocephalus exvacuo** or **hydranencephaly.** It may also result from increased production and/or decreased reabsorption of cerebrospinal fluid. Most commonly it occurs from mechanical obstruction in cerebrospinal fluid flow associated with central nervous system malformations, infections, or mass lesions. Excess cerebrospinal fluid enlarges the ventricles and results in increased intracranial pressure.

Congenital Hydrocephalus: Congenital hydrocephalus, which has an incidence of 1 in 1000 live births, may occur as an isolated defect. It may also be associated with other central nervous system malformations, neural tube defects, congenital infections, skeletal dysplasias, or multiple congenital anomalies. As an isolated defect, it is usually of sporadic or multifactorial etiology. Isolated congenital hydrocephalus may result from **stenosis or atresia of the aqueduct of Sylvius.** This form of congenital hydrocephalus is most often a multifactorial trait; it may also be inherited as an X-linked recessive disorder, which has been linked to the Xq28 region (MIM 307000). The **Dandy Walker syndrome** is characterized by malformations of the fourth ventricle and cerebellum that result in cystic transformation of the fourth ventricle and hydrocephalus. The majority of cases are sporadic; a familial form associated with polycystic kidneys and eye defects is inherited on an autosomal recessive basis (MIM 220200).

Defects Associated With Failure of Closure of the Neural Tube

Neural tube defects are common malformations associated with failure of closure of the neural tube between 24 and 29 days of fetal life. The defects, which may occur anywhere along the neural tube, are named by their site of occurrence and the type of tissues involved. All have bone defects of the skull or spine, and varying degrees of structural neural involvement.

Anencephaly: Anencephaly (MIM 206500) consists of complete or partial absence of the cerebral hemispheres, skull, and cranial vault. The defect results from failure of closure of the cranial (rostral) end of the neural type. Complete absence of the cerebrum occurs in 65% of cases. The defect may extend caudally into the cervical or upper thoracic areas. Two-thirds of affected patients are female. One-half of affected patients are stillborn, and the remainder usually die by 48 hours of age. The mean gestational age is 37.5 weeks. Polyhydramnios is noted 75% of the time. Twenty-one percent of affected patients have other malformations, especially facial and ear anomalies. Renal, cardiac, and gastrointestinal defects occur in as many as 16% of cases. Anencephaly may be noted on ultrasound after 14 weeks of gestation. The differential diagnosis includes amniotic band disruption sequence, which should be considered in those affected infants that survive longer than 2 days.

Spina Bifida Occulta: Spina bifida occulta, which occurs in at least 5% of the population, is usually asymptomatic. The condition, most commonly located in the lower lumbar area, results from failure of midline fusion of the vertebral arches. It may be found as an incidental finding on radiographs. Although isolated spina bifida occulta may be inherited as an autosomal dominant trait (MIM 182940), it is more often associated with underlying neurological defects **(occult spinal dysraphism),** meningoceles, or myelomeningoceles. An overlying skin abnormality, eg, a skin tag, area of hyperpigmentation, port wine stain, patch of hair, dimple, subcutaneous swelling, or sinus tract, may be noted. Underlying defects may include a tethered cord from fibrous bands or adhesions, diastematomyelia (longitudinal midline septum dividing the cord), or intraspinal lipomas, dermoids, or epidermomas. Varying motor and sensory neurological deficits may occur, which are related to the level and degree of spinal cord or nerve root involvement.

Encephaloceles: Encephaloceles involve herniation of the brain and meninges, or only meninges, through a defect, usually midline, in the skull. These defects are most frequently located in the occipital area, but may occur in the frontal and orbital areas and even extend into the nasopharynx. Encephaloceles, which occur in 1 in 5000 to 10,000 live births, are frequently associated with other congenital malformations.

Iniencephaly: Iniencephaly results from defects in the occipital area of the skull and the cervical and thoracic vertebrae. The defects allow the brain and cerebellum to be in contact with the cervicothoracic spine. The head is severely retroflexed and the neck absent. The defect may be open or covered with skin. An occipital encephalocele, anencephaly, or myelomeningocele may also be present. Iniencephaly is ten times more common in females than males. Affected infants with severe defects have a poor prognosis.

Meningocele: Meningocele, which consists of a midline protrusion of meninges without neural tissue, is usually accompanied by spina bifida. Many of the defects are asymptomatic; they are frequently covered with skin. They also may be associated with underlying neural defects as in spina bifida occulta. If the meningocele occurs in the high cervical or cranial areas, aqueductal stenosis, hydromyelia (distention of the central canal with compression of surrounding spinal cord structures), or Chiari (Arnold-Chiari) malformations may be associated. The Chiari type 2 malformation, frequently noted in patients with meningoceles and myelomeningoceles, consists of caudal displacement of the cerebellum and medulla, which results in obstruction of the flow of cerebral spinal fluid and hydrocephalus.

Myelomeningocele: Myelomeningocele, the most common neural tube defect, results from faulty closure of the caudal portion of neural tube. The defect consists of a midline protrusion of meninges and spinal cord and/or nerve roots with an associated spina bifida. The protrusion may consist of a sac covered with skin or a thin membrane or the defect may be exposed (myeloschisis). Although it may occur anywhere in the midline, myelomeningocele is most commonly found in the lumbosacral area. The location and extent of the defect will determine the degree of neurologic deficits. Lower lesions have a better prognosis. Weakness or flaccid paralysis of the legs, congenital dislocated hips, club feet, decreased range of motion of joints in the lower extremities, and varying degrees of bowel and bladder sphincter dysfunction occur. Eighty percent of affected patients have an associated Chiari malformation and hydrocephalus. Secondary scoliosis is common.

Defects associated with failure of closure of the neural tube occur in 2–3 per 10,000 live births. They are seen most frequently in the United Kingdom and Ireland and are less common in Asians and persons of African background. Most cases are sporadic and associated with mutlifactorial or polygenic inheritance. Some cases, however, are inherited as autosomal or X-linked recessive (MIM 301410) traits. Ten percent occur as part of a syndrome or with a chromosomal abnormality. There are also important environmental causes. The risk of occurrence is approximately 20 times that of the general population when the mother has insulin dependent diabetes mellitus. An increased risk also occurs with valproic acid or carbamazepine treatment for maternal seizures. An increased risk has been associated with maternal folic acid deficiency.

The risk of recurrence for sporadic cases of neural tube defects of any type is 4–8%. This figure increases to 10% with a second affected child. The risk is 3% if a parent is affected. The subsequent affected child may have the same or a different type of defect. Prenatal screening for the defects occurs by determination of maternal serum alpha-fetoprotein (MSAFP) levels, which are often routinely measured between 16 and 18 weeks of pregnancy. Alpha-fetoprotein (AFP) is produced by the yolk sac and the fetal liver cells and gastrointestinal tract. Increased AFP levels in maternal serum and in amniotic fluid may be found with neural tube defects, as well as with multiple gestations, open defects such as gastroschisis, congenital nephrosis, or fetal death. Decreased levels have been associated with chromosomal abnormalities, eg, trisomy 21. MSAFP can detect 80–90% of neural tube defects, including 95–100% of cases of anencephaly and 70–80% of cases of myelomeningocele. After detection of an elevated MSAFP, the family should be offered measurement of amniotic fluid AFP levels and detailed ultrasound to confirm the diagnosis. Amniocentesis and detailed ultrasound should also be offered to mothers with the increased environmental risks discussed earlier and to families

with prior affected children. Daily intake of 0.4 mg of folic acid has been shown to decrease the risk of recurrence by as much as 80%.

MENTAL RETARDATION

Psychomotor retardation occurs in 2–3% of the general population, and is 25% more common in males than females. Fifty percent of patients with severe psychomotor retardation (IQ less than 35) have genetic disorders. Down syndrome and Fragile-X syndrome are most commonly associated, along with other chromosomal abnormalities, developmental nervous system defects, and single gene disorders. Mild or moderate mental handicaps may be associated with multifactorial inheritance.

Fragile-X Syndrome

The Fragile-X syndrome (MIM 309550) is an X-linked disorder that occurs in 8% of males with mental handicaps. Approximately 1 in 1000 males have unstable cytosine-guanine-guanine (CGG) trinucleotide repeats (TNR) at the FMR-1 gene locus on the distal long arm of the X-chromosome (Xq27.3). Twenty percent of affected males will have a "premutation" that consists of 50–200 copies of the CGG TNR. Males with the "premutation" are usually asymptomatic and show no clinical manifestations of the disorder; they are detected by family studies of symptomatic affected patients. Eighty percent of affected males, however, will have more than 200 copies of the CGG TNR, or the "full mutation." Males with the "full mutation" have clinical findings known as the Fragile-X, or Martin-Bell, syndrome. The syndrome is characterized by varying degrees of mental retardation, large testes, an unusual facies, and often signs of connective tissue abnormalities. There is a wide spectrum of clinical manifestations. Mental handicaps may range from borderline normal to severe; most IQs fall into the 20–60 range, with a mean of about 30–45. Twenty percent of males with the "full mutation" have autistic-like mannerisms. Perseverative speech, language delay, and articulation problems are common. Some have attention deficit disorders. Poor coordination, generalized mildly decreased motor tone, increased reflexes, and seizures may be noted. Unusually large testes (over 30 ml), noted in 80–90% of affected males, are more frequently noted after puberty but may be present before. Testicular enlargement may be unilateral. Testicular function is normal. Although affected males are fertile, they very seldom reproduce. The characteristic facies includes a prominent forehead, jaw, and ears. The face is often long and narrow; the ears may also be long and posteriorly rotated. The nasal bridge is thickened and often extends down the nose. These features, like the enlarged testes, may not be apparent until late childhood or after puberty. Macrocephaly is common. Prenatal and postnatal growth may be increased. Occasionally a high arched palate or cleft palate occurs. Many affected males have signs suggestive of connective tissue involvement, eg, hyperextensible fingers, laxity of joints, skin striae, flat feet, inguinal hernias, pectus excavatum, and mitral valve insufficiency or prolapse.

Females with the "premutation" of 5–200 copies of the CGG TNR do not have clinical findings. Between 50–75% of females with the "full mutation" have varying degrees of mental handicaps that can be mild, eg, learning disabilities, or as severe as noted in affected males. Affected females may be diagnosed incorrectly as having infantile autism. Although most affected females usually do not have the dysmorphic features or abnormal connective tissue findings seen in affected males, occasionally they are noted.

Additional information concerning the molecular genetics of Fragile-X syndrome is included in the section on molecular pathology. Fragile-X testing should be considered in any individual, male or female, with unexplained mental retardation, attention deficit disorder, or autism.

Rett Syndrome

Rett syndrome (MIM 312750) is an X-linked disorder associated with mental handicaps and autistic features. It affects approximately 1 in 12,000 females. Because it has not been observed in males, it has been proposed that the trait is lethal to males during intrauterine life. Most girls appear normal during early infancy. They are often diagnosed between the ages of 6 and 18 months with what is thought to be infantile autism. Head growth slows or stops; communication skills decline. Affected girls usually develop generalized seizures; an independent multifocal spike and wave pattern is frequently noted on electrocephalograms. Development of characteristic stereotypic hand movements, eg, hand-wringing or hand-washing, and episodes of hyperventilation or periodic breathing point to the diagnosis of Rett syndrome. After a period of declining skills during childhood, the disorder appears to stabilize; the girls may live into adulthood. Scoliosis, which is common later in the disease, may require orthopedic intervention.

SEIZURES

Approximately 0.5 to 1.0% of the general population have recurrent seizures, or epilepsy. In addition, approximately 2.2% of the general population who do not have epilepsy have abnormal EEG patterns. Seizures are more common in young children, adolescents, and the elderly. Most epilepsy is idiopathic in nature. Genetic influences, however, may occur with any type of seizures, especially those that are generalized. Acquired seizures, from trauma or infec-

tions, or those associated with other genetic disorders, eg, metabolic or developmental defects, occur in approximately 20% of cases. Seizures may be the presenting sign in persons with tuberous sclerosis or neurofibromatosis. Table 11–1 gives the current classification of seizure disorders.

Family studies have shown an increased frequency of seizures and seizure disorders in relatives of persons with epilepsy, compared to that for the general population. This pattern is more commonly noted with generalized seizures. Siblings and offspring of persons with seizure disorders have an increased risk to develop seizures; the risk is approximately 1–10%. The risks for siblings and offspring with various types of seizures are shown in Table 11–2. Children of mothers with seizures are more likely to develop seizures than children of fathers with seizures. The risk for siblings of index cases further increases if the mother also has seizures; the risk is estimated to be 17–33% if both parents have seizure disorders. Twin studies have shown a higher concordance for seizures among monozygous twins (40–95%) than in dizygous twins (5–20%). These findings suggest that genetic influences are involved. For most types of seizures, polygenic or multifactorial factors exist. Only a small number of seizure disorders are inherited as autosomal, or very rarely, X-linked traits.

Three major types of seizure disorders occur: partial, generalized and unclassified.

Partial (Focal)

Partial (focal) seizures result from activation of a system of neurons limited to part of one cerebral hemisphere. With simple partial seizures, consciousness is not impaired; with complex partial seizures, consciousness becomes impaired. Partial seizures may evolve into generalized tonic-clonic convulsions. **Benign epilepsy of childhood,** a form of partial seizures, is associated with EEG spike foci in the Rolandic or centrotemporal region. Affected patients usually have focal (partial) motor seizures of the face

Table 11–1. Abbreviated international classification of seizure disorders.

Classification	Type
Partial (focal, local) seizures	Simple partial Complex partial Partial evolving to generalized tonic-clonic convulsions
Generalized (convulsive or nonconvulsive) seizures	Absence Myoclonic Clonic Tonic Tonic-clonic Atonic
Unclassified epileptic seizures	

Table 11–2. Risks for seizures in relatives of patients with idiopathic epilepsy.

Type in Proband	Percentage Risk for Siblings	Percentage Risk for Offspring
Partial seizures	1–4	7
Absence seizures	2–5	2–5
Infantile spasms	5–10	–
Generalized, tonic-clonic	4–8	9
Febrile seizures	9–22	8

that occur during sleep or on awaking. The onset usually occurs between 5–9 years of age. Although seizures usually cease after age 15, some affected patients continue to have seizures into adult life. The disorder is thought to be inherited as an autosomal dominant trait, expressed only during childhood. **Photosensitive epilepsy** (MIM 132100), an autosomal dominant form of partial seizures, is induced by flickering lights or unusual light patterns. **Reading epilepsy** (MIM 132300), also an autosomal dominant trait, is induced by reading or watching television.

Generalized Seizures

Generalized seizures involve neuronal discharges in both hemispheres. Consciousness may be impaired and motor manifestations are usually bilateral. Generalized seizures are subdivided into absence, myoclonic, clonic, tonic, tonic-clonic, and atonic (astatic) seizures. The following discussion includes those types of generalized seizure disorders with genetic features other than polygenic or multifactorial inheritance.

Absence (Petit Mal) Seizures: Absence seizures (petit mal) are usually noted between 4 and 8 years of age. Typical absence seizures are characterized by brief episodes of abrupt loss of consciousness, without change in postural tone. Absence seizures may be accompanied by mild clonic or tonic movements, loss of motor tone, automatisms, or autonomic phenomena. One-third of affected patients will develop a generalized, major motor seizure disorder. Absence seizures are associated with a characteristic symmetric, frontally predominant, 3 Hz spike and slow wave EEG pattern. One form of absence seizures, associated with a "centrecephalic" EEG pattern, may be inherited as an autosomal dominant trait with reduced penetrance for seizures, but almost complete penetrance for the EEG abnormalities (MIM 117110). The onset occurs between 4.5–16.5 years of age. Although 45% of siblings have an abnormal EEG, only 25% have seizures. Thirty-five percent of offspring have abnormal EEGs.

Myoclonic Seizures: Myoclonic seizures, a form of generalized seizures, are characterized by clinical myoclonic jerks and a characteristic EEG with a polyspike and wave pattern. Occasionally a spike and wave pattern or a sharp and slow wave pattern are

noted. **Infantile spasms (West syndrome)** are a form of myoclonic seizures that occurs in 1 in 5000. The onset is usually between 4–6 months of age. Males are more likely to be affected than females. Patients have a characteristic "salaam" attack with sudden, brief, nodding of the head, associated with extension or flexion of the trunk and extremities. Infantile spasms are associated with an EEG pattern (termed hypsarrhythmia) that consists of a very high-amplitude, slow, asynchronous, disorganized background with intermixed, independent, frequent multifocal spikes. Infantile spasms are often noted in patients with metabolic disorders, birth defects, tuberous sclerosis, and perinatal problems, eg, hypoxia.

Juvenile Myoclonic Epilepsy (Impulsive Petit Mal): Juvenile myoclonic epilepsy (impulsive petit mal, MIM 254770) has its onset between 6–22 years of age. Myoclonic jerks occur for 1–3 years before the onset of generalized tonic clonic seizures. Approximately one-third of affected patients also have absence seizures. Intellectual abilities are usually not affected. Most patients respond to anticonvulsant therapy. The disorder has been linked to the HLA-BF locus on the short arm of chromosome 6. Although the inheritance pattern is unclear, multifactorial, autosomal recessive, and autosomal dominant patterns of inheritance have been suggested.

Progressive Myoclonic Epilepsies: The progressive myoclonic epilepsies are associated with degenerative disorders of the central nervous system.

A. Progressive Myoclonic Epilepsy of Unverricht and Lundborg: Progressive myoclonic epilepsy of Unverricht and Lundborg (MIM 254800), also known as Baltic myoclonic epilepsy, is a rare autosomal recessive disease that has its onset between 6 and 13 years of age. Affected patients present initially with twitching that progresses to myoclonus. Dementia, dysarthria, and ataxia occur later in the disease. Abnormal giant somatosensory evoked potentials, delayed nerve conduction velocity, and abnormal electromyography consistent with denervation are indicative of peripheral nerve involvement. The metabolic defect is unknown. The disorder has been associated with a deletion at chromosome 21q22.3 in some families.

B. Lafora Body Disease: Lafora body disease (MIM 254780), an autosomal recessive disorder, is associated with generalized seizures that become more myoclonic in nature with time. The onset is usually between 10 and 18 years of age. Affected patients have a progressive seizure disorder with dementia and loss of vision; death usually occurs about 10 years after the onset. Lafora "bodies" are present in the substantia nigra, superior olive, dentate nucleus, globus pallidus, and sensorimotor cortex. They may also be found in skeletal muscle, heart, liver, and skin.

C. Hartung Myoclonic Epilepsy: Hartung myoclonic epilepsy (MIM 159600) is an autosomal dominant progressive disorder that has a slower course than the two disorders just discussed. The disorder is associated with sensorineural hearing loss and diffuse cortical atrophy. Lafora bodies are not found. The biochemical basis for the disorder is unknown.

Progressive myoclonic epilepsy may also be seen in Huntington disease and with biochemical genetic disorders, eg, mitochondrial encephalomyopathies, sphingolipidoses, sialidoses, biopterin deficiency, Wilson disease, and ceroid lipofuscinosis.

Benign Familial Neonatal Seizures: Seizures occur in 1% of all neonates. They are frequently associated with perinatal and metabolic problems, or with biochemical genetic disorders. Benign familial neonatal seizures are inherited as an autosomal dominant trait for which linkage has been established to chromosome 20q13 (MIM 121200). Multifocal or generalized seizures start between 2 and 15 days of life, frequently at age 2 or 3 days, and then disappear by 1–6 months of age. Psychomotor development is usually not affected.

Pyridoxine Dependency: Pyridoxine dependency (MIM 266100), an autosomal recessive disease, is associated with neonatal, and frequently, intrauterine seizures. The exact biochemical defect is unclear; the disorder may result from deficient activity of glutamate decarboxylase and reduced synthesis of GABA.

Febrile Seizures

Febrile seizures (MIM 121210), which occur between the ages of 6 months and 6 years, are associated with an elevation of temperature to 104° or more. Febrile seizures may be of any type, but are most often generalized tonic-clonic. The average age of onset is between 18 and 22 months. Febrile seizures occur more frequently in males than females. Most febrile seizures occur in otherwise normal children. Children with other neurological problems, however, may be more susceptible. One-third of affected patients will have a second febrile seizure; 1–3% will develop a chronic seizure disorder. Febrile seizures are often familial and associated with multifactorial or polygenic inheritance. Family studies have shown that up to 58% of patients have a

family history of seizures, usually febrile. Siblings have a 15% risk for a febrile seizure and a 1% risk for having a seizure of another type. If one parent also has febrile seizures, then the sibling's risk for a febrile seizure increases to 36%.

Because of the increased risk for birth defects in children of women with epilepsy who take anticonvulsants during pregnancy, such women optimally should have appropriate genetic and neurologic consultation before planning a pregnancy.

NEUROCUTANEOUS SYNDROMES

Neurocutaneous syndromes are commonly recognized genetic diseases that result from developmental anomalies of the skin and nervous system. The syndromes include neurofibromatosis, tuberous sclerosis, and von Hippel-Landau disease, which are also known as phakomatoses, a name derived from the Greek word phakos meaning spot, mole, or birthmark.

Neurofibromatosis

Neurofibromatosis (NF) consists of two distinct disorders, NF-1 and NF-2, that result from mutations in genes at two different genetic loci. Although both are autosomal dominant disorders in which affected patients have cafe-au-lait spots, the conditions should be considered as separate diseases. The diagnostic criteria for the two diseases, as established by a clinical conference at the National Institutes of Health in 1987, appear in Table 11–3.

Neurofibromatosis-1 (NF-1): Neurofibromatosis-1 (NF-1) (MIM 162200), also known as von Reckinghausen disease or peripheral neurofibromatosis, is an autosomal dominant disorder that occurs in 1 in 3000. NF-1 has a high mutation rate; 30–50% of patients represent new mutations in the gene, which is located at chromosome 17q11.2. The disease is highly penetrant, but has a wide variability in clinical expression even among members of the same family. The clinical manifestations become more apparent with age; confirmation of the diagnosis before puberty may be difficult. Many of the clinical manifestations are thought to be the result of abnormalities in cells derived from neural crest origin. Cafe-au-lait spots, the most common manifestation of the disease, occur in over 95% of affected patients. Cafe-au-lait spots are flat, pigmented macules, which often have irregular borders, and are named after their color of "coffee with milk." They may be present at birth, are most often found on the trunk, and increase in size and number with age, especially during puberty and pregnancy. Cafe-au-lait spots may also be noted in other genetic syndromes and in persons without NF. Cutaneous neurofibromas, soft tumors which develop from peripheral nerve sheaths, are usually not apparent until late childhood. Cutaneous neurofibromas are most common on the trunk; they frequently occur in the

Table 11–3. Diagnostic criteria for neurofibromatosis-1 and neurofibromatosis-2.

Disorder	Diagnostic Criteria
Neurofibromatosis-1 (NF-1) (Von Reckinghausen disease)	Two or more of the following: 1. Six or more cafe-au-lait macules over 5 mm in greatest diameter in prepubertal individuals and over 15 mm in greatest diameter in postpubertal individuals 2. Two or more neurofibromas of any type or one plexiform neurofibroma 3. Freckling in the axillary or inguinal regions 4. Optic pathway glioma 5. Two or more Lisch nodules (iris hamartomas) 6. A distinctive osseous lesion such as sphenoid dysplasia or thinning of long bone cortex with or without pseudoarthrosis 7. A first-degree relative (parent, sib, or offsping) with neurofibromatosis-1 by the above criteria
Neurofibromatosis-2 (NF-2) (Bilateral acoustic neurofibromatosis)	One of more of the following: 1. Bilateral eighth nerve masses seen with appropriate imaging techniques (eg, CT or MRI) 2. A first-degree relative with neurofibromatosis-2 and either: a. unilateral eighth nerve mass, or b. two of the following: neurofibroma, meningioma, glioma, schwannoma, or juvenile posterior subcapsular lenticular opacity

areolar area of affected females. Although they may become large or pedunculated with age, cutaneous neurofibromas rarely become malignant. Plexiform neurofibromas, however, may undergo malignant transformation to neurofibrosarcomas. Plexiform neurofibromas are usually larger, deeper lesions that arise from large major nerves. They may occur anywhere in the body and impair function of adjacent tissues. Plexiform neurofibromas frequently are noted in the orbital and periorbital areas. They may also result in limb hypertrophy or bowing of the long bones, especially the tibia. Demineralization, fractures, and pseudoarthroses may occur. Hyperpigmentation may be present in the skin overlying a plexiform neurofibroma. Freckling may be seen in the axillary or groin area. Optic gliomas, which can involve the optic nerves, chiasm, optic radiations, or hypothalamus, occur in 15–20% of patients with NF-1. Lisch nodules of the iris are noted in 10% of young children and 90% of adult patients with NF-1. Lisch nodules are hamartomas, often tan in color, that occur in any area of the iris. A slit-lamp examination may be needed to confirm their presence. The nodules usually do not interfere with vision. Congenital glaucoma, however, can result from involvement of the eye; it is often associated with a neurofibroma of the eyelid.

Specific osseous lesions are more commonly noted in NF-1. Scoliosis is common. Plexiform neuromas may involve the long bones, as described previously. Abnormalities in radiographs of the long bones may also result from subperiosteal neurofibromas. Skull radiographs may show a ballooning of the middle fossa, enlarged or J-shaped sella, abnormalities of the sphenoid wing, and bony defects of the orbit or lambdoid sutures. Enlargement of the optic nerve, other cranial nerves, or intervertebral foraminae may be noted. Approximately 6% of NF-1 patients de-

velop malignancies, which usually occur after 10 years of age. Affected patients have an increased risk to develop tumors of the nervous system, which include astrocytomas of the cerebrum and cerebellum, meningiomas, medulloblastomas, and ependymomas. Intraspinal tumors may also occur. Other malignancies that have been noted in NF-1 include leukemia, Wilms tumor, neuroblastoma, and the multiple endocrine neoplasia syndrome type II (includes pheochromocytoma and medullary carcinoma of the thyroid). There does not appear to be an increased risk for the acoustic neuromas seen in NF-2. Other findings commonly noted in NF-1 patients include macrocephaly and short stature. Approximately 40% of affected patients have learning disabilities or attention deficit disorders; 10% have mental retardation and seizures. Hypertension may result from involvement of small renal arteries. Ten percent of patients may have involvement of the gastrointestinal tract.

The gene for NF-1, which is very large, has been identified and cloned. The gene product, "neurofibromin," has a molecular weight of 250 kD. The NF-1 gene has significant homology to GAP, a known tumor-suppressor gene. Some mutations noted in the NF-1 gene indicate that inactivation of the gene occurs, which could explain the abnormalities in cell growth characteristic of this disorder. Molecular genetic testing may be used for prenatal and presymptomatic testing in informative families.

Neurofibromatosis-2 (NF-2): Neurofibromatosis-2 (NF-2) (MIM 101000) is also known as central or bilateral acoustic neurofibromatosis. NF-2, which occurs in 1 in 50,000 persons, is much less common than NF-1. Like NF-1, however, NF-2 is inherited as an autosomal dominant trait that is fully penetrant, but variably expressed. Acoustic neuromas, often bilateral, occur in 95% of affected patients by age 30 years. Acoustic neuromas are Schwann cell tumors that arise from the vestibular nerve. The neuromas are usually benign. They can, however, become very large, space occupying lesions that lead to increased intracranial pressure. The first clinical manifestation is usually hearing loss, which can be unilateral or bilateral. Approximately 50% of NF-2 patients have cafe-au-lait spots or cutaneous neurofibromas; these neurocutaneous lesions are usually less numerous than those seen with NF-1. Although posterior subcapsular cataracts are common, Lisch nodules are not noted. NF-2 patients may also develop tumors of the central nervous system, especially meningiomas or schwannomas that involve other cranial nerves or cervical nerve roots. The gene for NF-2, linked to the long arm of chromosome 22, is also thought to be a tumor-suppressor gene. Linkage analysis may be used for prenatal or presymptomatic testing in informative families.

Tuberous Sclerosis

Tuberous Sclerosis: Tuberous sclerosis (TS) (MIM 191100), in its classical description, consists of seizures, mental retardation, and facial angiofibromas. The disorder, however, is also associated with depigmented skin lesions and developmental hamartomas in multiple organ systems. Clinical manifestations may widely vary. TS, which occurs in 1 in 10,000 persons, is inherited as an autosomal dominant trait with high penetrance. Like neurofibromatosis, there is a high mutation rate. Approximately 50% of patients are thought to represent new gene mutations. The gene for TS has been linked to chromo-

some 9q34 in some families, and to 11q22–q23 in others. The criteria for the diagnosis of TS are shown in Table 11–4. Seizures, the most common clinical manifestation, usually start during the first year of life as infantile spasms or partial seizures. With age, TS patients develop other types of generalized seizures, which are often very difficult to control with anticonvulsant therapy. At least 50% of patients have psychomotor retardation that may be the only clinical manifestation of the disease. Psychomotor retardation is more commonly seen in those patients with TS that have early onset seizures. Cutaneous manifestations of TS include angiofibromas, previously known as adenoma sebaceum, which first appear between age 1 and 4 years as flesh, pink, or brown colored papules in patches, in a "butterfly pattern," on the malar areas of the face. Angiofibromas may increase with age; they are noted in 50% of older patients with TS. Hypopigmented skin areas of varying size, often present at birth, occur on the trunk and limbs. As with angiofibromas, they become more prominent with age. These hypopigmented skin areas, which are more easily seen with the use of an ultraviolet Wood lamp, may appear as an "ash-leaf spot" or in a "confetti" shaped arrangement of very small white macules. A characteristic "shagreen patch" of rough, leathery, skin may be noted on the eyelids or in the lumbosacral or gluteal areas. A "brown patch" on the forehead may be the first sign of the disorder in neonates or infants. Subungual or periungual fibromas, which more commonly involve the toenails than fingernails, may appear during teenage. Gingival fibromas and dental enamel pits are common. Retinal hamartomas, noted in 50% of

Table 11–4. Criteria for the diagnosis of tuberous sclerosis. Patients should have at least two clinical features.

Category	Clinical Feature
Dermatologic	Hypopigmented macules (ash-leaf spots) Fibroadenomas (adenoma sebaceum) Periungual fibromas Shagreen patches Brown patch on forehead
Dental	Dental enamel pits
Ophthalmic	Retinal hamartomas Hypopigmented defects of the iris
Neurologic	Periventricular tubers Cerebral astrocytomas Sacrococcygeal chordomas Nonspecific EEG abnormalities, including hypsarrhythmia
Cardiovascular	Cardiac rhabdomyomas Aortic and major artery constrictions
Renal	Renal angiomyolipomas
Pulmonary	Diffuse interstitial fibrosis

Adapted from Oski FA et al (editors); *The Principles and Practice of Pediatrics,* 2nd ed, JB Lippincott, 1994.

patients, may be seen as nodular (mulberry) shaped tumors in the area of the optic nerve, or as round or oval, gray-yellow glial patches, in central or peripheral regions. Fifty to eighty percent of patients develop renal cysts or angiomyolipomas. Children with TS are also known to develop cardiac rhabdomyomas. Adults, especially females, may develop pulmonary lymphangiomatosis; multicystic changes may lead to spontaneous pneumothorax or chronic lung disease.

The disorder is named for sclerotic tuberal areas that can be found in any area of the cerebral cortex. These cerebral "tubers" are hamartomas found most often in cortical gyri. Subependymal nodules occur on the ventricular walls and protrude into the ventricules. The nodules frequently become calcified after 5 months of age. Giant-cell astrocytomas, also hamartomas, often develop in the same location as the subependymal nodules. The nodules or harmartomas may grow large enough to cause ventricular obstruction and dilatation, and at times symptomatic hydrocephalus. Neuroimaging by CT or MRI is helpful in documenting the cerebral tubers, hamartomas, and ventricular size. Diffuse sclerosis and cystic-like changes in bones may also be noted. Because of the wide spectrum of clinical manifestations in TS, it is important that other family members be carefully examined for clinical signs of the disorder.

Von Hippel-Lindau Disease

Retinal angioma, cerebellar hemangioblastoma, and an increased risk for other tumors are characteristic of von Hippel-Landau disease (VHLD) (MIM 193399). The disorder is inherited as an autosomal dominant with incomplete penetrance and variable expression. The retinal angiomas, usually unilateral, are located in the retinal periphery where they can easily be overlooked without indirect examination. Retinal angiomas, which most often occur about 25 years of age, may be associated glaucoma, retinal detachment, and visual loss. Central nervous system hemangioblastomas, which most often occur after the third decade, are mainly found in the cerebellum. Hemangioblastomas may also occur in the medulla and spinal cord where they may be associated with syringomyelia. Very rarely, hemangioblastomas occur in the pituitary gland, third ventricle, or cerebral hemispheres. Cerebellar hemangioblastomas may become cystic or calcify. Cystic changes also may occur in the pancreas, kidneys, adrenal gland, and epididymis, and infrequently in the liver, spleen, or lungs. Affected patients have a higher than average incidence of renal cell carcinoma, pheochromocytoma, and epididymal cystadenoma. Twenty five percent of patients with VHLD develop renal cell carcinoma, which can be bilateral. Oat cell carcinoma of the lung and hepatocellular carcinoma of the liver have also been reported in patients with VHLD; these carcinomas, however, may be independent findings. The disorder has been linked to chromosome 3p.

Sturge-Weber Syndrome

Sturge-Weber syndrome (encephalofacial angiomatosis) (MIM 185300), a sporadic condition, is associated with congenital vascular lesions of the face, eye, and meninges. A facial hemangioma (port wine stain) usually involves the upper face and periorbital region, which may extend to other facial areas, the neck, trunk, or extremities. An associated leptomeningeal venous angioma occurs in the parietal or occipitoparietal regions and may be bilateral. Intracranial calcification of the angioma, which occurs during the first year of life, may appear as a linear, parallel configuration or in a convolutional pattern on radiographs. Between 25 and 30% of affected patients also have abnormal development of the choroidal membrane of the eye, which results in congenital glaucoma that is usually unilateral but may be bilateral. Between 2 and 7 months of age, 50% of patients develop partial or generalized seizures. One-fourth to one-half have hemiparesis; hemianopsia is common. Varying degrees of psychomotor retardation occur in approximately 50% of affected patients. Macrocephaly, colobomas of the iris, abnormal ears, coarctation of the aorta, and cutaneous xanthogranulomas also have been reported.

MYOPATHIES

Muscular Dystrophies
X-linked Recessive Muscular Dystrophies:
A. Duchenne Muscular Dystrophy: Duchenne muscular dystrophy (DMD) (MIM 310200) is an X-linked recessive disorder that affects 1 in 3700 live male births. The disorder usually becomes clinically apparent between ages 3 and 5 years, when gait abnormalities and weakness of the muscles of the pelvic girdle are noted. Pseudohypertrophy of calf muscles, lumbar lordosis, and contractions of the Achilles tendon occur. Weakness and atrophy of skeletal musculature progresses from proximal to distal involvement. Secondary contractions, kyphoscoliosis, and lumbar lordosis may be noted (Figure 11–1). Most affected boys lose their ability to climb stairs between 7 and 13 years of age; loss of ambulation occurs between 9 and 16 years of age. Intellectual ability is often low-normal; 25–30% of affected males have some degree of mental retardation. Cardiomyopathy occurs in 84%, and cardiac failure, from cardiomyopathy or respiratory insufficiency, is present in 95% of cases late in the disease. Most affected males die prior to 25 year of age.

DMD is associated with absent or very low levels of dystrophin. Dystrophin, a large protein, is found at the inner surface of the sarcolemma membrane in skeletal and cardiac muscle, and to a lesser extent in smooth muscle and brain. Lack of dystrophin appears to affect stability of the muscle membrane and may

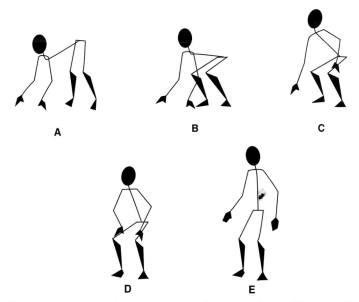

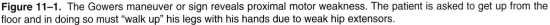

Figure 11–1. The Gowers maneuver or sign reveals proximal motor weakness. The patient is asked to get up from the floor and in doing so must "walk up" his legs with his hands due to weak hip extensors.

be associated with abnormal calcium binding and calcium influx into the muscle fibers leading to muscle necrosis. Dystrophin analysis of muscle biopsies is available in specialized laboratories. DMD patients also have low or absent muscle nebulin, a cytoskeletal protein that maintains alignment of contractile filaments during contraction. Lack of nebulin is thought to result in segmental tears and focal myofibrillar disruption. Muscle biopsy shows a characteristic pattern of fiber necrosis, degeneration, and regeneration. Variation in fiber size, phagocytosis, and replacement of muscle fiber by fat and endomysial connective tissue is also noted. High serum creatine phosphokinase (CK) levels, present from birth, become most elevated during the active phase of muscle necrosis.

The gene for dystrophin is located on the short arm of the X chromosome in the Xp2.3–p2.1 region. It is the largest human gene for which cDNA has been isolated; more than 60 exons are known to exit. Mutations at the dystrophin locus have been found with DMD, Becker muscular dystrophy (BMD), and intermediate forms of the disorder. Single or multiple exon deletions have been noted in 60–70% of affected males, and partial gene duplications in 6–10%. A point mutation has been found in one patient. Translocations with autosomes, involving the dystrophin gene locus, have also been reported. Molecular genetic techniques, eg, PCR or pulsed field gel electrophoresis (PFGE), which can detect more than 80% of the known mutations, may be used to establish the diagnosis in 65–70% of cases.

DMD has a very high mutation rate, which correlates with reduced reproductive fitness in affected

males. Approximately two-thirds of affected males inherit the disorder from their carrier mothers. In the remaining one-third of affected males, the disease results from new mutations in the dystrophin gene. In at least 75% of families with affected males, carrier detection for mothers and other female relatives may be accomplished by deletion analysis or RFLP. Approximately 8% of female carriers will be symptomatic; most have motor weakness. Affected females with more severe disease should be evaluated for X chromosomal abnormalities, eg, Turner syndrome or X-autosomal translocations.

Prenatal detection is available for informative families. Germ cell mosaicism has been reported in 5–15% of female carriers for DMD who may not be detected by carrier testing. For this reason, any woman with a son with DMD should be offered prenatal testing.

B. Becker Muscular Dystrophy (BMD): Becker muscular dystrophy (BMD), also known as late-onset X-linked muscular dystrophy, occurs in 3–6 per 100,000 male births. Clinical manifestations are similar to DMD, except that the onset is later, the findings are more variable, and the course is slower. Findings on muscle biopsy and serum CK elevations are less severe than DMD. In BMD, although dystrophin is frequently present in muscles, it may be reduced in concentration or have a smaller molecular weight and size than normal. Molecular deletions, which result in partial dystrophin function, are often smaller than those seen with DMD. About 10% of cases fall into an **intermediate clinical phenotype** between DMD and BMD, with correspondingly different molecular and dystrophin findings. BMD associated with contractures and cardiomyopathy, known as **Emery-Dreifuss syndrome,** is also inherited as an X-linked recessive disorder.

C. Microdeletion Syndromes: Two microdeletion syndromes involving the dystrophin gene and surrounding gene loci are known. One microdeletion syndrome involves, in gene order towards the centromere, congenital adrenal hypoplasia (AHC), glycerol kinase (GK), and DMD. Rarely the ornithine transcarbamylase (OTC) gene locus is also involved. The other microdeletion syndrome consists of DMD, McLeod red blood cell phenotype (XK), chronic granulomatous disease (CYBB), and the retinitis pigmentosa (RP) loci. Affected males present with various combinations of the associated diseases, depending upon the extent and position of the deletion.

D. Scapuloperoneal Dystrophy: Both myopathic and neurogenic forms of scapuloperoneal dystrophy occur, which are inherited as X-linked traits (MIM 312850). The myopathic forms presents between the second and fourth decade with a gait disturbance and degeneration of the scapular and deltoid muscles. Facial muscles are not involved; significant disability does not occur.

Autosomal Recessive Muscular Dystrophies:

A. Limb-girdle Muscular Dystrophy: Limb-girdle muscular dystrophy (MIM 253600), an autosomal recessive disorder, has its onset in late childhood or adolescence. The condition, which affects primarily the hip and shoulder girdles, is slowly progressive over a twenty year period. Loss of ambulation occurs between 15 and 50 years of age. Muscle dystrophin is normal; the etiology is unknown. In some families, the disorder appears to be an autosomal dominant trait; other cases appear to be sporadic.

B. Congenital Muscular Dystrophies: The congenital muscular dystrophies (MIM 253550–254130), a heterogeneous group of autosomal recessive conditions that present with weakness during the first few months of life, have muscle biopsy findings indicating a myopathy. These disorders, however, are usually not progressive. Most are characterized by proximal muscle weakness, hypotonia, hyporeflexia, and normal CK values. The disorders, which are classified according to the ultrastructural findings on muscle biopsy, include nemaline myopathy, central core disease, myotubular myopathy, and centronuclear myopathy. A severe variant, with mental retardation and seizures, occurs in Japan (Fukuyama type).

Autosomal Dominant Muscular Dystrophies:

A. Facioscapulohumeral Muscular Dystrophy: The onset of facioscapulohumeral muscular dystrophy (MIM 158900) occurs between 5 and 25 years of age. Weakness, which begins in the facial muscles, progresses to involve muscles of the shoulder girdle and extensors of the wrist and fingers. More severely affected patients may have involvement of the hip-girdle, anterior tibial, and peroneal muscles with associated foot drop, kyphoscoliosis, and lumbar lordosis. Intelligence and life span are normal. A very severe variant form of the disorder with onset in infancy, is associated with sensorineural deafness and exudative telangiectasis of the retina (Coats syndrome). The gene for the disorder has been localized to chromosome 4q35. Mutations in affected patients have included deletions and de novo rearrangements. All forms are inherited as autosomal dominant traits with variable penetrance.

B. Ocular Muscular Dystrophy: Ocular muscular dystrophy (MIM 158800), an autosomal dominant disorder, is characterized by ptosis, with or without weakness of other extraocular muscles. The onset may occur at any age, from infancy to older adulthood.

C. Oculopharyngeal Muscular Dystrophy: Oculopharyngeal muscular dystrophy, an autosomal dominant disorder, usually involves only the extraocular muscles in adults. It may occasionally affect the muscles of swallowing in children with the disorder. Some affected patients also have limb weakness and retinitis pigmentosa; in these patients, defects in mitochondrial oxidative phosphorylation may be involved.

D. Distal Muscular Dystrophy: Distal muscular dystrophy (MIM 158800), a rare autosomal dominant disorder, begins as weakness in the distal muscles of the hands and feet that progresses to involve the proximal muscles. Although most affected patients are adults, some patients have the onset of their disease during infancy.

Myotonic Dystrophies

Myotonia is characterized as muscle stiffness. An abnormality of the muscle fiber membrane leads to prolonged contractions in affected muscles. Affected patients have difficulty in relaxing the hand after a sustained grip. Percussion myotonia may be demonstrated by percussion of the thenar muscles, which results in a sustained flexion of the thumb in affected patients. Electromyography shows a characteristic pattern of high-frequency, repetitive discharge potentials that wax and wane in amplitude, producing a sound like that of a "dive bomber."

Myotonic Dystrophy: Myotonic dystrophy (MIM 160900), an autosomal dominant trait, affects adults and children and is estimated to occur in 1 in 8000 persons. Clinical findings are variable, even within families, and involve multiple organ systems. Two forms of the disorder exist: the classical form with adult onset, and a congenital form that occurs in neonates.

A. Classical Form: The classical form of myotonic dystrophy, which usually presents in young adults, may also be seen in childhood. Affected patients present with muscle weakness in the distal extremities, involving the hands and feet, and dystrophic atrophy of facial muscles. Myotonia may be demonstrated in the hands or tongue. Other clinical manifestations include cataracts, frontal balding, gonadal atrophy, diabetes mellitus, dysphagia, decreased bowel motility, pulmonary hyperventilation, craniofacial bony abnormalities including micrognathia, mild mental retardation, and a characteristic indifferent personality. Cataracts may be visible only by slit-lamp examination. Serious cardiac conduction abnormalities are common, including bradycardia and first-degree heart block, which may progress to complete heart block and sudden death. Muscle biopsy reveals type 1 fiber atrophy. Abnormalities in the distribution and arrangement of myofibrils and myofilaments are also noted. The age of onset and clinical involvement vary greatly among patients from the same family. Only about one-third of affected persons with known molecular abnormalities at the gene locus (described below) are symptomatic at any given time. Clinical abnormalities may not appear until age 50 or older. Figure 11–2 shows the facial involvement in myotonic dystrophy.

The gene for myotonic dystrophy is located on the long arm of chromosome 19. A cytosine-thymine-guanine (CTG) triplet repeat undergoes expansion in myotonic dystrophy patients. In normals, 5–27 copies of the triplet repeat are present. Myotonic dystrophy patients with mild symptoms have at least 50 repeats. Affected patients with severe presentation have a greatly increased number of repeats; segments as long as several kilobases in length occur. The repeat appears to expand as it is passed to younger generations; children frequently have more severe disease, with an earlier onset, than their parents.

B. Congenital Form: The congenital form of myotonic dystrophy occurs in 20% of neonates who inherit an abnormal number of CTG repeats from their mother. The mother may or may not be symptomatic; frequently the mother is diagnosed after the birth of the affected child. Affected neonates have severe hypotonia, facial diplegia with ptosis, and arthrogryposis. Lack of sucking, swallowing, and spontaneous respiration also occur. Cataracts may be noted; psychomotor retardation is common. A history of polyhydramnios or of decreased fetal movement may be obtained. Myotonia is not present in the neonatal period, but develops during childhood. Affected children later also develop the multisystem clinical manifestations seen with the classic form of the disorder. Muscle biopsy in the neonatal period is "immature," with abnormal arrangement of myofibrils. Type 1 fiber atrophy, as noted in the classic form, is not seen in the neonatal period but later develops. Mothers who have a child with congenital myotonic dystrophy have a high risk for a subsequent affected child.

Other Types of Myotonic Disease: Other types of myotonic disease are known to be inherited disorders. **Myotonia congenita Thompson** (MIM 160800), an autosomal dominant disorder, is associ-

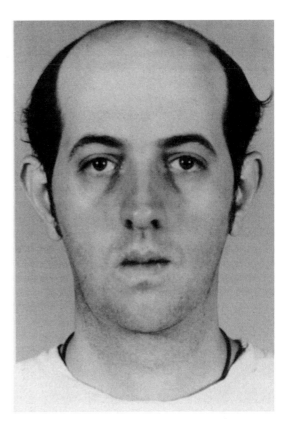

Figure 11–2. A 37-year-old man with myotonic dystrophy, showing frontal baldness, bilateral ptosis, and wasting of the temporalis, facial, and sternocleidomastoid muscles. (Photograph courtesy of R Griggs. Reproduced, with permission from Greenberg DA, Aminoff MJ, Simon RP: *Clinical Neurology,* 2nd ed, Appleton & Lange, 1993.)

ated with mild myotonia at birth, which diminishes with age and is limited to only a few muscle groups. **Autosomal recessive congenital myotonia** is clinically differentiated from congenital myotonic dystrophy by a later onset, between 4–12 years of age, and the absence of cataracts. Severe, distal, muscle atrophy and weakness occur in affected young adults. An altered fatty acid composition of muscle phospholipids has been reported. **Myotonic chondrodystrophy (Schwartz-Jampel syndrome)** (MIM 255800), an autosomal recessive variant of myotonic dystrophy, presents in early childhood with diffuse myotonia, muscle pseudohypertrophy, short stature, chondrodystrophy, joint abnormalities, and an unusual facies. **Paramyotonia congenita** (MIM 168300), an autosomal dominant disorder with onset during childhood, is characterized by generalized episodes of flaccid paralysis that may be precipitated by exposure to cold. Dystrophic findings do not occur. Serum potassium is normal during episodes, which differentiates this disorder from periodic paralysis.

MYASTHENIA GRAVIS

Myasthenia gravis (MIM 254200) is associated with abnormal function of the neuromuscular junction. The most common form of the disorder affects mainly adults, has an autoimmune basis, and is associated with the production of antibodies to acetylcholine receptors. Affected patients may have an ocular form of the disease, which affects primarily the eye muscles, or a generalized form that affects eye, facial, and limb muscles. Ptosis, diplopia, slurred speech, difficulty in chewing and swallowing, or weakness of the extremities are the most frequent presenting symptoms. Weakness progressively increases with exercise. Respiratory involvement may be severe enough to require assisted ventilation. Ten percent of adult patients have thymomas. Pupillary reflexes are normal; tendon reflexes are intact. Improved strength, usually with relief of ptosis, is noted following the careful intravenous injection of an anticholinesterase, eg, edrophonium chloride. Elevated concentrations of acetylcholinesterase receptor antibodies are found in 90% of patients. Approximately 3.5% of these cases are familial, but not inherited in any specific inheritance pattern. The HLA-B8 allele is noted in some affected families and in affected females with early onset disease.

Transient Neonatal Myasthenia: Transient neonatal myasthenia, seen in 10–15% of children born to mothers with generalized myasthenia gravis, results from passive transfer of antibodies from the mother, or from fetal synthesis of antibodies to the acetylcholine receptor. Unlike congenital myotonic dystrophy, transient neonatal myasthenia, is not inherited.

Inherited Myasthenias: The inherited myasthenias, which more frequently affect children, are not associated with antibodies to acetylcholine receptors. **Congenital myasthenia** (MIM 254210), an autosomal recessive disorder, is characterized by ptosis and/or ophthalmoparesis from birth. The disorder may result from a reduced number of acetylcholine receptors, end plate acetylcholinesterase deficiency, or reduced acetylcholine release. Affected patients frequently respond to anticholinesterase therapy. **Familial infantile myasthenia** (MIM 254210), a presumed autosomal recessive disease, presents with neonatal hypotonia that frequently requires assisted ventilation. Extraocular muscle weakness is not noted. Recurrent episodes of apnea and feeding difficulties occur. The disorder may result from a presynaptic defect in acetylcholine resynthesis. Most affected patients respond to anticholinesterase therapy. **Defects in postsynaptic acetylcholine-induced ion channels** are autosomal dominant disorders that have a variable age of onset, from infancy to adulthood. Progressive muscle involvement, which usually begins with ophthalmoparesis, is noted. Most affected patients do not respond to anticholinesterase therapy. **Limb-girdle myasthenia,** an autosomal recessive disorder of adolescents, is associated with proximal weakness that becomes worse with exercise. Ocular muscles are not involved. Most affected patients respond to anticholinesterase drugs.

DISEASES OF MOTOR NEURONS

Spinal Muscular Atrophies

Spinal muscular atrophies result from degeneration of motor neurons in the anterior horn cells in the spinal cord, medulla, and midbrain. Secondary denervation of muscle fibers results in muscular atrophy, progressive paralysis, and hyporeflexia or areflexia. The group of disorders is clinically and genetically heterogeneous with great variability in the age of onset and progression of the disorders. Autosomal dominant, autosomal recessive, and X-linked recessive forms exist. In general, the recessive forms tend to have little intrafamilial clinical variance, whereas the autosomal dominant forms may have wide intrafamilial variance. The diagnosis is established on the basis of clinical history and physical examination, along with findings on electromyography and muscle biopsy that are consistent with denervation. Creatine kinase may be elevated, but not to the extent seen with the muscular dystrophies. Table 11–5 gives characteristics of the spinal muscular atrophies. The listings and classification will change as molecular understanding of the disorders becomes known.

Spinal muscular atrophies of childhood, which occur in 1 in 14,300 live births, are the second most common fatal recessive genetic disorders, after cystic fibrosis. One in 40 persons of white Western European ancestry is a carrier for an autosomal recessive form of spinal muscular atrophy (SMA).

Werdnig-Hoffman Disease: The gene for Werdnig-Hoffman disease (MIM 253300), types I, II, and III, has been localized to chromosome 5q11.2–q13.1. Linkage analysis has shown mutations in the gene linked to the D5S39 locus for all three forms. The gene product and reason for the motor neuron loss is presently unknown. All types of the disorder are inherited as autosomal recessive traits. Prenatal diagnosis is feasible by linkage analysis in informative families. The different types of Werdnig-Hoffman disease vary in age of onset. In general, the earlier the onset, the more rapid the progression.

Type I, Acute Infantile Fatal SMA: Type I, Acute Infantile Fatal SMA, has its onset between birth and 2 months of age. One-third of cases have a history of decreased fetal movement in utero. Severe weakness of proximal muscles of the limbs and intercostal muscles occurs. Spontaneous movement may only be noted in the hands and feet. Affected patients have a narrow thorax with a pectus excavatum deformity and flaring of the lower ribs. Deep tendon re-

Table 11–5. Characteristics of the spinal muscular atrophies (SMAs).

Type of SMA		Incidence (Carrier Rate)	Inheritance Pattern	Age of Onset	Age of Death	Gene Location
I. Proximal (PSMA)						
1. Acute Early Infantile) PSMA Type I)	a. Werdnig-Hoffman (WH) Type I	1 in 25,700 (1 in 80)	AR	Birth–2 months	Less than 3 years	5q11.2q–13.1
2. Chronic Childhood (PSMA Type II)	a. WH Type II, Chronic Early Infantile	1 in 24,000 (1 in 90 for AR forms)	AR	2–12 months	7 months– 7 years	5q11.2–q13.1
	b. WH Type III, Late Infantile		AR	1–2 years	19 years	5q11.2–q13.1
	c. Kugelberg-Weland		AR	2–17 years	Adult	Unknown
	d. Others	Rare	AD	3–8 years	Normal life span	Unknown
3. Juvenile Onset (PSMA Type IV)		Rare	AD	6 months– 5 years	Normal life span	Unknown
4. Adult Onset PSMA	a. AR (PSMA Type III), Kugelberg-Weland	1 in 300,000 for all forms	AR	15–60 years	Normal life span	Unknown
	b. AD (PSMA Type V)		AD	25–65 years	20 years after onset	Unknown
	c. XLR		XLR	Adult		Unknown
II. Distal (DSMA)						
1. Autosomal dominant forms	a. Juvenile and adult onset	1 in 60,000 for all forms	AD	2–40 years	Normal life span	Unknown
2. Autosomal recessive forms	a. Severe infantile form		AR	Infancy	Less than one year	Unknown
	b. Juvenile forms		AR	4 months– 20 years	Normal life span	Unknown
III. Neurogenic						
1. Scapuloperoneal atrophy	a. Type I, AD	Rare	AD	4–70 years	May be reduced	Unknown
	b. Type II, AR	Rare	AR	2–5 years		Unknown
	c. X-linked	Rare	XLR			Unknown
2. Scapuloperoneal SMA with cardiomyopathy		Rare	AD	Childhood– young adult		Unknown
3. Fascioscapulohumeral muscular atrophy		Rare	AD	Before age 20 years		Unknown
IV. Other						
1. Adolescent SMA with hypertrophic calf muscles		Rare	XLR	Teenage		Unknown
2. Juvenile progressive bulbar palsy	a. Fazio-Londe (no deafness)	Rare	AR	Childhood	Rapid course	Unknown
	b. Vialleta-van Laere (with deafness)	Rare	AR	Less than 20 years	20–40 years	Unknown
3. Spinal bulbar SMA with androgen resistance	Kennedy disease	Rare	XLR	Adult		Xq12–q21 CAG TNR

AD = autosomal dominant; AR = autosomal recessive; XLR = X-linked recessive; CAG = cytosine-adenosine-guanine, TNR = trinucleotide repeat.

flexes are absent. Fasciculations of the tongue may be noted. Congenital dislocation of the hips and flexion deformities of the hands may be present. Autopsy reveals involvement of cranial nerve motor nuclei, and occasionally cerebellar hypoplasia, which may not be clinically apparent. Although motor milestones are affected due to the hypotonia, there appears to be no loss of innate intelligence. Most affected infants are social and interactive. Fairly rapid progression of motor weakness becomes generalized. Decreased ability to handle secretions occurs. The average age of death is 7–9 months. Most affected patients die from respiratory compromise or pneumonitis by 3 years of age.

Types II, Chronic Early Infantile, & III, Late Infantile SMA: Types II, the chronic early infantile type, and III, the late infantile type, are forms of chronic childhood SMA with later onset and less rapid progression than type I. Deep tendon reflexes may be present early in the disease, and later diminish or disappear.

Kugelberg-Welander Disease: Juvenile proximal hereditary muscular atrophy, or Kugelberg-Welander disease, occurs later and is more slowly progressive than type III Werdnig-Hoffman disease. The genetic locus is unknown. Although the disorder is usually inherited as an autosomal recessive trait (MIM 253400), autosomal dominant (MIM 158600) or X-linked recessive inheritance may also be involved.

Adult Forms of Proximal SMA: Adult forms of proximal SMA, which are less common than the childhood forms, may be inherited on an autosomal dominant (MIM 182980), autosomal recessive (MIM 271150), or X-linked recessive basis.

Distal SMA (DSMA): Distal SMA (DSMA) presents with distal hypotonia, in contrast to the proximal involvement of the other forms of SMA. Multiple types of DSMA exist, which have variable onset, from infancy to adulthood, and varying patterns of inheritance. The autosomal dominant forms (MIM 182960), which are highly penetrant, occur twice as frequently as the autosomal recessive forms. Affected patients have periods of relative arrest in progression of their disorder; life expectancy may not be shorted. The name, **neurogenic SMA,** distinguishes this group of disorders from the hereditary myopathies and sensorimotor neuropathies that have similar clinical presentations.

Kennedy Disease: X-linked spinal bulbar muscular atrophy (SBMA), also known as Kennedy disease (MIM 313200), is characterized by the adult onset of proximal muscle weakness and atrophy. Affected males frequently have signs of androgen insensitivity, eg, gynecomastia and infertility. Forty-three percent of patients have an increased number of cytosine-adenine-guanine (CAG) trinucleotide repeats in the first exon of the androgen receptor gene at chromosomal location Xq12–q21.

Familial Amyotrophic Lateral Sclerosis

Amyotrophic lateral sclerosis (ALS), a progressive degenerative disorder of adult onset, involves the alpha motor neurons of the spinal cord and lower cranial nerves and the upper motor neurons of the corticobulbar and corticospinal tracts. Although 60% of affected patients present with signs of both upper and lower neuron involvement, 20–25% have progressive bulbar and pseudobulbar palsies (primarily corticobulbar tract and bulbar motor neuron involvement), 7–15% have progressive muscular atrophy (spinal motor neuron involvement), and 5–10% have primary lateral sclerosis (pyramidal tract involvement). Progressive weakness and bulbar involvement lead to death from respiratory compromise, which usually occurs 2–3 years after the diagnosis. The diagnosis is established by clinical features, electromyography, muscle biopsy, and occasionally, autopsy findings. The incidence is between 1 in 70,000 and 1 in 100,000. Approximately 5–10% of cases are familial and inherited as an autosomal dominant trait (MIM 105400). A few cases of autosomal recessive inheritance have been reported (MIM 205100, 205200). Although the inherited forms usually have an earlier onset, often before 30 years of age, they are otherwise indistinguishable from sporadic cases unless there is a family history of the disorder. The gene for one of the familial forms of ALS has been localized to the long arm of chromosome 21.

HEREDITARY MOTOR AND SENSORY NEUROPATHIES

Hereditary Motor and Sensory Neuropathies (HMSN), or Charcot-Marie-Tooth Disease: The hereditary motor and sensory neuropathies (HMSN), or Charcot-Marie-Tooth disease, are genetically and clinically heterogeneous. All are associated with a progressive "peroneal" pattern of muscular atrophy and sensory involvement. HMSN are separated into two major types on the basis of pathophysiologic findings. HMSN type I, the **demyelinating, hypertrophic type,** is associated with segmental demyelination of nerve sheaths, proliferation of Schwann cells (termed an "onion bulb" formation), and reduced nerve conduction velocity (NCV). HMSN type II, or the **axonal or neuronal form,** is associated with axonal degeneration and normal or slightly slowed NCV, without hypertrophic changes on nerve biopsy. The autosomal dominant forms of the disorder occur in approximately 1 in 2800 persons, the autosomal recessive forms occur in 1 in 70,000, and X-linked forms occur in 1 in 28,000.

A. HMSN Type I: HMSN type I (MIM 118200), the most common hypertrophic form, presents in children or in young adults. Most patients become symptomatic in the first decade, and rarely after the age of 30 years. Males are usually more clinically affected than females. As many as 10% of affected patients have abnormal neurophysiologic studies but are clinically asymptomatic. Progressive distal wasting and weakness are noted in the peroneal nerve distribution, with associated foot drop, pes cavus, and hammer toes. Sixty percent of patients have decreased deep tendon reflexes. Sensation is usually impaired. As the disease progresses, weakness of the hands may appear. Action tremors and ataxia may be noted. One-third of patients have thickened peripheral nerves. Absent or markedly slowed NCV are noted; sensory nerve action potentials are undetected. The **Roussy-Levy phenotype** (MIM 180800), with prominent tremor and ataxia, may be seen in some cases of HMSN I. HMSN type I is most commonly inherited as an autosomal dominant trait with 100% penetrance, but variable age of onset and expressivity. HMSN type I is subdivided into type IA and type IB, which have different molecular characteristics.

1. HMSN Type IA: HMSN type IA has been associated with point mutations at the PMP22 locus, which is within the type IA gene locus on the short arm of chromosome 17 (17p21–p11.2). Large 1.5 mb (megabase) tandem duplications at the gene locus also occur. In **hereditary neuropathy with liability of pressure palsies (HNPP),** an autosomal dominant disorder also localized to chromosome 17p21–p11.2, large 1.5 mb deletions, which correspond to the 1.5 mb duplications seen with HMSN type IA, occur. This suggests that unequal crossovers during meiosis may be responsible for the generation of both diseases.

2. HMSN Type IB: HMSN type IB has been linked to the long arm of chromosome 1 (1q) and the Duffy blood group. Autosomal recessive forms of HMSN type I, with an earlier onset and more severe course than the autosomal dominant forms, are known. In one series of patients, an autosomal recessive form has been linked to chromosome 8q21.2–q13.

B. HMSN Type II: HMSN type II has similar clinical and neurophysiologic findings to type I, but different neuropathologic findings. Type II may also be inherited as an autosomal dominant or autosomal recessive trait. The autosomal dominant form has a later onset and slower progression than HMSN type I. The autosomal recessive forms (MIM 214400), which are rare and heterogeneous, may present as adolescent or severe childhood forms of the disease.

C. HMSN Type III (Dejerine-Sottas Disease): HMSN type III, also known as Dejerine-Sottas disease, is a rare, severe form of the disorder that presents with delayed motor development and hypotonia in infancy. Ataxia and peripheral nerve hypertrophy are common. The disorder is inherited as an autosomal recessive trait. Point mutations in the PMP22

gene locus on chromosome 17p21–p11.2, different from those noted in HMSN type IA, have been reported.

D. X-linked HMSN: X-linked HMSN (MIM 302800) occurs in males between the ages of 5–15. Most affected patients have segmental demyelination, while others have the axonal form of the disease. Affected individuals may also have deafness or mental retardation. Carrier females may have abnormal clinical or neurophysiologic findings. The disease has been linked to the DXYS1 and p58–1 loci on the long arm of the X chromosome (Xq13.1).

Carrier and prenatal testing are available for informative families for the types of HMSN with known genetic loci.

E. Complex Forms of HMSN: Other complex forms of HMSN are associated with optic atrophy, deafness, palmoplantar keratoderma, nail dystrophy, and pigmentary retinopathies.

The differential diagnosis for HMSN includes other genetic disorders, eg, Friedreich ataxia, Refsum disease, Fabry disease, distal SMA, leukodystrophies, abetalipoproteinemias, amyloidosis, porphyrias, and disorders of DNA repair.

HEREDITARY SENSORY NEUROPATHY (HSN)

HSN Type I, or Hereditary Radicular Neuropathy: HSN type I, or hereditary radicular neuropathy (MIM 162400), an autosomal dominant disorder of young adults, is associated with progressive symmetrical loss of distal pain and temperature perception, especially in the legs. Light touch may be preserved. Affected patients are at risk to develop ulcers, infections, and bony deformities of the feet. Deep tendon reflexes are decreased; mild weakness and ataxia may occur. Taste, sweating, lacrimation, and autonomic functions are normal.

HSN Type II, or Congenital Sensory Neuropathy: HSN type II, also known as congenital sensory neuropathy (MIM 201300), is inherited as an autosomal recessive trait, associated with severe, universal sensory loss in infancy. Autonomic function is intact; growth and intelligence are usually normal. Painless fractures and self-mutilation may begin as early as 4 months of age. Taste sensation is diminished; fungiform papillae are absent from the tongue. Corneal and gag reflexes may be depressed. Generalized hypotonia and absent deep tendon reflexes are seen.

HSN Type III, Riley-Day Syndrome, or Familial Dysautonomia: HSN type III, Riley-Day syndrome, or familial dysautonomia (MIM 223900), is a slowly progressive degenerative disorder of unknown etiology that affects sensory, autonomic, and motor functions. A developmental arrest of the sensory and autonomic nervous systems occurs. The disorder often presents at birth with intrauterine growth retardation. Affected infants are noted to have hypotonia, absent deep tendon reflexes, and poor responsiveness to painful stimuli. Dysphagia, drooling, and recurrent episodes of vomiting and aspiration pneumonia are common. Signs of autonomic involvement include labile blood pressure and temperature, excessive sweating, diminished lacrimation, and episodic transient skin blotching with eating or stress. Hypomotility and atony of the gastrointestinal tract or bladder may be present. Fungiform papillae of the tongue are absent. Older affected children have poor motor coordination. Seizures, EEG abnormalities, and scoliosis may occur. Initially there is decreased perception of temperature and of skin and bone pain. Visceral pain is usually intact. As the disease progresses, loss of proprioception results in gait abnormalities. Intelligence is usually normal. Only one-third of patients reach age 20 years. The diagnosis is made on the basis of clinical findings and abnormal responses to tests for sensory and autonomic dysfunction, eg, a lack of flare after intradermal histamine or the presence of pupillary constriction following the ocular application of mecholyl (methacholine) or pilocarpine. Urinary excretion of breakdown products of epinephrine and norepinephrine is reduced. The disorder, inherited as an autosomal recessive trait, is almost exclusively seen in persons of Eastern European Jewish (Ashkenazi) ancestry. In this subpopulation, the carrier rate is 1 in 30; 1 in 3700 infants are affected with the disorder. The gene has been linked to chromosome 9q33–q31. Prenatal diagnosis has been recently accomplished with linkage analysis.

HSN Type IV, Congenital Insensitivity to Pain and Absent Sweating: Congenital insensitivity to pain and absent sweating, HSN type IV (MIM 256800), which has its onset in infancy, may initially be confused with familial dysautonomia. The disorder, however, is not progressive; tearing is intact. Touch, as well as pain and temperature, sensation are diminished; affected patients may have self-inflicted injuries. Visceral sensation is usually also impaired. Most patients have psychomotor retardation. The disorder is inherited as an autosomal recessive trait. **Congenital insensitivity to pain with normal sweating** is a rare autosomal recessive disorder with clinical similarities to HSN type IV.

HSN Type V, Congenital Indifference to Pain: Congenital indifference to pain, or HSN type V (MIM 243400), is an autosomal recessive disorder that involves only pain perception. Other sensory modalities are intact and the autonomic nervous system is not involved. Except for injuries and secondary deformities from decreased lack of reaction to normal painful stimuli, most patients have a benign course.

Congenital Autonomic Dysfunction with Universal Pain Loss and Progressive Panneuropa- **thy with Hypotonia:** Congenital autonomic dysfunction with universal pain loss and progressive panneuropathy with hypotonia are rare disorders of infancy reported only in males; autosomal or X-linked recessive inheritance may be involved.

HEREDITARY ATAXIAS

Numerous types of **hereditary spinocerebellar ataxia (SCA)** exist. These rare disorders of idiopathic nature may be classified, on the basis of age of clinical presentation, into early onset ataxias, which are usually autosomal recessive disorders; or late onset types, which are usually autosomal dominant conditions.

Early Onset SCA:

A. Friedreich Ataxia: Friedreich ataxia (MIM 229300), the most common of the early onset hereditary ataxias, occurs in 1–2 per 100,000 persons. The disorder is associated with idiopathic degeneration of the spinocerebellar tracts, pyramidal tracts, and posterior columns of the spinal cord. Loss of large dorsal root ganglion cells and degeneration of large myelinated axons in peripheral nerves also occurs. For most affected patients, the onset of their disease occurs between 5 and 16 years of age. Initially there is a progressively ataxic gait, followed by ataxic involvement of all limbs. Dysarthria, nystagmus, impaired position and vibratory sensation in the legs, distal muscle weakness and atrophy, and absent deep tendon reflexes are common. Pes cavus, kyphoscoliosis, and extensor plantar responses are noted in over 90% of affected patients. Hand deformities may occur later in the disease. At least two-thirds of patients develop a progressive hypertrophic cardiomyopathy or serious cardiac arrhythmia. Insulin resistance and abnormal glucose tolerance are frequently noted; 10% of affected patients develop diabetes mellitus. Hearing impairment, cataracts, retinitis pigmentosa, or optic atrophy may occur. Most affected patients are unable to walk within 5 years of diagnosis; most die from cardiorespiratory complications about 25 years after the onset, usually between age 40–50 years. The diagnosis is established on the basis of MRI, electromyographic, and somatosensory evoked potential abnormalities, along with the clinical findings. The disorder is inherited as an autosomal recessive trait; the gene for the disorder has been localized to the pericentric region of chromosome 9 (9q21–q13). Prenatal diagnosis has been accomplished in some families.

B. Other Rare Forms of Early Onset SCA: Other rare forms of early onset SCA may have associated hypogonadism, myoclonus, pigmentary retinopathy, optic atrophy, cataracts, deafness, mental retardation, or extrapyramidal features. An X-linked recessive SCA also presents with early onset.

Late Onset SCA: Clinical symptoms usually occur after 20 years of age in late onset SCA. Approximately two-thirds of patients with late onset SCA are isolated cases that may or may not be inherited. Four types of the disorder are recognized, which are distinguished by the associated problems that occur in addition to the spinocerebellar ataxia.

A. Type I: Late onset SCA type I, an autosomal dominant disorder, is associated with opthalmoplegia, optic atrophy, dementia, and extrapyramidal features. The gene for SCA type I has been localized to chromosome 6p23–p22. Affected patients have expanded cytosine-adenine-guanine (CAG) trinucleotide repeats at the gene locus. Larger expansions are seen in patients with younger, frequently juvenile, onset of the disease.

B. Type II: SCA type II, also autosomal dominant, is associated with pigmentary retinopathy ophthalmoplegia, and extrapyramidal features. SCA type II has been linked to the long arm of chromosome 12.

C. Type III: SCA type III, which does not have other associated neurological features, has its onset after the age of 50.

D. Type IV: SCA type IV is associated with myoclonus and deafness. An autosomal dominant, periodic cerebellar ataxia has also been reported.

Ataxia may be a predominant clinical feature of many inborn errors of metabolism. It is also seen in disorders associated with defective DNA repair, eg, ataxia telangiectasia, xeroderma pigmentosum, and Cockayne syndrome.

DISORDERS OF BASAL GANGLION

Huntington Disease

Huntington disease (MIM 14310), an autosomal dominant disorder usually of adult onset, is associated with progressive dementia, personality change, and chorea. The disorder, which occurs in 1 in 24,000, is most common in persons of northern European background. It is rare in Asians and persons of African ancestry. Gradual loss of small interneurons occurs in the caudate and putamen. Atrophy of the cerebral cortex, thalamus, and cerebellum is also noted. Ventricular dilatation may be seen late in the disease. Interneurons that use gamma-amino-butyric acid (GABA) as a neurotransmitter appear to be most affected. The dopaminergic pathways are usually preserved.

Neurobiochemical studies have shown decreased levels of GABA, acetylcholine, substance P, dynorphin, glutamic acid decarboxylase, and occasionally of choline acetylase, in the basal ganglia of Huntington patients. Changes in binding have also been noted at excitatory N-methyl-D-aspartate receptors in the putamen. Relative overactivity of dopaminergic pathways, and a toxic effect of glutamate on striatal neurons, may be related to the chorea seen with the disease.

This does not explain other clinical features, however. It is also unclear whether these changes are primary or secondary in the pathogenesis of the disease. A better understanding of the function of "Huntingtin," the recently isolated product of the gene associated with the disease, may clarify the basic defect.

Most affected patients have an insidious onset of their disease between the ages of 35 and 45 years. Onset, however, may occur as early as infancy, or as late as the eighth decade. Restlessness, forgetfulness, mild postural changes, incoordination, and altered speech and handwriting are frequent early clinical findings. Changes in personality, depression, and other affective disorders are commonly noted. Some affected patients develop frank psychoses with hallucinations, delusions, or paranoia. As the disease progresses, the movement disorder becomes more apparent and choreic movements become incessant. Dystonia, ataxia, dysarthria, and dysphagia develop.

Most affected patients become totally disabled over a 10–25-year period. Deaths are usually related to cardiovascular and respiratory complications.

Approximately 10% of patients have the onset of disease before the age of 20 years. This **juvenile form** of the disease, also called the Westphal variant, is associated with less chorea, more rigidity, and a faster progression. Death occurs 8–10 years after onset. The juvenile form is more likely to be inherited from the father. Paternal inheritance has been noted in 92% of cases with onset less than 10 years of age, and in 56% of cases with onset between the ages of 10 and 20 years.

The gene for Huntington disease, IT-15, located at chromosome 4p16.3, has been recently isolated. The disease is associated with an increased number of cytosine-adenine-guanine (CAG) trinucleotide repeats at the 5′ end of the gene. A higher number of repeats is also associated with a younger onset of the disorder. The association of paternal inheritance with earlier onset appears to be independent from this finding.

Although the disease is almost 100% penetrant, cases apparently representing new mutations are known. In recent studies, clinically unaffected older relatives of apparent new mutation cases were noted to have CAG repeats in a number between normals and affecteds. This suggests a predisposition for the disease in the family, with expansion of the repeats in a subsequent generation as seen in myotonic dystrophy.

Presymptomatic testing is available for family members. Such testing, however, should be done with appropriate genetic and psychological counseling by clinics experienced with Huntington disease counseling. Prenatal diagnosis is possible.

Parkinson Syndrome

Parkinson syndrome, a disorder of adult onset, is associated with progressive resting tremor, muscular rigidity, slowness of movements, and loss of postural reflexes. Degeneration of pigmented cells in the substantia nigra and locus ceruleus, and atrophy of the globus pallidus and putamen occurs. Eosinophilic intraneural inclusion granules, termed Lewy bodies, are noted in the basal and sympathetic ganglia, brain stem, and spinal cord. Neurobiochemical changes include decreased levels of dopamine, homovanillic acid, norepinephrine, serotonin, tyrosine hydroxylase, dopamine decarboxylase, and glutamic acid decarboxylase.

The disorder, which occurs in 1 in 1000, usually has its onset between 40–70 years of age. Approximately 5–15% of cases are familial, in whom the onset is frequently earlier and course more severe. In most familial cases, the disorder is inherited as an autosomal dominant trait with variable penetrance. Autosomal recessive and X-linked inheritance are rare. A **juvenile onset variant** is usually inherited as an autosomal recessive trait, although some cases have been consistent with autosomal dominant inheritance.

Other forms of familial disorders affecting the basal ganglia are shown in Table 11–6.

PROGRESSIVE DEMENTIA

Alzheimer Disease

Alzheimer disease, a common disorder of progressive dementia, affects 2–3% of the population. The onset is usually between 50 and 75 years of age. Reduced activity of choline acetyltransferase in the cerebral cortex and hippocampus is noted. Degeneration of the nucleus basalis of Meynert, the main origin of cortical cholinergic innervation, and degeneration of the cholinergic septal-hippocampal tract occur. Pathologic findings also include neurofibrillary tangles in neuronal cell bodies, granulovacuolar degeneration, and extracellular neuritic (senile) plaques that contain beta-amyloid protein. Notably, patients with Down syndrome (trisomy 21) frequently have Alzheimer-like brain findings after the age of 40.

Familial Alzheimer Disease: Although most cases of Alzheimer disease are sporadic, familial Alzheimer disease may be inherited as an autosomal dominant trait. In earlier onset forms of the disease, with clinical symptoms before 60 years of age, autosomal dominant forms have been associated with mutations at two different chromosomal loci. Mutations are most commonly found at a loci linked to

Table 11–6. Hereditary disorders of the basal ganglia.

Disorder	Onset	Inheritance Pattern	Genetic Locus
Chorea			
Benign familial chorea	Childhood	AD, AR	Unknown
Familial paroxysmal choreoathetosis	Childhood	AD	Unknown
Familial paroxysmal dyskinesia	Childhood	AD, AR	Unknown
Familial calcification of the basal ganglia	Adult	AD	Unknown
Familial chorea and acanthocytosis	Adult	AR	Unknown
Huntington disease	Adult Juvenile	AD	4p16.3
Restless legs syndrome	Adult	AD	Unknown
Dystonia			
Idiopathic tortion dystonia	2–45 years	AD	9q32–q34
	4–16 years	AR	Unknown
	Adult	XLR	Xq21.3
Myoclonus			
Familial essential myoclonus	AD	Childhood	Unknown
Familial progressive myoclonus & ataxia	AD	Childhood	Unknown
Tics			
Tourette syndrome	AD, MF	2–13 years Males > females	Unknown
Tremors			
Benign essential tremor	AD	Any age	Unknown
Parkinson disease	AD	Adult	Unknown
Juvenile parkinsonism	AR	Childhood	Unknown

AD = autosomal dominant; AR = autosomal recessive; XLR = X-linked recessive; MF = multifactorial.

chromosome 14q24.3. About 2–3% of familial, early onset forms of the disorder have been associated with mutations in the gene coding for the amyloid-beta-protein precursor (APP), which is located on chromosome 21.

More recently, an increased risk for developing Alzheimer disease has been associated with apolipoprotein E4 (apoE4). The gene coding for apolipoprotein E genotypes is located on the proximal long arm of chromosome 19q13.1. ApoE functions as a ligand for the LDL receptor and the remnant receptor in lipoprotein metabolism. ApoE3/E3 is the normal, most common genotype. Homozygous apoE4/E4 is associated with type V hyperlipoproteinemia, a severe form of familial hypertriglyceridemia. ApoE4 is also known to bind to beta-amyloid. Alzheimer patients with apoE4 genotypes have greater amyloid deposition in the brain at autopsy. In some families with Alzheimer disease, the risk for development of the disease, and for an earlier onset of the disease, has been associated with the apoE4 genotype, which is dose related. That is, persons homozygous for apoE4/E4 have the highest risk, those heterozygous for apoE4 have an intermediate risk, and those with other isoforms of apoE (E2 and E3) have the least risk to develop the disease. Because 3% of the general population is homozygous for apoE4/E4, this genotype may play a major role in increasing the risk for the development of Alzheimer disease in families already predisposed to the disorder.

Pick Disease

Pick disease, clinically indistinguishable from Alzheimer disease, can only be differentiated by pathologic studies. Severe atrophy of the frontal and temporal lobes with reactive gliosis and ballooning of cells are found. Plaques or neurofibrillary changes as seen in Alzheimer disease do not occur. Most cases are sporadic, but some familial cases of autosomal dominant inheritance (MIM 172700) are known. The basic defect and genetic loci are unknown.

NEUROPSYCHIATRIC DISORDERS

Schizophrenia and mood disorders are known to have a higher incidence among family members than in the general population. The disorders appear to be related to polygenic and environmental factors.

Schizophrenia

Schizophrenia, which occurs in approximately 1% of the general population, affects males and females equally. Approximately 10% of primary relatives are also affected. A higher concordance of the disease occurs in monozygous twins, compared to dizygous twins. To date, linkage studies have not shown consistent information for a gene assignment of the disorder.

Affective Disorders

The major mood or affective disorders include unipolar disease, which is associated with major recurrent depressive episodes, and bipolar disease, which is associated with manic-depressive episodes.

Unipolar Disease: Unipolar disease, which is more common than bipolar disease, occurs in 4.3% of the population, more frequently in females than males. Unipolar disease is seen in 6–19% of primary relatives of index cases. Bipolar disease may also occur in relatives of patients with unipolar disease, but is less common and only occurs in 0.3–4.1% of primary relatives.

Bipolar Disease: Bipolar disease, which occurs in 0.5–1% of the general population, affects males and females equally. Both bipolar and unipolar disease may be noted in primary relatives of patients with bipolar disease, at rates of 3–18% and 6–28%, respectively.

Monozygous twins have a higher concordance than dizygous twins for both types of the disorder. Genetic linkage studies have not shown consistent or conclusive data.

The lifetime risks for the development of schizophrenia and mood disorders in family members are shown in Table 11–7. Children of two affected parents have a significant risk to develop the disorders. Genetic counseling for affected mothers should emphasize that lithium, and possibly other neuroleptics or antidepressants, may be fetal teratogens. These drugs may also be excreted in breast milk.

Table 11–7. Estimated lifetime risks for neuropsychiatric disease in relatives of affected patients.

Relative	Percentage Risk of Unipolar Disease	Percentage Risk of Bipolar Disease	Percentage Risk of Schizophrenia
Sibling	3–19	4–28	7–10
Dizygous twin (fraternal)	11	14	12–14
Monozygous twin (identical)	40	72	40–60
Child, one parent affected	20	9–27	8–16
Child, both parents affected	–	50–75	37–46

REFERENCES AND SUGGESTED READING

Bird TD. Epilepsy. In: *The Genetic Basis of Common Diseases,* King RA, Rotter JI, Motulsky AG, editors, Oxford University Press, 1992.

Bodensteiner JB, editor, Pediatric Neurology, The Pediatric Clinics of North America 1992;**39:**591.

Brosius J, Fremeau RT, editors, *Molecular Genetic Approaches to Neuropsychiatric Diseases,* Academic Press, 1991.

Conneally PM, editor, *Molecular Basis of Neurology,* Blackwell Scientific, 1993.

Dyck PJ, Thomas PK, Griffin JW, Low PA, Poduslo JF, editors, *Peripheral Neuropathy,* 3rd ed, WB Saunders, 1993.

Emery AE, Rimoin DL, editors, *Principles and Practice of Medical Genetics,* 2nd ed, Churchill Livingstone, 1990.

Gershon ES, Cloninger CR, *Genetic Approaches to Mental Disorders,* American Psychiatric Press, 1994.

Greenberg DA, Aminoff MJ, and Simon RP, *Clinical Neurology,* 2nd ed, Appleton & Lange, 1993.

Ionasescu V, Zellweger H, *Genetics in Neurology,* Raven Press, 1983.

Robinson A, Linden MG, *Clinical Genetics Handbook,* 2nd ed, Blackwell Scientific, 1993.

Rosenberg RN, *Neurogenetics,* Principles and Practice, Raven Press, 1986.

Rubenstein AE, Korf BR, *Neurofibromatosis,* Thieme Medical Publishers, 1990.

Swaiman KF, editor, *Pediatric Neurology,* 2nd ed, Mosby, 1994.

Endocrine System

12

The pituitary develops from two sources of primitive ectoderm. During the fourth and fifth week of fetal development, Rathke's pouch, a diverticulum in the roof of the primitive posterior pharynx, elongates and grows toward the brain, where it fuses with an outgrowth of the floor of the diencephalon called the saccus infundibulum. Cells derived from Rathke's pouch become the adenohypophysis or anterior lobe of the pituitary. Cells from the infundibulum become the neurohypophysis, which includes the posterior lobe of the pituitary, the hypophyseal stalk, and the median eminence.

Pituitary hormones are regulated by hypothalamic releasing and inhibitory hormones. These regulatory hormones bind to specific high affinity cell membrane receptors of the appropriate pituitary cell type. Anterior pituitary hormones, except for prolactin, are also under feedback regulation by hormones secreted by their target glands. The anterior pituitary secretes seven hormones: (1) growth hormone (hGH), (2) thyrotropic hormone (TSH), (3) adrenocorticotropic hormone (ACTH), (4) leutinizing hormone (LH), (5) follicle stimulating hormone (FSH), and (6) prolactin (Pr). The posterior pituitary secretes vasopressin (AVP, or antidiuretic hormone, ADH) and oxytocin.

Panhypopituitarism
Embryonic Defects
A. Congenital Absence of the Pituitary: Congenital absence of the pituitary, an autosomal recessive disorder, results in severe neonatal adrenal insufficiency, hypothyroidism, and hypoglycemia. In children with this condition, the anterior pituitary is absent; the posterior pituitary may be present or absent. Affected male infants may have hypogonadism and micropenis. Unless recognized and treated early, most affected infants die in the neonatal period.

B. Familial Pituitary Dwarfism with an Abnormal Sella Turcica: Familial pituitary dwarfism with an abnormal sella turcica (MIM 262700), also inherited as an autosomal recessive trait, may be a mild variant of congenital absence of the pituitary. Affected patients have a very small sella turcica that is located in a morphologically abnormal sphenoid bone.

C. Familial Hypopituitarism with a Large Sella Turcica: Familial hypopituitarism with a large sella turcica (MIM 262710) is an autosomal recessive disorder associated with growth hormone, thyrotropin, and gonadotropin deficiencies.

D. Empty Sella Syndrome: Empty sella syndrome, which may be seen as early as childhood, results from a defect in the diaphragma sella that allows extension of the subarachnoid space into the sella turcica. The disorder, which can be familial and possibly inherited as an autosomal recessive trait, is associated with proportionate short stature, an unusual facies, spinal anomalies and delayed sexual maturation. Empty sella syndrome can also occur with pituitary tumors and postpartum pituitary infarctions (Sheehan syndrome), or after pituitary trauma, radiation therapy, or surgery.

Midline Structural Defects of the Face or Brain: Varying degrees of panhypopituitarism may occur with other midline structural defects of the face or brain.

A. Cleft Lip and Palate: Patients with cleft lip and palate have been reported to have congenital aplasia of the pituitary. Approximately 4% of patients with isolated cleft lip and palate will have growth hormone deficiency.

B. Solitary Maxillary Central Incisor: A solitary maxillary central incisor has been associated with short stature and isolated growth hormone deficiency. Because relatives of affected patients have been reported to have holoprosencephaly, solitary maxillary central incisor may be the mildest manifestation of the autosomal dominant form of holoprosencephaly (see Chapter 11).

C. Holoprosencephaly: Patients with holoprosencephaly, which may occur as an isolated defect or associated with chromosomal abnormalities, may have varying degrees of panhypopituitarism.

D. Anencephaly: Anencephaly is usually associated with complete absence of the hypothalamus, absence or severe hypoplasia of the posterior pituitary, and variable degrees of pituitary insufficiency.

E. Trans-sphenoidal Encephalocoeles: Trans-sphenoidal encephalocoeles may have variable degrees of pituitary dysfunction.

F. Septo-optic Dysplasia Sequence: Malformations of anterior midline structures of the brain comprise septo-optic dysplasia sequence. Varying degrees of agenesis of the septum pellucidum, hypoplasia of the optic chiasma and nerves, and hypoplasia of the hypothalamus and pituitary infundibulum occur. Pituitary insufficiency, which ranges from isolated growth hormone deficiency to complete panhypopituitarism, results from deficiencies in one or more hypothalamic releasing hormones. Visual impairment, partial to complete amblyopia, pendular nystagmus, visual field defects, and hypoplastic optic discs with an aberrant vascular pattern are noted. Severely affected patients present in the neonatal period with hypoglycemia, hypotonia, seizures, and prolonged jaundice. Milder cases may present later with short stature or visual abnormalities. The disorder is usually sporadic in occurrence, but a few familial cases are known (MIM 182230).

Familial Panhypopituitary Dwarfism: Familial panhypopituitary dwarfism is associated with growth hormone deficiency and one or more additional pituitary tropic hormone deficiencies. Most cases are sporadic, but two genetic forms exist that are inherited either on an autosomal recessive (type I, MIM 262600) or on an X-linked recessive (type II, MIM 312000) basis. All forms are clinically and endocrinologically indistinguishable. Growth hormone deficiency, most often associated with gonadotropin deficiency, may also be associated with ACTH and TSH deficiencies. Most affected patients have clinical signs of primary growth hormone deficiency and sexual immaturity. Affected males may have small testes and micropenis.

Pituitary deficiencies may also be noted with the CHARGE association and with syndromes that have midline facial or brain involvement. Panhypopituitarism has also been associated with 18p- and 20p- chromosomal defects, gonadal dysgensis, Fanconi anemia, hemoglobinopathies, histiocytosis X, hemochromatosis, and neurofibromatosis.

Disorders of Human Growth Hormone

Human growth hormone (hGH or somatotropin), the most abundant hormone in the pituitary, is synthesized by somatotrophs in the anterior pituitary. Human growth hormone is secreted by the anterior pituitary in response to hypothalamic growth hormone releasing hormone (GHRH or somatocrinin); hGH release is inhibited by somatostatin. Stimulation of growth hormone receptors, located on hepatic cells and in other tissues, results in the release of somatomedin, or insulin-like growth factor (IGF-I), which stimulates growth and anabolism in tissues. IGF-I (somatomedin C), which is highly dependent on circulating hGH levels, is synthesized in the liver and other tissues. The gene for hGH (GH1) is part of a gene complex at chromosome 17q24–22 that includes two genes for growth hormone (GH1 and GH2), two genes for human chorionic somatomam-

motropin, hCS (CSH1 and CSH2), and one hCS-like pseudogene (CSHP1). The gene locus for IGF-I has been mapped to chromosome 12q24.1–22, for IGF-II to chromosome 11p15.5, for GHRH to chromosome 20p, and for somatostatin to chromosome 3q28.

Isolated Growth Hormone (hGH) Deficiency: Isolated growth hormone (hGH) deficiency occurs in 1 in 4000 to 1 in 10,000 births. Clinical findings include proportionate short stature, increased subcutaneous adipose tissue, a relatively small face with high forehead, fine wrinkled skin, and a relatively high-pitched voice. Fasting hypoglycemia may occur. Growth velocity is delayed. Length and height, which progressively fall further away from the normal mean with time, are usually significantly decreased by 2 years of age. Bone age is delayed and proportionate to the delay in stature. Normal secondary sexual development may occur, or it may be delayed in onset. Most cases of isolated hGH deficiency are sporadic or associated with trauma, infections, tumors, or birth defects of the central nervous system. Approximately 12 percent of cases are familial.

Type IA hGH Deficiency: Type IA hGH deficiency (MIM 262400), an autosomal recessive disorder, is associated with complete deficiency of hGH and deletions in the GH1 gene locus. This is the most severe form of hGH deficiency. Affected neonates may have a shortened length and hypoglycemia. These patients initially respond to hGH replacement therapy, but then develop anti-hGH antibodies and a diminished response.

Type IB hGH Deficiency: The most common form of the disorder, type IB hGH deficiency (MIM 262400), is an autosomal recessive disease that is presumed to result from faulty GHRH synthesis or secretion. Some affected patients have spontaneous hypoglycemia in infancy. Plasma hGH levels are deficient but rise with GHRH stimulation. Affected patients usually respond to treatment with hGH.

Type II (Pituitary) hGH deficiency: Pituitary deficiency of hGH, or type II hGH deficiency (MIM 173100), an autosomal dominant disorder, results in clinical manifestations that may be milder than other forms of hGH deficiency. Affected patients, however, have an increased tendency to develop hypoglycemia; they also vary in their response to hGH replacement therapy.

Type III hGH Deficiency: Type III hGH deficiency (MIM 307200), an X-linked recessive disorder, is characterized by hGH deficiency associated with varying degrees of hypogammaglobulinemia and reduced levels of circulating B lymphocytes. The disorder may result from a contiguous gene deletion syndrome involving loci for immunoglobulin production and hGH expression on the X chromosome.

Pituitary Dwarfism with Biologically Inactive hGH: Patients with pituitary dwarfism with biologically inactive hGH (MIM 262650) have normal levels of circulating hGH but low levels of somatomedin. Affected patients may respond to hGH replacement therapy. The inheritance pattern for the disorder is uncertain, but may be autosomal recessive.

Laron Dwarfism: Laron dwarfism (MIM 26250), an autosomal recessive disorder, results from abnormal hGH receptors on liver cells and deficient IGF-1 (somatomedin C) production. Affected patients have features of severe hGH deficiency; males may have micropenis. Plasma levels of hGH may be normal or elevated; IGF-1 levels are low. Affected patients do not usually respond to hGH replacement therapy.

Pituitary Dwarfism with Somatomedin Unresponsiveness: Patients with pituitary dwarfism with somatomedin unresponsiveness have normal plasma levels of hGH and elevated levels of IGF-1. The defect in peripheral unresponsiveness to IGF-1 appears to be at the IGF-I receptor or post-receptor level in target tissues. Reduced IGF binding to 50% of normal has been shown in cultured skin fibroblasts from an affected patient.

Other Genetic Diseases
of Anterior Pituitary Function

Isolated deficiencies of other anterior pituitary hormones will be covered in the sections that discuss their target organs.

Genetic Diseases
of Posterior Pituitary Hormones

Familial Central Diabetes Insipidus (Hereditary Vasopressin-sensitive Diabetes Insipidus): Familial central diabetes insipidus (hereditary vasopressin-sensitive diabetes insipidus) results from aplasia or degeneration of the magnocellular neurosecretory cells of the supraoptic and paraventricular nuclei that secrete vasopressin (AVP) and oxytocin. Affected patients have polydipsia and polyuria. When they cannot keep up with their large fluid requirement, these patients are at risk to develop severe dehydration and hypernatremia. Plasma AVP levels are very low or absent; affected patients respond to treatment with exogenous vasopressin. Oxytocin secretion may or may not be affected. The onset is usually in infancy but may not be apparent until late childhood or adolescence. The disorder is usually inherited as an autosomal dominant trait with variable expression (MIM 125700), but can be X-linked recessive (MIM 304900). Another X-linked recessive form of the disorder, which has intact neurosecretory cells, is thought to be caused by failure of AVP synthesis.

Wolfram Syndrome, or DIDMOAD: Wolfram syndrome, or DIDMOAD (MIM 222300), is an autosomal recessive disorder characterized by **d**iabetes **i**nsipidus, **d**iabetes **m**ellitus, **o**ptic **a**trophy and **d**eafness. Juvenile onset diabetes mellitus usually precedes the other symptoms. Optic atrophy may be associated with a peripheral pigmentary retinopathy. A bilateral sensorineural, high-frequency hearing loss may be mild and detected only by audiograms. Most affected patients have a neurogenic bladder; some have ataxia, sideroblastic anemia, or hyperalaninuria. One-third of patients have central vasopressin-responsive diabetes insipidus. The basis for the disorder is unknown.

Familial Nephrogenic Diabetes Insipidus Type I: Patients with familial nephrogenic diabetes insipidus type I (MIM 304800), an X-linked disorder, have renal tubular unresponsiveness to AVP. AVP normally binds to V_2 receptors on the basolateral surface of hormone-responsive renal epithelial cells; the V_2 receptors activate the formation of cAMP with a resultant increase in renal concentrating ability and water and salt permeability. The disorder is associated with a defect in the V_2 receptor signal transduction pathway in both the kidney and in extrarenal tissues. Affected patients present in the neonatal period with severe polydipsia, polyuria, and persistent hypotonic urine. These infants, preoccupied with water ingestion, have poor weight gain from a decreased caloric intake. Dilation of the urinary tract and renal insufficiency may occur. They are at risk for severe dehydration, hypernatremia, hyperthermia, and seizures. Plasma levels of AVP are normal or elevated; there is no response to exogenous vasopressin. The genetic locus for the disorder is at chromosome Xq28.

Familial Nephrogenic Diabetes Insipidus Type II: Familial nephrogenic diabetes insipidus Type II (MIM 125800) is a rare, autosomal dominant disorder with an intact cAMP response. The disorder is thought to result from a post-receptor defect in recognition of the cAMP signal.

Nephrogenic diabetes insipidus may also be seen with other renal disorders, sickle cell anemia, and autosomal dominant hypoparathyroidism.

GENETIC DISORDERS
OF THYROID FUNCTION

Embryonic Defects

At 24 days of fetal life, the thyroid gland starts to develop from midline endoderm of the floor of the primitive pharynx. The developing thyroid moves down into the neck, to a position anterior to the trachea, and in so doing creates a thyroglossal duct that normally closes.

Thyroglossal Duct Cyst or Sinus: Failure of the duct to close may lead to a thyroglossal duct cyst or sinus, which most commonly occurs just inferior to the hyoid bone.

Ectopic Thyroid Gland: Failure of the thyroid to descend properly can result in an ectopic thyroid gland, which is frequently smaller than normal and results in hypothyroidism. Ectopic thyroids may be found at the base of the tongue (lingual thyroid), anywhere along the path of the thyroglossal duct, or in the anterior thorax.

Thyroid Hormones

The thyroid hormones T_3 (3,5,3´ triiodothyronine) and T_4 (tetraiodothyronine or thyroxine) are synthesized by the thyroid gland follicular cells from tyrosine and iodine in response to TSH (thyroid stimulating hormone). TSH binds to receptors on the follicular cells, activating a cAMP second messenger system. Hypothalamic thyrotropin releasing factor (TRF or TRH) stimulates pituitary TSH synthesis and secretion. TSH synthesis and release are inhibited by circulating thyroid hormone levels in classical feedback regulation. T_4 is transported by thyroxine-binding globulin (TBG), thyroxine-binding prealbumin (TBPA), and albumin. In tissues T_4 is converted to T_3, which is three to four times more metabolically active than T_4, or to rT_3 (reverse T_3), which is biologically inactive. T_3 levels are low during fetal life but increase after birth. Thyroid hormone effects on tissues are mediated by the hormones binding to specific nuclear receptors. The receptors have a higher affinity for T_3 than for T_4. Genetic defects may occur at any of the steps involved with thyroid hormone synthesis, transport, or binding in peripheral tissues.

Congenital Hypothyroidism

Congenital hypothyroidism may be associated with hypothalamic or pituitary dysplasias, as discussed with the disorders associated with panhypopituitarism. **Familial isolated TSH deficiency** rarely has been reported.

Thyroid Dysgenesis: Thyroid dysgenesis (MIM 218700), the most common cause of congenital hypothyroidism, occurs in 1 in 4000 live births and is most often sporadic. The disorder is more frequent in children of Hispanic and Far Eastern background and less common in children of African descent. Females are two times more likely to be affected than males. The disorder usually results from thyroid aplasia or hypoplasia, but may be due to an ectopic thyroid gland. Although all states currently screen newborns for congenital hypothyroidism, cases may be missed; the clinician should evaluate any infant who shows clinical signs of the disease. Affected young infants have large fontanelles, immature facial bones, delayed bone age, and poor linear growth. They frequently display decreased activity, feeding problems, delayed passage of meconium, constipation, abdominal distention, umbilical hernias, prolonged hyperbilirubinemia, and hypothermia. Decreased circulation results in mottling, and dry skin that may be cold to touch. Myxedema is associated with a hoarse cry, enlarged muscle mass and tongue, and a fullness of the subcutaneous tissues, that is most often noted in the lower eyelids. Psychomotor retardation occurs

from delayed myelination of the central nervous system. Treatment with thyroid hormone replacement therapy will improve all clinical findings, except for the retardation, which is irreversible. Thus, it is important that cases detected by newborn screening be confirmed and treated promptly to prevent psychomotor retardation.

Defects in the Synthesis and Release of Thyroid Hormones: Defects in the synthesis and release of thyroid hormones are rare, autosomal recessive traits that result in congenital hypothyroidism.

A. Iodide Concentrating Defects: Iodide concentrating defects (MIM 264400) are associated with faulty transport and concentration of iodide in the thyroid gland, where it is used for thyroid hormone synthesis.

B. Organification Defects: Organification defects (MIM 274500, 274700) result from deficiency of peroxidase enzyme activity or peroxidase generation that is needed for oxidation of thyroidal iodide, iodination of thyroglobulin-bound tyrosine, or "coupling" of mono- and diiodotyrosines to form thyroid hormones.

C. Iodotyrosine Deiodinase Defects: Iodotyrosine deiodinase defects (MIM 274800) are associated with deficient activity of iodotyrosine dehalogenase, which results in iodine wasting rather than recycling.

D. Defects in Thyroglobulin Synthesis: Because normal thyroglobulin is needed for "coupling" of iodotyrosines, defects in thyroglobulin synthesis (MIM 274900) result in decreased thyroid hormone synthesis.

E. Pendred Syndrome: The Pendred syndrome (MIM 274600), an autosomal recessive disorder associated with a defect in organification, affects 1 in 14,000 persons with variable degrees of congenital deafness, goiter, and hypothyroidism.

Disorders of TSH Unresponsiveness: Disorders of TSH unresponsiveness (MIM 275200), rare autosomal recessive traits, result from defects in homone-receptor binding or post-receptor stimulation of thyroid follicular cells. Congenital hypothyroidism with low thyroid hormone levels occurs.

Decreased Peripheral Responsiveness to Thyroid Hormones: Decreased peripheral responsiveness to thyroid hormones is also probably related to abnormal receptor binding. Affected patients have elevated free T_3 and free T_4, normal TSH levels, goiter, stippled epiphyses, retarded bone age, and deafness. With age, the hormone levels and epiphyses normalize; the goiter disappears. Intelligence is usually normal. The disorder is inherited as an autosomal recessive trait in some families (MIM 274300) and as an autosomal dominant trait in others (MIM 188570).

Immunoglobulins may be implicated in some cases of congenital hypothyroidism. For example, thyroid dysgenesis has been occasionally associated with thyroid growth-blocking immunoglobulin. TSH-binding inhibitor immunoglobulin (TBII), in association with maternal chronic lymphocytic thyroiditis, may be the cause of familial cases of congenital hypothyroidism or transient neonatal hypothyroidism.

Disorders of Thyroid Hormone Transport: Disorders of thyroid hormone transport are associated with abnormalities of thyroid hormone-binding serum proteins.

A. Thyroid-binding Globulin (TBG) Deficiency: Thyroid-binding globulin (TBG) deficiency (MIM 314200), an X-linked trait, occurs in 1 in 5000–12,000 newborns. It is thought to result from defective hepatic TBG synthesis or from instability of TBG. T_4 binding capacity is very low in affected males and approximately one-half normal in carrier females. Serum T_4 levels are proportionately reduced; free T_4 and free T_3 levels are normal, however, and the patients are euthyroid. Partial TBG deficiencies are also known. TBG deficiency may also occur with the carbohydrate-deficient glycoprotein (CDG) syndrome, an autosomal recessive disorder, discussed with the inborn errors of metabolism. Although these patients do not have congenital hypothyroidism, newborn screening tests will frequently give false positive testing results in affected infants.

Elevated levels of TBG, TBPA, or an abnormal serum albumin in familial dysalbuminemic hyperthyroxinemia, are genetic disorders that are all associated with elevated serum T_4, normal free T_4, and euthyroid states.

Autoimmune Thyroid Disease

Graves Disease: Graves disease (MIM 27500), a multifactorial disorder that occurs in 0.4% of the population, is the most common cause of hyperthyroidism. Although most frequently seen in adults, the disorder may present at any age from birth to old age; it is 7–10 times more common in women than men. Graves disease is characterized by thyrotoxicosis and diffuse goiter, which result from stimulation of thyroid follicular cells by thyroid-stimulating immunoglobulins (TSIs). Cell-mediated immunity is also abnormal; a defect in suppressor T cell function has been postulated. Serum T_3 and T_4, free T_3 and T_4, and thyroid hormone binding ratios are elevated; thyroid stimulating hormone (TSH) is low. An infiltrative opthalmopathy with exophthalmos, weakness of the extraocular muscles, and periorbital edema is present in 50% of patients. Five to ten percent of patients also have an infiltrative dermopathy, which most often occurs as violaceous plaques of induration over the pretibial areas and dorsum of the feet. The disorder, which is known to occur more frequently in relatives of affected patients, is strongly associated with certain HLA haplotypes. Graves disease in Caucasians is associated with HLA-B8 and HLA-DR3 haplotypes; in African Americans it is associated with the HLA-DRw6 haplotype. Transplacental passage of maternal TSIs may result in Graves disease in neonates.

Hashimoto Thyroiditis: Hashimoto thyroiditis (MIM 140300), also a common multifactorial disorder, is characterized by chronic lymphocytic thyroiditis and goitrous hypothyroidism. Like Graves disease, it is more common in females and adults, is autoimmune mediated, and is frequently seen in relatives of index cases. Lymphocytic infiltration and nontender enlargement of the thyroid gland are noted. A phase of hyperthyroidism, similar to Graves disease, may occur prior to the development of hypothyroidism. Affected patients have high levels of circulating antithyroglobulin and antimicrosomal antibodies. The disease is associated with HLA-B8, HLA-DR3 and HLA-DR5 haplotypes. Patients with Down syndrome have an increased incidence of Hashimoto thyroiditis; the disorder has been reported in patients with Turner, Klinefelter, and Noonan syndromes.

GENETIC DISORDERS OF PARATHYROID FUNCTION

Embryonic Defects

The parathyroid glands develop from epithelial proliferation of the dorsal parts of the third and fourth pharyngeal pouches during the fifth week of fetal life. As they develop, the primitive parathyroid glands descend with the primitive thyroid and thymus into the neck to become situated on the dorsal surface of the thyroid gland.

Ectopic Parathyroid Gland: Ectopic parathyroid glands may result from failure of the glands to descend or to properly separate from the primitive thyroid and thymus. Ectopic parathyroid tissue may be found near the bifurcation of the common carotid artery or anywhere near or within the thyroid or thymus glands in the neck and upper thorax. Occasionally more than four glands are formed.

Congenital Absence of a Parathyroid Gland: Congenital absence of a parathyroid gland may result from failure of a gland to differentiate or from atrophy during development. The parathyroid glands become functionally active during fetal life in regulating fetal calcium metabolism.

Parathyroid Hormone

Parathyroid hormone (PTH) is synthesized by "active" chief cells of the parathyroid gland. PTH secretion is mainly influenced by serum calcium and calcitriol levels. The primary function of PTH is to maintain physiologic concentrations of calcium in body fluids. PTH, through the renal production of active vitamin D metabolites, stimulates reabsorption of calcium by the kidney, calcium resorption from bone, and calcium absorption from the gut. PTH also affects body fluid phosphorus levels by a direct phosphaturic action on the kidney and through bone resorption. PTH receptor actions in bone and kidney are mediated by cAMP.

Hypoparathyroidism

Neonatal Hypoparathyroidism: Neonatal hypoparathyroidism, when it occurs as an isolated disorder, can be inherited as an autosomal recessive (MIM 241400), autosomal dominant (MIM 146200), or more commonly as an X-linked recessive disease (MIM 307700). Hypoparathyroidism is associated with hypocalcemia, hyperphosphatemia, irritability, and seizures. Neonatal hypoparathyroidism may also occur in association with malformations of the third and fourth branchial arches, eg, the DiGeorge sequence (see immunology and cardiology sections), or be secondary to suppression of the fetal parathyroids by maternal hypercalcemia from maternal hyperparathyroidism.

Primary hypoparathyroidism is also seen in the polyendocrine syndrome type I.

Hyperparathyroidism

Neonatal Hyperparathyroidism: Neonatal hyperparathyroidism (MIM 239200), a rare autosomal recessive disorder, is characterized by hyperplasia of the parathyroid glands and severe hypercalcemia at birth. The disorder may also be secondary to maternal hypoparathyroidism.

Hereditary Primary Hyperparathyroidism: Hereditary primary hyperparathyroidism (MIM 145000), an autosomal disorder with onset near puberty, results from hyperplasia of the parathyroid glands or adenomas in one or more of the glands.

Hyperparathyroidism is also associated with the multiple endocrine neoplasia syndromes.

Hereditary Hypocalciuric Hypercalcemia: Hereditary hypocalciuric hypercalcemia (MIM 145980), an autosomal dominant disorder, is associated with hypercalcemia and a lowered renal clearance of calcium from birth. The etiology for the disease is unknown; affected patients are frequently asymptomatic. Although not classically a form of hyperparathyroidism, this disorder should be considered in the differential diagnosis of any patient who presents with hypercalcemia.

Pseudohyperparathyroidism (PHP)

Elevated PTH levels, because of end-organ unresponsiveness to PTH, occurs in pseudohyperparathyroidism (PHP) (MIM 103580).

A. Type Ia: Type Ia of the disorder is associated with a generalized resistance to hormones and other agents that stimulate adenylate cyclase. The disorder results from deficient activity of the Gs (guaninenucleotide binding) protein, which is needed for receptor stimulation of adenylate cyclase. In addition to PTH, thyrotropin, gonadotropin, glucagon, and

isoproterenol stimulation of cAMP production is also affected. Patients with type Ia PHP have serum calcium levels that may be normal or low, depending upon other distal factors that influence serum calcium levels, eg, calcitriol and renal function. Hypocalcemia, if it occurs, most often develops during early childhood. Elevated serum phosphorus and PTH levels usually precede hypocalcemia. Hypothyroidism and hypogonadism are common; distal responses to glucagon and isoproterenol are normal. Affected patients also have physical findings known as the **Albright osteodystrophy phenotype,** which includes short stature, obesity, a rounded face, short fourth and occasionally fifth metacarpals and metatarsals, psychomotor retardation, seizures, and subcutaneous ossifications. The disorder is inherited as an autosomal dominant trait. Affected family members may have the clinical features of PHP Ia, or that of pseudopseudohyperparathyroidism (PPHP). Although patients with PPHP also have the Albright osteodystrophy phenotype and elevated levels of PTH, they have a normal rise in cAMP excretion in response to PTH and do not develop hypocalcemia. PPHP patients, however, also have Gs deficiency; the reason for their normal cAMP response is unclear.

B. Type Ib: Type Ib PHP is associated with normal Gs activity, decreased cAMP excretion in response to PTH, and a normal physical appearance. The defect is unknown but may be in the PTH receptor. Type Ib is rare and may be sporadic or familial.

C. Type II PHP: Type II PHP (MIM 203330), a rare disease, is usually not familial and may be acquired. The disorder is characterized by hypocalcemia, hyperphosphatemia, elevated PTH levels, normal cAMP excretion in response to PTH, normal renal function, and a normal appearance. The defect is unknown.

GENETIC DISORDERS OF ADRENAL FUNCTION

The adrenal cortex and medulla have different embryonic origins. The fetal cortex, and later the permanent cortex, develop from the mesodermal epithelial lining of the posterior abdominal wall. The medulla develops from an adjacent sympathetic ganglion, and is of neural crest origin.

Hormone Synthesis and Regulation of the Adrenal Cortex

The adrenal cortex is composed of 3 zones. The outer zona glomerulosa, which produces aldosterone, is regulated by the renin-angiotensin system and potassium. The middle zona fasciculata and inner zona reticularis, which are regulated by ACTH, produce glucocorticoids, mineralocorticoids, androgens, and estrogens. The adrenal steroid hormone biosynthetic pathway is shown in Figure 12–1.

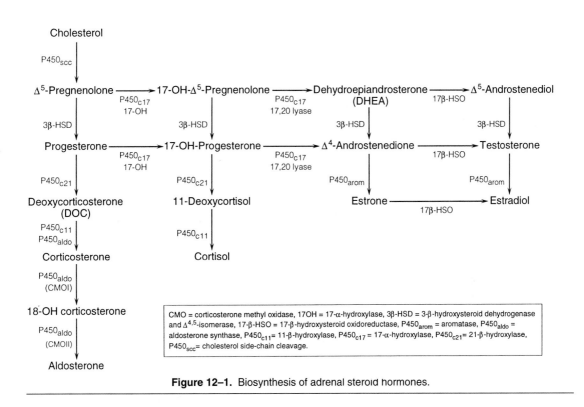

Figure 12–1. Biosynthesis of adrenal steroid hormones.

Glucocorticoids: Most enzymes involved with adrenal steroid hormone production belong to the family of cytochrome P450 oxygenases. Cholesterol is the precursor molecule for all of these steroid hormones. Conversion of cholesterol to pregnenolone is the rate-limiting step and the major site of ACTH action on the adrenal gland.

Pituitary ACTH is released in response to hypothalamic corticotropin-releasing hormone. ACTH binds to high-affinity plasma membrane receptors on the adrenocortical cells, which by cAMP-mediated intracellular phosphoprotein kinases, stimulate the production and secretion of cortisol, adrenal androgens, and deoxycorticosterone (DOC). Glucocorticoids bind to specific cytosolic receptors, which are present on most tissues, and interact with nuclear chromatin acceptor sites, resulting in the transcription of proteins that facilitate hormone response. Glucocorticoids in general inhibit DNA and protein synthesis and accelerate protein catabolism and lipolysis to provide substrates for intermediary metabolism. In the liver, however, glucocorticoids stimulate RNA and protein synthesis in order to promote hepatic gluconeogenesis.

Mineralocorticoids: Renal juxtaglomerular cells of the afferent arteriole of the glomerulus secrete renin, which acts on its substrate angiotensinogen to form angiotensin I (inactive form); angiotensin I is then converted to angiotensin II (active form). Angiotensin II: (a) acts directly on the adrenal cortex to stimulate aldosterone production and secretion, (b) stimulates release of catecholamines from the adrenal medulla, and (c) has a direct renal effect to promote sodium retention. The net effect is to maintain normal serum electrolytes. Mineralocorticoids act on their target tissues by combining with cytosolic receptors. The hormone-receptor complexes then move to the nucleus and increase the transcription of proteins that result in activation of the Na^+- K^+ ATPase pumps and permease in target tissues, eg, the renal tubules. Although aldosterone and DOC have approximately equal affinity for mineralocorticoid receptors, aldosterone, which is less bound to transport proteins, is quantitatively more available. Cortisol also has a mineralocorticoid effect and may bind mineralocorticoid receptors. Cortisol, however, which is usually degraded to inactive cortisone in target tissues, normally does not contribute significantly to the regulation of sodium and potassium balance.

Disorders of Adrenal Cortical Insufficiency

In primary diseases of the adrenal cortex that result in glucocorticoid deficiency, affected patients present with weakness, fatigue, weight loss, anorexia, nausea, or vomiting. If there is chronic insufficiency, hyperpigmentation of the skin and mucous membranes may occur from increased pituitary ACTH and β-lipotropin secretion. The hyperpigmentation is most marked in exposed and pressure areas of the skin. If the adrenocorticoid deficiency is secondary to ACTH deficiency, eg, pituitary or hypothalamic disorders, hyperpigmentation will not be present. Severe hypoglycemia may occur in affected children. In affected adults, hypoglycemia may occur with periods of decreased intake or fasting. Amenorrhea and loss of axillary and pubic hair may be seen in affected females. Vitiligo may occur with autoimmune forms of the disorder. If an associated mineralocorticoid deficiency also occurs, renal salt wasting and potassium retention may lead to hyponatremia, hyperkalemia, acidosis, dehydration, salt craving, hypotension, or abdominal pain. Affected patients are also at risk to develop an acute adrenal crisis with hypovolemic shock at times of infections, trauma, surgery, or dehydration.

Autoimmune Addison Disease: Autoimmune Addison disease is associated with lymphocytic infiltration of the adrenal cortex and adrenal insufficiency. The disorder may occur alone but most often occurs as part of the inherited polyendocrine autoimmune syndromes.

Adrenal insufficiency may be seen with anencephaly and panhypopituitarism.

X-linked Adrenoleukodystrophy: Adrenal insufficiency may be a presenting symptom with X-linked adrenoleukodystrophy, a peroxisomal disorder discussed with the inborn errors of metabolism.

Microdeletion Syndrome on the X Chromosome: Adrenal insufficiency may also occur with a microdeletion syndrome on the X chromosome, which also involves varying combinations of Duchenne muscular dystrophy, glycerol kinase deficiency, and ornithine transcarbamylase deficiency.

Familial Glucocorticoid Deficiency: Adrenocortical unresponsiveness to ACTH results in familial glucocorticoid deficiency. Degenerative changes in the zona fasciculata and zona reticularis are noted that do not include a lymphocytic infiltrate. Affected patients have elevated ACTH levels and decreased adrenocortical glucocorticoid secretion. Mineralocorticoid production may be normal or partially deficient. The onset occurs during childhood with seizures, hypoglycemia, muscle weakness, and hyperpigmentation.

Glucocorticoid Resistance: Glucocorticoid resistance (MIM 138040), a rare autosomal dominant disorder, is associated with the formation of abnormal glucocorticoid receptors in peripheral tissues. Point mutations in the receptor gene have been reported. Elevated ACTH levels result from lack of feedback regulation. Cortisol production is increased but does not lead to clinical signs of Cushing syndrome. Increased ACTH stimulation results in the increased production of DOC and corticosterone, which cause hypertension, hypokalemia, and suppressed production of renin and aldosterone.

Hypoaldosteronism

Primary Congenital Hypoaldosteronism: Primary congenital hypoaldosteronism is a rare, autosomal recessive disorder associated with deficient activity of corticosterone 18-methyl oxidase II, an enzyme involved in the conversion of corticosterone to aldosterone. Low levels of aldosterone and elevated plasma 18-hydroxycorticosterone and urinary tetra-18-hydroxy-11-dehydrocorticosterone are noted. Affected patients have chronic hyperkalemia, hyponatremia, renal salt wasting, and elevated renin levels.

Pseudohypoaldosteronism: Pseudohypoaldosteronism (MIM 264350), a rare autosomal recessive disorder of infancy, is characterized by renal insensitivity to mineralocorticoids that may be a result of abnormal mineralocorticoid receptors. Affected patients have hyponatremia, hyperkalemia, and elevated renin levels. The disorder may also be seen in premature infants and patients with obstructive uropathies.

Hyporeninemic Hypoaldosteronism: Impaired renin release by the kidney, or hyporeninemic hypoaldosteronism, has been reported in patients with sickle cell anemia.

Pseudohyperaldosteronism

Pseudohyperaldosteronism is associated with decreased mineralocorticoid secretion as a result of low or insufficient renin production.

11-β-Hydroxysteroid Dehydrogenase Deficiency: 11-β-Hydroxysteroid dehydrogenase deficiency is characterized by hypertension, hpokalemia, suppressed renal and aldosterone production, but normal cortisol levels during childhood. Reduced conversion of cortisol to inactive cortisone in tissues results in cortisol occupying mineralocorticoid receptors and cortisol-induced apparent mineralocorticoid excess (AME).

Liddle Syndrome: Liddle syndrome (MIM 177200), is a rare, autosomal dominant disorder associated with a generalized increase in activity of Na^+-K^+ ATPase pumps. Affected patients have hypertension, hypokalemia, renal potassium wasting, metabolic alkalosis, and suppressed renin activity and aldosterone production.

Congenital Adrenal Hyperplasias

The congenital adrenal hyperplasias are autosomal recessive disorders associated with defects in adrenal hormone synthesis that result in cortisol deficiency. Chronic ACTH stimulation leads to hyperplasia of the adrenal glands. Cortisol deficiency may manifest as hypoglycemia, a poor response to stress, or an acute adrenal crisis. Depending upon the site of the synthetic block, aldosterone production may also be affected and salt-wasting occur. In some forms of the disorder, hypertension results from elevated levels of adrenal metabolites with potent mineralocorticoid activity. Because some of the enzymes involved are also needed for gonadal sex steroid hormone synthesis, incomplete masculinization and sexual infantilism may occur in males. In other forms, chronic

ACTH stimulation results in increased production of adrenal androgens and androgen precursors, which causes masculinization of female fetuses and hyperandrogenic effects in both males and females. Increased ACTH stimulation may also result in hyperpigmentation.

The fetus will undergo sexual differentiation into a female unless the sex-specific region, including the sex-determining region (SRY), is present on the Y chromosome. The SRY gene produces a "testis determining factor" that results in the differentiation of the primitive gonad into a testis between 43 and 50 days of gestation. Normal male differentiation requires that the Leydig cells of the fetal testis produce testosterone by about 6 to 7 weeks of gestation, and that the Sertoli cells produce anti-Mullerian hormone (AMH) at 8 weeks. AMH results in involution of the Mullerian duct system and allows development of the Wolffian ducts into male internal genitalia. In the absence of AMH, the Mullerian ducts develop into female internal genital organs. Because AMH production is normal in fetuses with congenital adrenal hyperplasia (CAH), the internal structures develop normally in both male and female affected fetuses. The external genitalia in male fetuses with certain forms of CAH will be incompletely masculinized or ambiguous (male pseudohermaphroditism), due to the absence of testosterone production during fetal life. In female fetuses with other forms of CAH, elevated adrenal androgen and androgen precursor levels prior to 12 weeks of gestation results in masculinization of the external female genitalia, which may also be ambiguous (female pseudohermaphroditism). Elevated adrenal androgen levels during fetal life may also cause penile or clitoral enlargement. Continued adrenal androgen elevation after birth results in advanced bone and somatic growth, early closure of the epiphyses and short adult height, early development of pubic and axillary hair, acne, sexual im-

maturity, small testes, and gynecological problems in females. The clinical manifestations vary with the site of the enzymatic defect and the severity of the disorder. Table 12–1 shows the characteristics of the congenital adrenal hyperplasias.

P450$_{c21}$ 21-α-Hydroxylase Deficiency (MIM 201910)

One mild and two severe forms of the disorder are known.

A. Classic, or Salt-Wasting Form: In its severe classic, or salt-wasting form, 21-α-hydroxylase deficiency occurs in approximately 1 in 14,000 live births. Seventy five to eighty percent of patients with severe 21-α-hydroxylase deficiency will present with this form of the disorder. Reduced synthesis of both cortisol and aldosterone result in hypoglycemia, hyponatremia, hyperkalemia, and acidosis, most often during the first 2 weeks of life. Some affected infants who develop an acute adrenal crisis with dehydration and vascular collapse, may die if the disorder is unrecognized. Increased ACTH secretion from lack of cortisol feedback results in elevation of cortisol precursors and their conversion to adrenal androgens. At birth, affected females have varying degrees of virilization and ambiguous external genitalia. Affected males may appear normal or have an enlarged phallus. Untreated cases in both sexes have continued androgen excess after birth, resulting in advanced bone age and growth. Acne, increased muscular development, pubic and axillary hair, and phallic enlargement may occur during childhood. Suppression of the pituitary-gonadal axis may lead to failure of maturation of the testes and sexual immaturity. Affected females may have menstrual irregularities. Due to early epiphyseal closure, patients who are large as children may become short adults. Elevated levels of plasma 17-hydroxyprogesterone, 21-deoxycortisol, androstenedione, testosterone, and renin are noted. Urine pregnanetriol, 11-keto-pregnanetriol, and 17-

Table 12–1. Characteristics of the congenital adrenal hyperplasias.

Enzyme Deficiency	Salt-wasting	Hypertension	Female External Genitalia at Birth	Male External Genitalia at Birth	Post-natal Virilization
1. P450$_{c21}$ 21-α-Hydroxylase					
a. Classic form	Yes	No	Ambiguous	Male	Yes
b. Simple virilizing	No	No	Ambiguous	Male	Yes
c. Late-onset	No	No	Female	Male	Yes
2. P450$_{c11}$ 11-β-Hydroxylase	No	Yes	Ambiguous	Male	Yes
3. P450$_{scc}$ Cholesterol side chain cleavage defect	Yes	No	Female	Female	No
4. 3-β-Hydroxysteroid dehydrogenase/Δ^{4,5}-isomerase	Yes	No	Mild virilization	Ambiguous	Yes
5. P450$_{c17}$ 17-α-Hydroxylase	No	Yes	Female	Female, ambiguous	No

ketosteroids are also elevated. Plasma cortisol and aldosterone levels are low. Measurement of 17-hydroxyprogesterone levels in dried blood filter paper spots may be used for newborn screening; programs are currently available in some states. Treatment includes steroid replacement therapy with glucocorticoids and mineralocorticoids, and additional dietary salt. Acute adrenal crises must be treated vigorously with glucose, electrolytes, fluids and higher glucocorticoid doses. Plastic surgery repair of ambiguous genitalia should be completed prior to one year of age.

B. Simple Virilizing Form: The simple virilizing form of 21-α-hydroxylase deficiency occurs in 1 in 60,000 live births. Approximately 25% of patients with the severe form of 21-α-hydroxylase deficiency present with the simple virilizing form. The disorder is similar to the classical form, except that there is usually sufficient aldosterone production to prevent salt-wasting. Acute neonatal adrenal crises are uncommon; plasma renin levels are normal. Masculinization of females may be less severe than in the classic form.

C. Late Onset, or Asymptomatic "Cryptic" Forms: Milder, non-classical, late onset, or asymptomatic "cryptic" forms of the disorder occur more often than the classic and simple virilizing forms. The late onset form, which is extremely common, is estimated to occur in 1 in 1000 individuals. It is most common in persons of Eastern European Jewish background, where the prevalence is 1 in 27. In Hispanics it occurs in 1 in 53 persons, in Yugoslavs 1 in 63, and in Italians 1 in 333. Females with late onset 21-α-hydroxylase deficiency have normal external genitalia at birth, but develop mild virilization during childhood. Affected females may also have acne, hirsutism, premature pubic and axillary hair, menstrual irregularities, amenorrhea, or polycystic ovarian disease. Males with the late onset form may have acne, premature pubic and axillary hair, premature beard growth, inappropriately small testes, and infertility. Plasma levels of 17-hydroxyprogesterone may be borderline, but become elevated with ACTH stimulation. Patients with the asymptomatic form of the disorder are frequently relatives of patients with late onset forms.

The gene for 21-α-hydroxylase is located on the short arm of chromosome 6 between the HLA-B and HLA-DR loci. HLA-linkage studies have shown that the HLA-A3, Bw47, DR7, and Bw60 have a high degree of association with the salt-losing form; HLA-B51 is associated with the simple virilizing form; and HLA-B14 and DR1 are associated with the non-classical form of the disorder. Two genes, designated P450c21A (or CYP21P) and P450c21B (or CYP21), are associated with 2 loci for C4 (fourth component of complement), C4A and C4B. The respective gene order is C4A-P450c21A-C4B-P450c21B. P450c21A is a pseudogene that does not produce a functional protein; P450c21B encodes for a protein with 21-α-

hydroxylase activity. Exchange of genetic material between the active gene and the pseudogene during meiosis (gene conversion) may result in loss of 21-α-hydroxylase activity. Patients with gene conversions and complete deletion of the P450c21B gene are known, as are patients with point mutations and other molecular defects. Most affected individuals are compound heterozygotes for two different molecular defects. The clinical severity of the disease is roughly correlated to the severity of the mutations involved and the degree of reduction in enzymatic activity. Prenatal diagnosis for 21-α-hydroxylase deficiency has been accomplished by measurement of 17-hydroxyprogesterone levels in amniotic fluid. Chorionic villus sampling may be used for HLA typing or molecular genetic analysis.

P450$_{c11}$ 11-β-Hydroxylase Deficiency (MIM 202010): 11-β-Hydroxylase deficiency, which occurs in 1 in 100,000 live births, is found in 5–8% of cases of CAH. The disorder is most common among persons of Middle Eastern Jewish background. The 11-β-hydroxylase locus is located on the long arm of chromosome 8. Two tandemly duplicated genes of high homology exist. One gene is active in the zona fasciculata and the zona glomerulosa, encodes for 11-β-hydroxylase activity, and catalyses the formation of corticosterone and cortisol from deoxycorticosterone and 11-deoxycortisol. The other gene, also known as aldosterone synthase (P450$_{aldo}$), is active in the zona glomerulosa, encodes for 18-hydroxylation and 18-oxidative activity in addition to 11-hydroxylase activity, and catalyzes the formation of aldosterone from deoxycorticosterone. The 18-hydroxylase activity of P450$_{aldo}$ is also known as corticosterone methyl oxidase I (CMO I); the 18-oxidase activity (18-dehydrogenase) of P450$_{aldo}$ is also termed CMO II. The classic form of the disorder is associated with elevated plasma 11-deoxycorticosterone (11-DOC), 11-deoxycortisol, and adrenal androgens. Elevated urine metabolites of these compounds, eg, tetrahydro-11-deoxycortisol, may be noted with or without ACTH stimulation testing. Plasma renin is decreased. Virilization of affected female infants occurs secondary to increased fetal adrenal androgen production. Clinical signs of continued elevation of adrenal androgens after birth may be seen in both affected males and females. Hypertension, which distinguishes this disease from 21-β-hydroxylase deficiency, results from elevated 11-DOC or its metabolites. Hypertension may not be noted until late childhood or adolescence. Marked variability in hormonal and clinical findings results in mild, late onset, and asymptomatic forms of the disorder. Salt-wasting has been noted in young patients who have mutations involving P450$_{aldo}$, both of the P450$_{c11}$ genes, or with isolated CMO II deficiency.

P450$_{scc}$ Cholesterol Side Chain Cleavage Defect (Cholesterol Desmolase Deficiency) (MIM 201710): P450$_{scc}$ (desmolase), the first step in the biosynthesis of adrenal and gonadal steroid hormones, catalyzes the conversion of cholesterol to pregnenolone. Deficient activity of P450$_{scc}$ is a rare disorder that results in severe deficiency of cortisol, aldosterone, and gonadal hormones. Markedly elevated plasma ACTH levels lead to large, lipid-laden adrenals that may displace the kidney. Most affected patients present in the neonatal period with failure to thrive, vomiting, dehydration, hyponatremia, and hyperkalemia. Two-thirds die in early infancy. Affected male neonates have female or ambiguous genitalia; affected females have normal external genitalia. The gene for P450$_{scc}$, located on chromosome 15, has been cloned.

3-β-Hydroxysteroid Dehydrogenase and Δ^{4,5}-Isomerase Deficiency (MIM 201810):

3-β-Hydroxysteroid dehydrogenase and Δ^{4,5}-isomerase deficiency is the only one of the congenital adrenal hyperplasias that is not associated with deficiency of a P450 enzyme. The affected enzyme catalyzes both the dehydrogenation and isomerization of 3-β-hydroxy-Δ^5-steroids to 3-keto-Δ^4-steroids in the adrenals and gonads. At the chromosome locus on the short arm of chromosome 1, two highly homologous genes exist. One gene is expressed in the adrenals and gonads, while the other is expressed in the placenta and peripheral tissues. Deficient activity of 3-β-hydroxysteroid dehydrogenase/Δ^{4,5}-isomerase results in severe deficiencies of aldosterone, cortisol, testosterone, and estradiol. Salt wasting and adrenal crises may occur in the neonatal period. Affected males are incompletely masculinized or have ambiguous genitalia at birth. Females may have clitoral enlargement from elevated dehydroepiandrosterone (DHEA) levels or conversion of DHEA into testosterone in other tissues. Elevated plasma levels of pregnenolone, 17-hydroxypregnenolone, DHEA, and DHEA-sulfate occur. Urinary pregnenetriol, 16-pregnenetriol, and the ratio of Δ^5 to Δ^4 steroids are elevated. A milder form, which is not associated with salt-wasting or adrenal crises, presents in females with premature pubic hair, hirsuitism, or oligomenorrhea. Late onset forms are also known.

P450$_{c17}$ 17-α-Hydroxylase Deficiency (MIM 202110):

The gene for P450$_{c17}$, located on chromosome 10, encodes for both 17-α-hydroxylation and 17,20 lyase activities in the adrenal gland and the gonads. The combined deficiency of both enzymes is the most common form of the disorder, which occurs in 1 in 50,000 live births. Isolated deficiencies of either 17-α-hydroxylase or 17,20 lyase are also known. Affected patients with deficiency of both enzymes have reduced synthesis of cortisol and sex steroid hormones. Most patients present in adolescence with sexual infantilism and hypertension. Elevated plasma levels of DOC and corticosterone result in hypertension, hypokalemia, and alkalosis. Secondary suppression of renin and aldosterone secretion occurs. Because levels of the weak glucocorticoid corticos-

terone are elevated, clinical signs of cortisol deficiency do not usually occur. Affected male neonates have female or ambiguous external genitalia; females are normal. In both sexes, impaired androgen and estrogen production results in sexual immaturity after birth. Plasma levels of progesterone, pregnenolone, corticosterone, and DOC are elevated, as are the urinary metabolites of these compounds.

P450$_{arom}$ Aromatase Deficiency:

Deficiency of P450$_{arom}$ results in decreased estrogen production and virilization of the female fetus. If it occurs in the placenta, the deficiency may also lead to virilization of the mother as well as the fetus during pregnancy.

Disorders of the Adrenal Medulla

Synthesis of the catecholamines epinephrine and norepinephrine from tyrosine by the adrenal medullary chromaffin cells is regulated by the sympathetic nervous system. Pheochromocytomas are rare catecholamine-producing tumors which are usually derived from chromaffin cells. In addition to epinephrine and norepinephrine, the tumors may also secrete other bioactive peptides.

Familial Pheochromocytoma: Familial pheochromocytoma (MIM 171300) may occur as an isolated, autosomal dominant trait or with the multiple endocrine neoplasia (MEN) syndromes type 2A and 2B.

GENETIC DISORDERS OF SEX STEROID HORMONE METABOLISM

Male Pseudohermaphroditism: Male pseudohermaphroditism results from deficient testosterone secretion or response during fetal life. Affected males have testes, but the external genitalia are not masculinized. The disorder can result from testicular aplasia or hypoplasia, unresponsiveness of the fetal Leydig cells to placental human chorionic gonadotropin or fetal pituitary leutinizing hormone, impaired biosynthesis of testosterone, or defects in testosterone recognition at target tissues.

Some of the defects involved in impaired biosynthesis of testosterone are discussed with the congenital adrenal hyperplasias. Deficient testosterone biosynthesis can occur with **isolated P450$_{c17}$ 17,20 lyase deficiency,** which results in a deficiency of testosterone and estradiol precursors. Affected male neonates have female or ambiguous external genitalia. Affected females have sexual infantilism. Similar clinical findings can occur with **deficient activity of 17-hydroxysteroid oxidoreductase (dehydrogenase).** Both of these biochemical steps are shown in Figure 12–1.

Both testosterone and dihydrotestosterone (DHT) bind with nuclear androgen receptors in their target tissues, which results in the transcription of proteins that produce androgenic effects. For testosterone to have certain biological actions, it must first be converted to DHT by 5-α-reductase in the cells of the target tissues. Testosterone regulates the secretion of leutinizing hormone and results in virilization of the Wolffian ducts during fetal life. DHT causes development of the external male genitalia and prostate during fetal life as well as male secondary sexual characteristics at puberty.

Deficient Activity of 5-α-Reductase: Deficient activity of 5-α-reductase (MIM 264500) results in incomplete masculinization of the urogenital sinus and external male genitalia during fetal life. A characteristic pattern of abnormalities known as **pseudo-vaginal perineoscrotal hypospadias syndrome** are noted at birth. The disorder is inherited on an autosomal recessive basis; the gene is located on chromosome 2. Most affected males are compound heterozygotes for two different molecular mutations.

Testicular Feminization: Defects involving the androgen receptors of androgen-dependent target tissues (androgen resistance) result in testicular feminization (MIM 313700). During fetal life, the Wolffian ducts do not differentiate properly into internal male genitalia, and the external male genitalia are not masculinized. Because there is secretion of anti-Mullerian hormone, female internal genital development is suppressed. The "complete" testicular feminization phenotype is characterized by males with a 46,XY karyotype, female external genitalia, and bilateral testes that may occur in the abdomen, inguinal canal, or labia. Affected males have absent or rudimentary female and male internal genital structures. Female secondary sexual characteristics develop at puberty from increased production of estradiol from testosterone. However, menses do not occur and pubic and axillary hair are scant or absent. The gene for the androgen receptors has been localized to chromosome Xq11–q13; the disorder is inherited as an X-linked recessive trait. Molecular defects may result in failure of formation of the receptors, unstable receptors, receptors with impaired binding, or post-receptor binding defects. **Incomplete forms** of the disorder, including **Reifenstein syndrome** (MIM 312300), are associated with varying degrees of testicular feminization and infertility.

GENETIC DISORDERS OF THE PANCREAS AND INSULIN

Embryonic Defects

During the fourth week of fetal life the dorsal and ventral pancreatic buds develop from endothelial cells of the primitive foregut, in the area that will become the proximal duodenum. The buds later fuse to form the definitive pancreas. The islet cells also develop from these endothelial cells; insulin and glucagon secretion starts at about 20 weeks.

Annular Pancreas: An annular pancreas, which may result from improper fusion of the pancreatic buds, can cause obstruction of the second part of the duodenum in the neonatal period.

Accessory Pancreas: An accessory pancreas may occur on the wall of the stomach or duodenum or in a Meckel diverticulum.

Congenital Absence of the Pancreas or Islet Cells: Only very rarely does congenital absence or hypoplasia of the pancreas or congenital absence of the islet cells occur.

Insulin Resistance

Insulin is produced and secreted by the B cells of the pancreas. The human insulin gene is located on the short arm of chromosome 11. Pre-proinsulin is transformed by microsomal enzymes into proinsulin (86 amino acids), which is subsequently divided to form insulin (51 amino acids) and C-peptide (31 amino acids). Insulin receptors are present in most tissues. Insulin binding to receptors in fatty tissues, the liver, and muscles is associated with biological responses that promote growth and result in utilization of substrates for fuel. Genetic defects in insulin receptors or in post-receptor processes result in insulin resistance and glucose intolerance, or in clinical diabetes. Most insulin resistance syndromes also have associated acanthosis nigricans and hyperandrogenism.

Type A Syndrome of Insulin Resistance: Type A syndrome of insulin resistance (MIM 243090) is a heterogeneous group of disorders associated with extreme insulin resistance, acanthosis nigricans, and hyperandrogenism. Lipoatrophy or obesity are not noted. The disorder is associated with mutations in the insulin receptor gene that result in a decreased number of receptors or the synthesis of abnormal receptors that affect receptor binding or post-receptor functioning. The inheritance pattern is unclear but may be autosomal dominant.

Leprechaunism: Leprechaunism (MIM 246200), an autosomal recessive disorder, is also associated with mutations in the insulin receptor gene. Patients have intrauterine and postnatal growth retardation, an abnormal "leprechaun" facies, paradoxical fasting hypoglycemia, hyperplasia of the islet cells, hyperinsulinemia, decreased adipose tissue (lipoatrophy), mild hirsutism, and hyperandrogenism. Most affected infants do not live past 2 years of age. In some patients, responses to IGF-1, EGF and other growth factors are also decreased. The reason for the dysmorphic phenotype and severity, compared to type A insulin resistance, is unknown.

Lipoatrophic Diabetes (Seip-Berardinelli Syndrome): Lipoatrophic diabetes (Seip-Berardinelli syndrome) (MIM 269700), an autosomal recessive disorder, is associated with insulin resistance, glucose intolerance, atrophy of subcutaneous fat, hypertriglyceridemia, hepatomegaly, acanthosis nigricans, and hyperandrogenism. The **Brunzell type** of lipoatrophic diabetes also has associated cystic angiomatosis of the soft tissues and bones. The defect for these disorders is unknown.

Diabetes Mellitus, Type I

Ten to twenty percent of diabetes in North America and Europe have type I diabetes mellitus, or insulin-dependent diabetes mellitus (IDDM). The disorder most often occurs in children and young adults. Untreated IDDM is associated with severe glucose intolerance and ketosis. Affected patients have essentially no circulating insulin and require the administration of exogenous insulin for control of their disease. In the United States, IDDM occurs in about 0.26% of Caucasians under the age of 20 years. It is less common in persons of Asian or African-American background. Family studies have shown that a familial tendency exists, but it is less than that seen with type II or non-insulin dependent diabetes (NIDDM). For IDDM, the concordance rate for monozygous twins is less than 50%, which suggests that factors in addition to genetics are involved with the etiology of the disease.

Type I diabetes is associated with an increased incidence of specific HLA haplotypes that vary according to ethnic background. In Caucasians, HLA-DR3 and HLA-DR4 haplotypes, or both, are noted in 95% of IDDM patients, which is a higher frequency than that noted in the non-diabetic population. Certain HLA-DQ haplotypes are associated with an increased risk for development of the disorder; other haplotypes are associated with a decreased risk. Seventy to ninety percent of IDDM patients with HLA-DR4 also have HLA-DQw3.2 (DQw8 by recent nomenclature). HLA-DQw3.1 (DQw7) appears to be protective.

Autoimmune destruction of pancreatic B cells from circulating antibodies to islet cells is thought to play a major role in development of the disease. IDDM patients with HLA-DR3 are more likely to have pancreatic islet cell antibodies; patients with HLA-DR4 are more likely to have antibodies to insulin. Thus, although the disease is not classically inherited, the susceptibility to develop the disease may be. Pancreatic islet cell antibodies are noted in 60–85% of patients with IDDM. Thirty to sixty percent also have antibodies to insulin prior to therapy. These antibodies may also be found in IDDM patients prior to the onset of clinical disease. The autoimmune process may be initiated by environmental factors such as toxins or infectious agents. Most pancreatic islet cell antibodies appear to be directed against glutamic acid decarboxylase (GAD), which is located in pancreatic B cells. Coxsackie B_4 virus contains a sequence of 24 amino acids that has considerable homology to GAD; bovine serum albumin has a region of homology with a pancreatic B cell surface protein, p69. This "molecular mimicry" may be a reason that the immune system also targets the pancreatic B cells when it responds to an environmental agent. IDDM patients show infiltration of both helper and cytotoxic T lymphocytes in the pancreatic islet cells at the onset of their disease. The concept of autoimmune destruction of pancreatic B cells is also supported by the fact that immune suppression therapy may delay the progression to insulin dependency in some newly diagnosed patients with IDDM. Patients with type I diabetes have an increased incidence of other autoimmune endocrine disorders, including polyendocrine autoimmune syndrome type I.

The risks for the development of IDDM in family members of affected patients is higher than that for the general population. Siblings have a 5–10% risk and monozygous twins a 33% risk to develop the disease. The risks for children of an affected parent are higher if the father has IDDM (4–6%) than if the mother has IDDM (2–3%). HLA typing of at-risk family members may help to further define their risks.

Diabetes Mellitus, Type II

Type II diabetes mellitus, or non-insulin dependent diabetes mellitus (NIDDM), is a common disease that occurs predominately over the age of 40. In contrast to type I insulin-dependent diabetes mellitus, which has an autoimmune basis, type II is more likely to be associated with genetic factors. Type II diabetes mellitus is also not linked to specific HLA haplotypes as is type I diabetes mellitus. Although the exact mode of inheritance is unknown, the concordance rate for monozygous twins is 45–96% for clinical disease, and for older monozygous twins approaches 100% for glucose intolerance. The concordance rate for dizygous twins for clinical disease is much lower, at 3–37%. Other primary relatives have a 10–15% risk to develop clinical diabetes mellitus, and a 20–30% risk for abnormal glucose intolerance. Children of affected patients have a 33% risk to develop the disorder.

Maturity-onset Diabetes of the Young, MODY: Maturity-onset diabetes of the young, MODY (MIM 12585), an autosomal dominant condition, is characterized by mild hyperglycemia in older children or young adults. Some patients have mutations in the glucokinase gene, located on chromosome 7. Glucokinase is critical in determining the threshold of plasma glucose at which the pancreatic B cells secrete insulin. In other families, the disorder has been linked to chromosome 20. Another **atypical form of early onset NIDDM,** inherited as an autosomal dominant trait, occurs in African Americans; acute insulin dependency is followed by a period of non-insulin dependence. Other cases of early onset, familial, type II diabetes mellitus may result from the inheritance from both parents of two diabetogenic genes for late-onset diabetes mellitus.

Mutations in the Insulin Gene: Mutations in the insulin gene, located on the short arm of chromosome 11 (MIM 176730), may or may not be associated with glucose intolerance or clinical disease. The mutations may result in decreased synthesis of insulin, decreased processing and persistence of proinsulin, or decreased insulin receptor binding. Mutations in the insulin receptor gene are discussed with insulin resistance.

Diabetic Progeny

Diabetic progeny have an increased risk for congenital malformations, which is related to the degree of control of maternal diabetes during the pregnancy. The overall risk for major congenital malformations in diabetic pregnancies is 6%; the risk may be over 20% if there is poor control during the first trimester. Mothers with insulin-dependent diabetes mellitus have the highest risk; those with non-insulin dependent diabetes have an intermediate risk; women with gestational diabetes have a lower risk for malformations in their offspring. Malformations most often involve the renal, cardiovascular and central nervous systems. Table 12–2 lists the malformations that have been reported in diabetic pregnancies. There is an 8% risk for transposition of the great vessels. In addition, 16% of cases of the caudal regression syndrome are associated with maternal diabetes during pregnancy.

Caudal Regression Syndrome: Caudal regression syndrome (MIM 182940) is associated with variable degrees of incomplete development of the sacrum and lumbar vertebrae; agenesis of the body of the sacrum; extreme lack of growth in the caudal region; disruption of the distal spinal cord with associated neurological impairment of the legs and bowel and bladder control; flexion contractures of the hips and knees; and deformities of the feet. Renal agenesis, imperforate anus, myelomeningocoele, cleft lip, cleft palate, and microcephaly also occur.

Femoral Hypoplasia–Unusual Facies Syndrome: Femoral hypoplasia–unusual facies syndrome (MIM 134780), a sporadic disorder, is also seen more frequently in diabetic progeny. The syndrome has some features in common with caudal regression syndrome including dysplastic sacrum, vertebral anomalies, bony abnormalities of the pelvis, and hypoplasia or absent femurs and fibulae. Unusual facial features include a short nose with hypoplastic alae nasi, long philtrum, thin upper lip, micrognathia, and upward slanting palpebral fissures. Cleft palate, hypoplasia of the humeri, scoliosis, inguinal hernias, small external genitalia, polycystic or absent kidneys, and an abnormal urinary collecting system occasionally occur. Short stature results from shortening of the legs.

Genetic counseling prior to conception and prenatal monitoring should be offered to women with diabetes of any type.

Nesidioblastosis

Nesidioblastosis, or hyperplasia of pancreatic B cells, results in neonatal hyperinsulinemia and hypoglycemia. The condition commonly occurs in infants of diabetic mothers.

Familial Nesidioblastosis: Familial nesidioblastosis may occur as an autosomal recessive disorder (MIM 256450), or in association with Beckwith (Beckwith-Wiedemann) syndrome (MIM 130650).

POLYENDOCRINE (GLANDULAR) AUTOIMMUNE SYNDROMES

The polyendocrine or polyglandular autoimmune syndromes consist of varying combinations of diseases that are of autoimmune etiology. Non-autoimmune diseases may also be associated. Table 12–3 lists the disorders that occur in type I and type II polyendocrine syndrome.

Type I Polyendocrine Syndrome: Type I polyendocrine syndrome (MIM 240300), which has

Table 12–2. Malformations reported with diabetic pregnancies.

Site	Malformation
Brain/central nervous system	Anencephaly Hydrocephalus Myelomeningocoele
Heart	Transposition of the great vessels Ventricular septal defect Atrial septal defect
Body cavity/viscera	Situs inversus
Kidney/ureter	Renal agenesis Cystic kidney Duplicated ureters
Pelvis/legs	Caudal regression syndrome Femoral hypoplasia-unusual facies syndrome
Anus	Anal/rectal atresia

Table 12–3. Type I and type II polyendocrine autoimmune syndromes and associated disorders.

Syndrome	Characteristics	Commonly Associated Disorders	Less Commonly Associated Disorders
Type I	Onset in infancy and childhood Autosomal recessive No HLA association	Adrenal insufficiency Mucocutaneous candidiasis Hypoparathyroidism Alopecia Malabsorption Chronic active hepatitis Pernicious anemia Primary hypogonadism Primary hypothyroidism	Vitiligo Primary hyperthyroidism (Graves disease) Keratoconjunctivitis Hypophysitis Insulin-dependent diabetes mellitus
Type II	Onset in adults Autosomal dominant HLA-B8, HLA-DR3 associated	Primary hyperthyroidism (Graves disease) Atrophic thyroiditis Insulin-dependent diabetes mellitus Adrenal insufficiency (Addison disease) Celiac disease Myasthenia gravis Primary hypogonadism	Hypoparathyroidism, geriatric type Goitrous thyroiditis Pernicious anemia Vitiligo Alopecia Hypophysitis Serositis Parkinson disease

its onset in infancy or childhood, is inherited on an autosomal recessive basis with no HLA association. Mucocutaneous candidiasis and hypoparathyroidism are usually noted in early infancy; adrenal insufficiency later develops.

Type II Polyendocrine (Schmidt) Syndrome: Type II polyendocrine (Schmidt) syndrome (MIM 269200), which occurs in middle-aged adults, is an autosomal dominant disorder with variable clinical presentation; the disorder is associated with HLA-B8 and HLA-DR3 haplotypes. Type II polyendocrine syndrome has also been associated with Sjogren syndrome, selective immunoglobulin A deficiency, juvenile dermatomyositis, systemic lupus erythematous, chronic active hepatitis, and dermatitis herpetiformis. Because of variable clinical presentation, siblings of affected patients with type I polyendocrine syndrome, and first-degree relatives of patients with type II, should be evaluated for the respective disorder.

MULTIPLE ENDOCRINE NEOPLASIA (MEN) SYNDROMES

Multiple Endocrine Neoplasia (MEN) Syndromes: Multiple endocrine neoplasia (MEN) syndromes are autosomal dominant disorders associated with the development of endocrine tumors. The tumors, which produce polypeptide or biogenic amines, are composed of cell types derived from embryonic neuroectoderm. These cell types are also known as amine precursor uptake and decarboxylation cells, or APUD cells. The tumors, frequently multicentric in origin, initially are characterized by hyperplasia that may progress to an adenoma or carcinoma, depending on the cell type involved. Three forms of the disorder, MEN-1, MEN-2A and MEN-2B, are currently recognized, which differ according to the combination and type of tumors involved. Type MEN-1 patients also may have lipomas; type MEN-2B patients have characteristic mucosal neuromas which are not APUD cell type. Although the index cases in families most often present during adulthood, MEN-2A and MEN-2B may be seen in early childhood. The disorders are highly penetrant but vary in expression. MEN-1 has been mapped to chromosome 11q13. Studies of tumors from MEN-1 patients show loss of the chromosome 11 allele inherited from the normal parent; this suggests that the disease most probably results from deletion of a regulatory gene involved with tumor suppression. MEN-2A and MEN-2B are associated with mutations in the RET proto-oncogene, located at chromosome 10q11.2. Primary family members should be evaluated and monitored closely, especially those at-risk for MEN-1 and MEN-2A in which the new mutation rate is low. Children of affected parents with all types of MEN have a 50% chance to develop the disorder. Presymptomatic at-risk family members may be diagnosed as gene carriers by using linkage studies in MEN-1 and by molecular genetic techniques in MEN-2A or 2B, eg, RFLP or direct mutational analysis. Table 12–4 lists the characteristics of the MEN syndromes and the recommendations for monitoring at-risk family members.

Multiple Endocrine Neoplasia Syndrome Type 1 (MEN-1): Multiple endocrine neoplasia syndrome

Table 12–4. Characteristics of multiple endocrine neoplasia (MEN) syndromes.

Characteristic	MEN-1	MEN-2A	MEN-2B
Chromosomal location (Gene)	11q13 (MEM1)	10q11.2 (RET proto-oncogene)	10q11.2 (RET proto-oncogene)
Inheritance pattern	Autosomal dominant	Autosomal dominant	Autosomal dominant
New mutation rate	Low	Low	High
Associated hyperplasia or neoplasia	Parathyroid hyperplasia or adenoma Pancreatic islet cell Pituitary Carcinoid tumors Adrenocortical adenomas	Medullary thyroid carcinoma Pheochromocytoma Parathyroid hyperplasia or adenoma	Medullary thyroid carcinoma Pheochromocytoma Multiple mucosal neuromas
Other associated clinical features	Lipomas, subcutaneous or visceral	Cutaneous lichen amyloidosis	Marfanoid habitus
Recommended testing for at-risk family member	Genetic: Family linkage studies Endocrine: Ionized serum calcium Serum prolactin	Genetic: RFLP or direct mutation analysis Endocrine: Pentagastrin test with serum calcitonin measurements Timed urine for epinephrine & norepinephrine Ionized serum calcium	Genetic: RFLP or direct mutation analysis Endocrine: Pentagastrin test with serum calcitonin measurements Timed urine for epinephrine & norepinephrine
Recommended endocrine testing after gene carrier status established	Above plus: Serum gastrin Imaging of pituitary	As above Consider total thyroidectomy	As above Consider total thyroidectomy

type 1 (MEN-1; MIM 13110), previously known as Wermer syndrome, consists of familial cases of parathyroid, pancreatic islet cell, and pituitary hyperplasia or neoplasia. Index cases most often present between 20 and 30 years of age. Approximately 60% of patients will develop two tumors; 20% will develop three or more.

Hyperparathyroidism, the most common finding, noted in 80–88% of patients, may be detected as early as 17 years of age. Multicentric, hyperplasia of the parathyroid glands occurs, which can progress to adenoma formation.

Pancreatic islet cell tumors, found in 75–81% of patients with MEN-1, are multicentric and may become malignant and metastasize. Serum concentrations of gastrin, pancreatic polypeptide, glucagon, insulin, C-peptide, somatostatin, and calcitonin may be elevated. Gastrinomas, or gastrin secreting tumors, comprise 50–60% of the pancreatic islet cell tumors; insulinomas comprise 25–35%; glucagonomas are less common. Excess gastrin production may cause peptic ulcers and the Zollinger-Ellison syndrome. A "watery diarrhea syndrome" associated with elevated levels of vasoactive intestinal polypeptide (VIP) may also occur.

Pituitary adenomas are noted in 50–65% of patients with MEN-1. Prolactinomas are the most com-

mon form, which are associated with galactorrhea and amenorrhea. Non-functioning chromophobe adenomas are also common. Fifteen to twenty five percent of pituitary adenomas in MEN-1 are eosinophilic growth hormone producing tumors which result in acromegaly. Acromegaly may also result from the production of growth hormone releasing hormone by pancreatic islet cell or other endocrine tumors. Very infrequently, Cushing syndrome may result from excess corticotropin (ACTH) production by a basophilic pituitary tumor or a carcinoid tumor. Cushing syndrome may also result from ectopic production of corticotropin-releasing hormone.

Tumors of mixed cell type are known. **Carcinoid tumors,** uncommon in the MEN syndromes, occur more often with MEN-1 than with MEN-2. Carcinoid tumors most often arise from the thymus, but also can occur in the lung, stomach, or duodenum. They are often asymptomatic, but may produce serotonin, calcitonin or corticotropin; approximately 50% are locally invasive or metastatic. Adrenocortical adenomas have also been reported. Occasionally subcutaneous or visceral lipomas are noted in patients with MEN-1.

Multiple Endocrine Neoplasia Syndrome Type 2A (MEN-2A, Sipple Syndrome): Multiple endocrine neoplasia syndrome type 2A (MEN-2A,

Sipple syndrome; MIM 171400) is associated with medullary thyroid carcinoma, unilateral or bilateral pheochromocytoma, and parathyroid hyperplasia or adenomatosis. The mean age of diagnosis for index cases is 33 years of age. Because of family counseling and monitoring, the average age for diagnosis in affected family members is younger, between 7–13 years of age. Most patients (97%) with MEN-2A present with thyroid C-cell hyperplasia. The multicentric hyperplasia may progress to nodular hyperplasia and **medullary thyroid carcinoma** which can metastasize. There are increased serum levels of calcitonin, calcitonin-related peptide, somatostatin, dihydroxyphenylalanine decarboxylase, and chromogranin-A. Because C-cell hyperplasia has been noted as early as 20 months of age, and medullary thyroid carcinoma as early as 3 years, monitoring and genetic evaluation of at-risk relatives should start at age 1–2 years. In that there is a greater than 90% risk that a gene carrier will develop medullary thyroid carcinoma, total thyroidectomy should be considered in an individual found to be a gene carrier for MEN-2A.

Pheochromocytoma occurs in 30–50% of patients, which may be single or multiple, unilateral or bilateral. Only very rarely does adrenomedullary carcinoma occur. Patients are frequently symptomatic from the increased production of catecholamines.

Hyperparathyroidism, which occurs in 10–50% of patients, is similar to that seen in patients with MEN-1. **Cutaneous lichen amyloidosis,** occasionally reported with MEN-2A, consists of multiple, pruritic, infiltrative papules overlying a well-demarcated plaque that occurs in the scapular area of the upper back.

Multiple Endocrine Neoplasia Syndrome Type 2B (MEN-2B): Multiple endocrine neoplasia syndrome type 2B (MEN-2B; MIM 162300), also known as MEN-3 in other classifications, is characterized by the combination of medullary thyroid carcinoma, pheochromocytomas, and multiple mucosal neuromas. MEN-2B patients have characteristic **mucosal neuromas** which occur on the tongue, lips, buccal mucosa, eyelids, subconjuctival areas, and throughout the gastrointestinal tract. Hypertrophied corneal nerves may be seen on slit-lamp examination. Ganglioneuromatosis of the gastrointestinal tract can result in swallowing problems, constipation, megacolon, or colic-like illnesses with diarrhea. The presence of mucosal neuromas should alert the physician to MEN-2B and the risk of medullary thyroid carcinoma. Ninety percent of patients have bilateral, multicentric C-cell hyperplasia; **medullary thyroid carcinoma** may occur, which has an earlier onset and is more aggressive than that seen with MEN-2A. Because the thyroid carcinoma may metastasize prior to 1 year of age, monitoring of at-risk family members should start at birth. As with MEN-2A, total thyroidectomy should be considered in individuals found to be gene carriers for MEN-2B. Occasionally medullary thyroid carcinoma will occur in an affected family member as an isolated finding without the other associated problems.

Unilateral or bilateral **pheochromocytomas** occur in 45–50% of patients. Sixty-five percent of affected patients have a **marfanoid habitus** with a tall, thin body build and long, thin extremities. Lax joints, pectus excavatum, pectus carinatum, and a high-arched palate are frequently noted; dislocated lens do not occur.

REFERENCES AND SUGGESTED READING

Emery AE, Rimoin AL, editors, *Principles and Practice of Medical Genetics,* 2nd ed, Churchill Livingstone, 1990.

Greenspan FS, Baxter JD, *Basic and Clinical Endocrinology,* 4th ed, Appleton & Lange, 1994.

King RA, Rotter JI, Motulski AG, editors, *The Genetic Basis of Common Diseases,* Oxford University Press, 1992.

Mahoney CP, ed, Current Issues in Pediatric and Adolescent Endocrinology, Ped Clin of N America, December 1990, 37:1229.

Scriver CR, Beaudet AL, Sly WS and Valle D, *The Metabolic Basis of Inherited Disease,* 6th ed, McGraw-Hill, 1989

Wilson JD and Foster DW, *Williams Textbook of Endocrinology,* 8th ed, WB Saunders, 1992.

SECTION III.
Inborn Errors of Metabolism

Amino Acid & Organic Acid Metabolism

13

INTRODUCTION TO INBORN ERRORS OF METABOLISM

Inborn errors of metabolism are genetically determined disorders that affect the biochemical pathways in the body. They may result from deficient activity of essential enzymes, deficiencies of cofactors or activators for the enzymes, or faulty transport of compounds. The clinical findings are usually related to the type and toxicity of the metabolites that accumulate or to deficiencies of products of the biochemical reactions that are impaired. Defects occur in the cytosol of cells as well as in organelles such as mitochondria, lysosomes, and peroxisomes. The disorders may result from mutations in the nuclear or mitochondrial DNA. Often, the genetic mutation will correspond to the clinical phenotype. Although DNA analysis may be used to establish the diagnosis of some of the disorders, not all patients will have a previously recognized mutation. In some families, a distinctive pattern of restriction fragment length polymorphisms (RFLP) is present at the genetic locus for the disorder; this RFLP pattern can be used for carrier or prenatal testing (informative family). Although the majority of inborn errors of metabolism are inherited as autosomal recessive traits, some of the disorders are inherited as X-linked traits, while others are associated with maternal (mitochondrial) patterns of inheritance. For family counseling and carrier and prenatal testing, an accurate diagnosis, with either enzymatic or DNA confirmation of the disorder, is usually needed.

With certain exceptions, inborn errors of metabolism have been classically considered disorders of children. However, delayed or milder presentation during late teenage or adult life can occur for almost all of the disorders. If the pattern of clinical and laboratory findings suggests a certain disorder, the age of the patient should not exclude the disorder from being included in the differential diagnosis. Adults are being increasingly recognized to have hyperammonemia from urea cycle defects, severe acidosis from or-

ganic acidemias, and central nervous system degeneration from lysosomal storage disorders or defects in mitochondrial oxidative phosphorylation.

Newborn screening for phenylketonuria occurs in all states. Screening for homocystinuria, maple syrup urine disease, galactosemia, and biotinidase deficiency routinely occurs in some areas of the United States. Pilot newborn screening programs are being conducted for other inborn errors of metabolism. Clinicians should be aware of which disorders are included in the newborn screening programs in their location and the fact that not all cases of these diseases will be detected by newborn screening, especially homocystinuria. Any child suspected of having one of the disorders on the basis of clinical findings should receive an evaluation for the disorder even if newborn screening for the disorder has been done.

This section is written to provide a basic understanding of the inborn errors of metabolism. The reader is encouraged to consult with a person experienced in clinical biochemical genetics for additional assistance in the evaluation and treatment of a patient. The disorders have been classically grouped as to the type of compounds involved, eg, amino acids or organic acids, or the subcellular location of the abnormality, eg, peroxisomal disorders. Table 13–1 gives the clinical features of the major types of inborn errors of metabolism.

DISORDERS OF AMINO ACIDS AND ORGANIC ACIDS

Disorders of amino acids and their metabolites, organic acids, have widely varying clinical presentations. Some of the disorders are associated with acute episodes of severe metabolic acidosis, eg, methylmalonic acidemia, while others, eg, phenylketonuria, result in progressive mental retardation. Distinctive odors, which occur from the accumulation of abnormal organic acids in some of the patients (eg, "sweaty feet" with isovaleric acidemia) are shown in

Table 13–1. Clinical Findings in Inborn Errors of Metabolism

Clinical Manifestations Laboratory Findings	General Type of Disorder to Consider								
	A	B	C	D	E	F	G	H	I
Episodic nature	++	++	++	++	+	+	–	–	–
Poor feeding	++	+	++	+	+	+	+	–	–
Abnormal odor	+	+	–	+	–	–	–	–	–
Lethargy, coma	+	+	+	+	+	+	–	–	–
Seizures	+	+	+	–	+	+	+	–	+
Developmental regression	+	+	+	–	+	–	+	++	+
Hepatomegaly	+	+	+	+	+	+	+	+	+
Hepatosplenomegaly	–	–	–	–	–	–	–	+	+
Splenomegaly	–	–	–	–	–	–	–	–	+
Hypotonia	+	+	+	+	+	+	+	–	+
Cardiomyopathy	–	+	–	+	+	+	–	+	–
Coarse facies	–	–	–	–	–	–	–	++	–
Birth defects	–	+	–	–	+	–	+	–	–
Hypoglycemia	+	+	–	+	+	+	–	–	–
Acidosis	+	++	–	+	+	+	–	–	–
Hyperammonemia	+	+	++	+	+	–	–	–	–
Ketosis	+	+	+	–	–	+	–	–	–
Hypoketosis	–	–	–	+	–	–	–	–	–

Abbreviations: A = amino acidopathies; B = organic acidopathies; C = urea cycle defects; D = fatty acid oxidation defects; E = mitochondrial disorders; F = carbohydrate disorders; G = peroxisomal disorders; H = mucopolysaccharidoses; I = spingolipidoses; ++ = usually present; + = may be present; – = usually not present. (Reproduced, with permission from Wappner RS, Biochemical Diagnosis of Genetic Diseases, *Pediatric Annals* 1993:**22**:283)

Table 13–2. Some of the disorders may be detected by newborn screening programs. Spot screening tests may be done on random urine samples and include the ferric chloride test (detects oxoacids, also known as ketoacids), dinitrophenylhydrazine test (oxoacids), nitrosonaphthol (tyrosine metabolites), sodium cyanide-nitroprusside or silver nitroprusside test (sulfhydryls), and a sulfite paper strip test. Urine spot screening tests, however, may produce either false-positive or false-negative results. All screening tests should be followed by additional testing with quantitative determinations of metabolites and enzymatic assays, when available, to confirm the presumed or suspected disorder. Quantitative determination of plasma and urine amino acid levels is done by ion-exchange chromatography or occasionally by high performance liquid chromatography. Organic acids may be identified by gas chromatography combined with mass spectrophotometry (GC/MS). Short chain volatile organic acids may be determined by gas chromatography. The results from patients should be compared to normal individuals of the same age. Medications, eg, antibiotics and valproic acid, and diet, eg, medium chain triglyceride oil, may interfere with interpretation of the results. It is most important

that the laboratory doing the determinations be informed of the clinical findings, age of the patient, medications, and diet for proper interpretation of the results. The majority of the disorders are inherited as autosomal recessive traits, while a few are associated with X-linked inheritance patterns. The molecular

Table 13–2. Characteristic urine odors associated with various disorders resulting from inborn errors of metabolism.

Urine Odor	Disorder
Acid, sweaty feet	Glutaric acidemia type II
Cabbage	Tyrosinemias
Cat's urine	3-Methylcrotonyl-CoA carboxylase deficiency
Maple syrup, burnt sugar	Maple syrup urine disease (2-oxo-3-methylvaleric acid)
Mousy	Phenylketonuria
Sweaty feet	Isovaleric acidemia
Sweet	2-Methylacetoacetyl-CoA thiolase deficiency

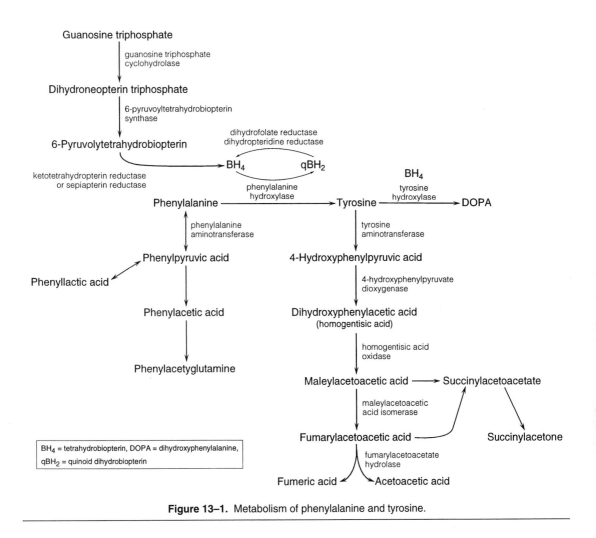

Figure 13–1. Metabolism of phenylalanine and tyrosine.

genetic abnormalities are known for many of the disorders. Carrier and prenatal testing for families with affected individuals vary with the disorder involved.

DISORDERS OF PHENYLALANINE AND TYROSINE METABOLISM

The metabolic pathways for phenylalanine and tyrosine are shown in Figure 13–1. Phenylalanine is considered an essential amino acid in that it cannot be synthesized in the body. Because tyrosine can be synthesized from phenylalanine, tyrosine is a nonessential amino acid. Both phenylalanine and tyrosine are present in natural foods, especially those high in protein content.

Hyperphenylalaninemias

Phenylketonuria (PKU): Phenylketonuria (PKU), perhaps the most recognized of the inborn errors of amino acid metabolism, results from deficient activity of phenylalanine hydroxylase. It is an autosomal

recessive disorder, most frequent among Caucasian populations, that occurs in one in 12,000 births. Patients with PKU are normal at birth. During the first year of life untreated PKU patients gradually develop irreversible severe pyschomotor retardation, pigment dilution, eczematoid-like rashes, autistic-like behavior, microcephaly, seizures, and hyperreflexia. Prior to newborn screening, most affected children were diagnosed after 6 months of age, usually during an evaluation for psychomotor delay. Untreated PKU patients have markedly elevated levels of phenylalanine and its abnormal metabolites phenylpyruvate and phenylacetate. Elevated levels of phenylpyruvate will give a blue-green color with ferric chloride urine spot testing. A distinctive "mousy" odor may be noted from the increased levels of phenylacetate. Serum phenylalanine levels are usually above 20 mg/dl. Levels of tyrosine are normal or low-normal. Because the enzyme is only expressed in the liver, enzymatic testing for phenylalanine hydroxylase is usually not performed to confirm the disease. The gene, however, located at chromosome 12q22–q24, has been cloned, and DNA mutation analysis may be accomplished with peripheral leukocytes. Multiple mutations have been found at the phenylalanine hydroxylase locus; most patients with PKU are compound heterozygotes for two different mutations.

Newborn screening for PKU occurs in all of the United States. Neonates with positive screening should be promptly referred for evaluation and therapy, in that the best outcomes have occurred in infants in whom control of phenylalanine levels was achieved prior to 1 month of age. Treatment for PKU consists of a lowered phenylalanine diet which includes the use of special dietary supplements, either devoid or low in phenylalanine, and measured amounts of natural foods that are low in protein. Optimum therapeutic blood levels of phenylalanine are 2–6 mg/dl for PKU children under 8 years of age. Frequent monitoring of blood phenylalanine levels and diet adjustments must be individualized for the PKU patient and should be done by experienced clinicians. Although most PKU children have intelligence quotients that are within 5 points of their unaffected siblings, a significant number of treated PKU individuals have learning disabilities and behavioral difficulties. Dietary treatment should continue for the life of the PKU individual. Older children and adults with PKU who have stopped dietary control have developed bizarre personality changes, behavioral problems, loss of intellectual functioning, changes in the cerebral white matter with neuroimaging of the brain, and occasionally, an acute progressive demyelinating encephalopathy. Many of these problems respond to reintroduction of dietary therapy and control of phenylalanine levels.

Hyperphenylalaninemia: Patients with mild variants of PKU, known as hyperphenylalaninemia, have elevated blood phenylalanine levels that are lower than those seen with classical PKU. Patients with hyperphenylalaninemia often do not need special dietary supplements in that their phenylalanine levels may be controlled with a natural, but not excessive, protein intake.

Maternal PKU Syndrome: Untreated maternal PKU during pregnancy results in a high percentage of miscarriages, fetal cardiac malformations, midfacial underdevelopment, growth retardation, and damage to the developing fetal brain. The findings in offspring of untreated PKU mothers are known as maternal PKU syndrome and are similar to that seen with fetal alcohol exposure. Because maternal PKU syndrome results from disease in the mother, effects occur regardless of whether the fetus is affected or unaffected with PKU. Women with hyperphenylalaninemia may also have a risk for maternal PKU effects on the fetus during pregnancy if their blood phenylalanine levels are over 6 mg/dl.

Defects in the Synthesis or Recycling of Tetrahydrobiopterin: Approximately 1–2% of patients with elevated phenylalanine levels will have defects in the synthesis or recycling of tetrahydrobiopterin, which is a cofactor for phenylalanine hydroxylase. In addition, because tetrahydrobiopterin is also a cofactor for tyrosine hydroxylase and tryptophan hydroxylase, these patients will also have deficient production of dopamine and 5-hydroxytryptophan which results in progressive neurological deterioration during infancy. All patients with positive newborn screening for PKU should be evaluated for tetrahydrobiopterin defects, which can be done by measuring urinary biopterin metabolites. Untreated, most patients with tetrahydrobiopterin synthesis or recycling defects die by 1 year of age. Treatment with tetrahydrobiopterin and neurotransmitters, in addition to lowered phenylalanine diets, has resulted in varying outcomes.

Tyrosinemias

Tyrosinemia Type I: Tyrosinemia type I, hepatorenal or hereditary tyrosinemia or tyrosinosis, is an autosomal recessive disorder associated with deficient activity of fumarylacetoacetate hydrolase. The disorder was named after the markedly elevated levels of tyrosine and its metabolites that occur in affected patients. However, the disorder is now known to involve a metabolic block further in the tyrosine metabolic pathway. Deficient activity of fumarylacetoacetate hydrolase results in the accumulation of succinylacetone and succinylacetoacetone, which are thought to be responsible for many of the clinical findings. The disorder occurs in approximately 1 in 100,000–1 in 120,000 births. It is most common in the Lac-St. Jean region of Quebec where it has an incidence of 1 in 685 births. Patients with complete lack of fumarylacetoacetate hydrolase often have an acute form of presentation with progressive liver dysfunction leading to hepatic failure before 1 year of age. A cabbage-like odor may be noted. A chronic form of the disease is more often seen in patients with some residual activity of the hydrolase. Patients with the chronic form of tyrosinemia type I usually have multisystem involvement, which can include chronic hepatic dysfunction, Fanconi-type renal tubular dysfunction, hypertrophic cardiomyopathy, and peripheral and central nervous system involvement. Because succinylacetone inhibits Δ-aminolevulinic acid dehydratase, there are increased levels of Δ-aminolevulinic acid and episodes of visceral and neurological impairment as seen with acute intermittent porphyria. Approximately one-third of patients develop hepatoma as a late complication of their disorder.

Laboratory findings in patients with tyrosinemia type I will include elevated blood and urine levels of succinylacetone and succinylacetoacetate. Special organic acid procedures are needed to detect these two compounds. Blood and urine tyrosine, methionine, and tyrosine metabolites, 4-hydroxyphenylpyruvate and 4-hydroxyphenyllactate, will be elevated. Liver function tests will be abnormal. Elevated alpha-feto-protein levels are usually present from birth. A generalized aminoaciduria will be present. Renal tubular loss of phosphorus may result in rickets. Urine Δ-aminolevulinic acid will be elevated. Treatment includes a lowered tyrosine, phenylalanine, and methionine diet, which is accomplished with special dietary supplements and limited amounts of natural foods that are low in protein. Dietary therapy, however, may not prevent progression of the disease or lower the risk for hepatoma. Although liver transplantation may be considered for children with advanced liver dysfunction, this may not eliminate the succinylacetone production. Treatment with 2-(2-nitro-4-trifluoromethylbenzoyl)-1,3-cyclohexanedione (NTBC), an inhibitor of 4-hydroxyphenylpyruvate dioxygenase which decreases succinylacetone production, has shown promise if started early in the course of the disease. Newborn screening is carried out in Quebec by measuring the activity of fumarylacetoacetate hydrolase and levels of succinylacetone in dried blood filter paper cards. Deficient activity of the hydrolase may also be shown in erythrocytes, lymphocytes, cultured skin fibroblasts, and liver biopsy samples. Prenatal diagnosis is available.

Tyrosinemia Type II: Tyrosinemia type II, or the Richner-Hanhart syndrome, is an autosomal recessive disorder that results from deficient activity of tyrosine aminotransferase. Blood and urine levels of tyrosine are markedly elevated. Elevated levels of tyrosine metabolites will be noted on organic acid determinations including 4-hydroxyphenylpyruvate, 4-hydroxyphenyllactate, 4-hydroxyphenylacetate, N-acetyltyrosine, and tyramine. Oculocutaneous symptoms develop during early infancy and include corneal erosions, ulcerations, opacities, and plaques. The cutaneous manifestations consist of pruritic blisters or erosions on the palms and soles which become crusted and then keratotic. Some patients have psychomotor retardation. Most patients respond to treatment with lowered tyrosine and phenylalanine diets. Special supplements low in tyrosine and phenylalanine will often be needed for adequate total protein intake.

Deficient Activity of 4-Hydroxyphenylpyruvic Acid Dioxygenase (Hydroxylating Oxidase): Patients with deficient activity of 4-hydroxyphenylpyruvic acid dioxygenase (hydroxylating oxidase), a rare condition, have seizures, pyschomotor retardation, or episodes of acute ataxia and lethargy. Plasma levels of tyrosine are variably elevated. Urine organic acids will show elevated 4-hydroxyphenyllactate, 4-hydroxyphenylacetate, and 4-hydroxyphenylpyruvate. Hepatic and oculocutaneous manifestations do not occur. Deficient activity of 4-hydroxyphenylpyruvic acid dioxygenase may be shown in liver or kidney biopsy samples.

Transient Neonatal Tyrosinemia: Transient neonatal tyrosinemia, noted in as many as 10% of premature infants, is thought to result from physiologic immaturity of 4-hydroxyphenylpyruvic acid dioxygenase. Levels of tyrosine and phenylalanine are elevated. Many of the infants display lethargy, prolonged jaundice, feeding problems, and occasionally metabolic acidosis. The disorder is seen more frequently in populations where there is less breast feeding and more feeding of infant formulas which are higher in protein than breast milk. Many patients respond to a lowered protein intake and supplemental vitamin C.

Alcaptonuria

Alcaptonuria is a rare disorder which results from deficient activity of homogentisic acid oxidase. Elevated levels of homogentisic acid (2,5-dihydroxyphenylacetic acid), a metabolite of tyrosine, lead to pigment deposition in connective tissue throughout the body (ochronosis). The pigment is a polymer derived from homogentisic acid. Deposition of pigment is usually first noted between 20 and 30 years of age in the sclera and ear cartilage. Gray or slate blue colored deposits are noted in the sclera near the insertions of the rectus muscles between the cornea and the canthi. Deposition in the ear cartilage is first noted in the antihelix and concha areas. Urine from affected patients which has been left standing (autooxidation) or has been alkalinized will turn a dark brown color. If cloth diapers from affected infants are washed with alkaline cleaning solutions there will be an increase in intensity of the dark brown staining. The pigment is also present in perspiration and can stain clothing. Brownish discoloration may be noted in the axillary and inguinal areas of affected individuals.

In later adult life gradual deposition of homogentisic acid in the large joints and lumbosacral spine results in decreased range of motion and ankylosis. Acute inflammatory episodes frequently occur. The disorder should be considered in the differential diagnosis of rheumatoid arthritis and osteoarthritis. Radiograms, however, will be different from these two disorders. There is narrowing and increased calcification of the intervertebral disc space; osteophytes are not usually seen. On tissue biopsies, gray to bluishblack pigment deposition is evident. Quantitative measurements of homogentisic acid may be done in blood, urine, or tissue samples. Urine spot testing for reducing substances will be positive. Treatment with ascorbic acid may delay the onset and reduce the severity of clinical symptoms.

DISORDERS OF METHIONINE METABOLISM

Dietary protein contains methionine, an essential amino acid, which is metabolized to homocystine, cystine, and ultimately to inorganic sulfur which is

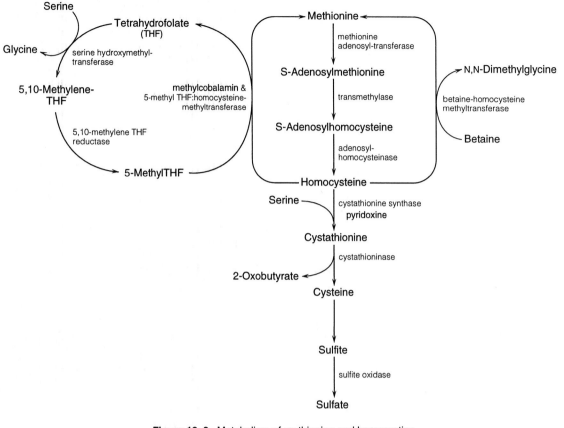

Figure 13–2. Metabolism of methionine and homocystine.

excreted from the body (Figure 13–2). S-adenosyl-methionine, an intermediate in the conversion of methionine to homocystine, is an important source of methyl groups that are needed for neurotransmitter, myelin, and phospholipid metabolism, and in DNA and RNA modification. In that the demand for methyl groups is frequently higher than the dietary methionine supply, approximately one-half of the homocystine produced is remethylated back to methionine by two pathways which use either 5-methyltetrahydrofolate or betaine as the methyl donors.

Hypermethioninemia

Elevated blood and urine levels of methionine, or hypermethioninemia, which occur without elevation of other methionine metabolites, are thought to be benign and result from deficient activity of methionine S-adenosyltransferase.

Homocystinuria

Classical Homocystinuria: Elevated levels of both methionine and homocystine are noted in patients with classical homocystinuria who have deficient activity of cystathionine synthetase. The disorder, inherited as an autosomal recessive trait, is

estimated to occur in 1 in 335,000 births. Affected patients appear normal at birth and develop clinical signs of their disorder during early childhood. The elevated levels of homocystine interfere with the cross-linkage of collagen and result in dislocated lens, osteoporosis, scoliosis, and a Marfanoid body habitus with tall stature, thin and long extremities, and a high-arched palate (Figure 13–3). In contrast to Marfan syndrome, patients with homocystinuria often have decreased range of motion of the elbows and knees and may develop a pes cavus foot deformity. Elevated levels of homocystine also disrupt the vascular endothelium and lead to thrombus formation, which can occur at any age and in any vessel. Affected patients develop hypertension, pulmonary emboli, myocardial infarctions, and cerebrovascular accidents. By age 20 years, 25% of the patients will have had a major thromboembolic event, and by age 28 years, 50% will be affected. Patients with classical homocystinuria develop psychomotor handicaps; the average intelligence quotient is 64. Many patients also have unusual personalities and behavioral or psychiatric disturbances. Quantitative amino acid determinations will show elevated blood and urine levels of methionine, homocystine, and other homo-

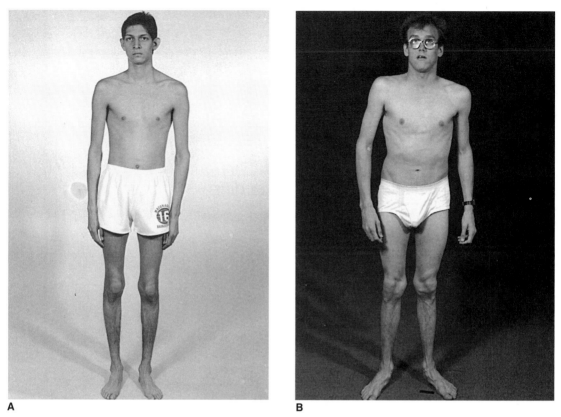

Figure 13–3. Homocystinuria. **(A)** Teenage boy who presented with a pulmonary embolus; **(B)** young adult. (Reproduced, with permission from: Oski FA et al: *Principles and Practice of Pediatrics,* 2nd ed, JB Lippincott, 1994.)

cystine metabolites. Measurement of cystathionine synthetase may be done with mitogen-stimulated lymphocytes or cultured skin fibroblasts. Prenatal diagnosis and carrier detection are available. Treatment includes a diet reduced in methionine, pyridoxine (vitamin B_6, a cofactor for cystathionine synthetase), betaine and folate (remethylation of homocystine to methionine), and cystine (which has become an essential amino acid because it is the product of the reaction that is affected). Effective treatment will change the natural course of the disorder, but will not improve the psychomotor handicaps or structural changes that have occurred as a result of the collagen disruption or vascular disease.

Pyridoxine-responsive Homocystinuria: Approximately 50% of patients with homocystinuria have milder clinical findings and some residual activity of cystathionine synthetase. They will usually show a clinical response to large doses (250–900 mg per day) of pyridoxine. Many of these pyridoxine-response homocystinuric patients have normal intelligence.

Newborn screening for homocystinuria, by means of measuring methionine in dried blood filter paper spots, is being done in some areas during the first few days of life. However, most patients with either classical or pyridoxine-responsive homocystinuria will not be detected by newborn screening because of the slow rise in methionine levels in affected patients at this early age. Patients with benign hypermethioninemia, however, are frequently detected by newborn screening. Elevated levels of methionine in the newborn period may also be seen with the tyrosinemias, untreated galactosemia, and other causes of liver dysfunction.

Defects in the Remethylation of Homocystine to Methionine: Homocystinuria can also result from defects in the remethylation of homocystine to methionine. Patients with this form of homocystinuria will have elevated homocystine levels, but reduced levels of methionine. Defects in the remethylation of homocystine can result from nutritional deficiencies in folate or cobalamin (vitamin B_{12}) or from defects in the transport or activation of folate or cobalamin. **Deficient activity of 5,10-methylenetetrahydrofolate reductase** results in deficient levels of 5-methyltetrahydrofolate, the major transport form of folate (Figure 13–4). Other patients will have a **functional deficiency of 5-methyltetrahydrofolate:homocystine methyltransferase** as a result of

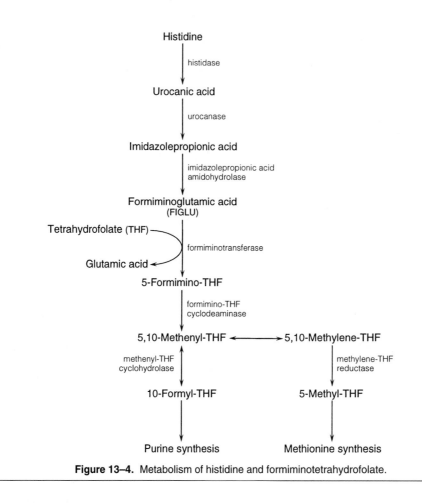

Figure 13–4. Metabolism of histidine and formiminotetrahydrofolate.

failure of formation of its cofactor methylcobalamin. Defects in cobalamin activation may result in **homocystinuria combined with methylmalonic aciduria;** these disorders are discussed in further detail with methylmalonic acidemia. Patients with remethylation defects usually have progressive central nervous system degenerative disorders in addition to the findings seen with cystathionine synthetase deficiency. Some will respond to high dose therapy with folate, pyridoxine, betaine, and hydroxycobalamin.

Sulfite Oxidase Deficiency

Sulfite oxidase deficiency, a rare autosomal recessive disorder, is characterized by the accumulation of sulfite and S-sulfocysteine, dislocated lens, and a severe, progressive demyelinating central nervous system disorder. Although isolated sulfite oxidase deficiency can occur, it more often results from a deficiency of its molybdenum cofactor. Because the molybdenum cofactor is also needed for enzymatic activity of xanthine dehydrogenase and aldehyde oxidase, patients with molybdenum cofactor deficiency will have low levels of uric acid and elevated urinary xanthine and hypoxanthine in addition to sulfite and

S-sulfocysteine accumulation. Deficient activity of sulfite oxidase or xanthine dehydrogenase may be shown in liver biopsy samples or cultured skin fibroblasts. There is no effective treatment. Prenatal diagnosis is possible.

DISORDERS OF HISTIDINE METABOLISM

Histidine appears to be an essential amino acid, especially in young infants and children, that is needed for nitrogen retention and growth. Histidine is metabolized to formiminoglutamic acid (FIGLU) which is a donor for the formyl groups utilized in the metabolism of tetrahydrofolic acid. (Figure 13–4)

Histidinemia

Histidinemia, an autosomal recessive disorder that occurs in 1 in 10,000 births, is associated with deficient activity of histidase (histidine ammonia lyase). Patients have elevated levels of plasma and urine histidine. Elevated urine histidine metabolites, including imidazolepyruvic acid, imidazolelactic, and imidazoleacetic acids, will produce a positive urine ferric chloride test and a green color which can be confused with the blue-green color seen with ferric chloride testing in PKU. Reduced activity of histidase can be shown in liver or uncultured skin biopsies. On the basis of results from newborn screening programs for histidinemia, it has been concluded that most patients with histidinemia do not have clinical findings as a result of their disorder. However, approximately 1% of affected individuals have been noted to have psychomotor retardation and speech difficulties, which suggests that the elevated histidine levels may play a role in the development of these problems by enhancing the effects of other factors, eg, perinatal hypoxia, at an early age. The elevated histidine levels will respond to special diets low in histidine.

Urocanic Acidemia

Urocanic acid, a metabolite of histidine, is markedly elevated in the urine of patients with urocanic acidemia. The disorder results from deficient activity of urocanase which can only be measured in liver biopsy samples. As with histidinemia, it is unclear whether the biochemical findings are related to the psychomotor retardation and growth retardation noted in some patients.

Other Disorders
of Histidine Metabolism

Elevated levels of histidine and formiminoglutamic acid (FIGLU), a metabolite of histidine, have been noted with deficient activity of **formininotransferase,** most probably a benign disorder, and with **deficient activity of formiminotetrahydrofolate cyclodeaminase,** which results in hypotonia, cortical atrophy, seizures, and psychomotor retardation. Because the enzymes are only expressed in liver and detailed studies in patients have not been done, the correlation between clinical and biochemical findings is still unclear.

Formiminoglutamic acid (FIGLU) is important in the metabolism of folate acid. **Deficient activity of methylenetetrahydrofolate reductase** results in reduced production of 5-methyltetrahydrofolate, which serves as a methyl donor in the remethylation of homocystine to methionine. Affected patients with methylenetetrahydrofolate reductase deficiency are discussed with homocystinurias. Failure to reactivate (recycle) tetrahydrofolate from dihydrofolate due to **deficient activity of dihydrofolate reductase** is associated with one of the biopterin deficient forms of phenylketonuria.

DISORDERS OF
THE UREA CYCLE

The urea cycle converts excess nitrogen, in the form of ammonium ions, into urea, which can be excreted in the urine (Figure 13–5). Metabolic blocks in the urea cycle occur in approximately one in 60,000 births. Defects in the urea cycle are associated with elevated ammonia levels that are extremely toxic and lead to encephalopathies, cerebral edema, and often death. Infants with the severe neonatal forms of the disorders usually appear normal for the first 24–48 hours of life. Affected patients then develop poor feeding, irritability, temperature instability, vomiting, seizures, and lethargy which progresses to coma and circulatory collapse. Plasma ammonia levels are markedly elevated, often above 1000 μM. Patients with milder and late onset forms of the disorders often have a history of protein avoidance, intermittent episodes of vomiting and lethargy, behavioral changes, seizures, psychomotor retardation, or other neurological deficits.

The diagnosis of a specific disorder of the urea cycle is established by the pattern of elevation of amino acids, the presence or absence of urinary orotic acid, and ultimately enzymatic or DNA testing. Initial treatment may require dialysis, preferably hemodialysis. Intravenous use of phenylacetate and benzoate, which combine with excess amine groups of ammonia precursors to form nontoxic products, may be used if the plasma ammonia levels are only mildly or moderately elevated, eg, less than 350 μM. The outcome is inversely related to the degree of hyperammonemia and the time in coma. Only 30–50% of patients with massive neonatal hyperammonemia will survive the episode. All patients who have been rescued from severe neonatal hyperammonemia have significant psychomotor handicaps and neurological deficits. If the patient survives, maintenance treatment includes restricted protein intake, special formulas which are low in protein and contain only essential amino acids, and supplemental L-citrulline or L-arginine, which have become essential amino acids for the urea cycle due to the metabolic block. Oral or enteral phenylbutyrate, which is metabolized in the body to phenylacetate, or combined phenylacetate and benzoate therapy are usually continually needed to control the ammonia levels. Despite successful initial control of their disorder, patients with urea cycle defects are at risk to develop subsequent episodes of acute hyperammonemia with intercurrent illnesses or protein excess. The disorders are inherited as autosomal recessive traits except for ornithine transcarbamylase deficiency, which is inherited as an X-linked disorder. The availability of carrier and prenatal testing varies with the specific disorder involved. The genes for many of the disorders have been cloned or isolated, and molecular diagnostic testing can often be used for carrier and prenatal testing in informative families.

Non-inherited, Transient Neonatal Hyperammonemia: Some neonates will have non-inherited, transient neonatal hyperammonemia, which may be as severe as that seen with defects of the urea cycle.

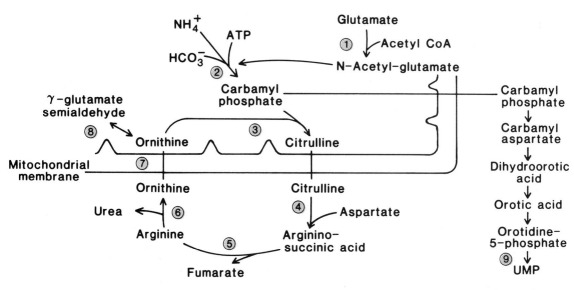

Figure 13–5. The urea cycle. 1 = N-acetyl-glutamate synthetase (NAGS); 2 = carbamyl phosphate synthetase I (CPS I); 3 = ornithine transcarbamylase (OTC); 4 = argininosuccinate synthetase (AS); 5 = argininosuccinate lyase (AL); 6 = arginase; 7 = mitochondrial ornithine transport defect (HHH); 8 = ornithine aminotransferase; 9 = decarboxylase, site of allopurinal block in the pyrimidine pathway; ATP = adenosine triphosphate; CoA = coenzyme A; UMP = uridine monophosphate. (Reproduced, with permission from: Oski FA et al: *Principles and Practice of Pediatrics,* 2nd ed, JB Lippincott, 1994.)

These patients are often premature infants who become symptomatic before 48 hours of age, which is earlier than the onset seen with inherited disorders of the urea cycle. Therapy and evaluation should proceed as for a urea cycle defect in that the neurological outcome of neonatal massive hyperammonemia may be the same.

Secondary Hyperammonemia: Secondary hyperammonemia may occur with any of the organic acidurias and may be the presenting sign. Patients with neonatal presentation of propionic acidemia, methylmalonc acidemia, and maple syrup urine disease may have elevated ammonia levels as high as those seen in primary defects of the urea cycle. The organic acids, especially propionic acid, inhibit the activity of N-acetylglutamate synthetase. Modest elevation of plasma ammonia is also frequently noted in patients with disorders of mitochondrial fatty acid oxidation. Urinary organic acid profiles are indicated as part of the evaluation in any patient with hyperammonemia. Secondary hyperammonemia may also occur with liver dysfunction and valproate anticonvulsant therapy.

Deficient Activity of N-acetylglutamate Synthetase: Deficient activity of N-acetylglutamate synthetase is a very rare disorder of the urea cycle which usually has its onset in the neonatal period. Plasma ammonia levels are markedly elevated. Plasma levels of citrulline and arginine and urine levels of orotic acid are usually normal. Treatment includes supplements of arginine (an activator of N-acetylglutamine synthetase), N-carbamylglutamate (a congener of

N-acetylglutamate), lowered protein special diets, and phenylbutyrate or combined phenylacetate and benzoate. Deficient activity of N-acetylglutamate synthetase may be shown in liver biopsy samples.

Deficient Activity of Carbamyl Phosphate Synthetase I (CPS I): Deficient activity of carbamyl phosphate synthetase I (CPS I) usually presents in the neonatal period with hyperammonemic coma. Milder affected patients who have 10–25% of normal residual enzymatic activity may have a later onset of their disease. Plasma levels of ammonia are markedly elevated. Plasma levels of citrulline and arginine are low; urinary orotic acid is normal. Treatment includes supplements of L-citrulline, lowered protein special diets, and phenylbutyrate or combined phenylacetate and benzoate. Deficient activity of CPS I may be shown in liver, rectal, or duodenal biopsy samples. Molecular diagnostic testing may be used for prenatal diagnosis in informative families.

Deficient Activity of Ornithine Transcarbamylase (OTC): Deficient activity of ornithine transcarbamylase (OTC), which is inherited as an X-linked trait, is one of the more common disorders of the urea cycle. Affected males usually present in the neonatal period with hyperammonemic coma. Ammonia levels are massively elevated, frequently over 1000 µM and as high as 3000 µM. As many as 70% of affected males do not survive the neonatal period. Plasma citrulline levels are low; urinary orotic acid is markedly elevated. Transaminases and uric acid levels are often elevated. The enzymatic deficiency may be shown in liver biopsy samples. Milder affected males with 10–25% of normal residual enzymatic activity have a milder course and later onset, which can be even as late as during adult life. Treatment includes supplements of L-citrulline, lowered protein special diets, and phenylbutyrate or combined phenylacetate and benzoate. Liver transplantation will correct the metabolic disorder, but any residual neurologic problems that have resulted from hyperammonemia will remain.

Approximately 20% of **females who are carriers for OTC deficiency** are clinically symptomatic. In symptomatic carrier females, random inactivation of one of the two X chromosomes during early embryonic life (Lyonization) results in a significant number of their hepatocytes having the remaining active X chromosome being the X with the abnormal OTC gene. These women usually have only 10–20% of normal OTC activity. Symptomatic female carriers may present at any age with a history of protein avoidance or intolerance, or with symptoms of acute or chronic hyperammonemia or its sequelae. Neurological problems are common and include encephalopathies, cerebral atrophy, and cerebral vascular accidents. Some women have become acutely hyperammonemic in the post-partum period. At least three symptomatic females have died with hyperammonemia in the neonatal period. Treatment varies with the degree of severity and is similar to that for hemizygous affected males. Carrier detection for female relatives of affected patients is available by means of measuring urinary orotic acid or orotidine, which become elevated while taking allopurinol (Figure 13–5). Carrier and prenatal testing are also available by molecular genetic techniques in informative families.

Citrullinemia: Deficient activity of argininosuccinate synthetase results in markedly elevated citrulline levels and the disorder known as citrullinemia. Most affected infants have a severe form of the disorder and neonatal hyperammonemic coma. Plasma citrulline levels are usually greater than 1000 μM; urinary orotic acid may be moderately increased. Mild and adult forms of the disorder also occur. Treatment includes a reduced protein diet, supplemental L-arginine, and phenylbutyrate or combined phenylacetate and benzoate. The disorder may be confirmed by measurement of argininosuccinate synthetase in cultured skin fibroblasts or liver biopsy samples. Prenatal diagnosis may be done with enzymatic assay. Carrier and prenatal testing may also be done with molecular genetic techniques in informative families.

Argininosuccinic Aciduria: Deficient activity of argininosuccinase, or argininosuccinate lyase, results in argininosuccinic aciduria. There are neonatal, mild, and asymptomatic forms of the disorder. The neonatal form may present as late as 2 weeks of age with hyperammonemic coma. Milder cases have been identified during infancy and childhood with presenting signs of hepatomegaly, psychomotor delays, and abnormal, friable, kinky hair (trichorrhexis nodosa). Liver biopsy will show fatty infiltration and fibrosis. Mildly elevated transaminases are common. Asymptomatic cases have been detected by newborn screening. Urine argininosuccinic acid levels are markedly elevated; plasma citrulline levels and urinary orotic acid levels will be moderately increased. Patients with argininosuccinic aciduria usually respond to treatment with a lowered protein diet and L-arginine supplements. Phenylacetate and benzoate therapy are usually only needed to control acute hyperammonemic episodes. The disorder is confirmed by demonstrating deficient activity of argininosuccinase in erythrocytes, cultured skin fibroblasts, or liver biopsy samples. Prenatal diagnosis is available by enzymatic assay. Carrier and prenatal testing may be done with molecular genetic techniques in informative families.

Argininemia: Argininemia, which results from deficient activity of arginase, is a very rare disorder associated with elevated plasma arginine levels (usually over 500 μM) and moderate hyperammonemia. Most affected patients have the onset of episodic vomiting, irritability, seizures, cerebral atrophy, psychomotor retardation, and a progressive spastic quadriparesis during early infancy. Hepatomegaly, multifocal hydropic changes on liver biopsy, and abnormal liver function testing may occur. Urine levels of orotic acid, other pyrimidines, and arginine are elevated. High levels of urinary arginine result in elevated urinary levels of the other dibasic amino acids (lysine, ornithine, and cystine) due to competition for shared renal transport mechanisms. Treatment includes supplements of lysine and ornithine, lowered protein diets, and phenylbutyrate or combined phenylacetate and benzoate. The disorder may be confirmed by measurement of arginase activity in erythrocytes, leukocytes, or liver biopsy samples. Carrier testing is available, but prenatal testing is not.

Ornithine Aminotransferase Deficiency: Ornithine aminotransferase deficiency is associated with elevated levels of ornithine and a characteristic progressive gyrate atrophy of the choroid and retina. It is a very rare condition which is more common in persons of Finnish background. Hyperammonemia does not occur. Urinary levels of the dibasic amino acids (ornithine, arginine, lysine, and cystine) may be increased. Most patients present during childhood with myopia, night blindness, and reduced peripheral vision. Posterior subcapsular cataracts also develop. Chorioretinal degeneration progresses and complete visual loss occurs between the ages of 20 and 50 years. Treatment may be attempted with supplemental lysine or α-aminoisobutyric acid, pyridoxine, and a lowered dietary protein intake.

Patients with lysinuric protein intolerance and the hyperammonemia-hyperornithinemia-homocitrullinuria syndrome may also have hyperammonemia

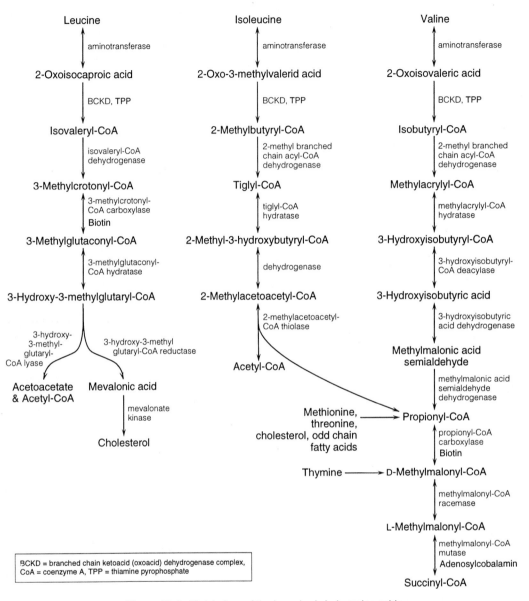

Figure 13–6. Metabolism of the branched chain amino acids.

on the basis of defective transport of amino acids needed for proper functioning of the urea cycle. These disorders are discussed with the disorders of amino acid transport.

DISORDERS OF GLYCINE METABOLISM

Non-ketotic Hyperglycinemia (NKH): Non-ketotic hyperglycinemia (NKH) is an autosomal recessive disorder associated with markedly elevated levels of glycine, especially in the cerebrospinal fluid. The

disorder results from deficient activity of the mitochondrial glycine-cleaving enzyme complex. Affected patients present at birth or early in the neonatal period with severe hypotonia and central nervous system depression. Affected patients frequently require assisted ventilation. Most have major motor or myoclonic seizures which are difficult to control and associated with independent multifocal spike discharges or hypsarrythmia patterns on electroencephalograms. There is essentially no psychomotor development, and the patients that survive the neonatal period are profoundly handicapped. Most patients die prior to 1 year of age, but prolonged survival, even into the late teens, is known. There is no effective treatment; however, benzoate or dextromethorphan therapy may improve seizure control. Valproic acid anticonvulsant therapy should be avoided in that clinical deterioration has been noted in some patients while taking valproate. The disorder is confirmed by simultaneous measurement of cerebrospinal fluid and plasma glycine levels. An increased cerebrospinal fluid glycine to plasma glycine ratio is noted in affected infants. Activity of the glycine-cleaving enzyme complex may be determined in liver biopsy samples. Recent cloning of the genes for the glycine-cleaving enzyme complex will allow accurate carrier and prenatal diagnosis for informative families. The disorder is estimated to occur in one in 250,000 births, but many patients may die unrecognized in the newborn period.

Markedly elevated levels of glycine also may be noted in patients with organic acidemias, eg, propionic aciduria and methylmalonic aciduria. The elevated levels of organic acids inhibit the activity of the glycine-cleaving enzyme complex. Patients taking valproic acid for anticonvulsant therapy will also have elevated glycine levels.

DISORDERS OF LYSINE

Familial Hyperlysinemia: Familial hyperlysinemia is a benign autosomal recessive condition that is associated with reduced activity of the bifunctional enzyme α-aminoadipic semialdehyde synthase. The bifunctional enzyme consists of the activities of lysine ketoglutarate reductase and saccharopine dehydrogenase. Individuals with the disorder have been found to have elevated blood and urine levels of lysine and often mildly increased urinary levels of saccharopine. There appear to be no associated clinical findings. The enzymatic defect can be shown in cultured skin fibroblasts.

Saccharopinuria: Saccharopinuria is a rare variant of familial hyperlysinemia which has reported to occur in patients with psychomotor retardation who have markedly elevated urine levels of saccharopine. In one patient who had enzymatic studies, there was no activity of saccharopine dehydrogenase and only partial reduction in lysine ketoglutarate reductase.

Glutaric Acidemia Type I: Glutaric acidemia type I is an autosomal recessive disorder that is estimated to occur in 1 in 30,000 births. The disorder is associated with deficient activity of glutaryl-CoA dehydrogenase. Glutaryl-CoA, an intermediate in the metabolism of lysine, hydroxylysine, and tyrptophan, is normally metabolized to crotonyl-CoA by the action of glutaryl-CoA dehydrogenase. Patients with glutaric acidemia type I have a progressive macrocephaly from birth. During the first 2 years of life they develop a movement disorder with dystonia, dyskinesis, rigidity, functional hypotonia, and hyper-

reflexia. Neuroimaging will show cerebral atrophy with white matter changes and neuronal degeneration of the caudate and putamen. Some of the patients have acute episodes of metabolic ketoacidosis, often precipitated by an intercurrent illness, which are associated with hypoglycemia, elevated transaminases, hyperammonemia, coma, and seizures. Acute episodes usually respond to intravenous glucose, hydration, and bicarbonate. Urine organic acid determinations will show elevated levels of glutaric and 3-hydroxyglutaric acids. With an acute episode, levels of glutaconic acid and dicarboxylic acids will also be increased. Deficient activity of glutaryl-CoA dehydrogenase may be shown in leukocytes or cultured skin fibroblasts. Treatment consists of a lowered protein diet and special supplements low in lysine and tryptophan. Some patients have been reported to respond to large doses of riboflavin, which is a cofactor for glutaryl-CoA dehydrogenase. L-carnitine therapy is also indicated in that plasma levels of free carnitine will be low. The best outcomes have been reported in patients who were started on treatment prior to the changes in the caudate and putamen and development of the dystonia. Prenatal and carrier testing is available.

Glutaric acidemia type II is discussed with the disorders of fatty acid oxidation. Lysinuric protein intolerance is included with the disorders of amino acid transport.

DISORDERS OF BRANCHED CHAIN AMINO ACIDS

The branched chain amino acids, leucine, isoleucine, and valine, are essential amino acids that are utilized for protein synthesis or metabolized to products that can be used for energy production (Figure 13–6). Most disorders involving the metabolism of the branched chain amino acids are associated with the accumulation of abnormal metabolites of the amino acids which are known as organic acids. Markedly elevated levels of organic acids can cause significant metabolic acidosis. In addition, elevated levels of organic acids, especially propionic acid, may inhibit the activity of N-acetylglutamate synthetase, an enzyme involved in the first step of urea synthesis. The resultant secondary hyperammonemia can be as severe as that found with primary defects in the urea cycle. Inhibition of the glycine-cleaving enzyme complex by the organic acids may result in hyperglycinemia. The elevated organic acid levels may also cause bone marrow depression and lead to neutropenia, thrombocytopenia, or pancytopenia. During acute episodes of metabolic decompensation there will be patterns of elevation of specific organic acids which suggest the defect involved. Nonspecific elevation of lactate and 3-hydroxybutyrate also frequently occurs. Between acute episodes some of the disorders of branched chain amino acid metabolism are associated with the continued production of abnormal organic acids; in other disorders this does not occur. Neurological symptoms such as seizures and encephalopathies, poor feeding, emesis, and failure to thrive are common. Many patients die with acute episodes of ketoacidosis. Those who survive often have psychomotor handicaps.

Screening urine spot tests for oxoacids, such as the ferric chloride and dinitrophenylhydrazine (DPNH) tests, may be positive in affected patients. Newborn screening for maple syrup urine disease and biotinidase deficiency is available in some locations. Blood and urine determination of quantitative amino acids will show elevation of the branched chain amino acids in maple syrup urine disease and the branched chain aminotransferase deficiencies. Patients with metabolic defects further into the pathways (after the dehydrogenase steps) will not show elevation of the precursor branched chain amino acids because the prior metabolic steps are not reversible. Patients with defects throughout the pathways, however, will have characteristic patterns of abnormal urine organic acids. Enzymatic confirmation of the disorders should be done when available. Many of the assays can be performed with leukocytes or cultured skin fibroblasts and liver biopsy samples are only infrequently required.

All of the disorders are inherited as autosomal recessive traits except for the cardiac-neutropenia form of 3-methylglutaconic aciduria, which is inherited as an X-linked trait. Prenatal diagnosis is available for some of the disorders by means of enzymatic testing, molecular genetic studies, or the determination of abnormal metabolites in amniotic fluid.

The branched chain amino acids are converted to their corresponding α-ketoacids (oxoacids) by cytosolic aminotransferases prior to being transported into the mitochondria for oxidative decarboxylation. Most mammalian tissues have only one aminotransferase, which acts on all three branched chain amino acids. However, there have been reports of one patient with isolated **hypervalinemia** and three patients with combined **hyperleucinemia and hyperisoleucinemia,** without elevation of valine, who presented in early infancy with neurological impairments and failure to thrive. These cases suggest that there may be two aminotransferases which are substrate specific, one for valine and one for both leucine and isoleucine.

Maple Syrup Urine Disease (MSUD)

Maple syrup urine disease (MSUD) occurs in 1 in 200,000 births. It is most common among the Mennonites of North America in whom it has an incidence of 1 in 176. The disorder is associated with deficient activity of the branched chain amino α-ketoacid dehydrogenase complex. The complex is composed of three major components, E_1, E_2, and E_3. Activity of the complex is regulated by a kinase and phosphatase which influence the activity of E_1. E_1 is a decarboxylase which has a thiamine pyrophosphate (TPP) cofactor. E_2 is a dihydrolipoyl acyltransferase which transfers the branched chain acyl groups formed by E_1 to coenzyme A (CoA). E_3 is comprised of lipoamide dehydrogenase which requires FAD and NAD^+. The E_3 component of the branched chain α-ketoacid dehydrogenase complex is identical to the E_3 component of the pyruvate dehydrogenase complex and the E_3 component of the α-ketoglutarate dehydrogenase complex. The net result of the activity of the branched chain α-ketoacid dehydrogenase complex is the production of branched chain acyl-CoA, CO_2, and NADH. The genes for the separate components of the complex, which have separate chromosomal locations, have been cloned. Mutations in all three major components of the complex have been found in patients with MSUD. Mutations of E_2 are the most common; many patients are compound heterozygotes for two different molecular mutations.

Patients with untreated MSUD have markedly elevated levels of the branched chain amino acids and their corresponding oxoacids (ketoacids) in the blood, urine, and spinal fluid. Plasma leucine levels are the most elevated and often are above 1000 μM. The presence of alloisoleucine, a metabolite of 2-oxo-3-methylvalerate, appears to be unique to MSUD and its presence should alert the clinician to the diagnosis. Urine organic acid profiles will show elevated levels of 2-oxoisocaproic, 2-oxo-3-methylvaleric, 2-oxoisovaleric, 2-hydroxyisovaleric, 2-hydroxyisocaproic, and 2-hydroxy-3-methylvaleric acids. The disorder is named after the burnt-sugar or maple-sugar odor produced by 2-oxo-3-methylvaleric acid. Deficient activity of the branched chain α-ketoacid dehydrogenase complex may be shown with leukocytes or cultured skin fibroblasts.

There are four forms of MSUD which are characterized by the age of onset, severity, and responsiveness to thiamine (vitamin B_1), a cofactor for the E_1 component of the branched chain α-ketoacid dehydrogenase complex.

Classical Form: The classical form of MSUD has its onset during the first week of life. Patients have poor feeding, irritability, lethargy, hypotonia or hypertonia, abnormal movements, and seizures, which progress to cerebral edema and coma. Severe metabolic acidosis and ketosis occur which are often accompanied by hyperammonemia and hypoglycemia. Initial treatment includes intravenous hydration, glucose, and bicarbonate to correct the acidosis. Dialysis, preferably hemodialysis, may be required. Increasing caloric intake to suppress catabolism by the use of special formula supplements or special amino acid mixtures, which are devoid of protein or the branched chain amino acids, has also been successful in controlling the disorder. Maintenance therapy includes special dietary preparations which are missing the branched chain amino acids and measured amounts of natural protein foods. Supplements of thiamine should also be given until it is clear that the patient is not thiamine-responsive. Even with control of their disease, the patients are at risk for acute episodes of ketoacidosis, which can be life-threatening, for the remainder of their lives.

Intermediate Form: The intermediate form of MSUD usually presents after the newborn period with failure to thrive, vomiting, ataxia, and psychomotor handicaps. These patients will have biochemical findings similar to, but milder than classical MSUD.

Intermittent Form: An intermittent form of MSUD may also present at any age after the neonatal period with acute episodes of ketoacidosis that are often associated with intercurrent illnesses or increased protein intake. In patients with the intermittent form of MSUD, the abnormal levels of amino acids and organic acids are usually only present during an acute episode.

Thiamine-response Form: Patients with a thiamine-response form of MSUD usually have milder clinical and biochemical findings and respond to large doses of thiamine. Patients with the intermediate, intermittent, and thiamine-responsive forms of MSUD have some residual activity of the branched chain α-ketoacid dehydrogenase complex, which allows the later onset and less severe clinical picture.

In addition to the four recognized forms of MSUD, three patients have been reported with a combined deficiency of the branched chain α-ketoacid dehydrogenase, pyruvate dehydrogenase, and α-ketoglutarate dehydrogenase complexes. There is a defect in the common E_3 subunit of all three complexes. Affected patients are neonates or young infants who have ketolactic acidosis, ataxia, and progressive extrapyramidal tract signs. There are elevations of lactic acid and α-ketoglutarate in addition to the biochemical findings of MSUD.

Patients with MSUD are often symptomatic at the time the results of newborn screening testing are known. Asymptomatic patients with positive newborn screening for MSUD should be immediately evaluated. Although many patients with the classical form of MSUD have severe psychomotor handicaps, there are patients with classical MSUD who have had normal psychomotor outcomes. The best outcomes have occurred in patients who have been started on therapy within 24 hours of the onset of symptoms, and in affected infants born into families where the disease has already occurred. Prenatal diagnosis is available using enzymatic assays in chorionic villi samples or cultured amniocytes. Carrier testing and prenatal diagnosis are also available through molecular genetic techniques.

Disorders of Leucine Metabolism

Isovaleric Acidemia: Isovaleric acidemia, a disorder of leucine metabolism, results from deficient activity of isovaleryl-CoA dehydrogenase. There are two forms of the disorder. In the **severe neonatal form,** infants present within the first 2 weeks of life with poor feeding, vomiting, lethargy, seizures, and hypothermia, which progress to coma. Affected infants have a severe metabolic ketoacidosis and frequently marked secondary hyperammonemia. The elevated organic acid levels may also cause bone marrow depression and lead to neutropenia, thrombocytopenia, or pancytopenia. Approximately one-half of severely affected infants do not survive the neonatal period. In the **chronic intermittent form,** the onset is delayed until later during the first year of life. There is a history of episodes of acute ketoacidosis, vomiting, lethargy, and coma with intercurrent illnesses or increased protein intake. Many patients with the chronic intermittent form have not had significant psychomotor handicaps.

With acute episodes, patients with either form of the disorder will have a characteristic offensive odor described as "sweaty feet" which occurs due to elevated isovaleric acid levels in body fluids. Elevated urine levels of isovalerylglycine, the conjugation product of isovaleryl-CoA and glycine, will be noted at all times on organic acid analysis. With episodes there will also be elevations of 3-hydroxyisovaleric and 4-hydroxyisovaleric acids, in addition to other oxidation and conjugation products of isovaleric acid. Elevated plasma or serum isovaleric acid levels can be detected with short chain organic volatile acid profiles. Carnitine determinations will show lowered free and total, and elevated esterified fractions due to the binding of free carnitine by isovaleryl-CoA. Initial therapy should include intravenous hydration, glucose, and bicarbonate, and supplements of glycine and/or L-carnitine. Patients with the neonatal form may require dialysis, preferably hemodialysis. Maintenance therapy includes diets lowered in protein, special dietary formulas devoid of leucine, and glycine and/or L-carnitine supplements. Deficient activity of isovaleryl-CoA dehydrogenase may be shown with leukocytes or cultured skin fibroblasts. Prenatal diagnosis is available by enzymatic assay in cultured amniocytes or by measuring isovalerylglycine levels in amniotic fluid with stable isotope dilution analysis.

Deficient Activity of 3-Methylcrotonyl-CoA Carboxylase: Deficient activity of 3-methylcrotonyl-CoA carboxylase most often present in early infancy with poor feeding, vomiting, irritability, lethargy, seizures, and hypotonia which may progress to coma. Affected patients have a metabolic acidosis often accompanied by hypoglycemia. With acute episodes of acidosis there may be a characteristic odor described as "cat's urine." Urine organic acid analysis will show elevated levels of 3-methylcrotonylglycine and 3-hydroxyisovaleric acid. Treatment is similar to that for isovaleric acidemia. Deficient activity of 3-methylcrotonyl-CoA carboxylase may also occur as part of holocarboxylase synthetase deficiency or biotinidase deficiency which are discussed later in this section. Because of this, children should also receive supplemental biotin (10 mg daily) until the exact diagnosis is established. Deficient activity of 3-methylcrotonyl-CoA carboxylase may be shown in leukocytes or cultured skin fibroblasts. Prenatal diagnosis is possible.

3-Methylglutaconic Aciduria: 3-Methylglutaconic aciduria exists in multiple forms. The **mild form** is characterized by delayed language development, macrocephaly, and elevated urinary levels of 3-methylglutaconic acid, 3-hydroxyisovaleric acid, and 3-methylglutaric acid. The mild form results from deficient activity of 3-methylglutaconyl-CoA hydratase, which can be measured in leukocytes or cultured skin fibroblasts.

At least two additional forms of the disorder are not associated with deficient activity of the hydratase; the exact biochemical basis remains unknown. In the **severe form,** elevated urinary levels of 3-methylglutaconic and 3-methylglutaric acids are noted in patients with a slowly progressive encephalopathy characterized by hypotonia, spastic quadriparesis, optic atrophy, and psychomotor regression. A third form of the disorder is associated with a dilated cardiomyopathy and neutropenia. Patients with the **cardiac-neutropenia form** of the disorder have elevated urinary levels of ethylhydracrylic acid in addition to elevation of 3-methylglutaconic acid and 3-methylglutaric acid. Elevation of 3-hydroxyisovaleric acid does not occur with the severe and cardiac-neutropenia forms. The mild and severe forms are inherited as autosomal recessive traits; the cardiac-neutropenia form appears to be inherited on an X-linked basis. Affected patients may respond to treatment with a lowered protein diet, special supplements low in leucine, and L-carnitine supplements.

3-Hydroxy-3-Methylglutaric Aciduria: 3-Hydroxy-3-methylglutaric aciduria results from deficient activity of 3-hydroxy-3-methylglutaryl-CoA lyase deficiency. Affected patients present before two years of age with vomiting, lethargy, hypotonia, seizures, metabolic acidosis, and often severe hypoglycemia. One-half of the patients have hyperammonemia and elevated transaminases. Because of the site of the metabolic block, ketosis does not occur. There will be elevated urinary levels of 3-hydroxy-3-methylglutaric acid, 3-hydroxyisovaleric, 3-methylglutaconic acids, and 3-methylglutaric acid. Initial therapy will require intravenous hydration, glucose, and bicarbonate to correct the acidosis. Affected patients may respond to treatment with a lowered protein diet, special supplements low in leucine, and L-carnitine supplements. In addition, fasting should be avoided in that it may precipitate hypoglycemia. Deficient activity of 3-hydroxy-3-methylglutaryl-CoA lyase may be shown in leukocytes or cultured skin fibroblasts.

Mevalonic Aciduria: Mevalonic aciduria is a rare disorder associated with deficient activity of mevalonate kinase. Although the defect is in the leucine metabolic pathway, it is also a defect in the first step in the synthesis of cholesterol and related compounds. Affected patients present with dysmorphic features, severe failure to thrive, cataracts, hepatosplenomegaly, anemia, hypotonia, and cerebral atrophy in early infancy. Milder affected patients may not have dysmorphic features. Plasma cholesterol levels may be normal or slightly low. Urinary organic acid profiles will show markedly elevated levels of mevalonic acid. Deficient activity of mevalonate kinase may be shown in leukocytes or cultured skin fibroblasts. Prenatal diagnosis is available by measuring mevalonate kinase in cultured amniocytes or measuring levels of mevalonic acid in amniotic fluid with stable isotope dilution analysis. There is no effective therapy; patients with the more severe forms have died in infancy.

Disorders of Isoleucine Metabolism

2-Methylacetoacetyl-CoA Thiolase (β-ketothiolase) Deficiency: Patients with 2-methylacetoacetyl-CoA thiolase (β-ketothiolase) deficiency present with wide variations in the clinical severity of their disorder. They may present as early as the neonatal period with severe metabolic ketoacidosis or be diagnosed as adults. In the more severe form patients usually present between 1 and 2 years of age with acute episodes of vomiting, diarrhea, coma, and metabolic ketoacidosis associated with times of intercurrent illnesses or increased protein intake. The patients may have a "sweet" odor. Urine organic acid profiles will show elevated levels of 2-methyl-3-hydroxybutyric acid, and often elevated 2-methylacetoacetic acid, 2-butanone, and tiglylglycine. Treatment of acute episodes should include intravenous hydration, glucose, and bicarbonate. A lowered protein diet may reduce the frequency of acute episodes. Carnitine deficiency does not usually occur. Deficient activity of 2-methylacetoacetyl-CoA thiolase may be shown in leukocytes or cultured skin fibroblasts. Prenatal diagnosis is possible.

Mitochondrial Acetoacetyl-CoA Thiolase Deficiency and Cytosolic Acetoacetyl-CoA Thiolase Deficiency: Mitochondrial acetoacetyl-CoA thiolase deficiency and cytosolic acetoacetyl-CoA thiolase deficiency are very rare disorders associated with chronic ketolactic acidosis, faulty utilization of acetoacetate, and neurological dysfunction. Elevated levels of 3-hydroxybutyrate and acetoacetate occur even when not fasting. The enzymatic deficiencies may be shown in cultured skin fibroblasts or liver biopsy samples.

Disorders of Propionate Metabolism

Propionic Acidemia: Propionic acidemia results from deficient activity of propionyl-CoA carboxylase. Propionyl-CoA, a metabolite of isoleucine, valine, methionine, threonine, odd-chain fatty acids, and cholesterol, is normally metabolized to methylmalonyl-CoA and subsequently to succinyl-CoA which enters the tricarboxylic acid cycle. Deficient activity of propionyl-CoA carboxylase may occur as an isolated disorder. Propionic acidemia may also be seen with multiple carboxylase deficiency, which results from defects in the metabolism of biotin, a cofactor for propionyl-CoA carboxylase and three other carboxylases.

Isolated Propionyl-CoA Carboxylase Deficiency: Most patients with isolated propionyl-CoA carboxylase deficiency present in the neonatal period with poor feeding, emesis, hypotonia, and lethargy, which progress to coma. Seizures and hepatomegaly may also be present. There is severe metabolic acidosis and ketosis. Secondary hyperammonemia may occur from inhibition of the urea cycle and can be as severe as that seen with primary disorders of ammonia metabolism. The elevated organic acids may also cause bone marrow depression leading to neutropenia, thrombocytopenia, or pancytopenia. Patients with less severe forms of the disorder, who often have some residual enzymatic activity, present after the neonatal period with recurrent episodes of ketoacidosis, protein avoidance, psychomotor handicaps, seizures, or failure to thrive. Urine organic acids will show markedly elevated levels of metabolites of propionic acid, including 3-hydroxypropionate, methylcitrate, and tiglylglycine. Elevated plasma or serum propionate levels can be shown with short chain volatile organic acid determinations. Quantitative amino acid testing will reveal markedly elevated levels of glycine which result from inhibition of the glycine-cleaving enzyme complex by the elevated propionyl-CoA levels. Prior to our understanding organic acid metabolism, this disorder was known as one of the ketotic hyperglycinemias. Plasma levels of free and total carnitine will be low and levels of esterified carnitine will be elevated. Acyl-carnitine or acyl-glycine determinations will also show an abnormal profile characteristic of the disorder.

Treatment of acute ketoacidotic episodes will require intravenous hydration, glucose, and bicarbonate. Dialysis, preferable hemodialysis, may be needed. Intravenous carnitine and increasing caloric intake with special formulas which lack the precursor amino acids for propionyl-CoA have been shown to improve control of acute ketoacidotic episodes. Biotin (10 mg daily) should also be given until a diagnosis of multiple carboxylase deficiency is excluded. Even with aggressive therapy, many patients with neonatal onset of their disorder do not survive and those that do have psychomotor handicaps. Affected patients are also at risk for repeated episodes of ketoacidosis which can be life-threatening. The outcome is better for the milder forms of the disorder and for those patients who are subsequently found to have multiple carboxylase deficiency. Deficient activity of propionyl-CoA carboxylase may be shown with leukocytes or cultured skin fibroblasts. Prenatal diagnosis has been accomplished by measurement of methylcitrate in amniotic fluid and by direct enzymatic assay or ^{14}C-propionate fixation using cultured amniocytes.

Multiple Carboxylase Deficiency and Biotinidase Deficiency

Biotin is an essential, water soluble, B vitamin which is found in many dietary sources of plant and animal origin. It can also be synthesized by intestinal microflora. Nutritional biotin deficiency is exceedingly rare. Biotin deficiency, however, has been reported in patients on prolonged total parenteral hyperalimentation without biotin and in patients who have been on chronic anticonvulsant therapy with phenytoin, primidone, or carbamazepine. Deficiency of biotin results in cutaneous and neurological symptoms. The cutaneous manifestations include alopecia, an erythematous perioral rash, dry skin, and secondary superficial *Candida* infections. Neurological symptoms include depression, apathy, myalgia, hyperesthesia, or paresthesia.

Biotin functions as a cofactor for four carboxylases. The carboxylases include cytosolic acetyl-CoA carboxylase, which is involved with the biosynthesis of long chain fatty acids; mitochondrial β-methylcrotonyl-CoA carboxylase, which is involved with the metabolism of leucine; mitochondrial pyruvate carboxylase, which is involved with the pathways of gluconeogenesis; and mitochondrial propionyl-CoA carboxylase, which is involved with the metabolism of four amino acids, odd-chain fatty acids, and cholesterol. Isolated deficiencies for the three mitochondrial carboxylases are discussed elsewhere in this section and result from mutations at the genetic locus for the carboxylase involved. Only one patient with cytosolic acetyl-CoA carboxylase deficiency has been reported. Patients with the isolated carboxylase deficiencies do not respond to biotin therapy.

The carboxylases are synthesized as inactive apoenzymes. Biotin becomes covalently attached to the apoenzymes by the action of holocarboxylase synthetase. The biotin-apoenzyme complex is termed a holocarboxylase and has enzymatic activity. Free biotin, which can be recycled, is released during intracellular proteolytic degradation of the holocarboxylases by the action of biotinidase.

Multiple Carboxylase Deficiency: Two disorders, holocarboxylase synthetase deficiency and biotinidase deficiency, are associated with metabolic defects in biotin metabolism. Both disorders result in reduced activity of the carboxylases, which require biotin as a cofactor. These disorders, known as multiple carboxylase deficiency, result in clinical and biochemical findings which are a combination of those seen with the isolated individual disorders. Patients with multiple carboxylase deficiency, whether due to holocarboxylase synthetase deficiency or biotinidase deficiency, will respond to biotin therapy.

Holocarboxylase Synthetase Deficiency: Holocarboxylase synthetase deficiency usually becomes evident in the newborn period and is less common than biotinidase deficiency. Affected patients present as neonates or young infants with poor feeding, vomiting, lethargy, hypotonia, and seizures which can progress to coma. Patients with later onset of the disorder may also have alopecia, perioral rashes, dermatitis, psychomotor handicaps, ataxia, hearing impairment, and optic atrophy. A metabolic ketosis and lactic acidosis will be present which is often accompanied by secondary hyperammonemia and bone marrow depression. Urine organic acid profiles will show elevated levels of 3-hydroxyisovaleric acid, 3-methylcrotonylglycine, 3-hydroxypropionate, methylcitrate, tiglylglycine, and lactate. Initial management of the patient should include intravenous hydration, glucose, and bicarbonate if the acidosis is significant. Patients respond to biotin therapy at an initial dose of 10 mg daily. The outcome will vary with the degree of acidosis and hyperammonemia during the initial presentation. Residual neurological problems may occur. The disorder is confirmed by showing reduced activity of propionyl-CoA carboxylase, pyruvate carboxylase, and 3-methylcrotonyl-CoA carboxylase in leukocytes (before biotin therapy) or cultured skin fibroblasts. Biotinidase activity will be normal. Prenatal diagnosis is available by means of enzymatic assay of the carboxylases in cultured amniotic fluid cells or by measurement of 3-hydroxyisovaleric acid and/or methylcitrate levels in amniotic fluid by stable isotope dilution analysis.

Biotinidase Deficiency: Biotinidase deficiency is more common than holocarboxylase synthetase deficiency and usually presents after 3 months of age and prior to age 3 years. Biotinidase deficiency occurs in approximately one in 61,000 births and is most common among French Canadians. Newborn screening for biotinidase deficiency occurs in some areas of the United States. Although acute metabolic acidosis with secondary hyperammonemia and bone marrow depression may occur, the disorder is more often associated with chronic dermatologic and neurologic problems. Psychomotor delay, ataxia, myoclonic seizures, hypotonia, hearing loss, visual problems, or optic atrophy are common. Partial or complete alopecia, perioral rashes, conjunctivitis, and other forms dermatitis are often noted. Patients

with a milder case, with residual biotinidase activity, may develop only alopecia or dermatitis. Urine organic acid profiles will show elevated levels of 3-hydroxyisovaleric acid, 3-methylcrotonylglycine, 3-hydroxypropionate, methylcitrate, tiglylglycine, and lactate. Initial therapy should include intravenous hydration, glucose, and bicarbonate if there is a significant metabolic acidosis. All patients have shown a clinical response to biotin at an initial dose of 10 mg daily. Residual neurological deficits, especially hearing loss and optic atrophy, may continue. The disorder is confirmed by demonstrating deficient activity of biotinidase in serum, leukocytes, or cultured skin fibroblasts. Because the activities of the carboxylases in leukocytes may be lowered prior to biotin therapy, and thus be misleading, simultaneous measurements of biotinidase and leukocytes carboxylase activity should be done on all patients suspected of having either of the disorders associated with multiple carboxylase deficiency. Activity of the carboxylases will be normal in cultured skin fibroblasts. Prenatal diagnosis is possible by measurement of biotinidase activity in cultured amniocytes.

Disorders of Methylmalonate and Cobalamin Metabolism

Methylmalonyl-CoA, a metabolite of propionyl-CoA and thymine, is normally metabolized to succinyl-CoA by the actions of methylmalonyl-CoA racemase and methylmalonyl-CoA mutase. Methylmalonyl-CoA mutase is produced as an apoenzyme that requires adenosylcobalamin, an active form of cobalamin (vitamin B_{12}), as its cofactor. Cobalamin is widely distributed in animal tissues and synthesized by microorganisms in soil, water, rumen, or the intestine. Dietary deficiency of cobalamin results in the disease known as pernicious anemia, which is associated with a megaloblastic anemia and cerebellar and posterior column neurological abnormalities. After absorption, dietary cobalamin, as hydroxocobalamin, is transported bound to transcobalamin II into the lysosomes of hepatic cells by absorptive endocytosis. While in the lysosome, the hydroxocobalamin is released from transcobalamin II and then actively excreted from the lysosome. The hydroxocobalamin is then converted to either methylcobalamin in the cytosol, or taken up into the mitochondria for conversion to adenosylcobalamin by the actions of two reductases and an adenosyltransferase (Figure 13–7). Methylcobalamin is a cofactor for N^5-methyltetrahydrofolate:homocysteine methytransferase, which catalyzes the remethylation of homocystine to methionine. Adenosylcobalamin is a cofactor for methylmalonyl-CoA mutase. Table 13–3 lists the various forms of methylmalonic acidemia and homocystinuria and their corresponding metabolic defects.

Isolated Methylmalonic Acidemia: Isolated methylmalonic acidemia results from deficient activity of methylmalonyl-CoA mutase. The disorder may result from mutations at the genetic locus for methylmalonyl-CoA mutase or from defects in the metabolism of hydroxocobalamin which result in failure of the formation of adenosylcobalamin, the cofactor for methylmalonyl-CoA mutase. There are four forms of isolated methylmalonic acidemia which have been characterized on the basis of the biochemical defects involved or by complementation groups found with studies of cultured skin fibroblasts from affected patients. Patients with the **mut⁰ form** of the disorder have essentially no mutase activity, whereas patients with the **mut⁻ form** translate a structurally abnormal mutase which has some residual enzymatic activity. Patients with **cblA** and **cblB** forms of the disorder have defects in the formation of adenosylcobalamin, the cofactor for methylmalonyl-CoA mutase. The cblA form is associated with reduced activity of the mitochondrial cobalamin reductase and the cblB form with reduced activity of mitochondrial cobalamin adenosyltransferase. Approximately one-third of patients with methymalonyl mutase deficiency will have the mut⁰ form, 31% will

have the cblA form, 25% will have the cblB form, and 11% will have the mut⁻ form of the disorder.

In general, the four forms are clinically indistinguishable except that the mut⁰ patients will present earlier than patients with the other forms. Most patients present within the first week of life with poor feeding, lethargy, vomiting, hypotonia, and respiratory distress which progress to coma. Hepatomegaly may be present. In older patients, psychomotor delays and failure to thrive are commonly seen. All forms will have a severe metabolic ketoacidosis with secondary hyperammonemia. Depression of the bone marrow may result in neutropenia, thrombocytopenia, or pancytopenia. The patients do not have a megaloblastic anemia. Serum cobalamin (vitamin B_{12}) levels will be normal. Urine organic acids will show markedly elevated levels of methylmalonic acid in addition to metabolites of propionyl-CoA such as 3-hydroxypropionate and methylcitrate. Quantitative amino acids will show elevated levels of glycine due to inhibition of the glycine-cleaving enzyme complex. Plasma levels of free and total carnitine will be low-

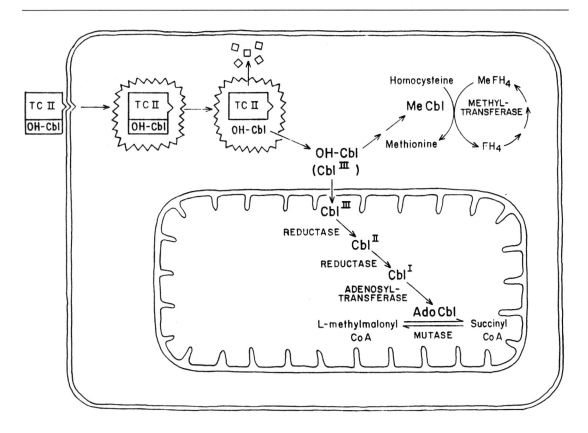

Figure 13–7. General pathway of the cellular uptake and subcellular compartmentation of cobalamins, and of the intracellular distribution and enzymatic synthesis of cobalamin coenzymes. Abbreviations: TC II = transcobalamin II; OH-Cbl = hydroxocobalamin; MeCbl = methylcobalamin; AdoCbl = adenosylcobalamin; CblᴵᴵᴵI, CblᴵᴵI, CblᴵI = cobalamins with cobalt valences of 3⁺, 2⁺, and 1⁺, respectively. (Reproduced with permission from: Scriver CR et al: *The Metabolic and Molecular Bases of Inherited Disease,* 7th ed, McGraw-Hill, 1995.)

Table 13–3. Metabolic defects in methylmalonic acidemia and homocystinuria.

Disorder	Metabolic Defect	Mechanism of Defect
Methylmalonic acidemia	Methylmalonyl-CoA mutase deficiency	1. Form mut°; mutation at genetic locus which results in no enzymatic activity 2. Form mut⁻; structurally abnormal enzyme
	Defects in the formation of adenosylcobalamin	1. Form cblA*; defect in mitochondrial cobalamin reductase 2. Form cblB; defect in mitochondrial cobalamin adenosyltransferase
Combined methylmalonic acidemia and homocystinuria	Defects in the formation of both adenosylcobalamin and methylcobalamin	1. Form cblC; unknown defect in cytosolic hydroxocobalamin metabolism 2. Form cblD; unknown defect in cytosolic hydroxocobalamin metabolism 3. Form cblF; defect in exit of hydroxocobalamin from lysosomes

Homocystinuria	Defects in the remethylation of homocystine to methionine	1. Defects in the synthesis of methylcobalamin (functional N^5-methyltetrahydrofolate:homocysteine methyltransferase deficiency)
		  a. Form cblE; exact defect unknown
		  b. Form cblG; exact defect unknown
		2. Defects in folate metabolism
		  a. 5,10-Methylenetetrahydrofolate reductase deficiency

	Cystathionine synthetase deficiency	1. Mutations at genetic locus which result in reduced enzymatic activity

* The cbl (cobalamin) forms are designated on the basis of complementation groups found in studies of affected patients.

ered and esterified carnitine fractions elevated. Initial treatment should include intravenous hydration, glucose, and bicarbonate to correct the acidosis. Occasionally dialysis, preferably hemodialysis, may be needed. Diets lowered in protein, special supplements low in the precursor amino acids (isoleucine, valine, methionine, and threonine) as for propionic acidemia, and carnitine are used for maintenance therapy. All patients should also receive daily intramuscular injections of hydroxocobalamin. Although patients with the mut° and mut⁻ forms will not respond to hydroxocobalamin, 90% of patients with the cblA form and 40% of the cblB form will respond. Measurement of the activity of methylmalonyl-CoA mutase and complementation or radiolabeled cobalamin studies may be done with cultured skin fibroblasts. It is important to know the exact form of the disorder for long-term management of the patients. Prenatal diagnosis is available by measurement of methylmalonic acid levels in amniotic fluid and by enzymatic determination of methylmalonyl-CoA mutase activity in cultured amniotic fluid cells. Levels of methylmalonic acid in midtrimester maternal urine have also been used to predict an affected pregnancy, but are not diagnostic by themselves.

Methylmalonic Acidemia Combined With Homocystinuria: Methylmalonic acidemia may also occur in combination with homocystinuria as a result of defects in the metabolism of cobalamin which result in the failure of formation of both adenosylcobalamin and methylcobalamin. Activities of both methylmalonyl-CoA mutase and N^5-methyltetrahy-drofolate:homocysteine methyltransferase (methionine synthetase) are deficient. Three forms of this rare disorder, named **cblC, cblD,** and **cblF,** have been identified by complementation studies. In types cblC and cblD, the exact defect is unknown, but it occurs after lysosomal processing and during the cytosolic metabolism of hydroxocobalamin. The cblF form results from a defect in the process by which hydroxocobalamin exits the lysosomes. The cblC form is most common and usually presents in infants less than 2 months of age. Clinical symptoms include failure to thrive, poor feeding, lethargy, hypertonicity, and progressive neurological dysfunction. Affected patients with a later onset will have cortical atrophy and myelopathies. The cblC patients usually do not have the severe metabolic ketoacidosis, secondary hyperammonemia, or hyperglycinemia as seen with mutase deficient forms of methylmalonic acidemia. A megaloblastic, macrocytic anemia is often present which may be accompanied by hypersegmented polymorphonuclear leukocytes and thrombocytopenia. Levels of cobalamin and folate will be normal. Urine organic acids will show elevations of methylmalonic acid, but less than that noted with methylmalonyl-CoA mutase deficiency. Quantitative amino acids will show elevated homocystine and cystathionine levels, but lowered methionine levels, consistent with a defect in the remethylation of homocystine to methionine.

Treatment includes large intramuscular doses of hydroxocobalamin, lowered protein diets, and betaine, which facilitates the remethylation of homocystine to methionine. Many patients do not respond to therapy and die in infancy. Those that survive often have severe psychomotor handicaps. The enzymatic diagnosis is confirmed by complementation or radiolabeled cobalamin studies in cultured skin fibroblasts. Prenatal diagnosis may be accomplished by measurement of methylmalonic levels in amniotic fluid. The two other forms of the disorder, cblD and cblF, are very rare and appear to be not as severe as the cblC form.

Two additional rare forms of cobalamin defects, **cblE** and **cblG,** are associated with defects in the formation of methylcobalamin, a cofactor for N^5-methyltetrahydrofolate:homocysteine methyltransferase (methionine synthetase). Affected patients have reduced activity of N^5methyltetrahydrofolate:homocysteine methyltransferase and a defect in the remethylation of homocystine to methionine. Most affected patients present in infancy with poor feeding, lethargy, hypotonia, and delayed development. They have homocystinuria, reduced methionine levels, and megaloblastic anemias. They do not have methylmalonic acidemia. Cobalamin and folate levels are normal. The exact defect in the formation of methylcobalamin in the cblE and cblG forms is unclear but the two forms are differentiated by complementation and radiolabeled cobalamin studies. Affected patients will respond to large doses of intramuscular hydroxocobalamin, folinic acid, and betaine therapy. However, neurological problems may remain. Prenatal diagnosis is possible. One patient with the cblE form was diagnosed prenatally, treated from birth with hydroxocobalamin, and has developed normally.

DISORDERS OF PROLINE
AND HYDROXYPROLINE METABOLISM

Proline and hydroxyproline, also known as imino acids, are nonessential amino acids. Proline and its metabolite pyrroline-5-carboxylate are important regulators of cellular metabolism which are linked to protein synthesis and the production of phosphoribosyl pyrophosphate and purine nucleotides. Proline may be synthesized from ornithine or glutamate. Hydroxyproline exists mainly bound to peptides (iminopeptides) in collagen; little hydroxyproline exists as the free amino acid. Hydroxyproline is formed by the hydroxylation of proline in procollagen and degraded to glyoxylate and pyruvate.

Elevated levels of proline and hydroxyproline may be noted with the hyperprolinemias (types I and II) and hyperhydroxyprolinemia. Elevated urinary glycine, in addition to elevated urinary proline and hydroxyproline (iminoglycinuria), may occur as a result of a defect in a shared renal tubular transport mechanism for these three amino acids. Patients with these findings do not appear to have any significant clinical problems.

Deficient Activity of Prolidase (Peptidase D):
Elevated levels of urinary iminopeptides which contain proline and hydroxyproline, especially glycylproline, result from deficient activity of prolidase (peptidase D). This enzyme is important in conserving proline and hydroxyproline from dietary sources or during collagen turnover. The disorder is a rare autosomal recessive condition that is associated with a chronic erythematous dermatitis on the face, palms, and soles, or with severe progressive ulcerations on the lower legs. Two-thirds of affected patients also have psychomotor retardation and recurrent infections. Occasional patients have been reported to have splenomegaly, prominent sutures, an abnormal shape of the skull, ptosis, or ocular proptosis. Other patients, detected by newborn screening programs, have been asymptomatic. The age of onset is variable from birth to adult life; the average age at diagnosis is 7 years. Deficient activity of prolidase may be shown in erythrocytes, leukocytes, or cultured skin fibroblasts. Prenatal diagnosis is possible.

DISORDERS OF THE γ-GLUTARYL CYCLE

The synthesis and degradation of glutathione (L-γ-glutamyl-L-cysteinyl-glycine) occurs in the γ-glutamyl cycle (Figure 13–8). Glutathione is a component of many important metabolic reactions. Glutathione is involved with the formation and maintenance of sulfhydryl groups of proteins and enzymes (eg, coenzyme A), provides reducing capacity for several reactions (eg, the formation of deoxyribonucleotides), and functions in the detoxification of peroxides, free radicals, some medications, and other compounds. Glutathione is also involved with the transport of amino acids across cell membranes. High levels of membrane-bound γ-glutamyl transpeptidase are found in tissues involved with amino acid transport such as the kidney, small intestine, choroid plexis, and the ciliary body. The enyzme γ-glutamyl transpeptidase catalyzes the formation of γ-glutamyl-amino acids from glutathione and extracellular amino acids, most often cystine, glutamine, methionine, and other neutral amino acids at the outer border of the cell membrane. Then the amino acids are transported as γ-glutamyl-amino acids across the cell membrane into the cytosol. Once inside the cells, the amino acids are released from the γ-glutamyl-amino acids with the formation of 5-oxoproline (pyroglutamate), a ring formation. 5-Oxoproline is then converted to glutamic acid (straight chain amino acid) by 5-oxoprolinase.

Five inherited disorders of the γ-glutamyl cycle are known. Three are associated with reduced synthesis of glutathione and two result from defects in glutathione degradation. All of the disorders are inherited as autosomal recessive traits.

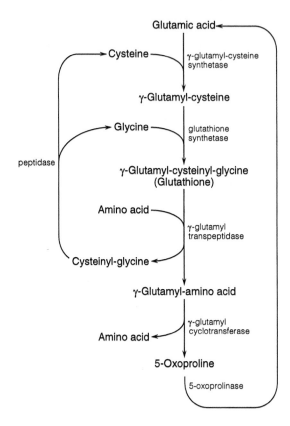

Figure 13–8. The γ-glutamyl cycle.

5-Oxoprolinuria (Pyroglutamic Aciduria): Generalized deficiency of glutathione synthetase results in 5-oxoprolinuria (pyroglutamic aciduria). Affected patients have the onset in infancy of chronic metabolic acidosis, mild hemolytic anemia, progressive psychomotor retardation, and cerebellar dysfunction. Neutropenia, defective granulocyte function, and increased susceptibility to bacterial infections have also been reported. Patients display markedly elevated blood and urine 5-oxoproline levels and reduced levels of erythrocyte glutathione. The low cellular levels of glutathione, and lack of normal feedback inhibition of γ-glutamyl-cysteine synthetase, lead to the overproduction of γ-glutamyl-cysteine, which is converted to 5-oxoproline. The 5-oxoproline may be detected by organic acid analysis. Measurement of glutathione synthetase activity may be shown in erythrocytes and cultured skin fibroblasts. Acute episodes of acidosis are treated with intravenous hydration and bicarbonate. Bicarbonate

or other buffers are often needed for maintenance therapy. Patients with 5-oxoprolinuria should avoid medications that require glutathione in their metabolism. Acetaminophen should be specifically avoided. Affected patients should also avoid therapeutic oxygen and radiation, or any other situation that may result in the formation of free radicals. Vitamin E may improve erythrocyte survival and granulocyte function.

Deficiency of Glutathione Synthetase Limited to Erythrocytes: Deficiency of glutathione synthetase limited to erythrocytes is associated with lowered levels of erythrocyte glutathione and a compensated hemolytic anemia. Occasionally splenomegaly may occur. There is no central nervous system involvement or 5-oxoprolinuria.

Deficient Activity of γ-Glutamyl-cysteine Synthetase: Deficient activity of γ-glutamyl-cysteine synthetase results in mild hemolytic anemia, spinocerebellar degeneration, peripheral neuropathies, myopathies, and a generalized amino aciduria in young adults. There is a generalized deficiency of glutathione and decreased formation of γ-glutamyl compounds. Elevated levels of 5-oxoproline do not occur. Deficient activity of γ-glutamyl-cysteine synthetase and reduced levels of glutathione may be shown in erythrocytes.

Deficient Activity of γ-Glutamyl Transpeptidase: Deficient activity of γ-glutamyl transpeptidase has been reported in young adults with psychomotor handicaps. Blood and urine glutathione, γ-glutamyl-cysteine, and cysteine levels are elevated. Hemolytic anemia does not occur. The enzymatic deficiency may be shown in cultured skin fibroblasts.

Deficient Activity of 5-Oxoprolinase: Deficient activity of 5-oxoprolinase results in elevated blood and urine levels of 5-oxoproline. There do not appear to be any related clinical problems. Deficiency of glutamic acid does not occur, in that it is present in foods and can also be synthesized from α-ketoglutarate.

Elevated levels of 5-oxoproline may also occur as a result of intestinal bacterial cyclization of glutamate or with the use of artificial diets. Elevation of 5-oxoproline may also be seen in patients with severe burns, Stevens-Johnson syndrome, or homocystinuria.

DISORDERS OF OXALATE METABOLISM

Both forms of hyperoxaluria, type I and type II, are autosomal recessive conditions that result in elevated urinary levels of oxalate and other organic acids. Because oxalate is relatively insoluble in water, affected patients develop nephrocalcinosis, calcium oxalate stones in the urinary tract, and extrarenal deposition of calcium oxalate crystals.

Type I Hyperoxaluria: Type I hyperoxaluria, more common than type II, is associated with deficient activity of peroxisomal alanine:glyoxalate aminotransferase and increased urinary excretion of oxalate, glyoxalic and glycolic acids. (See disorders of peroxisomes.)

Type II Hyperoxaluria: Type II hyperoxaluria, a rare condition, is associated with deficient activity of D-glyceric dehydrogenase which is extraperoxisomal in location. Patients excrete elevated levels of oxalate and L-glyceric acid. The exact mechanism for the hyperoxaluria in type II hyperoxaluria is unclear, however a defect in hydroxypyruvate metabolism is proposed which may indirectly increase the synthesis of oxalate from glyoxylate. Patients usually develop urinary tract stones by age 2 years, although more severely affected patients may develop stones during the first year of life. Other presenting signs include hematuria, nephrocalcinosis, urinary tract obstruc-

tion, renal colic, urinary tract infection, or renal failure. Renal failure is less common in type II compared to type I hyperoxaluria. Calcium oxalate deposition can also occur in the joints, leading to arthritis; in the heart, resulting in conduction defects; in the testes; and rarely, in the eye. The diagnosis is established by measuring oxalate excretion in a 24-hour urine collection. Urine organic acid determinations using isotope dilution analysis will show elevated L-glyceric acid levels. Treatment is directed at reducing the concentration of oxalate in the urine by increasing fluid intake, by avoiding natural foods high in oxalate (eg, spinach, rhubarb, cocoa, tea), and by alkalinizing the urine to increase the solubility of oxalate. Surgical removal of stones may be needed. Analysis of the stones may suggest the diagnosis. Deficient activity of D-glyceric dehydrogenase may be shown in leukocytes.

Secondary Hyperoxaluria: Secondary hyperoxaluria is not uncommon and may occur from ingestion of ascorbic acid or ethylene glycol, or from pyridoxine deficiency, increased intake of natural foods high in oxalate, and hyperabsorption of oxalate due to inflammatory bowel disease, disorders associated with fat malabsorption, or surgical intestinal resections. Urinary glycolic, glyoxalic, and L-glyceric acids are not increased with secondary hyperoxaluria.

DISORDERS OF AMINO ACID TRANSPORT

Inherited defects in each of three high capacity transport systems are associated with the decreased intestinal absorption and increased renal excretion of amino acids. The systems involve the transport of the dibasic, neutral, and iminoglycine groups of amino acids. Defective transport of the dibasic amino acids occurs in cystinuria; defective transport of the neutral amino acids results in Hartnup disease. A defect in the third transport system involving the iminoglycine group of amino acids (proline, hydroxyproline, and glycine) results in increased renal excretion of these amino acids in otherwise normal individuals and is not associated with clinical disease. Two additional disorders, lysinuric protein intolerance and hyperammonemia-hyperornithinemia-homocitrullinuria syndrome, are associated with hyperammonemia as a result of defective transport of amino acids essential for proper functioning of the urea cycle.

Cystinuria: Cystinuria is an autosomal recessive disorder estimated to occur in 1 in 7000 births. Cystinuria results from a defect in the high affinity renal tubular and intestinal transport system for cystine and the dibasic amino acids, lysine, arginine, and ornithine. Because the normal renal reabsorption of these amino acids does not occur, there are markedly elevated urine levels of cystine, lysine, arginine, or-nithine, and the mixed disulfide cysteine-homocys-teine. In addition, increased renal secretion of cystine may also occur. Cystine is extremely insoluble at high concentrations which leads to the formation of multiple recurrent renal calculi at any age, but most often during the second and third decades. Patients with cystinuria may present with acute abdominal pain from movement of a stone within the urinary tract, hydronephrosis or other obstruction of the uri-nary tract, urinary tract infections, hematuria, or re-nal failure. Affected patients may also have a history of passing very small stones known as "gravel." Cys-tine crystals have been observed in the diapers of af-fected infants. Usually the stones are radiopaque; they may form staghorn-shaped calculi. Microscopic urine examination will reveal cystine crystals in the shape of characteristic hexagonal plates. Urine spot testing with cyanide-nitroprusside will be positive. Analysis of a urinary tract stone may be helpful in suggesting the diagnosis. Although urinary lysine levels are the most elevated of the four amino acids involved, they do not result in clinical symptoms. Plasma levels of the amino acids involved may be lowered but are not of clinical significance.

Treatment is aimed at reducing the concentration of urinary cystine, and thus the stone formation. Most patients respond to increased oral intake of fluids, al-kalization of the urine (which increases the solubility of cystine), and reduced protein intake. Some patients will require the use of D-penicillamine (β,β-dimethyl-cysteine), N-acetyl-D-penicillamine, or 2-mercapto-propionyl glycine, which form cysteine-disulfides that are more soluble than cystine. Surgical removal of the urinary tract stones may be needed. Patients with ad-vanced renal disease may require renal transplant.

There are three allelic forms of cystinuria which dif-fer in the extent of intestinal defect in affected ho-mozygotes and whether or not heterozygous carriers have increased urinary excretion of the amino acids. Type I affected homozygotes have reduced intestinal transport of cystine, lysine, and arginine; type II ho-mozygotes have decreased lysine and variably reduced cystine intestinal transport; type III homozygotes dis-play a variable reduction in both lysine and cystine intestinal transport. Type I heterozygote carriers do not have increased urinary excretion of the amino acids, whereas type II and type II heterozygotes do. Many affected patients have been found to be com-pound heterozygotes for the different types of cysti-nuria.

Hartnup Disease: Hartnup disease results from defective renal and intestinal transport of the "neu-tral" amino acids. There is increased urinary and fe-cal excretion of alanine, serine, threonine, valine, isoleucine, leucine, phenylalanine, tyrosine, histidine, glutamine, asparagine, and most importantly, trypto-phan. Plasma levels of these amino acids are normal or reduced. Bacterial degradation of fecal tryptophan

results in the increased formation of indican and in-dolic acids, which are absorbed from the intestine and excreted in the urine of affected patients. Malab-sorption of tryptophan, a precursor for nicotinic acid (niacin) and nicotinamide, appears to be responsible for the clinical manifestations which are similar to those seen with nutritional niacin deficiency, or pel-lagra. A photosensitive, erythematous rash appears on exposed skin areas, which becomes desquamated and often depigmented. Intermittent episodes of ataxia occur, which can be associated with tremors, nystagmus, diplopia, increased motor tone and re-flexes, and nonspecific changes in electroencephalo-gram patterns. Affected patients may also have psy-chological problems, behavioral changes, or mild psychomotor handicaps.

On the basis of results from newborn screening programs, Hartnup disease is estimated to occur in one in 24,000 births. It is inherited as an autosomal recessive trait. Clinically symptomatic patients will respond to supplemental nicotinamide at a dose equal to that of twice the recommended dietary intake for age. Because individuals with Hartnup disease who have been detected by newborn screening programs are usually asymptomatic, it appears that additional environmental factors, eg, diarrhea or a lowered pro-tein intake, or other genetic factors may be involved with the development of clinical symptoms. In addi-tion, symptomatic patients are rarely seen in devel-oped countries, which have niacin-fortified cereals and grains and adequate protein diets.

Lysinuric Protein Intolerance (LPI): Lysinuric protein intolerance (LPI), which occurs most often in persons of Finnish background, is associated with a defect in the intestinal, hepatic, and renal tubular transport of the dibasic amino acids (lysine, arginine, ornithine) and cystine. These patients show marked elevation of urinary lysine levels. Elevation of uri-nary arginine and ornithine, but only slightly in-creased urinary cystine occurs, which distinguishes the disorder from cystinuria. Plasma values of lysine, arginine, and ornithine are low. Many of the clinical findings are related to lysine deficiency which results in impaired collagen production. Urea synthesis is impaired as a result of the deficiencies of arginine and ornithine. Moderate elevation of plasma ammo-nia (usually in the range of 100–300 µM), elevated plasma citrulline, and elevated urinary orotic acid usually occur only after eating meals that contain protein. Patients with LPI present during infancy or childhood with protein avoidance, vomiting, diar-rhea, short stature, lenticular opacities, hepatospleno-megaly, interstitial lung disease, hyperelastic skin, hyperextensible joints, osteoporosis, sparse hair, hy-potonia, psychomotor delays, and pancytopenia. A lowered protein diet and supplemental L-citrulline are recommended for treatment. L-Citrulline is a pre-cursor of L-arginine and is not transported by the same system as L-arginine or L-ornithine.

Hyperammonemia-hyperornithinemia-homocitrullinuria (HHH) Syndrome: Hyperammonemia-hyperornithinemia-homocitrullinuria syndrome, or HHH syndrome, results from defective transport of ornithine into the mitochondria, where it is needed for urea synthesis. Most patients present during the first year of life with intermittent episodes of hyperammonemia, and moderate elevation of plasma ornithine. Patients display increased urinary levels of the dibasic amino acids and homocitrulline, a metabolite of lysine. Urinary orotic acid may be elevated. Treatment includes ornithine supplements and a lowered protein diet.

REFERENCES AND SUGGESTED READING

See Page 256 and Appendix II.

14   Carbohydrate Metabolism

DISORDERS OF GALACTOSE METABOLISM

Classic Galactosemia: Classic galactosemia, an autosomal recessive condition that affects 1 in 62,000 births, is associated with deficient activity of galactose-1-phosphate uridyl transferase (Figure 14–1). Affected infants are normal at birth, but with the ingestion of galactose develop symptoms usually within the first week of life. Vomiting, diarrhea, poor weight gain, and prolonged hyperbilirubinemia are common. Hepatomegaly, hepatic dysfunction, nuclear cataracts, and generalized renal tubular dysfunction develop. With continued ingestion of galactose the infants become increasingly encephalopathic and may develop hepatic failure and septicemia, especially with *Esherichia coli.* If not recognized and treated, most will die by 6 weeks of age. There may be a non-glucose reducing substance present in the urine, provided that there has been sufficient intake of galactose, which may not occur in those that are ill or receiving intravenous fluids. Blood and tissue levels of galactose-1-phosphate are elevated and thought to be toxic to the liver, kidneys, and central nervous system. The conversion of elevated galactose to galactitol, an osmotic compound, is thought to be responsible for swelling and disruption of lenticular fibers, which leads to cataract formation. The disorder can be confirmed by demonstrating reduced activity of galactose-1-phosphate uridyl transferase in erthrocytes or cultured skin fibroblasts. Although treatment with dietary restriction of galactose will result in clinical improvement, many patients will later have learning disabilities, and females frequently have ovarian atrophy. Those who experience septicemia and meningitis often have additional residual defects. Newborn screening for galactosemia is being carried out in many states. Most testing employs measurement of blood galactose or galactose-1-phosphate levels. Given the severity of this disorder, infants identified as presumptive positives by newborn screening should be immediately switched to a formula free of galactose until the definitive testing is completed. Continued restriction of galactose, in the form of foods and in medications, should be continued for life. Milder forms of classical galactosemia are known which may not become symptomatic until after 4 months of age.

There are numerous mutant alleles at the galactose-1-phosphate uridyl transferase (transferase) locus which may or may not result in clinical symptoms. The most common of these is the Duarte variant, which results in a 50% reduction of enzymatic activity. Heterozygotes for the Duarte allele occur in 8–13% of the general population. Approximately 1 in 4000 newborns are compound heterozygotes for the Duarte allele (D) and the allele for classic galactosemia (G). Infants with **D/G galactosemia** have about 25% of normal transferase activity and will usually be detected by newborn screening. Most have elevated levels of galactose-1-phosphate and require dietary restriction of galactose for the first 6–12 months of life. The Duarte and other variants are confirmed by characteristic banding patterns noted on starch-gel eletrophoresis, in addition to measurement of erythrocyte transferase activity. The genes for classic galactosemia and many of the variants have been cloned. Carrier detection and prenatal diagnosis are available.

Galactokinase deficiency: Galactokinase deficiency, an autosomal recessive disorder, occurs in 1 in 150,000 births and is associated with increased galactose levels and cataracts. The other systemic features of classic galactosemia do not occur. Although cataracts usually regress with dietary galactose restriction, surgical removal may be needed.

Generalized Uridine Diphosphate Galactose-4-Epimerase Deficiency: Generalized uridine diphosphate galactose-4-epimerase deficiency is a rare, autosomal recessive disorder, which presents with clinical features similar to those seen in classic galactosemia. The disorder will be detected by newborn screening programs that measure blood galactose or galactose-1-phosphate levels and should be considered in patients with symptoms of classic galactosemia who have normal transferase activity.

Deficiency of Uridine Diphosphate Galactose-4-Epimerase, Confined Only to Leukocytes, Lymphocytes and Erythrocytes: Deficiency of uridine diphosphate galactose-4-epimerase, confined only to leukocytes, lymphocytes and erythrocytes, occurs in 1 in 46,000 births and is not associated with clinical abnormalities. The disorder is mentioned because it may result in positive newborn screening in those programs that measure erythrocyte galactose-1-phosphate levels.

DISORDERS OF FRUCTOSE METABOLISM

Fructose-1-Phosphate Aldolase B Deficiency: Fructose-1-phosphate aldolase B deficiency, or **he-**

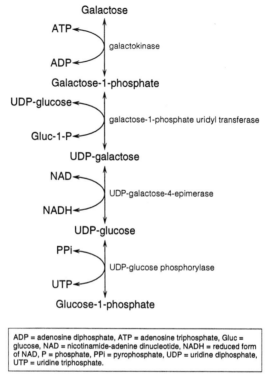

ADP = adenosine diphosphate, ATP = adenosine triphosphate, Gluc = glucose, NAD = nicotinamide-adenine dinucleotide, NADH = reduced form of NAD, P = phosphate, PPi = pyrophosphate, UDP = uridine diphosphate, UTP = uridine triphosphate.

Figure 14–1. Metabolism of galactose.

reditary fructose intolerance, is an autosomal recessive trait that is estimated to occur in 1 in 20,000 individuals. The disorder appears to be most common in persons of European ancestry. Clinical manifestations appear only after the ingestion of dietary fructose or sucrose, a disaccharide composed of fructose and glucose. Thus, in infancy, symptoms appear after weaning or with the introduction of foods naturally high in fructose, eg, fruits, juices, and vegetables, or formulas or other foods that contain sucrose. Many patients, even infants, will avoid foods that are sweet in taste. Symptoms are more severe in young infants than in older children and adults and may occur as acute episodes or chronic findings. With acute fructose ingestion, sweating, trembling, emesis, lethargy, coma, seizures, and shock may occur due to hypoglycemia and the depletion of intracellular Pi and ATP. At the time of an acute episode, there will be lowered levels of blood glucose and phosphate, and elevated levels of magnesium, potassium, and lactic acid. With sufficient fructose intake there may be elevated urinary fructose levels which will give a positive test for non-glucose reducing substances; elevated urinary fructose levels can also be shown by sugar chromatography. Chronic ingestion of fructose and elevated levels of fructose-1-phosphate lead to irritability, failure to thrive, vomiting, diarrhea, hepatomegaly, progressive hepatic dysfunction with cirrhosis, and a Fanconi type renal tubular dysfunction. Diffuse steatosis, scattered areas

of hepatic necrosis, periportal and intralobular fibrosis, and cirrhosis will be seen in liver biopsies. Kidney biopsies will show granulation and vacuolization of the epithelial cells and dilated proximal renal tubules. Deficient activity of aldolase B may be shown in liver or small intestinal biopsies. An intravenous—never oral—fructose tolerance test may be performed once the clinical condition has stabilized. Testing should be done by experienced clinicians and with careful observation of the patient. However, DNA diagnostic testing has also recently become available for individuals with common mutations of aldolase B. Such testing may eliminate the need for tolerance testing. Proven or suspected patients with hereditary fructose intolerance should not receive fructose in any form, including foods and medications. Most patients will show prompt clinical improvement, although those with advanced liver disease may have continued hepatic failure and require liver transplantation. Carrier and prenatal testing using DNA analysis in informative families will probably become available in the near future.

Fructose-1,6-Diphosphatase Deficiency: Fructose-1,6-diphosphatase deficiency is a rare, autosomal recessive disorder, associated with severe hypoglycemia, lactic acidosis, and ketosis which is precipitated by fasting or decreased carbohydrate intake. Many affected infants have their first episode before four days of age. Moderate hepatomegaly and hypotonia may occur; fructosuria is not seen. Liver or jejunal biopsy samples may be obtained to show deficient activity of fructose-1,6-diphosphatase. Carrier testing and prenatal diagnosis are not available. Clinical improvement is usually noted with a restriction of fructose intake, frequent feedings, and avoidance of fasting.

GLYCOGEN STORAGE DISORDERS

Glycogen storage disorders are associated with metabolic defects in the synthesis and degradation of glycogen (Figure 14–2). Glycogen is the principal storage form of carbohydrate in humans and found primarily in the liver and muscles. Stores of hepatic glycogen serve as a reserve for blood glucose during times of fasting, whereas muscle glycogen serves as a reserve for substrates needed for ATP production during exercise. Clinical and biochemical findings in the glycogen storage disorders are related to the type of defect involved, its effect on glycogen synthesis and/or degradation, and the site of glycogen storage. Table 14–1 lists the disorders, their associated biochemical defects, and clinical findings.

Hepatic Glycogen Storage Disorders

Hepatic glycogen storage disorders are estimated to occur in 1 in 60,000 births. The disorders are associated with varying degrees of hepatomegaly and fasting hypoglycemia. Functional testing, such as the response to glucagon or administration of other carbohydrates, may help to distinguish between the disorders, but should be done only with close observation of the patient and by experienced clinicians. In many of the disorders, the diagnosis may be established with enzymatic assays in erythrocytes, leukocytes, or cultured skin fibroblasts. Liver biopsy, preferably open, is required for enzymatic diagnosis for other disorders and can be also used for measuring total glycogen content and for glycogen structural analysis. All of the hepatic

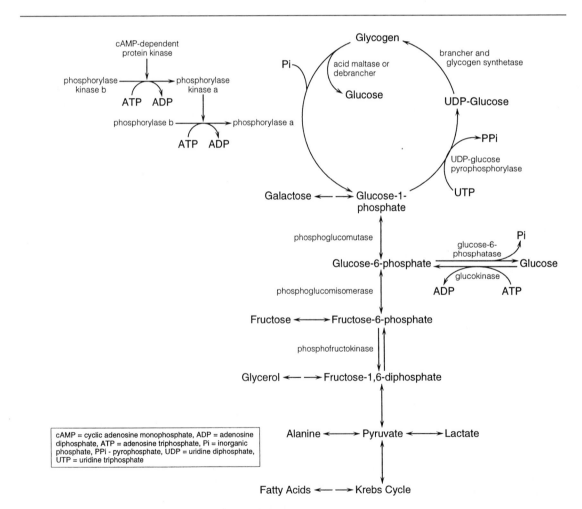

Figure 14–2. Glycogen metabolism.

Table 14–1. Glycogen storage disorders.

Type	Enzyme Affected	Major Tissue Involved	Clinical Features
0	Glycogen synthetase	Liver	Hypoglycemia, ketosis, no hepatomegaly
Ia	Glucose-6-phosphatase	Liver, kidney, intestine	Hypoglycemia, lactic acidosis, hepatomegaly, growth retardation
Ib	Transport defect of glucose-6-phosphate	As in Ia, plus neutrophils	As in Ia, plus recurrent infections, Crohn disease
Ic	Transport defect of inorganic phosphate	As in Ia	As in Ia, plus juvenile diabetes
II	Lysosomal α-glucosidase	Muscle, generalized	Progressive myopathy, cardiomyopathy, hepatomegaly
III	Debrancher	Liver, muscle	Mild type Ia, cirrhosis, ketosis, +/– hypotonia, +/– cardiomyopathy, +/– renal tubular dysfunction
IV	Brancher	Liver, muscle	Hepatomegaly, cirrhosis, failure to thrive, +/– hypoglycemia, +/– hypotonia, +/– cardiomyopathy
V	Muscle phosphorylase	Muscle	Weakness, cramps, myoglobinuria, muscle atrophy
VI	Hepatic phosphorylase	Liver	Hepatomegaly, ketosis, +/– hepatic fibrosis
VII	Muscle and erythrocyte phosphofructokinase	Muscle, erythrocytes	Weakness, cramps, myoglobinuria, muscle atrophy, +/– mild hemolytic anemia
Viii	Loss of activation of phosphorylase	Liver, brain	Hepatomegaly, progressive central nervous system dysfunction
IX	Phosphorylase kinase	Liver, +/– muscle	Hepatomegaly, ketosis, +/– mild hypotonia
X	cAMP-dependent kinase	Liver, muscle	Hepatomegaly, ketosis, +/– mild hypotonia
XI	Unknown	Liver, kidney	Hepatomegaly, renal tubular dysfunction, growth retardation

Adapted from Oski FA et al (editors), *Principles and Practice of Pediatrics,* 2nd ed, JB Lippincott, 1994.

glycogen storage disorders are inherited as autosomal recessive traits except for type IXb, which is inherited as an X-linked recessive trait. Carrier detection and prenatal diagnosis varies with the defect involved and the site of enzymatic expression.

Type Ia Glycogen Storage Disease (GSD): Type Ia glycogen storage disease (GSD), or von Gierke disease, is also known as hepatorenal GSD. The disorder results from deficient activity of glucose-6-phosphatase in the liver, kidneys, and intestine. Because glucose-6-phosphatase catalyzes the formation of free glucose from glycogen or any other source, these patients are totally dependent on a constant exogenous free glucose source and present with marked fasting hypoglycemia, lactic acidosis, and massive hepatomegaly during early infancy. Although the fasting hypoglycemia may be profound, patients often do not have clinical symptoms of hypoglycemia and are "tolerant" of the low glucose levels due to the ability of young infants to use alternative substrates in the brain. The infants demand frequent feedings, are often overweight, and have a "cherub" facies. Other findings include hypotonia, vomiting, diarrhea, and failure to thrive.

Fasting hypoglycemia occurs with only 2–3 hours of fasting. Glucose-6-phosphate, formed from dietary carbohydrate sources or during gluconeogenesis, cannot be converted to free glucose and instead is metabolized to lactic acid or stored as glycogen. In untreated patients, stimulation of glycolysis and gluconeogenesis results in elevated levels of triglycerides, free fatty acids, lactic acid, and uric acid. Atherosclerosis, xanthomas, gout, and uric acid nephropathy may occur. Sexual maturity is delayed. Abnormal bleeding tendencies result from decreased platelet adhesiveness related to the hypoglycemia.

Liver, kidney, and intestinal total glycogen content is elevated and of normal structure. Light microscopy will show glycogen, and often lipid, accumulation in the hepatocytes with glycogen present in the nuclei. Fibrosis is usually not present. Regenerative adenomatous nodules may be present in older patients, which can undergo malignant transformation. Measurement of glucose-6-phosphatase may be done with liver or intestinal biopsies. Recent cloning of the gene for type Ia GSD will allow DNA diagnosis, and carrier and prenatal testing for informative families in the near future.

The mainstay of treatment is to prevent hypoglycemia and reduce the stimulus for glycolysis and gluconeogenesis by supplying a constant source of exogenous glucose. This is accomplished by using formulas with glucose or glucose polymers as the only carbohydrate source. Small amounts of dietary galactose are allowed but there is strict elimination of fructose. Infants and young children usually require nocturnal drip feedings and frequent feedings during the day. Older children and adults respond to uncooked cornstarch slurries which can maintain blood glucose for 4–6 hours. With adequate treatment there is improvement in both the biochemical and clinical parameters and reduction in the liver size. The patients are at risk for significant acidosis and hypoglycemia with interruption of their exogenous glucose source for the remainder of their lives. Liver transplantation may be considered in older patients because of the risk for malignant transformation of the hepatic adenomas.

Type Ib Glycogen Storage Disease: Type Ib glycogen storage disease results from defective transport of glucose-6-phosphate across the microsomal membranes of hepatocytes and leukocytes. In addition to the clinical and biochemical features of type Ia GSD, patients with type Ib GSD have neutropenia and a defect in neutrophil mobility which leads to recurrent infections. Many also develop Crohn disease, which may be severe and require colectomy. Treatment of the glucose requirement is similar to that for type Ia GSD. Patients frequently require granulocyte colony-stimulating factor (GCSF) to control infections. Combined liver and bone marrow transplant may be considered in extreme cases.

Type Ic Glycogen Storage Disease: Type Ic glycogen storage disease results from a defect in the transport of inorganic phosphate across the microsomal membrane of hepatocytes. Patients have clinical and biochemical findings similar to type Ia GSD and may have insulin-dependent diabetes.

Type II Glycogen Storage Disease: Type II glycogen storage disease, also known as Pompe disease or generalized glycogenosis, is associated with deficient activity of lysosomal α-1,4-glucosidase (acid maltase) and generalized progressive lysosomal accumulation of glycogen. This disorder is discussed with the lysosomal storage disorders.

Type III Glycogen Storage Disease: Type III glycogen storage disease, or Cori disease, results from deficient activity of the debrancher enzyme, which removes the glucosyl residues in branched α-1,6-linkage from glycogen. The glycogen, which is stored in liver and muscle, has an abnormal structure with short outer chains. Affected patients present during the first year of life with fasting hypoglycemia, hepatomegaly, mild hypotonia, and growth retardation. Renal tubular dysfunction, mild inflammatory disease of the liver, cirrhosis, and cardiomyopathy may occur. The biochemical findings are similar to, but milder, than those noted with type Ia GSD. Lactate levels are usually not elevated with fasting, but can become elevated with glucose loading. Patients respond to glucagon in the fed state, but not in the fasted state. Gluconeogenesis is intact and galactose and fructose are converted to glucose. Most patients also have fasting ketonuria. With light microscopy, liver biopsies show more nuclear glycogen and less lipid droplets than noted with type Ia GSD; fibrous septa may be present. The disorder may be confirmed by measuring the debrancher enzyme in leukocytes and liver biopsy samples. Treatment consists of frequent feedings that are high in protein; there is no carbohydrate restriction. With age, many patients show improved tolerance of fasting.

Type IV Glycogen Storage Disease: Type IV glycogen storage disease, or Andersen disease, results from deficient activity of the brancher enzyme which attaches glucosyl residues in α-1,6, linkage and creates branching of the glucosyl chains during glycogen synthesis. There is storage of glycogen of abnormal structure which has less branch points and longer outer chains than normal. Storage of this less soluble form of glycogen is thought to be responsible for the cirrhosis seen in these patients. Affected patients present with hepatomegaly and failure to thrive in infancy. Fasting hypoglycemia, cardiomyopathy, hypotonia, muscular atrophy, and absent deep tendon reflexes may also occur. Many patients develop a progressive hepatic fibrosis, which may lead to hepatic failure. More severely involved patients may not live past 4 years of age. Milder cases have been reported—even patients in whom the clinical condition improves with age. With muscle or liver biopsies, glycogen content is normal, but the glycogen is of abnormal structure. The disorder may be confirmed by measurement of the brancher enzyme in leukocytes, cultured skin fibroblasts, and liver. Prenatal diagnosis has been accomplished.

Type VI Glycogen Storage Disease: Type VI glycogen storage disease, or Hers disease, results from deficient activity of hepatic phosphorylase which cleaves the outer glucosyl residues from the straight chains of glycogen during glycogen degradation. Affected patients present with often asymptomatic hepatomegaly and ketosis during early childhood. Hepatic fibrosis may occur; fasting hypoglycemia is uncommon. The disorder is confirmed by measuring hepatic phosphorylase in liver biopsy samples. Type IX and type X GSD may be clinically indistinguishable from type VI GSD.

Type VIII Glycogen Storage Disease: Type VIII glycogen storage disease is a very rare disorder associated with hepatomegaly and progressive central nervous system degeneration in young infants. Liver and brain biopsies show increased glycogen content. Although the basis for the disorder is unknown, impaired control of phosphorylase activation is thought to be involved.

Type IX Glycogen Storage Disease: Type IX glycogen storage disease results from deficient activity of the phosphorylase kinase which activates phosphorylase during glycogen degradation. Three forms of the disorder are known which differ in pattern of inheritance and the location of phosphorylase deficiency. Both type IXa GSD, inherited as an autosomal recessive trait, and type IXb GSD, inherited as an X-linked trait, are associated with decreased activity of hepatic phosphorylase kinase. Type IXc GSD, however, is associated with decreased activity of both hepatic and muscle phosphorylase kinase and is inherited as an autosomal recessive trait. Affected patients present with hepatomegaly and fasting ketonuria during childhood. Mild hypotonia may occur. In most cases the hepatomegaly improves with age, but some patients develop nodular cirrhosis and portal hypertension. The disorder may be confirmed by the measurement of phosphorylase kinase in erythrocytes, leukocytes, and liver and muscle biopsy (type IXc) samples.

Type X Glycogen Storage Disease: In type X glycogen storage disease, there is deficient activity of a cyclic AMP-dependent protein kinase, which is needed for the activation of phosphorylase kinase. Activities of hepatic and muscle phosphorylase are reduced and the phosphorylase is found only in the b or inactive form of the enzyme. Affected patients present with hepatomegaly, and occasionally mild hypotonia, during childhood.

Type XI Glycogen Storage Disease: Patients with type XI glycogen storage disease present with hepatomegaly, growth retardation, and proximal renal tubular dysfunction of the Fanconi type during childhood. There is glycogen storage in the liver and kidneys. The basis for the disorder is unclear, but is thought to be related to a functional deficiency of hepatic phosphoglucomutase.

Type 0 Glycogen Storage Disease: Type 0 glycogen storage disease is a rare disorder that results from deficient activity of hepatic glycogen synthetase. Affected patients present during the first year of life with fasting hypoglycemia and ketosis. Hepatomegaly does not occur and on liver biopsy there is reduced, but not absent glycogen stores.

Muscle Glycogen Storage Diseases

Type V GSD and **type VII GSD** involve only muscle and are clinically indistinguishable. The defects occur in the glycolytic pathway and result in decreased availability of substrates needed for ATP production in muscle during exercise. Most affected individuals present between 20 and 40 years of age with severe muscle cramps and myoglobinuria after strenuous exercise. Often there is a history of muscular fatigue with exercise during childhood or adolescence. With progression of the disorder, less cramping and myoglobinuria are noted, but muscular atrophy occurs. In general, type VII GSD is usually more severe than type V GSD. Blood levels of lactate dehydrogenase, aldolase, and creatine kinase become elevated. The myoglobinuria may be marked and result in acute renal failure. Venous lactate levels, mea-

sured before and after exercise in the same extremity, will fail to show the normal rise in levels. Electron micrographs of skeletal muscle will show glycogen deposition in the cytoplasm beneath the sarcolemma.

Deficient activity of muscle phosphorylase results in type V glycogen storage disease, or McArdle disease. And, type VII glycogen storage disease, or Tarui disease, is associated with deficient activity of muscle and erythrocyte phosphofructokinase. Type VII GSD patients may also have a mild hemolytic anemia. Deficient activity of either enzyme may be demonstrated in muscle biopsy samples.

OTHER DISORDERS OF CARBOHYDRATE METABOLISM

Glycerol Kinase Deficiency: Glycerol kinase deficiency is a rare X-linked disorder which presents with episodic vomiting, lethargy, and often significant metabolic acidosis during childhood. Elevated glycerol levels are noted on urinary organic acid determinations. Marked pseudohypertriglyceridemia will occur because most laboratories use a methodology for determining triglycerides that measures the amount of glycerol released with the hydrolysis of triglycerides. Episodes must be treated vigorously with intravenous hydration and bicarbonate. Maintenance therapy includes a lowered fat, high carbohydrate, frequent feeding diet. Many patients do well once their disorder is recognized. There is an adult, benign form of the disorder that may only be recognized when the pseudohypertriglyceridemia is noted. Glycerol kinase deficiency may also occur as a result of a microdeletion of the p21 region of the X chromosome. These patients have a more severe disorder that also involves various combinations of contiguous genes associated with congenital adrenal hypoplasia, Duchenne muscular dystrophy, and ornithine transcarbamylase deficiency.

Ketotic Hypoglycemia: Ketotic hypoglycemia, or substrate-limited hypoglycemia, is a common disorder that presents between the ages of 1 and 5 years with fasting hypoglycemia and ketosis. It is usually not an inherited condition, but affected siblings are known. The disorder is mentioned because many children who had been given this diagnosis in the past are now being found to have rare disorders of mitochondrial beta-oxidation of fatty acids. Others have been found to have metabolic defects in amino acid and organic acid metabolism. Along with an evaluation for the hormonal causes of hypoglycemia, testing of these children should also include quantitative amino acid, organic acid, and carnitine determinations in addition to acyl-carnitine or acyl-glycine profiles.

REFERENCES AND SUGGESTED READING

See Page 256 and Appendix II.

15 Mitochondrial Fatty Acid Oxidation

MITOCHONDRIAL FATTY ACID OXIDATION

Disorders of mitochondrial fatty acid oxidation are autosomal recessive conditions that are associated with impaired energy production, faulty formation of ketone bodies, and the accumulation of partially oxidized fatty acid metabolites during periods of fasting and stress. With fasting, fatty acids are mobilized from adipose tissue stores and transported to the liver and other tissues where they undergo beta-oxidation. Long chain (C10–C18) fatty acids are "activated" to form long chain acyl-coenzyme A (CoA) esters in the cytosol. The long chain acyl-CoA esters are then transported into the mitochondrial matrix as long chain acyl-carnitines (carnitine shuttle), which requires the actions of carnitine palmityl transferase (CPT) I, CPT II, and carnitine translocase. CPT I and CPT II function at the inner surfaces of the outer and inner mitrochondrial membranes, respectively, where they attach and subsequently remove carnitine from the long chain acyl-CoA esters by transesterification. Carnitine translocase is needed for the long chain acyl-carnitines to move across the inner mitochondrial membrane into the matrix. Medium (C6–C12) and short chain (C4–C6) fatty acids do not require carnitine-mediated transport into the mitochondrial matrix; they become "activated" to their CoA esters within the matrix.

The fatty acid acyl-CoA esters of varying lengths are then oxidized by the series of steps shown in Figure 15–1. The acyl-CoA esters are repeatedly cycled through the pathway; with each cycle the acyl-CoAs are reduced in length by two carbons and acetyl-CoA is formed, which may be converted to ketone bodies by the liver and kidney or enter the tricarboxylic cycle. A series of carbon chain length-specific dehydrogenases is involved in this process. For example, long chain acyl-CoA dehydrogenase (LCAD) catalyzes the reactions that involve fatty acid acyl-CoA esters with carbon lengths of C12–C18, medium chain acyl-CoA dehydrogenase (MCAD) those with C4–C14, and short chain acyl-CoA dehydrogenase (SCAD) those with C4 and C6. These acyl-CoA dehydrogenases are important components of the pathway in that they are flavoproteins that transport electrons produced by beta-oxidation of the fatty acids to the mitochondrial respiratory chain, where the electrons are used in the formation of ATP. Beta-oxidation of odd chain length fatty acids results in the additional formation of propionyl-CoA (3 carbon length). Carnitine-mediated transport is also required for the acetyl-CoA and acyl-CoA esters to exit the mitochondria.

Disorders of mitochondrial beta-oxidation of fatty acids are associated with symptoms that occur at times of fasting or decreased carbohydrate intake. Fasting, which increases lipolysis and fatty acid mobilization, results in elevated levels of free fatty acids and the production of abnormal levels of intermediates in the beta-oxidation pathways. The intermediates will be of a chain length comparable to the defect involved, eg, medium chain fatty acid metabolites (C6–C12) will accumulate with medium chain acyl-CoA dehydrogenase deficiency and long chain fatty acid metabolites (C12–C14) with long chain acyl-CoA dehydrogenase deficiency. The elevated metabolites can enter alternative pathways of oxidation in the microsomes (omega and omega-1 oxidation) and peroxisomes (beta-oxidation), which leads to excessive production of (omega-l)-hydroxy acids and dicarboxylic acids in the body fluids of affected patients. These acids can be detected by organic acid analysis using gas chromatography/mass spectrometry (GC/MS). The abnormal metabolites also form esters with either carnitine (acyl-carnitines) or glycine (acyl-glycines). Acyl-carnitine profiles as determined by fast atom bombardment with tandem mass spectrometry (FAB), or acyl-glycine profiles, using stable isotope dilution GC/MS, will show patterns consistent with the disorder involved. Acyl-carnitine profiles and acyl-glycine profiles are often abnormal between episodes, in contrast to urinary organic acids profiles, which may be abnormal only with acute episodes.

Carnitine (L-carnitine): Carnitine (L-carnitine) is an amino acid that functions in the carnitine-mediated transport of fatty acyl-CoA esters during mitochondrial beta-oxidation. Although endogenous carnitine may be synthesized from lysine, most carnitine is of dietary origin. Natural sources with high carnitine content include meats and dairy products; vegetable products have essentially no available carnitine. Carnitine deficiency has been reported to oc-

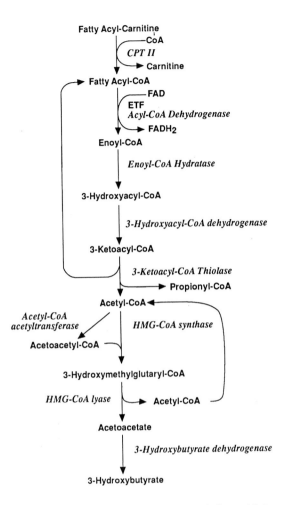

Figure 15–1. Hepatic mitochondrial metabolism of fatty acids. CPT = carnitine palmityl transferase; ETF = electron transport flavoprotein; HMG = 3-hydroxymethylglutaryl; CoA = coenzyme A; FAD = flavin adenine dinucleotide; $FADH_2$ = reduced form of FAD. (Adapted, with permission from Oski FA et al (editors): *Principles and Practice of Pediatrics,* 2nd ed, JB Lippincott, 1994.)

used for the treatment of seizure disorders. In disorders of fatty acid oxidation, other organic acidemias, or with the use of drugs that result in the accumulation of acyl-CoA compounds, abnormally high amounts of carnitine may become esterified and the levels of free, unbound, carnitine lowered to the point that beta-oxidation of fatty acids is impaired. Symptoms of **systemic free carnitine deficiency,** which may be a result of a disorder of fatty acid beta-oxidation or other causes, include intolerance of fasting, hypoglycemia, hypoketosis, hypotonia, myopathies, cardiomyopathies, and hepatic dysfunction. When used for treatment of carnitine deficiency, only the prescription form of L-carnitine should be used and the combined D-, L-form available in health food stores should be avoided.

DISORDERS OF MITOCHONDRIAL FATTY ACID BETA-OXIDATION

Medium Chain Acyl-CoA Dehydrogenase (MCAD) Deficiency: The prototype for the group of disorders is medium chain acyl-CoA dehydrogenase (MCAD) deficiency. The disorder is estimated to occur in 1 in 10,000 births and, thus, is as common as phenylketonuria. Although most patients present between 5 and 24 months of age, there are increasing reports of symptomatic patients at earlier ages, even during the newborn period. Episodes of vomiting, lethargy, hypotonia, and coma are seen with fasting or decreased carbohydrate intake. Mild hyperammonemia, hepatomegaly, and abnormal liver function testing are often noted. Many patients become hypoglycemic, which is not associated with ketosis and has led to the name of "hypoketotic hypoglycemia." The reason for the hypoglycemia is unknown, but may be related to the fact that during fasting in patients with MCAD deficiency, there is no increase in acetyl-CoA and ketone body production, which in normals would stimulate a gluconeogenic response. Some patients will make ketones with episodes, but the amount is considerably less than would be seen with patients with intact beta-oxidation of fatty acids. Prompt recognition of the disorder and treatment with intravenous glucose, hydration, and L-carnitine usually results in clinical improvement. However, some patients have a rapidly progressive course and develop cerebral edema and cardiorespiratory compromise. Is it estimated that 25% of patients die, often unrecognized, with their first episode. The highest mortality rates, up to 59% with an episode, occur between the ages of 15 and 26 months. Many patients appear to have Reyes syndrome; others have been considered cases of sudden infant death syndrome. But a careful history, clinical examination, and laboratory findings will often reveal differences that point to MCAD deficiency. Liver biopsy or au-

cur in persons on strict vegetarian diets, or with total parenteral nutrition. In the past, some infants given soy bean-based formulas also developed a carnitine deficient state; the formulas have been supplemented with carnitine since this was noted. Carnitine deficiency may also be seen with vitamin C and pyridoxine deficiencies (cofactors for carnitine synthesis), renal tubular disorders (renal loss), and hemodialysis (loss with hemofiltration).

Carnitine may also form carnitine esters with metabolites from other pathways, eg, propionyl-CoA in propionic acidemia, or isovaleryl-CoA in isovaleric acidemia. In this manner, carnitine may function as a "trap" for these abnormal compounds. Valproyl-carnitine esters are also formed when valproic acid is topsy specimens will show fatty infiltration of the liver which can be in either a macrovesicular or microvascular pattern. The mitochondrial ultrastructure is abnormal and inclusions may be present; the findings, however, are different from those seen with Reyes syndrome. Plasma free fatty acid levels will be elevated, but beta-hydroxybutyrate levels are inappropriately low. With episodes, urine organic acid profiles will show elevated dicarboxylic acids of medium chain length (C6–C12), including adipic, sebacic, and suberic acids. Between episodes urine organic acid profiles may be normal. Plasma and urinary acyl-carnitine and acyl-glycine profiles will be characteristically abnormal at all times. Plasma free carnitine levels will be low and esterified carnitine fractions high. Dried blood filter paper cards can be used for acyl-carnitine profiles and for DNA testing for MCAD deficiency. Deficient activity of MCAD may be shown with leukocytes or cultured skin fibroblasts. Treatment includes the avoidance of fasting. Supplemental oral L-carnitine also is recommended. Dietary intake of medium chain triglyceride (MCT) oil must be avoided. Long-term survival is known and many patients have normal intelligence.

Because of its relative frequency and good outcome with preventive treatment, the disorder may be considered for newborn screening in the future. All siblings should be evaluated for the disorder in that there is wide familial variation in the age of onset; presymptomatic siblings have often been identified after the diagnosis in a symptomatic sibling. Carrier testing and prenatal diagnosis are available with DNA analysis in informative families. Prenatal diagnosis has also been accomplished with radiolabeled enzymatic assays in cultured amniocytes.

Long Chain Acyl-CoA Dehydrogenase (LCAD) Deficiency: Compared to MCAD deficiency, the remainder of the known disorders of mitochondrial fatty acid oxidation are relatively rare. Long chain acyl-CoA dehydrogenase (LCAD) deficiency presents with clinical features similar to those seen with MCAD deficiency. However, the onset is earlier, usually before 6 months of age, the episodes are more severe, cardiomyopathies are common, and the mortality rate is higher. Patients with a milder clinical course and adults with episodes of myalgia and rhabdomyolysis are also known. Patients with the more severe forms may have portal fibrosis in addition to steatosis on liver biopsy. Urinary organic acid profiles may show elevated long chain dicarboxylic acids (C12–C14), as well as medium chain dicarboxylic acids, during acute episodes. However, the urinary organic acid profiles may not be abnormal in all patients with LCAD deficiency, and acyl-carnitine or acyl-glycine profiles may be needed to document abnormal findings. Plasma carnitine levels will show a lowered total and elevated esterified fractions. Defi-

cient activity of LCAD may be shown in leukocytes or cultured skin fibroblasts. Treatment includes the avoidance of fasting, and institution of a high carbohydrate diet, along with supplemental L-carnitine. In contrast to MCAD deficiency, medium chain triglycerides may be beneficial.

Long Chain 3-Hydroxyacyl-CoA Dehydrogenase (LCHAD) Deficiency: Long chain 3-hydroxyacyl-CoA dehydrogenase (LCHAD) deficiency presents in young infants, often before 9 months of age, with clinical findings similar to the infantile cases of LCAD deficiency. With episodes, the patients have elevations of 3-hydroxydicarboxylic acids and 3-hydroxymonocarboxylic acids. Severe metabolic acidosis may be present. Plasma and dried filter paper blood dot acyl-carnitine profiles are characteristic. The enzymatic deficiency may be shown in cultured skin fibroblasts. Treatment is similar to that for LCAD deficiency.

Trifunctional Enzyme Deficiency: Deficient activity of the "trifunctional enzyme" has been noted in patients with clinical findings similar to the infantile cases of LCAD and LCHAD deficiencies. The "trifunctional enzyme" includes the activities of long chain 3-hydroxyacyl-CoA dehydrogenase, 2-enoyl-CoA hydratase, and 3-ketoacyl-CoA thiolase. Patients have elevated levels of metabolites as noted with LCHAD deficiency, as well as other metabolites which accumulate due to the hydratase and thiolase deficiencies.

Deficient Activity of Short Chain Acyl-CoA Dehydrogenase (SCAD): Deficient activity of short chain acyl-CoA dehydrogenase (SCAD) is very rare. Because beta-oxidation of medium- and long chain fatty acids proceeds, these patients can make ketone bodies. Patients have poor feeding, failure to thrive, developmental delay, hepatomegaly, progressive hypotonia, and die during the neonatal period and early infancy. Fatty infiltration of the liver and a lipid myopathy are noted. Older patients with episodic weakness and deficiency of SCAD limited to muscle are also known. Patients will have abnormal organic acid determinations, as well as acyl-carnitine and acyl-glycine profiles, which show elevation of short chain fatty acid metabolites such as ethylmalonic acid. The enzymatic deficiency may be shown in cultured skin fibroblasts.

Deficient Activity of 2,4 Dienoyl-CoA Reductase: Deficient activity of 2,4 dienoyl-CoA reductase, which results in faulty beta-oxidation of only unsaturated fatty acids, has been reported in one patient with neonatal hypotonia, failure to thrive, microcephaly, and shortening of the trunk, arms, and fingers. Death occurred at 4 months of age. Hyperlysinemia and elevation of an unusual acyl-carnitine, 2-trans,4-cis-decadienoylcarnitine were noted. The enzymatic defect was confirmed in liver and muscle samples.

DISORDERS OF CARNITINE UPTAKE AND CARNITINE-MEDIATED TRANSPORT

Carnitine Plasma Membrane Transporter Deficiency: Four defects are associated with carnitine uptake or carnitine-mediated transport of acyl-carnitines. Carnitine plasma membrane transporter deficiency is the most common disorder of this group and is associated with a defect in the carrier protein responsible for sodium-dependent transport of carnitine across plasma membranes. Plasma and tissue levels of carnitine are extremely low. Urine organic acids and acyl-glycine and acyl-carnitine profiles will not be abnormal. Most patients present between 2 and 7 years of age with a progressive cardiomyopathy and hypotonia. Other patients present between 3 and 24 months of age with clinical findings similar to MCAD deficiency; hypoglycemia, hyperammonemia, hypotonia, hepatomegaly, and hepatic dysfunction occur prior to the onset of cardiac involvement. Treatment with L-carnitine usually results in a clinical response. The defect may be demonstrated in cultured skin fibroblasts.

Carnitine Translocase Deficiency: Carnitine translocase deficiency is a very rare disorder associated with clinical features similar to LCAD deficiency in infants. Total plasma carnitine levels are low and there is an increase in the esterified carnitine fraction. Plasma acyl-carnitine profiles will show elevation of medium and long chain metabolites.

Carnitine Palmityl Transferase (CPT) I Deficiency: Carnitine palmityl transferase (CPT) I deficiency presents in young infants with clinical features similar to those seen in MCAD deficiency. Because there is less muscular involvement than with CPT II deficiency, the disorder is also known as the "hepatic form" of CPT deficiency. Reduced activity of CPT I may be shown in cultured skin fibroblasts.

Carnitine Palmityl Transferase (CPT) II Deficiency: Carnitine palmityl transferase (CPT) II deficiency is more common than CPT I deficiency and has a variable clinical presentation. Most patients present as young adults with recurrent attacks of rhabdomyolysis that are precipitated by fasting, exercise, cold temperatures, or infections. These patients also have a high risk for anesthesia-related malignant hyperthermia. The activity of CPT II is reduced to 20–25% of normal. A severe, neonatal form of presentation has been reported with essentially no CPT II activity. Infants with approximately 10% residual activity of CPT II have presented with a "hepato-cardio-muscular" form and clinical findings similar to those with LCAD deficiency. Some of these patients have also had cardiac arrhythmias, renal cortical cysts, and central nervous system malformations. Deficient activity of CPT II may be shown in cultured skin fibroblasts. With both CPT I and CPT II deficiency, plasma carnitine levels usually show elevated total carnitine and esterified carnitine levels. Urine organic acid, acyl-carnitine, and acyl-glycine profiles are usually normal or not diagnostic.

DISORDERS OF ELECTRON TRANSFER FLAVOPROTEIN AND ELECTRON TRANSFER FLAVOPROTEIN-UBIQUINONE OXIDOREDUCTASE

Electron transfer flavoprotein (ETF) and electron transfer flavoprotein-ubiquinone oxidoreductase (ETF-QO) mediate the transfer of the electrons that are produced by flavin-containing enzymes, such as the dehydrogenases, to the mitochondrial respiratory chain. The activity of the acyl-CoA dehydrogenases involved in mitochondrial beta-oxidation of fatty acids, as well as other dehydrogenases involved with amino acid metabolism such as isovaleryl-CoA dehydrogenase, are affected.

Multiple Acyl-CoA Dehydrogenase Deficiency (MADD), or Glutaric Acidemia Type II: Deficiency of either ETF or ETF-QO has been associated with multiple acyl-CoA dehydrogenase deficiency (MADD), which is also known as glutaric acidemia type II. The most common and severe form of the disorder presents in the neonatal period with hypotonia, hepatomegaly, hypoglycemia, hyperammonemia, and metabolic acidosis. Patients also have a pervasive, acrid odor, similar to that of "sweaty feet" from elevated levels of isovaleric acid. Many of the patients have congenital anomalies in a pattern similar to Zellweger syndrome, including such features as a high forehead, hypoplastic midfacial area, hypertelorism, low-set ears, and cystic kidneys. Other anomalies have included rocker-bottom feet, muscular defects in the abdominal wall, anomalies of the external genitalia, and central nervous system malformations. Most patients do not survive the neonatal period, and those who do frequently develop cardiomyopathies. Occasionally, patients will present later than the neonatal period with milder clinical features. Organic acid determinations will show elevations of acids of varying chain length and origin, such as glutaric, ethylmalonic, 3-hydroxisovaleric, 2-hydroxyglutaric, 5-hydroxyhexanoic, adipic, suberic, and dodecanedioic acids. Plasma short chain volatile organic acid levels of isovaleric, isobutyric, and 2-methylbutyric acids are elevated. Acyl-carnitine and acyl-glycine profiles will show the presence of corresponding abnormal compounds. Ketonuria is usually not present. Quantitative urine amino acid determinations will show elevated proline and hydroxyproline. Prenatal diagnosis is available for the severe forms of multiple acyl-CoA dehydrogenase deficiency.

Ethylmalonic-Adipic Aciduria: Ethylmalonic-adipic aciduria is the mildest form of the disorder, which may present at any time from infancy to adulthood, with recurrent episodes of vomiting, hypoglycemia, acidosis, and occasionally hepatomegaly and/or myopathy. Urinary organic acid profiles will show a similar, but milder, pattern to that seen with the severe forms of the disorder. Plasma and urine sarcosine and esterified carnitine levels may also be elevated. The disorder may respond to treatment with riboflavin, carnitine, and dietary restriction of protein and fat.

REFERENCES AND SUGGESTED READING

See Page 256 and Appendix II.

Lactic Acidosis & Mitochondrial Oxidative Phosphorylation

16

DISORDERS OF PYRUVATE METABOLISM

Pyruvate is an important central intermediate in the glycolytic and gluconeogenic pathways (Figure 16–1). Pyruvate can be derived from glucose in the fed state or alanine during fasting. Pyruvate is usually converted to lactate during anaerobic metabolism in the muscles and other tissues. The lactate is then returned to the liver for gluconeogenesis or entry into the Krebs cycle. Lactic acidosis most commonly occurs with hypoxia, poor perfusion, hepatic dysfunction, sepsis, and other clinical states that interfere with the delivery of oxygen to tissues. Secondary lactic acidosis also may be seen with disorders that interfere with the production of acetyl-CoA or coenzyme A, such as the organic acidemias and disorders of fatty acid oxidation. Primary lactic acidosis is less common and results from defects in gluconeogeneis, the Krebs cycle, or oxidative phosphorylation. Lactic acid is only produced from pyruvate through the actions of cytosolic lactate dehydrogenase; the step is reversible and allows for both lactate and pyruvate levels to become elevated in the disorders that affect pyruvate metabolism. The lactate to pyruvate ratio is usually less than 25. The ratio will become elevated with disorders of oxidative phosphorylation (O/P), defects of the Krebs cycle, or with a variant of pyruvate carboxylase deficiency associated with hyperammonemia and citrullinemia. Because pyruvate may also be reversibly converted to alanine by alanine aminotransferase, elevated levels of alanine will also occur.

Deficient Activity of Pyruvate Carboxylase

Pyruvate carboxylase catalyzes the conversion of pyruvate to oxaloacetate, which can be used for gluconeogenesis or enter the Krebs cycle. Deficient activity of pyruvate carboxylase, a rare autosomal recessive disorder, presents between birth and 5 months of age with mild metabolic acidosis, hypoglycemia, hepatomegaly, and psychomotor delay. Episodes of severe lactic acidosis and renal tubular dysfunction may also occur. Most patients die by their fifth birthday. Computed tomography of the brain will show poor myelination, atrophy of the cerebral cortex, and a thinning corpus callosum. An increase in density and granularity of the mitochondrial matrix may be noted on liver biopsy samples. Some of the patients may have the Leigh syndrome phenotype as discussed with complex IV (cytochrome c oxidase) deficiency later in this chapter. Affected patients have elevated lactate, pyruvate, and alanine levels. Elevated levels of proline and α-ketoglutarate are also noted. Deficient activity of pyruvate carboxylase may be shown in cultured skin fibroblasts. Prenatal diagnosis is possible.

Variant of Pyruvate Carboxylase Deficiency: A variant of pyruvate carboxylase deficiency is associated with severe neonatal metabolic acidosis, hypoglycemia, and hepatomegaly. Affected patients will have severe lactic acidosis and increased levels of ammonia and citrulline in addition to elevated lactate, pyruvate, alanine, proline, and α-ketoglutarate. The lactate to pyruvate ratio will be elevated. Many of the clinical signs are thought to result from depletion of aspartate and oxaloacetate needed for proper functioning of the urea cycle as well as the Krebs cycle. Most patients do not live past 3 months of age.

Multiple Carboxylase Deficiency: Pyruvate carboxylase requires biotin as a cofactor. Pyruvate carboxylase deficiency also occurs as part of the multiple carboxylase deficiency that is associated with holocarboxylase synthetase deficiency or biotinidase deficiency. Affected patients have deficient activity of propionyl-CoA carboxylase and 3-methylcrotonyl-CoA carboxylase in addition to pyruvate carboxylase deficiency. These disorders are discussed in detail with propionic acidemia, holocarboxylase synthetase deficiency, and biotinidase deficiency in Chapter 13.

Deficient Activity of Phosphoenolpyruvate Carboxykinase

This deficiency is a very rare autosomal recessive disorder associated with lactic acidosis, hypoglycemia, hypotonia, hepatomegaly, and failure to thrive. It has variable clinical severity and may lead to death in infancy or later during childhood.

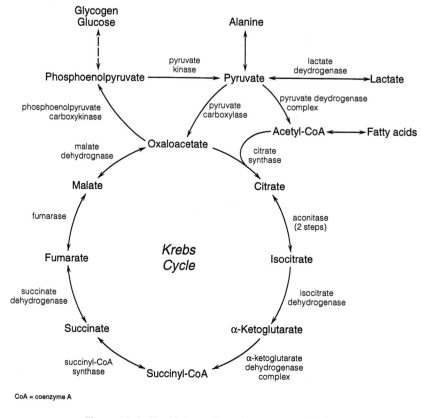

Figure 16–1. The Krebs cycle and pyruvate metabolism.

Deficient Activity of the Pyruvate Dehydrogenase Enzyme Complex

The pyruvate dehydrogenase enzyme complex catalyzes the conversion of pyruvate to acetyl-CoA. The pyruvate dehydrogenase enzyme complex is composed of: (1) three subunits, which include E_1 (pyruvate dehydrogenase), E_2 (dihydrolipoyl transacetylase) and E_3 (dihydrolipoyl dehydrogenase); (2) a lipoic acid-containing component "X"; and (3) a regulatory phosphorylase and kinase. The E_1 subunit requires thiamine pyrophosphate as a cofactor and consists of two subunits, alpha (α) and beta (β). The E_3 subunit of the pyruvate dehydrogenase enzyme complex is very similar to the E_3 subunits of the α-ketoglutarate and the branched chain α-ketoacid dehydrogenase complexes.

Defect in the $E_1\alpha$ Subunit: Deficient activity of the pyruvate dehydrogenase enzyme complex is one of the most common genetic causes of lactic acidosis in young infants and children. Most cases are new mutations which involve the $E_1\alpha$ subunit locus at chromosome Xp22.1. In this X-linked disorder, both hemizygous affected male and symptomatic affected heterozygous female patients have been reported to have varying degrees of clinical severity.

In the severe form of the disorder, a neonatal se-

vere lactic acidosis occurs that is often refractory to treatment. The affected infants are neurologically abnormal from birth, have lowered Apgar scores, and often require assisted ventilation. A history of poor intrauterine growth, low birth weight for gestational age, hypotonia, lethargy, and feeding problems are common. Some patients will have a dysmorphic facies with a high forehead, narrow face, enlarged fontanels, macrocephaly, low set small ears, wide nasal bridge, thin upper lip, and long philtrum. Other congenital malformations have included a shortening of the proximal extremities (rhizomelia), transverse palmar creases, and hydronephrosis. Computed tomography of the brain will show complete or partial agenesis of the corpus callosum, cerebral atrophy with compensatory increase in ventricular size, or cystic lesions in the cortex, brain stem, basal ganglia, or cerebellum. Blood levels of lactate and pyruvate and cerebrospinal fluid lactate levels will be elevated. Treatment with bicarbonate, or even dialysis, may not control the acidosis. Most patients that are severely affected from birth do not survive the neonatal period or early infancy.

Other less severely affected neonates will have mild to moderate chronic lactic acidosis, a progressive central nervous system degeneration, microcephaly, and profound mental handicaps. Most patients will have generalized seizures. Occasionally infantile spasms or a hypsarrhythmia electroencephalographic pattern will be noted. Death usually occurs before three years of age. Many of these patients will have a clinical course similar to that seen in the Leigh syndrome phenotype discussed later with complex IV (cytochrome c oxidase) deficiency of the respiratory chain.

Still other affected patients will have only ataxia, which can be episodic, and may or may not be accompanied by psychomotor retardation. In these patients, elevated levels of blood and cerebrospinal fluid lactate may only be noted at the times of the ataxic episodes. Many of these milder affected patients live longer, even to the adult years.

Measurement of pyruvate dehydrogenase enzyme complex activity may be done with muscle or liver biopsy or tissue samples and with cultured skin fibroblasts. Patients have been reported to have 0–60% of normal enzymatic activity. Reduced enzyme activity may be tissue specific; the defect may not be found if only cultured skin fibroblasts are measured. Because of the tissue specificity and residual activity, carrier and prenatal testing often cannot accurately be accomplished with enzymatic activity. However, laboratories proficient in molecular genetic techniques may successfully conduct carrier and prenatal testing in some families.

Currently, treatment is mainly symptomatic and supportive. Patients with significant lactic acidosis may require bicarbonate or citrate buffers. Dichloracetate, an investigational new drug that increases the activity of the pyruvate dehydrogenase complex, may be helpful in treating some patients affected with the more moderate or milder forms of the disorders, especially during the acute episodes of lactic acidosis.

In general, hemizygous affected male patients are more severely affected clinically than symptomatic heterozygous females. As with other X-linked genetic disorders, there is considerable clinical heterogeneity among symptomatic heterozygous females which is related to the relative degree of Lyonization, or early random inactivation of one of their two X chromosomes early in fetal life. In tissues which are highly dependent upon pyruvate metabolism, such as the liver and brain, symptomatic affected females usually have an unfavorable Lyonization with relatively more of the remaining "active" X chromosomes being the ones with the abnormal $E_1\alpha$ locus. Many heterozygous females may not be clinically affected. Because the family history is usually negative, it is thought that most cases result from new mutations in the parental gametes or germ cell lines.

Defect in the E_3 Subunit: Patients with a rare defect in the E_3 subunit, common to the pyruvate dehydrogenase, α-ketoglutarate dehydrogenase, and branched chain α-ketoacid dehydrogenase complexes, present as neonates or young infants with ke-

tolactic acidosis, ataxia, and progressive extrapyramidal tract signs. As a result of deficient activity of all three complexes, affected patients have elevations of lactic acid, α-ketoglutarate, and the amino acids and organic acids that accumulate with maple syrup urine disease.

DISORDERS OF THE KREBS CYCLE

Isolated Deficiency of the α-Ketoglutarate Dehydrogenase Complex

Isolated deficiency of the α-ketoglutarate dehydrogenase complex occurs as a rare disorder of childhood characterized by hypotonia, ataxia, choreoathetosis, and psychomotor retardation. Affected patients have markedly elevated levels of α-ketoglutarate and a mild lactic acidosis. Deficient activity of the α-ketoglutarate dehydrogenase complex may also occur with the combined deficiency of the α-ketoglutarate, pyruvate, and branched chain α-ketoacid dehydrogenase complexes as discussed with pyruvate dehydrogenase deficiency and maple syrup urine disease.

Deficient Activity of Fumarase

Deficient activity of fumarase (fumarate hydratase) has been reported in neonates or young infants with apnea, lethargy, hypothermia, microcephaly, psychomotor delay, and failure to thrive. Computed tomography will show cerebral atrophy. Affected patients have increased levels of lactic acid and increased lactate to pyruvate ratios. Urine organic acid profiles will reveal elevated Krebs cycle intermediates including fumarate, succinate, citrate, oxaloacetate, and α-ketoglutarate. Deficient activity of fumarase may be shown in cultured skin fibroblasts or liver biopsy samples.

DISORDERS OF MITOCHONDRIAL OXIDATIVE PHOSPHORYLATION (RESPIRATORY CHAIN)

Mitochondrial Oxidative Phosphorylation

Mitochondrial oxidative phosphorylation (O/P) produces most of the ATP which is needed by the cells for energy. The O/P system, also known as the respiratory chain, is located at the inner mitochondrial membrane (Figure 16–2). This system consists of five enzyme complexes (I–V), coenzyme Q_{10} (CoQ_{10}, ubiquinone), and transitional metal compounds, eg, iron-sulfur clusters. Electrons (as hydrogen ions in NADH and FADH) which are produced by the oxidation of pyruvate (glycolytic pathway), fatty acids (mitochondrial β-oxidation), and the Krebs cycle, enter the respiratory chain through Complexes I and II. The electrons are then trans-

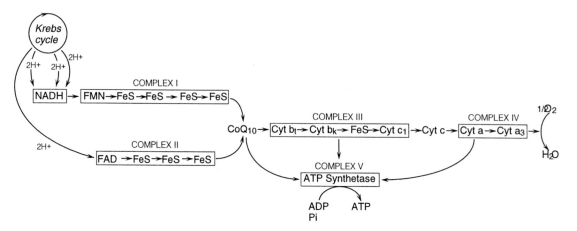

Figure 16–2. Mitochondrial respiratory chain (oxidative phosphorylation). Of the eight electrons that enter the respiratory chain from the Krebs cycle, six enter through NADH and Complex I. The other two, which are generated from succinate, enter through Complex II. Of the over 100 polypeptides that comprise the five complexes of the respiratory chain, 13 are encoded by mitochondrial DNA (see text). ADP = adenosine diphosphate; ATP = adenosine triphosphate; Cyt = cytochrome; CoQ_{10} = coenzyme Q, ubiquinone; FAD = flavine adenine dinucleotide; FeS = iron-sulfur cluster; FMN = flavine mononucleotide; H^+ = electron; NADH = reduced form of nicotinamide-adenine dinucleotide; Pi = inorganic phosphate. (Adapted from DeVivo DC, Brain and development, 1993:**15**:1.)

ferred sequentially to CoQ_{10}, Complex III, Complex IV, and ultimately to molecular oxygen. During the process, protons are pumped across the inner mitochondrial membrane and create a transmembrane proton energy gradient that is used by ATP synthase (Complex V) in the production of ATP. The net result of mitochondrial O/P is the production of ATP and water (oxygen consumption). More than 100 polypeptides are involved with mitochondrial O/P: Most are encoded by nuclear DNA (nDNA); 13 are encoded by mitochondrial DNA (mtDNA). The proteins of nDNA origin are synthesized on cytosolic ribosomes and must be "imported" into the mitochondria. This occurs as a result of "leader" or "chaperone" proteins, which are attached to the apoprotein precursors of the proteins at the time of synthesis and target the apoproteins for intramitochondrial location. The targeting proteins are removed once the apoproteins have reached their intramitochondrial location.

The Mitochondrial Genome and Mitochondrial Inheritance

The mitochondrial genome and its inheritance have been discussed in Chapter 2. Mitochondrial DNA (mtDNA) is a circular, double-stranded structure without introns; mutations in mtDNA disrupt oxidative phosphorylation. Since the number of mitochondria per cell and the number of copies of mtDNA per mitochondrion vary with the energy requirement of the cell, mtDNA mutations are usually expressed in tissues with high energy requirements. Because most of the subunits of the enzymes of oxidative phosphorylation are encoded by nuclear

genes, classical Mendelian inheritance is seen with many disorders associated with dysfunction of the respiratory chain. Mutations in mtDNA itself also occur and are inherited cytoplasmically (maternally). With cell division and replication, the mutant and normal type mtDNA of a heteroplasmic cell are *randomly segregated* to the daughter cells. In this manner, certain daughter cells will receive more, and others less of the mutant mtDNA of a heteroplasmic parent cell. With continued cell division, the relative amounts of normal and abnormal mtDNA may change, a pattern that has been noted in cell cultures from affected patients or in the patients themselves. This change may explain why some disorders apparently progress as more cell lines receive a relative increase in the amount of abnormal mtDNA. There also appears to be a *threshold effect* involved with the clinical expression of mtDNA mutations. Usually, a high percentage, eg, over 85%, of mutant mtDNA must be present for cellular function to be affected. The threshold will vary with:

1. The severity of the mutation
2. Its effect on energy production by the respiratory chain
3. The energy requirement of the tissues involved
4. The age of the individual.

The brain and muscles have a relatively higher demand for energy than other tissues. Growing children have a higher energy requirement than adults. In certain patients, the amount of heteroplasmy will allow adequate energy production except during times of stress or increased energy demand. In general, more severe mutations have a lower threshold and are clinically expressed earlier than milder mutations of the mtDNA. Milder mtDNA mutations also tend to be more variable and may only be expressed when other factors (eg, environmental toxins, aging, or nDNA mutations) have additive effects. Although most of the currently recognized disorders associated with mutations in mtDNA appear to be relatively rare, it is anticipated that mtDNA mutations will play an important role in future medicine, especially in regard to the process of aging.

Defects in the Function of the Respiratory Chain

Because the brain and muscle are highly dependent on mitochondrial energy production, many of the known clinical phenotypes associated with defects in O/P will have muscle and neurological dysfunction. Myopathies, cardiomyopathies, ophthalmoplegia, encephalopathies, and encephalomyopathies are common. Renal tubular, hepatic, pancreatic, or other endocrine dysfunction may occur. Disorders of O/P should be considered in the differential diagnosis of any patient with unexplained multisystem involvement which includes progressive myopathic or neurological dysfunction.

Routine Laboratory Evaluation: Routine laboratory evaluation may reveal hypoglycemia or abnormal liver function testing. Blood, urine, and cerebrospinal fluid lactate levels are elevated with some of the disorders. An elevated lactate to pyruvate ratio (over 25) suggests a defect in O/P. Urine organic acid profiles should be done to rule out other disorders which may clinically be indistinguishable, especially the organic acidemias and disorders of fatty acid oxidation.

Cerebral Imaging: Cerebral imaging may be helpful in evaluating a patient suspected of having a defect of O/P. Patients may have bilateral, symmetric, areas of low attenuation in the posterior medial nucleus of the thalamus and basal ganglia (Leigh phenotype) or unifocal or multifocal areas of cerebral edema or infarction (MELAS; mitochondrial encephalomyopathy, lactic acidosis, and stroke-like episodes). Electromyography will show nonspecific myopathic changes. Nerve conduction velocities are occasionally slowed. Electroencephalography will be abnormal in patients with seizures, but will otherwise not show any characteristic or specific changes.

Muscle Biopsies: Muscle biopsies usually provide valuable information in the evaluation of a patient suspected of having a disorder of mitochondrial O/P. The hallmark of mitochondrial disorders is the finding of "ragged red" fibers (RRF) in muscle biopsies from affected patients. The RRF consist of aggregates of abnormal mitochondria in the peripheral or intermyofibrillary areas that appear as red or purple patches with modified Gomori trichrome staining. The muscle fibers will usually lack cytochrome c oxidase activity. RRF are commonly found in patients

that have defects associated with the synthesis of mitochondrial proteins, such as the multiple mtDNA deletion and depletion syndromes, and with point mtDNA mutations that affect mitochondrial transfer RNA (tRNA). With electron microscopy, an increase in the size or number of mitochondria, or abnormal density or orientation of the mitochondrial cristae may be noted. The presence of mitochondrial paracrystalline, lattice-shaped inclusions or electron-dense globular bodies may also be observed. Muscle biopsies will often have nonspecific accumulation of glycogen or lipid droplets. Histochemical staining can be used to show deficient activity of enzymes such as cytochrome c oxidase or succinate dehydrogenase. Immunochemical studies may be done with antibodies to many of the respiratory chain components.

Muscle or liver biopsy samples or cultured skin fibroblasts may also be used for measuring enzymatic assay for many components of the respiratory chain. Muscle or liver biopsies, or tissues obtained at autopsy, should be fresh or quick frozen without preservative. Many patients have tissue-specific disorders and not all tissues will always express the defect. Molecular genetic studies may also be done with biopsy samples, cultured skin fibroblasts, or peripheral leukocytes and platelets. However, cultured fibroblast or leukocyte cell lines may lose abnormal mitochondria through replicative segregation. Muscle biopsies also may be needed for molecular studies if the findings in cultured cell lines are not abnormal.

The disorders of O/P have been in the past classified on the basis of clinical findings. Many acronyms were formed for some of the symptoms complexes, eg, MERRF (myoclonic epilepsy with ragged red fibers). However, now that the molecular basis for many of the disorders are known, they are more appropriately classified on the basis of the associated molecular defects. As with the prior classification, there is still considerable overlap in the etiology of the clinical syndromes, eg, the Leigh phenotype may result from both nuclear and mitochondrial DNA mutations. Thus, biochemical and molecular studies on patients will be needed for appropriate genetic counseling for the families of affected individuals. Further understanding of the biochemical and molecular basis for the disorders will hopefully clarify the classification in the future.

Defects in O/P That Result from Abnormalities in Nuclear DNA (nDNA)

These disorders are inherited as Mendelian traits and will have autosomal dominant, autosomal recessive, or X-linked patterns of inheritance. The defects and clinical phenotypes are shown in Table 16–1. The molecular defects associated with the disorders are unknown at the present time.

Deficiency of Complex I (NADH:ubiquinone oxidoreductase): Complex I is the largest of the complexes of the O/P system. Of the at least 35 polypeptides of complex I, only 7 are encoded by mtDNA and the remainder are encoded by nDNA. The 7 subunits encoded by mtDNA are termed ND1, ND2, ND3, ND4, ND4L, ND5, and ND6. Patients with defects in complex I have presented with three clinical phenotypes:

A. Myopathy: A myopathy with exercise intolerance, weakness, mild lactic acidosis, and occasionally cardiomyopathy or pigmentary retinopathy has been reported in children and young adults.

B. Fatal Infantile Multisystem Disorder: A fatal infantile multisystem disorder, characterized by severe lactic acidosis, hypotonia, psychomotor delay, cardiorespiratory failure, results in death during infancy.

C. Mitochondrial Encephalomyopathy: A mitochondrial encephalomyopathy may have its onset during childhood or adult life. Affected patients may also have ophthalmoplegia, pigmentary retinopathy, neurosensory hearing loss, movement disorders, sensory neuropathy, ataxia, seizures, and psychomotor regression.

Deficiency of Complex II (succinate:ubiqui-none oxidoreductase): Complex II contains 4 components which are encoded only by nDNA. Patients with complex II deficiency have been reported to have (A) **encephalomyopathies** or (B) **myopathies** with exercise intolerance, weakness, and myoglobinuria.

Deficiency of Complex III (ubiquinol:ferrocytochrome c oxidoreductase): Complex III contains 11 subunits; only 1, known as cytochrome b, is encoded by mtDNA. Patients with complex III deficiency have been reported with three clinical phenotypes:

A. Myopathy: A myopathy characterized by exercise intolerance followed by weakness has been reported in children and adults. The defect appears to be isolated to skeletal muscle.

B. Histiocytoid Cardiomyopathy of Infancy. A rare, fatal, histiocytoid cardiomyopathy of infancy appears to be limited to cardiac muscle.

C. Multisystem Encephalomyopathy: A multisystem encephalomyopathy may occur in a: (1) **fatal infantile form** which presents shortly after birth with lactic acidosis and hypotonia; or as a (2) **milder disorder** with onset during childhood or early adult

Table 16–1. Disorders of oxidative phosphorylation that result from defects in nuclear DNA (nDNA).

Disorder	Complex Subunits	Clinical Phenotypes
1. Deficiency of Complex I (NADH:ubiquinone oxidoreductase)	At least 35 polypeptides; seven encoded by mtDNA	1. Myopathy 2. Fatal infantile myltisystem disorder 3. Encephalomyopathy
2. Deficiency of Complex II (succinate:ubiquinone oxidoreductase)	Four components, encoded only by nDNA	1. Encephalomyopathy 2. Myopathy

3. Deficiency of Complex III (ubiquinol:ferrocytochrome c oxidoreductase)	11 subunits; one encoded by mtDNA	1. Myopathy
		2. Histiocytoid cardiomyopathy of infancy
		3. Multisystem encephalomyopathy
		   a. Fatal infantile form
		   b. Milder disorder

4. Deficiency of Complex IV (cytochrome c oxidase)	13 subunits; three encoded by mtDNA	1. Myopathic form
		   a. Fatal infantile myopathic form
		   b. Benign infantile myopathic form
		2. Encephalomyopathic form
		   a. Leigh syndrome
		   b. MNGIE syndrome
		   c. Alpers syndrome

5. Deficiency of Complex V (ATP synthase)	12–14 subunits; two encoded by mtDNA	1. Myopathy 2. Multisystem disorder
6. Deficiency of Coenzyme Q_{10} (CoQ_{10})		1. Myopathy and seizures
7. Defects in intergenomic signaling		
A. Depletion of mtDNA		1. Congenital infantile mitochondrial myopathy 2. Fatal infantile hepatopathy 3. Infantile or childhood myopathy
B. Multiple mtDNA deletions		1. AD form of CPEO

AD = autosomal dominant; CPEO = chronic progressive external ophthalmoplegia; Leigh syndrome = subacute necrotizing encephalomyopathy; MNGIE = mitochondrial neuropathy, gastrointestinal disorder, encephalopathy syndrome; mtDNA = mitochondrial DNA; nDNA = nuclear DNA.

life. Patients with the milder form may have varying combinations of hypotonia, short stature, pigmentary retinopathy, sensorineural hearing loss, peripheral neuropathy, pyramidal signs, ataxia, seizures, and psychomotor regression.

Deficiency of Complex IV (cytochrome c oxidase): Complex IV consists of 13 subunits; 3 subunits are encoded by mtDNA which include COI, COII, and COIII. Deficiency of complex IV, or cytochrome c oxidase (COX), has been reported in numerous patients. There are two major clinical phenotypes, a myopathy and a multisystem encephalomyopathy.

A. Myopathy: The myopathic form presents shortly after birth with severe generalized hypotonia, lactic acidosis, and respiratory distress. The myopathic form has two subgroups with very differing clinical outcomes.

1. Fatal infantile myopathy–The fatal infantile myopathic form is often accompanied by Fanconi-type renal tubular dysfunction and occasionally by a cardiomyopathy. Most infants develop respiratory insufficiency and die by one year of age.

2. Benign infantile myopathy–The benign infantile myopathic form, which presents initially with the same clinical features of its fatal counterpart, is associated with the spontaneous return of COX activity and clinical improvement by 1 to 3 years of age. This form of the disease may result from deficiency of an isoenzyme which is present only during early life.

B. Encephalomyopathy: The encephalomyopathic form of COX deficiency is a multisystem disorder that has been noted in some patients with Leigh syndrome, MNGIE (mitochondrial neuropathy, gastrointestinal disorder, encephalopathy) syndrome, and Alpers syndrome.

1. Leigh syndrome–Leigh syndrome (subacute necrotizing encephalomyopathy) is an autosomal recessive trait. Affected patients are normal in early infancy. Between 6 and 12 months of age there is a plateau in development followed by psychomotor regression. Optic atrophy, ophthalmoplegia, nystagmus, dystonia, dysphagia, tremors, ataxia, pyramidal signs, peripheral neuropathies, and a deceleration in head growth are common. Seizures may occur but are less common than with other disorders associated with the Leigh phenotype. Radioimaging studies will show focal, symmetrical areas of necrosis in the posterior medial nucleus of the thalamus, basal ganglia, and posterior columns of the spinal cord. Most affected patients have progressive deterioration and die by 4 to 5 years of age.

The Leigh phenotype may also be seen in some patients with deficient activity of pyruvate carboxylase, deficient activity of the pyruvate dehydrogenase (PDH) complex, mtDNA depletion syndromes, or with a point mutation in mtDNA associated with NARP (neuropathy, ataxia, and retinitis pigmentosa).

The Leigh phenotype that occurs with deficient activity of the PDH complex and mtDNA depletion usually presents in the neonatal period and is rapidly progressive. Seizures are more common in the Leigh phenotype associated with PDH complex deficiency and NARP. The pattern of inheritance of the Leigh phenotype will vary depending upon the basic defect involved. The Leigh phenotypes associated with pyruvate carboxylase deficiency, mtDNA depletion, and COX deficiency are autosomal recessive disorders. Deficiency of the PDH complex most often involves mutations in the $E_1\alpha$ subunit and is associated with an X-linked pattern of inheritance. And, the Leigh phenotype associated with NARP is associated with a maternal pattern of inheritance.

2. MNGIE syndrome–MNGIE syndrome is a multisystem disorder characterized by chronic progressive external ophthalmoplegia (CPEO), hypotonia, peripheral neuropathy, chronic diarrhea, intestinal pseudo-obstruction, leukodystrophy, lactic acidosis, and ragged-red fibers on muscle biopsy. The external ophthalmoplegia affects only the external ocular muscles and limits movements of the eye and eyelids. Some patients with MNGIE syndrome have been found to have partial COX deficiency. This form of the syndrome appears to be inherited as an autosomal recessive trait.

3. Alpers syndrome–Alpers syndrome (progressive poliodystrophy of infancy) has been associated with COX deficiency in two patients. Infants with Alpers syndrome present during the first year of life with seizures and a progressive atrophy and spongy degeneration of the cerebral cortex, cerebellum, basal ganglia, and brain stem. Some affected infants have progressive hepatic dysfunction with cirrhosis. Other patients with Alpers syndrome have had deficient activity of pyruvate carboxylase in the liver or deficient activity of the pyruvate dehydrogenase complex in the brain. For others, the basic defect is unknown.

Deficiency of Complex V (ATP synthase): Complex V is comprised of 12 to 14 subunits; 2 subunits are encoded by mtDNA, ATPase 6 and ATPase 8. Deficiency of complex V is rare and has been reported in patients with two clinical phenotypes: (A) a slowly progressive **myopathy** with ragged-red fibers; or with (B) a **multisystem disorder** characterized by hypotonia, ataxia, peripheral neuropathy, retinopathy, and dementia.

Deficiency of Coenzyme Q_{10} (CoQ_{10}): Deficiency of CoQ_{10} has been reported in two sisters with progressive limb weakness, exercise intolerance, myoglobinuria, and seizures. The patients showed a clinical response to CoQ_{10} therapy.

Defects in Intergenomic Signaling: These disorders result from mutations in nDNA genes which code for factors involved with the replication, transcription, or translation of mtDNA. Two types of disorders are known which are associated with generalized mtDNA depletion or with multiple deletions of mtDNA.

A. Autosomal Recessive Disorder with mtDNA Depletion: An autosomal recessive disorder with **mtDNA depletion** is thought to result from defects in nDNA genes which control mitochondrial replication. The absence of mtDNA has been noted in liver and muscle biopsies from affected patients. Affected patients have a severe mitochondrial myopathy with ragged-red fibers on muscle biopsy. Some patients have had decreased activity of more than one O/P component (eg, COX and cyt b). The disorder is associated with three clinical phenotypes:

1. Congenital Infantile Mitochondrial Myopathy: A congenital infantile mitochondrial myopathy (Leigh-like phenotype) is characterized by lactic acidosis, occasionally Fanconi-type renal tubular dysfunction, and death between 3 and 11 months of age. This form of the disorder may be clinically indistinguishable from other forms of the Leigh phenotype.

2. Fatal Infantile Hepatopathy: A fatal infantile hepatopathy, with lactic acidosis, cardiomyopathy, seizures, results in death between 4 and 9 months of age.

3. Infantile or Childhood Myopathy: An infantile or childhood myopathy has its onset at one year of age and usually results in death at 3 years.

B. Chronic Progressive External Ophthalmoplegia (CPEO): An autosomal dominant form of chronic progressive external ophthalmoplegia (CPEO) has been associated with **multiple mtDNA deletions**. Affected adults will have limited movement of the eye and eyelids, proximal limb weakness, vestibular areflexia, exercise intolerance, mild lactic acidosis, and ragged-red fibers on muscle biopsy. Cataracts, tremors, ataxia, and sensorimotor neuropathies may also occur. Children with multiple mtDNA deletions have been reported to have optic atrophy, hypotonia, peripheral neuropathies, myoglobinuria, and recurrent attacks of lethargy, coma, and ketoacidosis. The deletions occur in the areas of the mitochondrial genome associated with transcription and replication that are under the control of nDNA. The basis for the disorders is unknown.

Defects in the Coupling of O/P With ATP Synthesis

Luft Syndrome: Luft syndrome, or nonthyroidal hypermetabolism, is a sporadic disorder associated with elevated body temperature, heat intolerance, resting tachycardia, increased sweating, exercise intolerance and a generalized myopathy. Affected patients have the onset of this progressive disorder during their teens and usually die during middle age. Ragged-red fibers are present on skeletal muscle biopsy. It appears that the energy produced by the respiratory chain is not used for ATP synthesis but is dissipated as heat (uncoupled O/P).

Defects in O/P That Result from Abnormalities of Mitochondrial DNA (mtDNA)

Table 16–2 lists the disorders associated with defects in mitochondrial DNA.

Disorders Associated With Large-scale Rearrangements (Deletions or Duplications) of mtDNA: There are three disorders associated with large-scale arrangements. Kearns-Sayre syndrome and the Pearson syndrome are usually sporadic and not inherited. The syndrome of diabetes mellitus and deafness is associated with a maternal pattern of inheritance.

A. Kearns-Sayre Syndrome: Kearns-Sayre syndrome (KSS) is a sporadic disorder of childhood characterized by CPEO and retinitis pigmentosa. Most affected patients have the onset of their disease before age 20 and do not survive past the third or fourth decade. Other clinical findings include hearing loss, psychomotor retardation, poor coordination, and episodes of coma. Some patients will develop complete heart block, which may require a pacemaker or be associated with sudden death. Endocrine problems such as hypoparathyroidism, diabetes mellitus, and isolated growth hormone deficiency may occur. Increased lactate and pyruvate levels will be noted. Cerebral spinal fluid protein will be elevated. Some patients have had lowered cerebrospinal fluid levels of folic acid; these patients may benefit from folate therapy. Spongy degeneration of the brain will be noted with CT or MRI scanning. Calcification of the basal ganglia may occur, especially in those patients with hypoparathyroidism. Muscle biopsy will reveal ragged-red fibers. There are large scale rearrangements of mtDNA which are usually deletions, but may be duplications. The rearrangements involve more than one mtDNA gene. Because the disorder does not appear to be inherited, it is thought that the rearrangements occur after fertilization in the zygote and not in the germ cell line of the mother. "Incomplete" forms of KSS are known that may only have CPEO or CPEO associated with multisystem involvement (CPEO Plus). CPEO may also be seen with MELAS syndrome (associated with maternal inheritance and a point mutation in mtDNA, discussed later), and with autosomal dominant CPEO (an nDNA defect previously discussed).

B. Pearson Syndrome: Pearson syndrome is a sporadic, congenital disorder associated with refractory sideroblastic anemia, vacuolization of marrow precursors, and pancytopenia. Pancreatic fibrosis, which results in exocrine pancreatic dysfunction, frequently occurs. Affected patients occasionally have hepatic or renal problems. There are large-scale deletions or insertions of mtDNA as in KSS. Although some affected infants die, others will survive and recover bone marrow function. Some survivors have gone on to develop KSS. In these patients it is thought that there is selective loss or disadvantage of

Table 16–2. Disorders of oxidative phosphorylation associated with mutations in mitochondrial DNA.

Disorder	Clinical Phenotypes	Inheritance Pattern
A. Large-scale rearrangements (deletions or duplications) of mtDNA	a. Kearns-Sayre syndrome	Sporadic, not inherited
	b. Variants of Kearns-Sayre syndrome (CPEO and CPEO Plus)	Sporadic, not inherited
	c. Pearson syndrome	Sporadic, not inherited
	d. Diabetes mellitus and deafness	Maternal
B. Point mutations of mtDNA		
1. Structural mtDNA genes	a. LHON; Leber hereditary optic neuropathy	Maternal
	b. NARP; neuropathy, ataxia, and retinitis pigmentosa	Maternal
2. Synthetic mtDNA mutations [point mutations in mtDNA that affect transfer RNA (tRNA)]	a. MELAS; mitochondrial encephalomyopathy with lactic acidosis and stroke-like episodes	Maternal
	b. MERRF; myoclonic epilepsy and ragged-red fibers	Maternal
	c. MiMyCa; maternally inherited disorder with adult onset myopathy and cardiomyopathy	Maternal
	d. Maternally inherited diabetes mellitus and deafness	Maternal

CPEO = chronic progressive external ophthalmoplegia.

cell lines that have abnormal mtDNA during replication. The selective loss allows cells with normal mtDNA to repopulate the rapidly dividing bone marrow. Because of minimal or slower replication in the brain and muscles, the mutations are not lost, but persist, and with time lead to an encephalomyopathy.

C. Diabetes Mellitus and Deafness: A syndrome characterized by diabetes mellitus and deafness has been found to be associated with a large 10.4 kilobase deletion of mtDNA. Encephalomyopathy and CPEO do not occur. The disorder is associated with a maternal pattern of inheritance. It may also result from point mutations in mtDNA.

Disorders That Result From Point Mutations of mtDNA

In contrast to the sporadic disorders associated with large-scale rearrangements of mtDNA, the disorders associated with mtDNA point mutations are usually maternally inherited. Of the six clinical phenotypes described to date, two—Leber hereditary optic neuropathy (LHON) and neuropathy, ataxia, and retinitis pigmentosa (NARP)—are associated with defects in **structural mtDNA genes.** Patients with these two disorders do not usually have lactic acidosis or ragged-red fibers on muscle biopsy. The other four phenotypes are associated with point mutations in mtDNA that affect transfer RNA (tRNA) and are considered **synthetic mtDNA mutations.** Patients affected with the synthetic mtDNA mutations usually have lactic acidosis and ragged-red fibers on muscle biopsy. The four synthetic mtDNA mutation phenotypes include: (1) mitochondrial encephalomyopathy with lactic acidosis and stroke-like episodes (MELAS); (2) myoclonic epilepsy and ragged-red fibers (MERRF); (3) a maternally inherited disorder with adult onset myopathy and cardiomyopathy (MiMyCa); and (4) maternally inherited diabetes mellitus and deafness.

Leber Hereditary Optic Neuropathy (LHON): Leber hereditary optic neuropathy (LHON) is associated with bilateral visual loss in young adults. The onset may occur as early as 5 years of age or as late as 30. The loss of vision is often sudden, but may start unilaterally and progress to bilateral involvement. There is a retrobulbar neuropathy with central scotomas, edema of the disc, and a microangiopathy. Some affected patients will also have cardiac conduction defects, peripheral neuropathies, ataxia, or hyperreflexia. The disorder—associated with a maternal pattern of inheritance—should equally affect females and males. However, because more affected males than females are observed, other genetic or environmental factors may play a role in the development of the disease. At least 11 point mtDNA mutations have been associated with the LHON phenotype that have involved the ND1, ND2, ND4, ND5, and ND6 subunits of complex I, apocytochrome b of complex III, and COI of complex IV.

Neuropathy, Ataxia, and Retinitis Pigmentosa (NARP): Neuropathy, ataxia, and retinitis pigmentosa (NARP) is a multisystem disorder which can present at any age. Affected patients have retinitis pigmentosa, psychomotor retardation, ataxia, seizures, proximal weakness, and sensory neuropathies. An infantile form may present with a Leigh-type phenotype. Mutations in subunit ATPase 6 of complex V have been reported. The clinical severity is related to the relative amount of mutant mtDNA present.

Mitochondrial Encephalomyopathy With Lactic Acidosis and Stroke-like Episodes (MELAS): Patients with mitochondrial encephalomyopathy with lactic acidosis and stroke-like episodes (MELAS) have normal early development. This is followed, however, by exercise intolerance and a progressive encephalomyopathy with seizures and episodes which resemble strokes. Most patients have the onset of their symptoms before age 40 years. Many affected patients have migraine-like headaches which are preceded by nausea and vomiting. Seizures will often precede the stroke-like episodes. Hearing loss, short stature, learning difficulties, hypotonia, hemiparesis, and hemianopsia may occur. Approximately 10% of patients will have CPEO. All have lactic acidosis and ragged-red fibers on muscle biopsy. One-half will have elevated levels of cerebrospinal fluid protein. Radioimaging will show focal areas of cerebral edema or infarcts which are most commonly noted in the posterior temporal, parietal, and occipital lobes. One-third will have calcification of the basal ganglia. Two point mutations in mtDNA encoding for tRNA^{leu} and one mutation in tRNA^{lys} have been associated with the MELAS phenotype.

Myoclonic Epilepsy and Ragged-red Fibers (MERRF): Myoclonic epilepsy and ragged-red fibers (MERRF), which has its onset in childhood or adult life, is characterized by progressive generalized or myoclonic seizures, impaired coordination, psychomotor retardation, hearing loss, impaired deep sensation, and optic atrophy. Some affected patients have developed a cardiomyopathy and other features of MELAS. There is a spongy degeneration of the brain and degeneration of the posterior columns and spinocerebellar tracts. Lactic acid levels are elevated and ragged-red fibers are present on muscle biopsy. Some patients with MERRF have a mtDNA mutation at the tRNA^{lys} locus.

Maternally Inherited Disorder With Adult Onset Myopathy and Cardiomyopathy (MiMyCa): A maternally inherited disorder with adult onset myopathy and cardiomyopathy (MiMyCa) is usually limited to only muscular involvement. Affected patients have a lactic acidosis and ragged-red fibers on muscle biopsy. Mutations at the tRNA^{leu} locus, different from those found with MELAS, have been associated with this phenotype.

Other patients with mtDNA mutations have O/P phenotypes that presently do not fit into the above classifications. And some patients are being found to have acquired O/P disorders associated with environmental toxins and medications (eg, zidovudine).

Current treatment is mainly symptomatic and supportive. Patients with significant acidosis may require bicarbonate or citrate buffers. Dichloracetate, an investigational drug, increases the activity of the pyruvate dehydrogenase complex and may be helpful in treating some patients affected with the more moderate or milder forms of the disorders. Thiamine, riboflavin, CoQ$_{10}$, ascorbic acid, vitamin K analogs, and succinate may modify the course of disease in certain patients.

REFERENCES AND SUGGESTED READING

See Page 256 and Appendix II.

Peroxisomes

17

DISORDERS OF PEROXISOMES

Disorders of peroxisomes are a relatively recently described group of diseases that have an estimated combined incidence of 1 in 25,000. Peroxisomes are small, subcellular, single-membrane bound, electron-dense organelles that are so named because they contain catalase and are involved with peroxide-based respiration. They also contain enzymes responsible for the beta-oxidation of very long chain fatty acids (VLCFA), synthesis of plasmalogens and bile salts, and oxidation of phytanic and pipecolic acids.

The disorders are presently classified into three groups. Group 1 results from a defect in the formation of the peroxisomal membrane. Peroxisomes are absent or reduced in number in biopsies from affected patients; multiple peroxisomal functions are affected. Group 2 has intact peroxisomes, with more than one peroxisomal enzyme or function affected. Group 3 also has intact peroxisomes, but the disorders result from deficient activity of a single peroxisomal enzyme. Table 17–1 gives the present classification, the disorders involved, and their biochemical findings. This classification is expected to change with further understanding of the biochemical and molecular genetics involved. The disorders are inherited as autosomal recessive traits except for adrenoleukodystrophy (ALD) and adrenomyeloneuropathy (AMN), which are allelic X-linked traits.

Peroxisomal enzymes are responsible for the beta-oxidation of unsaturated VLCFA with carbon lengths greater than 22 and monosaturated long chain fatty acids (C22:1). Tetracosanoic acid (lignoceric acid; C24:0) and hexacosanoic acid (cerotic acid; C26:0) are markedly elevated in the plasma and tissues of affected patients. Patients with elevated VLCFA have reduced activity of peroxisomal lignoceroyl-CoA ligase and acyl-CoA oxidase. Plasmalogens, a type of ether-phospholipids, are major components of cell membranes and myelin. Two enzymes, dihydroxyacetone phosphate acyltransferase (DHAPAT) and alkyl dihydroxyacetone phosphate synthetase, are deficient in patients who have reduced plasmalogen synthesis. Reduced plasmalogen levels may be shown in erythrocytes from affected patients. The final steps in the biosynthesis of bile acids from cholesterol occur in the peroxisome. Patients with abnormal peroxisomal bile salt metabolism have increased body fluid levels of bile acid precursors such as 3α,7α-dihydroxy-5β-cholestanoic acid (DHCA) and 3α,7α,12α-trihydroxy-5β-cholestanoic acid (THCA). Abnormal levels of bile acid intermediates and VLCFA have been noted in patients with reduced activity of 3-oxoacyl-CoA thiolase, or the bifunctional enzyme, which functions as both enoyl-CoA hydratase and 3-hydroxyacyl-CoA dehydrogenase. Elevated levels of pipecolic acid, derived from lysine, occur as a result of deficient activity of pipecolic acid oxidase. Oxidation of phytanic acid, a long chain branched fatty acid of dietary origin, occurs in both the peroxisome and the mitochondria. Patients with faulty peroxisomal oxidation of phytanic acid have elevated levels of phytanic acid and pristanic acid, an intermediate in the oxidative process. Adult, or classical, Refsum disease was previously classified with the peroxisomal disorders but is now thought to result from defective mitochondrial phytanic acid oxidation. Adult Refsum disease is associated with progressive neurological dysfunction and the accumulation of phytanic acid, but not pristanic acid.

Group 1: Disorders Associated With Generalized Peroxisomal Dysfunction

Zellweger (Cerebrohepatorenal) Syndrome: The prototype for the groups of disorders is Zellweger (cerebrohepatorenal) syndrome (Figure 17–1). The clinical features of Zellweger syndrome are listed in Table 17–2. Patients present in the neonatal period with dysmorphic features, marked generalized hypotonia, and feeding and respiratory difficulties. Abnormal neuronal migration and fetal brain development result in macrogyria and polymicrogyria, failure of myelination and white-matter development, severe psychomotor retardation, seizures, and progressive neurological deterioration. Chondrodysplasia punctata, or punctate mineralization in the patellar and acetabular joint spaces, may be noted on radiograms. Radioimaging studies demonstrate the abnormal brain development, varying degrees of myelin abnormalities, renal cysts, and hepatomegaly. Although most affected infants do not live past 6 months of age, longer survival has been reported. Treatment is mainly symptomatic and sup-

Table 17–1. Characteristics of peroxisomal disorders.

	Enzymatic Deficiency or Biochemical Defect	Elevated VLCFA	Faulty Plasmalogen Synthesis	Abnormal Bile Acid Synthesis	Abnormal Phytanic Acid Oxidation	Elevated Pipecolic Acid	Other
Group 1: Generalized peroxisomal dysfunction due to faulty peroxisome biosynthesis							
Zellweger syndrome	Multiple	+	+	+	+/−	+	−
Neonatal ALD	Multiple	+	+	+	+/−	+	−
Infantile refsum disease	Multiple	+	+	+	+	+	−
Hyperpipecolic acidemia	Multiple	+	+	+	+/−	+	−
Group 2: Defects in more than one peroxisomal enzyme, intact peroxisomes							
Zellweger-like syndrome	Multiple	+	+	+	−	−	−
Rhizomelic chondrodysplasia punctata	Acyl-CoA:DHAPAT, phytanic acid α-oxidation	−	+	−	+	−	−
Group 3: Defect in a single peroxisomal enzyme, intact peroxisomes							
ALD/AMN	Lignoceroyl-CoA ligase	+	−	−	−	−	−
Pseudo-neonatal ALD	Acyl-CoA oxidase	+	−	−	−	−	−
Bifunctional enzyme deficiency	Bifunctional enzyme	+	−	+	−	−	−
Pseudo-Zellweger syndrome	3-Oxoacyl-CoA thiolase	+	−	+	−	−	+/−
Hyperoxaluria type I	Alanine:glyoxylate aminotransferase	−	−	−	−	−	+
Acatalasemia	Catalase	−	−	−	−	−	+
Glutaryl-CoA oxidase deficiency	Glutaryl-CoA oxidase	−	−	−	−	−	+

ALD = Adrenoleukodystrophy; AMN = Adrenomyeloneuropathy; CoA = coenzyme A; DHAPAT = dihydroxyacetone phosphate acyltransferase; VLCFA = Very long chain fatty acids; + = abnormal; − = normal.

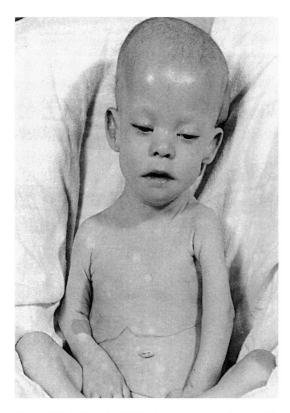

Figure 17–1. Classical Zellweger syndrome at age 8 1/2 months. (Reproduced, with permission from Oski FA et al (editors), *Principles and Practice of Pediatrics,* 2nd ed, JB Lippincott, 1994.)

portive. Multiple peroxisomal functions are affected. Elevated plasma levels of VLCFA, bile acid intermediates such as THCA and DHCA, and phytanic and pristanic acids, along with reduced plasmalogens in erythrocyte samples will support the clinical diagnosis. Enzymatic and DNA studies may be done with cultured skin fibroblasts. Prenatal diagnosis is available for at-risk families.

Neonatal ALD, Infantile Refsum Disease, and Hyperpipecolic Acidemia: The three other disorders presently in Group 1, neonatal ALD, infantile Refsum disease, and hyperpipecolic acidemia, have less severe but similar, clinical and biochemical features as those seen in Zellweger syndrome. The onset is later, dysmorphic features are variable, and renal cysts and chondrodysplasia punctata are not usually noted. The disorders may be differentiated on the basis of complementation groups with cultured skin fibroblast studies.

Group 2: Disorders Associated With Intact Peroxisomes and Defects in More Than One Peroxisomal Enzyme

Zellweger-like Syndrome: A Zellweger-like syndrome with intact peroxisomes has been reported in patients with dysmorphic features, abnormal VLCFA beta-oxidation, and defects in plasmalogen and bile salt synthesis. The exact metabolic defect is unknown.

Rhizomelic Form of Chondrodysplasia Punctata: Patients with the rhizomelic form of chondrodysplasia punctata present at birth with disproportionate short stature, shortening of the proximal extremities, frontal bossing, flattening of the nasal bridge, and joint contractures. Affected infants also have congenital cataracts, microcephaly, psychomotor retardation, ichthyosis, and failure to thrive. Most do not survive past infancy. Symmetrical epiphyseal and extraepiphyseal calcifications are more extensive than those seen with Zellweger syndrome; they may involve the vertebrae and extraskeletal tissues (Figure 17–2). Deficient activity of DHAPAT and phytanic acid oxidase results in faulty plasmalogen synthesis and elevated phytanic and pristanic acid levels, respectively. These patients also have an unprocessed form of 3-oxoacyl-CoA thiolase, as is noted in patients with defects in peroxisome biosynthesis, but the metabolism of VLCFA is normal.

Group 3: Disorders Associated With a Defect in a Single Peroxisomal Function

Adrenoleukodystrophy (ALD) and Adrenomyeloneuropathy (AMN): Adrenoleukodystrophy (ALD) and adrenomyeloneuropathy (AMN) are X-linked disorders associated with deficient activity of lignoceroyl-CoA ligase. Elevated levels of VLCFA accumulate in the ganglioside and cholesteryl ester fractions of cerebral white matter and the adrenal cortex. Figure 17–3 shows the leukodystrophy detected with MRI scanning of an affected patient. Boys with the childhood form of ALD have the onset of signs of progressive central and peripheral nervous system demyelination between 4 and 8 years of age. Dysarthria, dysphagia, and an abnormal gait are the usual presenting symptoms, that are followed by the gradual loss of psychomotor abilities, vision, and hearing. Adrenocortical insufficiency is common and may be present before the neurological symptoms develop. Most affected boys succumb to their disease between 3 and 5 years after the onset of symptoms. AMN is a milder, allelic, form of ALD that presents in young adult males. AMN patients may have primary hypogonadism in addition to adrenocortical insufficiency. Female carriers for ALD or AMN may also have symptomatic involvement. Replacement hormone therapy will correct the adrenocortical insufficiency. Treatment with dietary restriction of C26:0 along with supplemental glycerol trierucate (C22:1) and glycerol trioleate (C18:1) (Lorenzo's oil), has been shown to lower VLCFA levels and to result in clinical improvement in patients with AMN and in symptomatic female carriers for ALD. This treatment also may delay neurological deterioration

Table 17–2. Clinical features of Zellweger syndrome.

Category/System	Clinical Findings
Dysmorphic	High forehead, large anterior fontanel, hypoplastic supraorbital ridges, midfacial hypoplasia, epicanthal folds. Flattened occiput. High arched palate. External ear anomalies. Micrognathia. Redundant neck skin folds. Transverse palmar creases.
Neurologic	Abnormal neuronal migration, microgyria/pachygyria. Abnormal white matter. Seizures. Psychomotor retardation. Severe hypotonia, hyporeflexia/areflexia. Neurological deterioration.
Hepatic	Hepatomegaly, hepatic fibrosis, cholestasis, micronodular cirrhosis. Absent peroxisomes.
Renal	Cortical cysts, glomerular microcysts, albuminuria.
Adrenal	Lamellar inclusions; impaired response to ACTH.
Ophthalmic	Brushfield spots, congenital cataracts, congenital glaucoma, pigmentary retinopathy, optic nerve dysplasia/atrophy, nystagmus. Abnormal electroretinograms.
Cardiac	Ventricular septal defect, aortic abnormalities.
Skeletal	Chondrodysplasia punctata.
Other	Feeding problems, failure to thrive, impaired hearing.

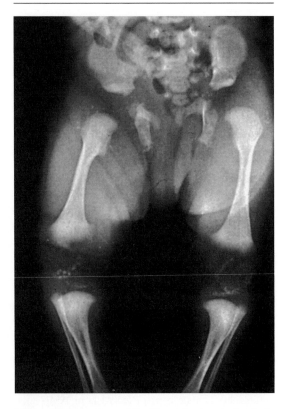

Figure 17–2. Radiograph in rhizomelic chondrodysplasia punctata. Note the extraepiphyseal calcifications. (Reproduced, with permission from Oski FA et al (editors), *Principles and Practice of Pediatrics,* 2nd ed, JB Lippincott, 1994.)

if started early, prior to the onset symptoms, in patients with childhood ALD identified as a result of family screening for the disease.

Pseudo-neonatal ALD and Deficiency of the Bifunctional Enzyme: Patients with pseudo-neonatal ALD and those with deficiency of the bifunctional enzyme present with hypotonia, seizures, and progressive central nervous system deterioration in early infancy or childhood. Dysmorphic features, like those seen with the Zellweger syndrome, are minimal in pseudo-neonatal ALD and usually absent in the bifunctional enzyme deficiency. In pseudo-neonatal ALD there is deficient activity of acyl-CoA oxidase and elevated levels of VLCFA. Deficiency of the bifunctional enzyme results in elevations of both VLCFA and THCA, a bile salt intermediate.

Pseudo-Zellweger Syndrome: Pseudo-Zellweger syndrome has clinical features similar to Zellweger syndrome except that intact peroxisomes are present. There is deficient activity of 3-oxoacyl-CoA thiolase and elevated levels of VLCFA, pipecolic acid, and bile acid intermediates.

Hyperoxaluria Type I: Hyperoxaluria type I, associated with deficient activity of alanine:glyoxylate aminotransferase, results in markedly increased urinary excretion of oxalic, glyoxylic, and glycolic acids. Although the age of onset is variable, affected children usually present by 5 years of age with recurrent nephrolithiasis, nephrocalcinosis, and chronic renal failure. Extrarenal accumulation of calcium oxalate may occur in other tissues, especially the bones, myocardium, and testes. Reduced dietary sources of oxalate and supplemental pyridoxine, phosphate, or magnesium may modify the outcome. Combined liver and renal transplantation may be considered in patients with advanced renal disease. Hyperoxaluria type II, less common than type I, is not a peroxiso-

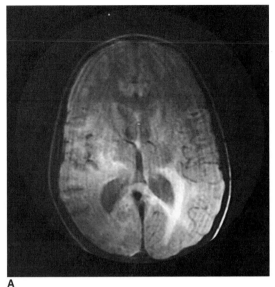
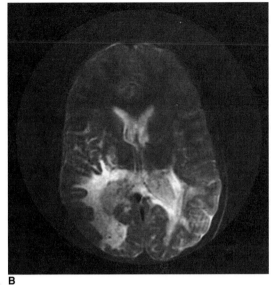

A
B

Figure 17–3. MRI of the brain in Adrenoleukodystrophy. **(A)** T1-weighted image; **(B)** T2-weighted image. Note the increased periventricular signal in the posterior areas. (Reproduced, with permission from Oski FA et al (editors), *Principles and Practice of Pediatrics,* 2nd ed, JB Lippincott, 1994.)

mal disorder. Type II, which usually presents with milder clinical findings than type I, is associated with deficient activity of D-glyceric dehydrogenase and elevated levels of urinary oxalic acid and L-glyceric acid.

Acatalasemia: Catalase deficiency, or acatalasemia, is usually asymptomatic. A severe variant in Japan, however, may be associated with varying degrees of ulcerating gangrenous lesions of the oral cavity during childhood.

Peroxisomal Glutaryl-CoA Oxidase Deficiency: Peroxisomal glutaryl-CoA oxidase deficiency has been found in one patient who presented with failure to thrive and vomiting. Elevated levels of urinary glutaric acid were noted that responded to riboflavin therapy.

REFERENCES AND SUGGESTED READING

See Page 256 and Appendix II.

18

Porphyrias

PORPHYRIAS

Porphyrias result from metabolic blocks in the heme biosynthetic pathway shown in Figure 18–1. Heme is an iron-containing compound found in hemoglobin, myoglobin, mitochondrial and microsomal cytochromes, and peroxisomal catalase and peroxidase. Biosynthesis of heme occurs in the liver and bone marrow. The biosynthesis of hepatic heme is feedback-regulated by the intracellular concentration of heme, which influences the level of activity of delta-aminolevulinic acid (ALA) synthetase, the first step in heme biosynthesis. In bone marrow, hematin stimulates heme synthesis in erythrocyte precursors by the induction of the heme biosynthetic enzymes.

The porphyrias are divided into erythropoietic and hepatic types, based on the site of overproduction of heme precursors. The heme precursors, known as porphobilinogens and porphyrins, accumulate and lead to clinical symptoms. The present classification of the porphyrias and their clinical and biochemical findings are shown in Table 18–1.

Photosensitivity: Photosensitivity occurs with the erythropoietic porphyrias and some of the hepatic forms. Porphyrins that are chelated with diamagnetic metals such as magnesium, zinc, selenium, and those that are metal-free have fluorescent properties. When present in elevated levels in the skin of patients and exposed to ultraviolet light, the porphyrins cause photodynamic cellular injury. Bullous formation in the epidermis, erythema, edema, pruritis, increased pigmentation, ulceration, and scarring may result. Hypotension and circulatory collapse have been reported in cases of extreme exposure with severe photosensitization. Treatment includes the avoidance of sunlight and the use of sunscreens and beta-carotene to improve light tolerance. Activated charcoal or cholestyramine may bind and retard the absorption of endogenous, enteral porphyrins.

Acute Neurovisceral Attacks: With the hepatic forms, acute neurovisceral attacks occur that are associated with increased levels of heme precursors. Attacks may be precipitated by exogenous drugs and chemicals, and by endogenous natural steroids that induce ALA synthetase activity. ALA and porphobilinogen (PBG) become markedly elevated in the urine of patients and result in a brown or reddish color to the urine on standing. During an acute attack, severe abdominal pain is followed by vomiting, weakness, and pain or discomfort in the chest, back, or extremities. Anxiety or depression, disorientation, and seizures may occur. Hypertension and tachycardia may be symptomatic. Attacks result from a neuropathy involving the anterior horn cells, dorsal root ganglion, splanchnic motor cells, cranial nerve nuclei, and the hypothalamus. Neuronal damage, axonal degeneration, and demyelination occur. With severe attacks, bulbar and respiratory paralysis may require assisted ventilation.

Carbohydrate loading, drugs that suppress heme production, and folic acid, a cofactor for PBG deaminase, may be used in the treatment of severe attacks. Other therapy is symptomatic and supportive. Neurological recovery is usually slow and may be partial or complete. Residual weakness is common. Although most patients are asymptomatic between attacks, increased urinary or stool levels of heme precursors are usually present in sufficient quantities for diagnostic testing. Because the attacks may be precipitated by environmental factors, eg, certain drugs, hormones, or ethanol, and by decreased carbohydrate intake, patients are advised to avoid these factors. Drugs that induce ALA synthetase activity have been associated with the attacks, in particular, barbiturates, other anticonvulsants, sulfonamides, griseofulvin, and synthetic estrogens or progestins. More complete lists are available for patients and their physicians.

Hepatic disease: Hepatic disease develops with some types of porphyria, most often as cirrhosis or focal hepatocellular necrosis.

All of the disorders are inherited either on an autosomal dominant or autosomal recessive basis, except for the sporadic and environmentally related cases of porphyria cutanea tarda (PCT). The autosomal dominant forms have a wide variation in clinical expression; many gene carriers are asymptomatic and considered "latent" cases. The diagnosis is usually established by the pattern of elevation of erythrocyte, urinary, and stool porphyrins. Determination of enzymatic activity in erythrocytes or cultured skin fibroblasts is available for some of these disorders.

The Erythropoietic Porphyrias
Congenital Erythropoietic Porphyria (CEP):
Congenital erythropoietic porphyria (CEP), an auto-

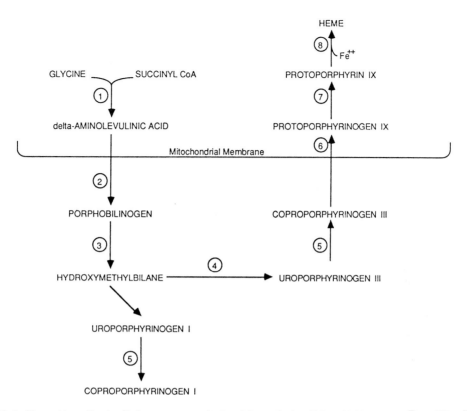

Figure 18–1. Heme biosynthesis. CoA = coenzyme A; 1 = delta-aminolevulinic acid (ALA synthetase); 2 = ALA dehydratase (PBG synthetase); 3 = porphobilinogen (PBG) deaminase; 4 = uroporphyrinogen III co-synthetase; 5 = uroporphyrinogen decarboxylase; 6 = coproporphyrinogen oxidase; 7 = protoporphyrinogen oxidase; 8 = ferrochelatase. (Reproduced, with permission from Oski FA et al (editors), *Principles and Practice of Pediatrics,* 2nd ed, JB Lippincott, 1994.)

somal recessive disorder, is associated with severe cutaneous photosensitivity that usually has its onset before the age of 5 years. Reddish brown or burgundy colored urine or diapers may be the first clinical manifestation in young infants. With ultraviolet light exposure, the skin becomes blistered and friable. The fluid in bullous vesicles may fluoresce. Skin infections and scarring are common and may lead to deformities of the eyelids, nose, ears, digits, and corneas. Reddish-brown discoloration of the teeth (erythrodontia) and hypertrichosis may also occur. Occasionally patients develop a hemolytic anemia with splenomegaly or cirrhosis. CEP results from reduced activity of uroporphyrinogen III co-synthetase, which may be determined in cultured skin fibroblasts or erythrocytes. CEP patients have increased porphyrins in the bone marrow, erythrocytes, spleen, urine, and stool. An adult-onset, milder form of CEP clinically resembles porphyria cutanea tarda (PCT).

Erythropoietic Protoporphyria (EPP): Patients with erythropoietic protoporphyria (EPP) develop photosensitivity during childhood, but it is usually milder than that seen with CEP. Affected patients

may also develop gallstones, cirrhosis, and hepatic failure. The disorder is inherited as an autosomal dominant trait with low penetrance. As many as 90% of gene carriers never have clinical symptoms. EPP results from decreased activity of ferrochelatase. Although the residual enzymatic activity of ferrochelatase in affected patients is lower than the 50% reduction that would be expected with an autosomal dominant trait, the assays used to measure the activity are tedious and may not accurately reflect that of intact cells. Affected patients have increased levels of heme precursors in erythrocytes, plasma, liver, bile, and stool.

Hepatoerythropoietic Porphyria (HEP): Hepatoerythropoietic porphyria (HEP) is an autosomal recessive trait associated with increased production of heme precursors in both the bone marrow and liver. Affected patients experience the onset of photosensitivity during or after childhood. Hepatic involvement and hemolytic anemia may also occur. The patients have markedly reduced activity of uroporphyrinogen decarboxylase and elevated porphyrins in erythrocytes, urine, and stool. HEP patients are thought to represent a homozygous affected form of porphyria

Table 18–1. Clinical and biochemical features of the porphyrias.

Type	Enzyme Affected (Percentage of Normal Activity)	Age of Onset	Photosensitivity	Acute Attacks	Hepatic	Genetics	Biochemical Findings
Erythropoietic porphyrias							
Congenital erythropoietic porphyria (CEP)	Uroporphyrinogen III co-synthetase (15)	Infancy	++++	–	–	AR	RBC—Uro, Copro, type I Urine—Uro, Copro, type I Stool—Copro, type I
Erythropoietic protoporphyria (EPP)	Ferrochelatase (10–25**)	Childhood	+++	–	+	AD	RBC—Proto IX Urine—normal Stool—Proto IX, +/– Copro
Hepatoerythropoietic porphyria (HEP)	Uroporphyrinogen decarboxylase (2–11)	Childhood to adult	++	–	+/–	AR	RBC—Proto Urine—Uro; 5-,6-,7-CP; +/– Copro Stool—Isocopro, Copro
Hepatic porphyrias							
Acute intermittent porphyria (AIP)	PBG deaminase (50)	After puberty	–	++++	–	AD	RBC—normal Urine—ALA, PBG Stool—normal
Porphyria cutanea tarda (PCT)	Uroporphyrinogen decarboxylase (40–65)	Before 20 years (40–60 yrs)*	++	–	++	AD (S,E)*	RBC—normal Urine—Uro; 5-,6-,7-CP; +/– Copro Stool—Isocopro, +/– Copro
Hereditary coproporphyria (HC)	Coproporphyrinogen oxidase (48–53)	Childhood	+/–	++	–	AD	RBC—normal Urine—PBG, ALA, Copro III, Uro Stool—Copro III
Variegate porphyria (VP)	Protoporphyrinogen oxidase (43–55)	After puberty	+/–	++	–	AD	RBC—normal Urine—PBG, ALA, Copro III Stool—X-porphyrins, Copro III
ALA dehydratase deficiency (ALAD)	ALA dehydratase (1–2)	Teenage Infancy	–	++	–	AR	RBC—Proto Urine—ALA, +/– PBG, Copro III Stool—normal

ALA = delta-aminolevulinic acid; Copro = coproporphyrins; CP = carboxyporphyrins; E = environmental; Isocopro = isocoproporphyrins; PBG = porphobilinogen; Proto = protoporphyrins; S = Sporadic; Uro = uroporphyrins; + = present; – = not present; ** = see text. Adapted from Wappner RS, Brandt IK. Inborn errors of metabolism. In: *Principles and Practice of Pediatrics*, Oski FA, DeAngelis CD, Feigin RD, Warshaw JB, editors, JB Lippincott, 1990.

cutanea tarda (PCT). PCT, an hepatic porphyria, is inherited as an autosomal dominant trait and associated with partial reduction of uroporphyrinogen decarboxylase.

Hepatic Porphyrias

Acute Intermittent Porphyria (AIP): Acute intermittent porphyria (AIP) is one of the more commonly recognized types of the disorders. The gene frequency may be as high as 1 in 10,000 to 1 in 20,000 persons. Affected patients have approximately 50% of normal activity of PBG deaminase (uroporphyrinogen I synthase). The disorder is characterized by acute neuroviseral attacks that most often occur after puberty. Only 10% of gene carriers have clinical symptoms, which are usually associated with the precipitating environmental factors discussed earlier. Women are more likely to have clinical expression of the disease than men. Acute attacks may occur with the hormonal changes of the menstrual cycle. Symptomatic patients have elevated urinary levels of ALA and PBG, which increase during attacks. Measurement of erythrocyte PBG deaminase activity is available in many laboratories. Overlap may occur, however, between the normal and affected ranges of enzymatic activity. Additional studies with mitogen-stimulated lymphocytes or cultured skin fibroblasts, along with quantitative urinary porphyrin measurements and family studies, may be needed for accurate detection of asymptomatic gene carriers.

Porphyria Cutanea Tarda (PCT): Porphyria cutanea tarda (PCT) may be inherited as an autosomal dominant trait. PCT may also occur sporadically or result from environmental hepatotoxins such as halogenated hydrocarbons, ethanol, estrogen, and iron. Patients with the autosomal dominant form of the disorder have a partial reduction in uroporphyrinogen decarboxylase activity in both erythrocytes and liver, whereas patients with the noninherited forms have decreased levels only in the liver. The inherited form usually has its onset before the age of 20 years, which is considerably earlier than that noted with the noninherited forms. Not all gene carriers have symptoms. Most symptomatic patients have skin photosensitivity that is not as severe as that of CEP. Affected patients develop small white plaques (milia) immediately after sunlight exposure, which are followed by the formation of vesicles and bullae. As with CEP, scarring, hypopigmentation, lichenification, and hypertrichosis

may occur. Adult patients also develop varying degrees of cirrhosis or focal hepatocellular necrosis. Hepatocellular carcinoma occasionally occurs. Because the majority of symptomatic patients have some degree of siderosis, repeated phlebotomy may be indicated to reduce iron stores. Elevated porphyrins may be found in the urine and stool. With the autosomal dominant form of PCT, uroporphyrinogen decarboxylase activity may be measured in erythrocytes.

Hereditary Coproporphyria (HC): Hereditary coproporphyria (HC) is characterized by acute neurovisceral attacks during childhood that are often precipitated by environmental factors. Photosensitivity, similar to that noted with PCT, occurs in 30% of symptomatic patients. During acute attacks, urinary ALA and PBG levels are elevated in addition to elevated levels of urine and stool coproporphyrin III. Between attacks, however, only stool coproporphyrin III levels are elevated. The disorder, which is inherited as an autosomal dominant trait, results from reduced activity of coproporphyrinogen oxidase. Homozygous affected patients have been reported with more severe clinical manifestations.

Variegate Porphyria (VP): Variegate porphyria (VP) results from reduced activity of protoporphyrinogen oxidase. It is most common in South African whites in whom it occurs in 1 in 330 persons. Affected patients become symptomatic after puberty with acute neurovisceral attacks that may be precipitated by environmental factors discussed earlier. Approximately 30% of the patients also have photosensitivity that may occur independently from the attacks. Hepatic involvement does not usually occur. ALA, PBG, and coproporphyrin III levels are increased in the urine during acute attacks. Between attacks, elevated stool porphyrins continue to be abnormal. Homozygous affected patients with marked reduction of enzymatic activity and severe clinical manifestations have been reported.

ALA Dehydratase Deficiency (ALAD): ALA dehydratase deficiency (ALAD) is a rare disorder characterized by acute neurovisceral attacks. Clinical symptoms start in infancy in some patients and during adolescence in others. Photosensitivity and hepatic dysfunction do not occur. The disorder, inherited as an autosomal recessive trait, results from a marked reduction in ALA dehydratase activity. Elevated urinary levels of ALA and coproporphyrin III, but usually not PBG, occur with acute attacks.

REFERENCES AND SUGGESTED READING

See Page 256 and Appendix II.

19

Purines & Pyrimidines

Disorders of purine and pyrimidine metabolism are rare inherited disorders that have a wide spectrum of clinical findings. Patients may have gouty arthritis, renal calculi, myopathies, immunodeficiencies, hemolytic anemias, or neurological problems with delayed development, autistic behaviors, and self-mutilation. In addition to being the basic elements of DNA (deoxyribonucleic acid) and RNA (ribonucleic acid), purine and pyrimidine metabolites are important constituents of other high-energy compounds and cofactors such as adenosine triphosphate (ATP) and nicotinamide-adenine dinucleotide (NAD). Although both purine and pyrimidine bases may be synthesized de novo from ribose-5-phosphate and carbamyl phosphate, respectively, there are "salvage" pathways of recycling and interconversion of the compounds that conserve the nucleosides and nucleotides and exert a negative feedback on de novo synthesis. Purines that are not recycled are degraded to uric acid, which is excreted by the kidney and intestine. Pyrimidines may be metabolized to β-alanine and β-amino-isobutyric acid. Figures 19–1 and 19–2 show the pathways of purine and pyrimidine metabolism.

DISORDERS OF PURINE METABOLISM

Primary Hyperuricemia (Gout)

Primary hyperuricemia, or gout, is associated with the increased synthesis of uric acid precursors and decreased renal excretion of uric acid. The disorder, which has its onset in adult life, is considered a polygenic, or multifactorial, trait in which genetic and environmental influences play a role in the development of clinical symptoms. Patients have elevated levels of plasma and urinary uric acid. Affected adults develop acute attacks of gouty arthritis which increase in frequency with time and may result in joint damage and deformity. Acute attacks of gouty arthritis may be precipitated by exercise, emotional stress, or trauma. The joint involvement is usually monoarticular and peripheral; the first metatarsophalangeal is most often affected. Deposition of crystals of monosodium urate monohydrate in the joints and surrounding tissues leads to an acute inflammatory reaction. The crystals may be found in joint fluid at the time of attacks. Usually the attacks will spontaneously resolve within a few days to weeks. Colchicine, steroids, and anti-inflammatory agents may be used for the treatment of acute gouty arthritis attacks. Affected patients may also develop deposits of monosodium urate crystals, known as gouty tophi, in the helix of the ears and over the points of insertion of tendons in the elbows, knees, or feet. Uric acid stones, as well as calcium oxalate stones, may form in the urinary tract. Renal failure may occur and be related to the urolithiasis or to underlying hypertension and renal vascular disease.

Treatment with allopurinol, which inhibits xanthine oxidase activity, will decrease purine biosynthesis and uric acid levels. Other treatment measures include increasing fluid intake, which will decrease the concentration of urinary uric acid; probenecid, which will increase uric acid clearance; and alkalinization of the urine, which will increase uric acid solubility. Patients should also avoid excessive intake of carbohydrates, ethanol, and purines, which may also result in the increased production and excretion of uric acid.

Primary hyperuricemia also occurs with disorders of purine metabolism such as the Lesch-Nyhan syndrome and overactivity of phosphoribosylpyrophosphate synthetase. Rarely, familial juvenile gout presents before the age of 25 years. Secondary gout may occur with other inborn errors of metabolism, such as type I glycogen storage disease, or with other clinical conditions associated with starvation, dehydration, lactic acidosis, and ketoacidosis. Secondary hyperuricemia may also occur with diabetes mellitus, hypothyroidism, hypoparathyroidism, hyperparathyroidism, Addison disease, idiopathic hypercalcuria, myeloproliferative disorders, renal failure, diuretic therapy, or during the treatment of malignancies.

Lesch-Nyhan Syndrome

Lesch-Nyhan syndrome is associated with *complete deficiency of hypoxanthine guanine phosphoribosyl transferase (HGPRT)*. There is decreased salvage of purines and loss of feedback inhibition of purine biosynthesis, which results in the overproduction and overexcretion of purines, especially uric acid. The disorder is inherited as an X-linked trait and is estimated to occur in one in 380,000 births.

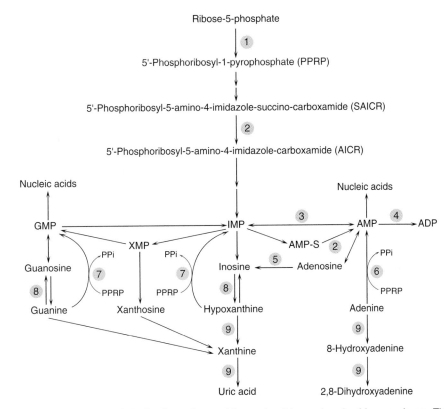

Figure 19–1. Purine metabolism. Only the ribose forms of the nucleosides and nucleotides are shown. The deoxyribose forms follow similar pathways. 1 = Phosphoribosylpyrophosphate synthetase; 2 = adenylosuccinase (adenylosuccinate lyase); 3 = adenylate deaminase; 4 = adenylate kinase; 5 = adenosine deaminase (ADA); 6 = adenine phosphoribosyl transferase (APRT); 7 = hypoxanthine-guanine phosphoribosyl transferase (HGPRT); 8 = purine nucleoside phosphorylase (PNP); 9 = xanthine oxidase. ADP = adenosine diphosphate; AMP = adenosine monophosphate; AMP-S = succinyladenosine (adenylosuccinic acid); IMP = inosine monophosphate; GMP = guanosine monophosphate; PPi = pyrophosphate; PPRP = phosphoribosyl pyrophosphate; XMP = xanthosine monophosphate.

Affected boys are normal at birth. Psychomotor delay is usually evident by 6 months of age, which is followed by the development of choreoathetosis, dystonia, and spasticity within the first year of life. Affected boys may also start to display compulsive self-mutilating behaviors during the first year. They will frequently bite their fingers and lips to the point of disfiguration. They also become verbally and physically aggressive and hostile towards others and often require dental extractions, restraints, and behavioral modification to protect themselves and their caretakers. Although most are moderately mentally handicapped, motor and expressive disabilities may make patients' innate intelligence appear lower than it really is. Most become wheelchair bound. Elevated urinary levels of uric acid occur in most patients at any age, whereas elevated serum levels of uric acid may not be apparent until after puberty. Yellow-orange urinary uric acid crystals may be noted as early as the first week of life. Renal failure and gouty arthritis may occur. Hypoxanthine will also be elevated in plasma and urine. Treatment with an increased fluid intake and carefully titrated doses of allopurinol may decrease the risk for urinary calculi, but will not improve the neurological manifestations. The diagnosis may be established by showing decreased levels of HGPRT in erythrocytes and cultured skin fibroblasts. The gene for the disorder, located at chromosome Xq26, has been cloned. Carrier and prenatal testing are available.

Partial Deficiency of HGPRT

Partial deficiency of HGPRT is associated with the development of gouty arthritis and renal calculi during teenage or early adult life. Twenty percent of affected males will also display cerebellar ataxia, spasticity, and mild psychomotor retardation. However, they do not develop the self-mutilating behaviors noted with the Lesch-Nyhan syndrome. Partial deficiency of HGPRT may be shown in erythrocytes and cultured skin fibroblasts. Treatment with allopurinol, increased fluid intake, and alkalinization of the urine may reduce the risk of gout and renal stone formation.

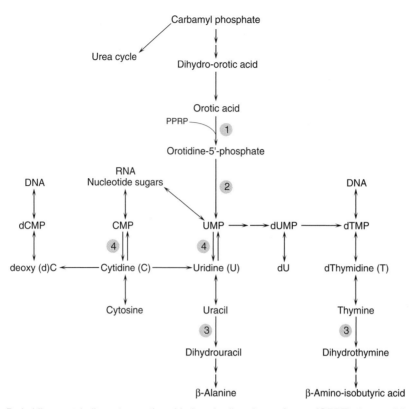

Figure 19–2. Pyrimidine metabolism. 1 = orotic acid phosphoribosyl transferase (OPRT); 2 = orotidine phosphate decarboxylase (OPD); 3 = dihydropyrimidine dehydrogenase; 4 = pyrimidine-5′-nucleotidase; DNA = deoxyribonucleic acid; MP = monophosphate; PPRP = phosphoribosylpyrophosphate; RNA = ribonucleic acid.

Phosphoribosylpyrophosphate Synthetase (PPRP-S) Overactivity

Phosphoribosylpyrophosphate synthetase (PPRP-S) overactivity is an X-linked disorder associated with increased de novo synthesis of purines, hyperuricemia, and hyperuricuria. The disorder is characterized by a loss of feedback inhibition of PPRP-S, the initial step in purine biosynthesis. Most affected males present during teenage years or as young adults with severe gout or renal stones. A more severe form of the disorder is associated with psychomotor retardation, autistic behaviors, hypotonia, and nerve deafness. Hearing impairment has been reported in female carriers for the severe form of the disorder. Patients have markedly elevated plasma and urine levels of uric acid. Treatment consists of increased fluid intake, allopurinol, and alkalinization of the urine. The defect may be demonstrated in erythrocytes, lymphocytes, and cultured skin fibroblasts.

Adenylosuccinase (Adenylosuccinate Lyase) Deficiency

Adenylosuccinase (adenylosuccinate lyase) deficiency is a rare, autosomal recessive disorder, as-

sociated with autistic behaviors, hypotonia, self-mutilation, cerebellar hypoplasia, and psychomotor retardation during childhood. Affected patients have elevated levels of succinyl aminoimidazole carboxamide riboside (SAICR) and succinyladenosine (AMP-S) in plasma, urine, and cerebrospinal fluid. Elevated levels of aspartic acid and glycine will also be noted on quantitative amino acid determinations. There is no effective therapy.

Adenine Phosphoribosyl Transferase (APRT) Deficiency

Adenine phosphoribosyl transferase (APRT) deficiency is a rare, autosomal recessive disorder characterized by increased urinary levels of 2,8-hydroxy-adenine, which is insoluble and results in the formation of renal calculi. Adenine is not salvaged but converted to 8-hydroxyadenine and 2,8-hydroxy-adenine by xanthine oxidase. The onset is variable and may occur during childhood or adult life. There is also a great variation in clinical severity. As many as 15% of patients are asymptomatic, while other severely affected patients may develop recurrent calculi and renal failure. Deficient activity of adenine phosphoribosyl transferase may be shown in erythrocytes, lymphocytes, and cultured skin fibroblasts. Treatment with an increased fluid intake, allopurinol, and reduced dietary intake of purines may decrease the incidence of renal calculi.

Deficient Activity of Xanthine Oxidase (Hereditary Xanthinuria)

Deficient activity of xanthine oxidase, or hereditary xanthinuria, is an autosomal recessive disorder with variable clinical expression. Affected patients will have markedly decreased levels of serum and urine uric acid and elevated urinary levels of xanthine and hypoxanthine. Only approximately 40–50% of affected patients will become symptomatic from renal calculi. Occasionally affected patients will develop chronic renal disease or renal failure. Deficient activity of xanthine oxidase may be shown in liver or intestinal biopsies. Combined deficiency of xanthine oxidase and sulfite oxidase may occur due to deficiency of a molybdenum cofactor which is needed for the function of both enzymes. Sulfite oxidase deficiency is discussed with the disorders of methionine metabolism.

Deficient Activity of Myoadenylate Deaminase

Deficient activity of myoadenylate deaminase is a rare, autosomal recessive, disorder associated with muscle cramping, myalgia, and elevated levels of creatine kinase after exercise. Most patients have the onset of their disorder during late childhood or in adolescence. There is deficient activity of the isoenzymes of adenylate deaminase which occur only in muscles. Levels of muscle ATP and total purines decrease to a greater extent than normal with exercise. There is also a failure of the normal rise in plasma ammonia with exercise. Affected patients may also have hypotonia, hyperuricemia, and gout. There is an increased risk for malignant hyperthermia with general anesthesia. Although there is no specific therapy, some patients have been reported to respond to ribose. Secondary myoadenylate deficiency is more common and may be noted with hypokalemic paralysis, muscular dystrophy, collagen vascular disorders including polymyositis, and other disorders with motor neuron involvement.

Other Disorders of Purine Metabolism

Other disorders of purine metabolism, such as purine-nucleoside phosphorylase (PNP) deficiency, are discussed in the Immunology section. Adenylate kinase deficiency is discussed in the Hematology section.

DISORDERS OF PYRIMIDINE METABOLISM

Hereditary Orotic Acidura

Hereditary orotic acidura is a rare, autosomal recessive disorder associated with deficient activity of uridine monophosphate synthetase. This bifunctional enzyme consists of activities of both orotic acid phosphoribosyltransferase and orotidine 5′-monophosphate decarboxylase which are involved with de novo pyrimidine biosynthesis. Affected patients have markedly elevated plasma and urinary levels of orotic acid and present during the first year of life with severe hypochromic anemia, megaloblastic changes in bone marrow, cellular immunodeficiency, psychomotor retardation, and failure to thrive. Birth defects, cardiac malformations, and occasionally, urinary tract obstruction from the crystalluria produced from massive orotic acid excretion may also occur. Treatment with uridine may result in clinical improvement. Deficient activity of uridine monophosphate synthetase may be shown in erythrocytes, leukocytes, lymphoblasts, liver biopsies, and cultured skin fibroblasts. Secondary orotic aciduria is more common and may be seen with defects in the urea cycle, Reyes syndrome, essential amino acid deficiency, and parenteral nutrition.

Other Disorders of Pyrimidine Metabolism

Deficient activity of pyrimidine-5′-nucleotidase is discussed in Chapter 6.

REFERENCES AND SUGGESTED READING

See page 256 and Appendix II.

COPPER METABOLISM

Wilson Disease

Wilson disease, an autosomal recessive disorder, is estimated to occur in 1 in 50,000 to 1 in 100,000 individuals. The disorder has been recently shown to be associated with reduced levels of a copper-transporting ATPase (Wc1 or pWD), which is normally present in the liver, kidney, and pancreas. Reduced incorporation of copper into ceruloplasmin and reduced biliary excretion of copper lead initially to hepatic copper storage, and later to storage in the central nervous system and other tissues. Copper is stored in a toxic form which can oxidize proteins and lipids of membranes, bind to proteins and nucleic acids, and result in free-radical production. Patients may present with either hepatic or central nervous system symptoms, or both.

Hepatic Presentation: The hepatic presentation, which most often occurs in children between the ages of 8 and 16 years, may be as acute or chronic liver dysfunction, usually in the form of cirrhosis. Some patients have acute, often recurrent, hemolytic crises that may result in renal tubular damage and hepatic necrosis. The crises are caused by the release of free copper from liver stores during a viral illness, stress, or an infarction of a regenerative nodule in a cirrhotic liver.

Central Nervous System Presentation: Patients with central nervous system presentation are usually adults between 20 and 40 years of age. Copper storage in the basal ganglia leads to movement disorders, dystonia, and dysarthria, which are often the presenting symptoms. With advanced disease, patients may also have seizures, intellectual deterioration, and pseudobulbar palsies. Neurological manifestations are rare before the age of 14 years. Nearly all patients with neurological manifestations will have yellow-brown or brown-green **Kayser-Fleischer rings,** which represent copper storage in the cornea. The rings, which appear just medial to the limbus, require slit lamp examination for detection in younger patients but may be seen directly in older affected individuals. Lenticular copper storage may result in "sunflower" cataracts.

Deposition of copper throughout the body may also lead to renal tubular damage, Fanconi syndrome, nephrocalcinosis, nephrolithiasis, pancreatic disease, cardiomyopathies, hypoparathyroidism, arthropathies, osteoporosis, neutropenia, thrombocytopenia, pancytopenia, or hemolytic anemia.

Routine laboratory testing will reveal reduced serum copper and ceruloplasmin. Serum non-ceruloplasmin (free) copper levels are actually elevated but are difficult to measure and not available on a routine basis. Urinary copper excretion will be elevated. Even higher elevations of urinary copper excretion will be noted after the administration of D-penicillamine. Not all patients, however, will be detected by this testing and the copper content of carefully handled liver biopsy samples may be needed to demonstrate elevated copper stores. The most sensitive diagnostic test demonstrates faulty in vitro incorporation of radiolabeled copper into ceruloplasmin. Treatment with D-penicillamine or trientine hydrochloride, as copper chelating agents, results in a gradual improvement in the hepatic and neurological symptoms. Zinc salts should be added with the chelating agents to prevent zinc deficiency and to induce the formation of metallothionein, which can sequester free copper. Acute hemolytic crises will require peritoneal dialysis or plasmapheresis to remove the massive elevation of free copper. In some cases, cirrhosis and portal hypertension persist; advanced liver disease may require liver transplantation.

Because the presentation has been variable among family members, all siblings of index cases should be evaluated for Wilson disease. Carrier testing for family members may include measurements of serum ceruloplasmin and D-penicillamine-augmented urinary copper excretion, but is best accomplished with in vitro radiolabeled copper studies. The genetic locus for Wilson disease is at chromosome 13q14.3. Carrier and prenatal testing may be done with linkage or molecular genetic studies in informative families.

Menkes Disease

Menkes Disease is an X-linked disorder that occurs in 1 in 50,000 to 1 in 100,000 male infants. The recently isolated gene for Menkes disease (MNK) appears to code for a copper-transporting ATPase (Mc1) that is normally present in all tissues except the liver. Affected patients have decreased intestinal absorption of copper and reduced copper content in the liver. Other tissues will show elevated levels of copper which, in contrast to Wilson disease, is stored in a nontoxic form. The clinical manifestations result from deficient activity of many enzymes that require copper for their synthesis, eg, cytochrome c oxidase (electron chain transport), superoxide dismutase (free radical detoxification), tyrosinase (melanin production), dopamine hydroxylase (neurotransmitter production), and lysyl oxidase (cross-linkage of elastin and collagen). Most affected patients present between the ages of two and three months of age with dysmorphic features, abnormal kinky or steely hair, and signs of central nervous system involvement. Table 20–1 lists the clinical manifestations of Menkes disease. The facies and hair are distinctive. Kinky or steely hair is sparse, brittle, depigmented, dull, short, and friable in the posterior and occipital areas. Upon microscopic examination the hair is noted to be twisted on the long axis (pili torti) and have an irregular caliber (monilethrix) and node-like fracture points (trichorrhexis nodosa). Radiographs show osteoporosis, widening and flaring of the metaphyses with spike-like protrusions, and Wormian bones in the skull. Hypsarrhythmia or multifocal spike patterns are noted on electroencephalograms. Arteriograms show tortuous, elongated arteries with areas of narrowing and dilatation. Radioimaging studies will reveal diffuse cerebral and cerebellar atrophy, often with areas of focal infarction or subdural hematomas. Affected patients develop feeding problems, failure to thrive, repeated infections, seizures, hypotonia, and progressive central nervous system deterioration. Most do not live past 3 years of age. Laboratory studies show reduced serum copper and ceruloplasmin levels. The copper content of liver biopsies is reduced, while that of intestinal biopsies is increased. There is increased uptake and decreased release of radiolabeled copper in cultured skin fibroblasts from affected patients. Patients with milder forms of Menkes disease present with similar clinical features and laboratory findings but at later ages. Treatment with parenteral copper histidinate has shown promise if started early in classical cases or if used in patients with mild forms of the disorder. In many cases, although the general condition improves, central nervous system involvement remains unchanged.

Some female carriers for Menkes diseases will have pili torti or mosaic skin pigmentation. Otherwise, carrier detection is difficult; not all carriers will be detected by radiolabeled copper studies in cultured skin fibroblasts. Fetal sex determination along with the measurement of the copper content of uncultured chorionic villi samples or with radiolabeled copper studies in cultured amniocytes may be used for prenatal diagnosis. The gene for the disorder is located on the X chromosome at q13.3. DNA diagnostic techniques have been recently developed and may be used for carrier and prenatal testing in informative families.

Occipital Horn Syndrome: The "occipital horn" syndrome has been described in children with mild clinical features of Menkes syndrome. Connective tissue findings are prominent in this disorder, which was previously known as X-linked cutis laxa and Ehlers-Danlos syndrome type IX. The disorder is named after the ossified occipital horns noted on radiographs. A hammer-like expansion of the lateral ends of the clavicles and a wavy outline of the cortex of long bones are also noted. The disorder is associated with a copper transport defect and has biochemical findings comparable to Menkes syndrome. The Occipital Horn syndrome is also inherited as an X-linked trait and may be allelic with Menkes syndrome or result from mutations in a closely-linked gene.

ZINC METABOLISM

Acrodermatitis Enteropathica

Acrodermatitis enteropathica is a rare, autosomal recessive disorder that most often presents during early infancy with a characteristic acrodermatitis, diarrhea, and failure to thrive. The clinical manifestations result from the intestinal malabsorption and severe systemic deficiency of zinc. Zinc functions as a

Table 20–1. Clinical features of Menkes syndrome.

System	Clinical Findings
Dysmorphic	Facies: cherubic face, pudgy cheeks, cupid-bow lips. Micrognatia. Inexpressive look. Oral: Gingival hyperplasia, high-arched palate.
Dermatologic	Hair: Kinky or steely; brittle, stubby, sparse; depigmented. Sparse eyebrows. Skin: Depigmented, seborrheic dermatitis.
Connective tissue	Lax skin, loose joints, hernias, tortuous arteries.
Ophthalmic	Retinal degeneration, optic atrophy, cataracts blindness, microcysts in iris.
Gastrointestinal	Feeding problems, gastroesophageal reflux, diarrhea.
Urologic	Bladder or ureteral diverticuli, hydroureter, hydronephrosis, uirinary reflux.
Neurologic	Developmental regression, hypotonia, seizures, strokes, subdural hematomas.
Skeletal	Wormian bones in skull, osteoporosis, fractures, pectus excavatus, club feet. Delayed bone age. Metaphyseal widening and flaring. Osteophytes, spurring.
Other	Hypothermia, lethargy, apnea, failure to thrive, recurrent infections, emphysema.

cofactor in many metabolic pathways and is needed for nucleic acid and protein synthesis, regulation of cell division, antioxidant function, hormone-receptor binding, wound healing, and a chemotactic response to infections. Because breast milk has more bioavailable zinc than infant formulas, affected infants who are breast fed will often present later than those fed commercial formulas and after the time of weaning. The acrodermatitis consists of irregular, vesicobullous plaques that have an erythematous base. The plaques are most often noted at the angles of the mouth, on the cheeks and eyelids, behind the ears, and in the antecubital, anterior knee, and diaper areas. Alopecia, paronychia, and dystrophic changes of the nails also occur. A corneal dystrophy, corneal opacities, photophobia, conjunctivitis, or blepharitis may be present. Patients have loose, watery stools and disaccharide intolerance. Repeated bacterial infections, superficial and systemic moniliasis, lethargy, irritability, tremors, ataxia, and cerebral atrophy occur. Anorexia and weight loss often lead to marasmus and death in untreated cases. Later-onset cases have been reported in older children and adults who may have neuropsychiatric complaints such as paranoia and depression. Some affected, untreated women have had repeated miscarriages, or infants born with anencephaly or skeletal dysplasias.

Laboratory testing shows markedly reduced zinc levels in most patients. Samples should be drawn so that contamination does not occur. An occasional patient initially will have a normal serum zinc level which then decreases with treatment and growth. Elevated plasma ammonia levels, reduced levels of alkaline phosphatase, and hypobetalipoproteinemia also may be noted. Replacement therapy with oral zinc salt preparations results in clinical improvement. Treated affected women have produced normal infants. No means for carrier or prenatal testing currently exists.

IRON METABOLISM

Familial (Idiopathic) Hemochromatosis

Familial (idiopathic) hemochromatosis, a relatively common disorder in whites of European background, is estimated to occur in 1 in 250 to 1 in 330 persons. The clinical manifestations result from excessive intestinal iron uptake and slowly progressive storage of iron as hemosiderin in the parenchymal cells of the liver, pancreas, heart, gonads, skin, and joints. Most patients present with clinical symptoms of iron overload after 20 years of age. The usual patient is a male, over 40 years of age, with cirrhosis or hepatomegaly. Younger patients often have car-

diomyopathies and arrhythmias. Other patients may present with an arthropathy and chondrocalcinosis. Other clinical features include increased skin pigmentation, hypogonadism secondary to gonadotrophin deficiency, abdominal pain, osteoporosis, and diabetes mellitus. Portal fibrosis and esophageal varices may occur. Affected females will have a later onset of symptoms due to the protective loss of iron through pregnancy and menses. Environmental factors that can result in an earlier presentation include alcoholism and an increased intake of dietary iron. The combination of bronze hyperpigmentation, diabetes mellitus, and cirrhosis—the classic triad associated with hemochromatosis—occurs late in course of the disease. It is now appreciated that most affected patients do not present in this manner. Untreated, 82% of symptomatic patients die within 5 years of their diagnosis, and 94% die within 10 years. Most deaths are from hepatic or cardiac failure or hepatoma. Patients with cirrhosis have an increased risk for the development of hepatoma; the risk ranges from 8 to 29% in various studies.

In most symptomatic patients laboratory testing shows elevated serum iron, transferrin saturation, and plasma ferritin. Asymptomatic affected patients, prior to the accumulation of significant iron storage, may not have elevated levels. Liver biopsies will show hemosiderin storage in hepatocytes and may be used for quantitative measurements to demonstrate elevated liver iron content. Computed tomography techniques can also be used to estimate the amount of hepatic iron overload.

Treatment consists of repeated, frequent phlebotomy which must be continued for life, although less often after the iron storage has been reduced. Most patients have an improved clinical status. The risk for the development of hepatoma continues, however. Therefore, it is important that all siblings of index cases be evaluated for the disorder, so that phlebotomy may be started before significant iron overload and cirrhosis occur. Patients who start treatment early (after elevation of serum ferritin, but before the development of organ damage and cirrhosis) have not shown an increased risk for hepatoma. The gene for familial hemochromatosis is located on the short arm of chromosome 6, near the HLA-A locus. Linkage studies have been used in informative families for the diagnosis of carriers and asymptomatic, homozygous affected individuals. All asymptomatic, affected relatives should be monitored periodically with serum iron, transferrin saturation, and ferritin levels. Monitoring should start after the age of 10 years in asymptomatic, affected male patients, and over the age of 20 in asymptomatic, affected females.

REFERENCES AND SUGGESTED READING

See page 256 and Appendix II.

Bone Mineralization

21

DISORDERS OF VITAMIN D ACTIVATION

To be physiologically active, vitamin D must be hydroxylated to its active metabolite 1,25-dihydroxyvitamin D. Vitamin D_2 (ergocalciferol) from nutritional sources or vitamin D_3 (cholecalciferol) from the photoconversion of 7-dehydrocholesterol in the skin are transported to the liver, where they undergo 25-hydroxylation by hepatic microsomal cholecalciferol-25-hydroxylase. The 25-hydroxyvitamin D (calcifediol) is then transported to the kidney, where a second hydroxylation occurs through the action of mitochondrial 25-hydroxyvitamin D-1-α-hydroxylase. The 1,25-dihydroxyvitamin D (calcitriol) that is formed then binds to 1,25-dihydroxyvitamin D receptors, which are located on the cell surface of many tissues throughout the body. After binding with its receptors, the activated vitamin D is transported into the nucleus of the cell, where it binds with DNA and induces translation of specific proteins, eg calcium-binding protein, which are responsible for the physiologic actions of vitamin D.

Vitamin D Deficiency

Vitamin D deficiency may result from inadequate nutritional intake of vitamin D. Because dairy products are fortified with vitamin D_2, most cases of nutritional vitamin D deficiency occur in patients with disorders associated with fat malabsorption, premature infants, or infants who are entirely breast fed and do not receive vitamin D supplementation or have inadequate exposure to sunlight. Patients with vitamin D deficiency will develop incomplete calcification of the bones, which is known as rickets in growing children or osteomalacia in adults. As the deficiency continues and secondary hyperparathyroidism develops, patients become hypocalcemic and may have hypocalcemic seizures (tetany). Lowered levels of serum phosphorus and elevated levels of serum alkaline phosphatase are also noted. Physical examination will reveal short stature and bowing of the legs from weight-bearing on the "softened" bones. Affected patients will also have widened wrists and knees, enlarged costochondral junctions (rachitic rosary), craniotabes of the skull (young infants), frontal bossing, and hypotonia. Failure to thrive, delayed motor milestones, repeated respiratory infections, and pneumonias from instability of ribs and chest muscles are also common. Pseudotumor cerebri will occasionally develop. Radiographs will show delayed bone growth, decreased mineralization, and widening of the growth plates. The growing ends of the metaphyseal areas become irregular, frayed, and appear concave or "cupped" due to an increase in the amount of uncalcified cartilage. Rickets may also occur from calcium deficiency (usually dietary), phosphorus deficiency (total parenteral nutrition, renal tubular dysfunction, or inherited defects), or from failure of the activation of vitamin D due to inherited disorders, renal disease, or by certain drugs, especially anticonvulsants.

Abnormalities in the Activation of Vitamin D

Two inherited disorders are associated with abnormalities in the activation of vitamin D. Both are autosomal recessive diseases associated with the development of hypocalcemia and rickets during infancy.

Hereditary Deficiency of 1,25-Dihydroxyvitamin D (Vitamin D Dependency Type I): Hereditary deficiency of 1,25-dihydroxyvitamin D, or vitamin D dependency type I, results from deficient activity of renal 1-α-hydroxylase. Affected patients are normal at birth and present between 2–24 months of age with hypocalcemia and rickets. Hypotonia is prominent. There are markedly reduced levels of 1,25-dihydroxyvitamin D and normal or increased levels of 25-hydroxyvitamin D. Serum calcium and phosphorus are lowered; parathyroid hormone and alkaline phosphatase are elevated. Radiographs will show florid rickets. Most patients respond to treatment with 1,25-dihydroxyvitamin D (calcitriol).

Generalized Resistance to 1,25-Dihydroxyvitamin D (Vitamin D Dependency Type II): Generalized resistance to 1,25-dihydroxyvitamin D, or vitamin D dependency type II results from defects in the interaction of 1,25-dihydroxyvitamin D and its receptors. There may be decreased receptor binding, defects in nuclear localization, or defects in DNA interaction of activated vitamin D. Affected patients are normal at birth and usually present between 2–8 months of age with hypocalcemia and rickets. Milder cases with later onset during childhood are known. Approximately 50% of more severely affected patients will have alopecia, which may be total or partial. Serum 1,25-dihydroxyvitamin D levels will be elevated despite the presence of hypocalcemia and secondary hyperparathyroidism. Treatment with various vitamin D preparations will result in clinical improvement in approximately one-half the patients. The others, usually severely affected, may not respond to even very high dose therapy.

FAMILIAL HYPOPHOSPHATEMIC RICKETS (FHR)

Familial hypophosphatemic rickets (FHR) is an X-linked dominant disorder that is also known as vitamin D-resistant rickets. It is associated with a defect in renal tubular, and probably intestinal, reabsorption of phosphorus and with abnormal regulation of renal 25-hydroxyvitamin D-1-α-hydroxylase activity. The lowered serum phosphorus levels in affected patients fail to stimulate an increase in renal 1-α-hydroxylase activity and synthesis of 1,25-dihydroxyvitamin D as is noted in normals. Affected patients present between 1–2 years of age with short

stature and bowing of the lower extremities (Figure 21–1). They have lowered serum phosphorus and elevated alkaline phosphatase levels. Because children have higher serum phosphorus and alkaline phosphatase levels than adults, it is important that the values of patients be compared to age-matched normal controls. In contrast to nutritional rickets or disorders of vitamin D activation, hypocalcemia, hypotonia, tetany, seizures, and significant secondary hyperparathyroidism do not occur. Blood calcium levels will be normal or slightly low, and parathyroid levels will be normal or only slightly elevated. Levels of 1,25-dihydroxyvitamin D will be normal or low, and 25-hydroxyvitamin D levels will be normal. Renal tubular reabsorption of phosphorus is markedly reduced. Other findings seen with Fanconi-type renal tubular dysfunction are not noted. Radiographs will show changes of rickets, such as fraying, widening, and cupping of the metaphyseal areas of the long bones. The radiographic changes are more prominent in the distal and proximal tibias, distal femurs, ulna, and radius (Figure 21–2). Untreated affected older

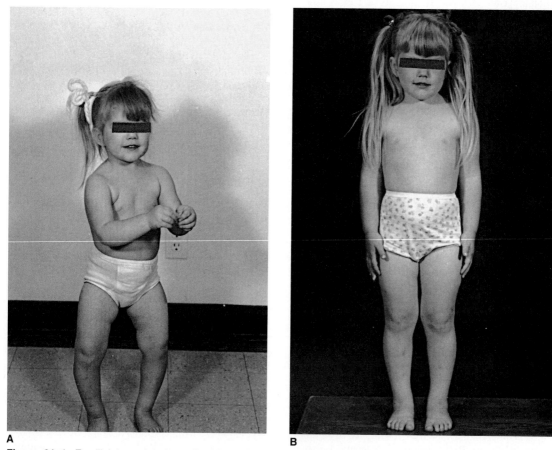

A **B**

Figure 21–1. Familial hypophosphatemic rickets: **(A)** before therapy; **(B)** after medical therapy and surgical osteotomies. (Reproduced with permission from: Oski FA et al (editors), *Principles and Practice of Pediatrics,* 2nd ed, JB Lippincott, 1994.)

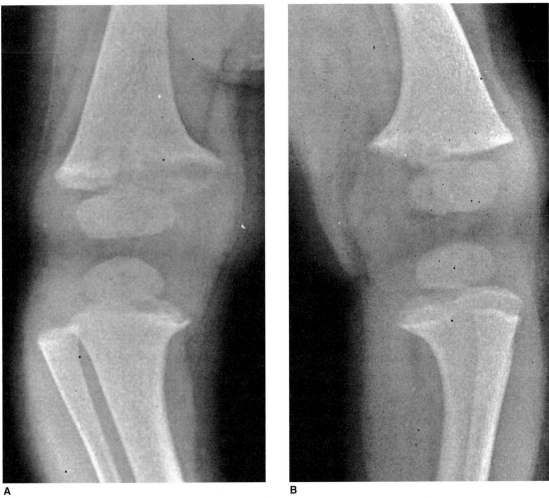

A   B

Figure 21–2. Familial hypophosphatemic rickets. **(A)** Radiogram of right knee. **(B)** Radiogram of left knee. Note the moth-eaten appearance of the epiphyses, especially on the medial aspects of the distal femurs and proximal tibias, and the varus deformities of the diaphyses of the tibias and femurs. (Reproduced, with permission from: Oski FA et al (editors), *Principles and Practice of Pediatrics,* 2nd ed, JB Lippincott, 1994.)

children and teenagers will have thickened cortices and coarse, dense trabecular bones. Although there is osteomalacia, an increase in the total mass of incompletely calcified osteoid may actually give elevated values with bone density measurements. Untreated affected adults may have calcification of tendons, ligaments, and joint capsules in the hands, hips, and pelvic areas. Osteophytes may be noted in the elbows, shoulders, and hips. Spinal ankylosis may develop. Affected patients also have delayed dental eruption, defects in dental enamel formation, and an increased risk for dental caries and abscesses. Treatment consists of titrated doses of neutral phosphorus preparations and 1,25-dihydroxyvitamin D. Careful monitoring of both blood and urine must be done to avoid hypercalcemia, hypercalcuria, and a secondary decrease in renal function. Most patients respond to

therapy with improvement in the rickets and linear growth. Many affected patients, especially affected males, will require surgical correction of the bowing.

Because the disorder is inherited as an X-linked dominant trait, both affected hemizygous males and heterozygous females will have lowered blood phosphorus levels. Almost all affected males will develop rickets. But, as many as 50% of affected females will not have clinical symptoms and will only have lowered blood phosphorus levels. The disorder has been linked to chromosome Xp22. Prenatal diagnosis is not possible at the present time.

DISORDERS OF ALKALINE PHOSPHATASE

Alkaline phosphatase is a pyrophosphatase, which releases phosphate ions needed for calcification of bone. It is contained within membrane-enclosed vesicles at sites of mineral deposition in the bone matrix and in cartilage. Inherited disorders associated with both decreased and elevated levels of alkaline phosphatase are known.

Hypophosphatasia

Hypophosphatasias are inherited disorders that are associated with lowered alkaline phosphatase levels. Because children have higher levels of alkaline phosphatase compared to adults, values from affected patients should be compared to age-matched controls. There will also be elevated blood and urinary levels of natural substrates for alkaline phosphatase, including pyridoxal-5-phosphate, inorganic pyrophosphate, and phosphoethanolamine. In addition, affected patients, especially those with the severe forms of the disorder, may develop significant hypercalcemia and hypercalcuria which may result in nephrocalcinosis and renal failure. There are four forms of the disorder which vary in the time of presentation and clinical severity.

Perinatal or Lethal Form of Hypophosphatasia: The perinatal or lethal form of hypophosphatasia is an autosomal recessive disorder in which there is almost complete lack of mineralization of the skeleton at birth. Radiographic findings are characteristic and may be distinguished from other forms of neonatal lethal bony dysplasia. Affected infants will have shortened, deformed extremities and severe craniotabes. Many infants are stillborn, while others usually die in the immediate neonatal period from respiratory insufficiency.

Infantile Form of Hypophosphatasia: The infantile form of hypophosphatasia is also an autosomal recessive disorder that presents before 6 months of age with severe generalized skeletal demineralization, short extremities, hypotonia, wide fontanels, and failure to thrive. Affected infants have marked hypercalcemia and hypercalcuria and frequently develop nephrocalcinosis. Premature synostosis of the skull may result in increased intracranial pressure and require surgical release. The premature synostosis may occur in demineralized osteoid and thus be present even without the usual radiographic changes noted in patients with cranial synostosis with normal mineralization. Treatment with reduced dietary intake of vitamin D and calcium, including the use of special dietary supplements low in calcium and vitamin D, may control the hypercalcemia. The use of sunscreens and reduced exposure to sunlight is also recommended. Careful monitoring is needed to prevent a superimposed vitamin D deficiency. Affected children will frequently require orthopedic intervention.

Childhood Form of Hypophosphatasia: The childhood form of hypophosphatasia usually presents before 5 years of age with premature loss of deciduous teeth and with short stature. This form of the disorder may be inherited as either an autosomal dominant or autosomal recessive trait. Radiographs will show demineralization, rachitic changes, and often characteristic focal areas of radiolucency which project from the growth plates into the metaphyses. Affected children may display clinical features suggestive of rickets including dolicocephaly, frontal bossing, bowed legs, prominent costochondral junctions, and widening of the distal long bones. Craniosynostosis may also develop and require surgical release. Varying degrees of severity and hypercalcemia and hypercalcuria are noted. Treatment is similar to that for the infantile form of the disorder.

Adult Form of Hypophosphatasia: The adult form of hypophosphatasia is the mildest form of the disorder which may be inherited as either an autosomal dominant or autosomal recessive trait. Affected adults will often have a history of early loss of deciduous teeth, repeated fractures, or rickets during childhood. Osteomalacia may result in stress fractures in the feet or legs. Pseudofractures are often noted in the lateral aspects of the proximal femoral shafts. Hypercalcemia and hypercalcuria are not usually clinically significant. Many affected patients are asymptomatic and only detected when screening blood panels are done which include alkaline phosphatase determinations.

Pseudohypophosphatasia: Pseudohypophosphatasia has been reported in patients with normal levels of alkaline phosphatase who have clinical and radiographic findings similar to the inherited hypophosphatasias. The basis for the disorder is unknown.

Hyperphosphatasia

Elevated levels of alkaline phosphatase may be noted with rickets, fractures, liver dysfunction, inherited genetic disorders, and during periods of accelerated growth. Serum alkaline phosphatase levels in children are approximately three times those of adults due to the increased levels of bone alkaline phosphatase associated with growth. In addition, many infants and children are noted to have *benign transient elevations of alkaline phosphatase* of unknown etiology between the ages of 2 months and 3 years. Most often the elevations are detected when screening blood panels are ordered that include determinations of alkaline phosphatase. Occasionally the patients will have intercurrent illness, especially diarrhea. Alkaline phosphatase levels will usually slowly normalize over a period of 4 months. Elevated alkaline phosphatase levels may also be noted with *benign familial hyperphosphatasia,* an autosomal dominant trait.

Hyperphosphatasemia with Osteoectasia (Juvenile Paget Disease): Elevated levels of alkaline phosphatase are also associated with hyperphosphatasemia with osteoectasia (juvenile Paget disease). This rare, autosomal recessive disorder of bone remodeling most often occurs in Puerto Rican and American Indian families. Affected children present between 1 and 3 years of age with increased head size, bowing of the femurs, fractures, and progressive skeletal deformities. Radiographs will show a cylindrical appearance to the long bones, with widened diaphyses, pseudocysts, irregular trabeculation, and dilated shafts (osteoectasia). Affected patients often die as adults from arterial complications of their disease. Some patients have shown a response to treatment with calcitonin.

REFERENCES AND SUGGESTED READING

See page 256 and Appendix II.

22

Other Recently Characterized Inborn Errors of Metabolism

SMITH-LEMLI-OPITZ SYNDROME

The Smith-Lemli-Opitz Syndrome is an autosomal recessive disorder that occurs in 1 in 20,000 to 1 in 40,000 births. The disorder was first described in 1964 and has been recognized as a discrete clinical entity characterized by a constellation of birth defects including an abnormal facies, hypogenitalism in males, moderately short stature, psychomotor retardation, and poor somatic growth. Table 22–1 lists the multiple dysmorphic features and other clinical findings of the Smith-Lemli-Opitz syndrome. The disorder is now known to result from a defect in cholesterol biosynthesis that results in markedly elevated levels of 7-dehydrocholesterol and other isomeric dehydrocholesterols, which are cholesterol precursors, and reduced levels of cholesterol. There is deficient activity of a 3β-hydroxysterol Δ^7-reductase which is responsible for the reduction of the double bond of 7-dehydrocholesterols during cholesterol synthesis. The biochemical abnormalities are thought to inter-fere with normal embryonic development, which leads to the multiple birth defects noted in affected patients.

The reduction in blood cholesterol levels in affected patients will not be apparent by standard laboratory procedures, which use colorimetric methods to measure cholesterol. This is because such methods will detect all 3β-hydroxysterols, including the abnormally elevated precursors. Measurement of neutral sterols in plasma, erythrocytes, or cultured skin fibroblasts by using a specific method which employs gas chromatography combined with mass spectrometry will show an abnormal pattern with elevated cholesterol precursors and lowered cholesterol. Evaluation of fecal bile acids by similar methods will also show abnormal patterns. Prenatal diagnosis will be possible by the measurement of 7-dehydrocholesterol in amniotic fluid. An investigational study of cholesterol supplementation is underway which will determine whether post-natal treatment will be effective in modifying the course of the disease.

Table 22–1. Dysmorphic and other clinical findings in Smith-Lemli-Opitz syndrome.

Category	Findings
Biochemical	Elevated 7-dehydrocholesterol and other isomeric cholesterol precursors. Reduced cholesterol by specific methodology.
Neurologic	Defects in brain morphogenesis. Hypoplasia of frontal lobes, cerebellum, brain stem. Abnormal neuronal organization. Irritability. Moderate to severe psychomotor retardation. Seizures. Microcephaly. Abnormal EEG. Hypotonia in infancy which changes to hypertonicity.
Other birth defects	Facies: Narrow, sloping, anterior forehead. Ptosis of eyelids, epicanthal folds. Flat nasal bridge, anteverted nares. Micrognathia. Low set, slanted, or posteriorly rotated ears. Eyes: Congenital cataracts, strabismus. Oral: Cleft palate, broad alveolar ridges. External genitalia: Hypoplastic labia, hypospadias, cryptorchidism. Extremities: Post-axial polydactyly, syndactyly of 2nd and 3rd toes, flexed fingers (camptodactyly), increased number of digital whorls, transverse palmar creases. Valgus deformity of the feet. Dislocated hips. Other: Congenital heart defects, hypoplasia of the thymus, renal anomalies, rectal anomalies, deep sacral dimple.
Other clinical	Stillbirth, breech delivery. Moderately small for gestational age; poor postnatal growth. Feeding problems. Pyloric stenosis. Inguinal hernias. Blond hair. Mildly elevated transaminases.

CARBOHYDRATE DEFICIENT GLYCOPROTEIN (CDG) SYNDROME

This disorder was first described in 1980 and the clinical spectrum of the disorder is still being defined. It is an autosomal recessive disease that occurs in 1 in 40,000 to 1 in 60,000 births in Sweden and has been reported in patients from western Europe, the United States and Japan. Affected patients have abnormal isoforms of glycoproteins which lack the normal terminal three sugars (trisaccharide) consisting of N-acetylglucosamine, galactose, and sialic acid. The compounds involved include serum glycoproteins, transport proteins, lysosomal hydrolases, and coagulation factors and inhibitors. Table 22–2 lists the proteins affected and whether there is a qualitative change in isoform pattern or reduced concen-

tration. The "marker" for the disorder is an abnormal transferrin isoform pattern which can be determined both qualitatively and quantitatively in serum and dried blood filter paper spots in specialized laboratories. Because of the lowered levels of thyroxine-binding globulin, many affected infants have positive newborn screening tests for hypothyroidism and are often identified in this way. Three variants of CDG syndrome, type I, and the recently discovered types II and III, are currently known.

Type I

At birth, neonates affected with CDG type I will be noted to have hypotonia and restricted movement of large joints. The skin and subcutaneous tissues are uneven in consistency, and either tough (peau d' orange), or puffy. The skin changes are most

Table 22–2. Abnormalities in serum proteins and enzymes in the carbohydrate-deficient glycoprotein syndrome.

Compound	Abnormal Isoforms	Quantitative Change
A. Glycoproteins and proteins		
Transferrin	Yes	
α-1-Antitrypsin	Yes	Reduced
α-1-Antichymotrypsin	Yes	
α-1-B Glycoprotein	Yes	
α-1-Acid glycoprotein	Yes	
Complement C1,C3a,C4a	Yes	
Ceruloplasmin	Yes	
Ferritin	Yes	
Albumin		Reduced
Haptoglobin		Reduced
Thyroxine-binding globulin		Reduced
Transcortin		Reduced
Apolipoproteins		Reduced
B. Lysosomal hydrolases		
N-acetylglucosaminidase	Yes	Elevated
Fucosidase	Yes	
Arylsulfatase A		Elevated
β-Galactosidase		Elevated
N-acetylglucosaminyltransferase		Reduced
C. Coagulation factors and inhibitors		
Factors IX and XI		Reduced
Antithrombin III		Reduced
Protein C		Reduced
Protein S		Reduced
Heparin cofactor II		Reduced
D. Other		
Carboxypeptidase N	Yes	

Modified from Hagber BA, et al: Carbohydrate-deficient glycoprotein syndromes: peculiar group of new disorders. Pediatr Neurol 1993;**9**:255.

evident over the thighs and buttocks. There may also be fat pads over the buttocks. Some patients will be noted to have lipoatrophic streaks or patches on the lower legs. Many patients have inverted, often laterally displaced, nipples. Some neonates develop lethargy, hypothermia, and poor feeding; occasionally generalized edema and cardiac failure occur.

During early infancy, failure to thrive, growth retardation, ataxia, and psychomotor delay become evident. All affected patients develop cerebellar atrophy and one-third will also have cerebral atrophy by radioimaging. It is also during early infancy that patients develop hepatic dysfunction or failure. Liver biopsy will show steatosis with slight to moderate fibrosis. On electron microscopy, there will be unusual lysosomal vacuoles, concentric membrane-like inclusions, and occasionally a small, rounded appearance to the enodoplasmic reticulum. Affected infants have also been reported to have cardiac involvement with thickening of the ventricular walls and pericardial effusions. Many of the infants die from hepatic or cardiac failure. Some of the patients have been noted to have proteinuria and large simple cysts or microcysts in the kidneys. A coagulopathy, with decreased levels of factors IX and XI, may develop. There may also be reduced levels of coagulation inhibitors such as antithrombin III, protein C, protein S, and heparin cofactor II.

Older infants and children will develop a slowly progressive peripheral neuropathy and retinitis pigmentosa. They may also have episodes of stupor, coma, or strokes with seizures, loss of vision, and hemiplegia. The episodes are often precipitated by intercurrent infections and may in some way be related to the abnormal coagulation factors. Many of the patients spontaneously recover from the episodes. The cardiac and hepatic problems of early infancy do not progress and are, in fact, less common in older patients. As teenagers and young adults, the patients often develop severe deformities of the thoracic spine, eg, scoliosis and kyphosis. Osteopenia is common. Most patients are moderately to severely mentally handicapped and are usually not ambulatory.

Types II and III

Types II and III of CDG were recently reported. Two patients with more severe psychomotor retardation, but no peripheral neuropathy or cerebellar atrophy, and differing patterns of transferrin isoforms have been designated as having CDG type II. An additional two patients with very severe neurological involvement, less severe cutaneous manifestations, and transferrin isoform patterns different from type I and type II, have been designated as having CDG type III.

REFERENCES AND SUGGESTED READING

See page 256 and Appendix II.

Lysosomal Storage Disorders

23

Lysosomes are cytoplasmic, single membrane-bound organelles that are involved with a variety of metabolic processes. The lysosomal storage disorders are a heterogeneous group of diseases characterized by progressive lysosomal accumulation of compounds including macromolecules such as mucopolysaccharidoses, sphingolipids, and glycoproteins, as well as small molecules such as cystine or sialic acid. The disorders result from deficient activity of lysosomal acid hydrolases that are involved with the degradation of macromolecules, failure of lysosomal localization of the hydrolases, or defects in the transport of compounds from the lysosomes. Loss of enzymatic activity may result from mutations in the genes coding for the enzymes or from mutations in genes coding for protective proteins or activators for the enzymes involved. The clinical manifestations are usually related to the type of compound that is stored and its natural distribution. Although most lysosomal storage disorders present during childhood, some of the disorders may not be clinically apparent until later in adult life. Neonatal, infantile, juvenile, and adult forms of the same disorder exist. The majority of the disorders are inherited as autosomal recessive traits, while a few are X-linked. The molecular basis for many of the lysosomal storage disorders is known. Often the variation in clinical presentation for a disorder can be correlated with the different molecular defects involved. An exact enzymatic diagnosis, and occasionally the molecular diagnosis, is needed for accurate carrier and prenatal testing for families with affected individuals.

MUCOPOLYSACCHARIDOSES

Mucopolysaccharides (MPSs), or glycosaminoglycans, are large macromolecules composed of repeating, frequently sulfated, disaccharide units attached to a protein core. A series of lysosomal acid hydrolases degrades the MPSs by stepwise removal of the sulfates and carbohydrate residues. Deficient activity of a specific lysosomal acid hydrolase associated with MPS degradation will result in only partial degradation of the compounds and progressive lysosomal storage of residual fragments. Partially degraded MPSs can be noted in the urine of affected patients. The diagnosis, however, is best established by enzymatic testing. Prenatal diagnosis is available for all of the MPS storage disorders. Accurate carrier detection is available for some, but not all, of the disorders.

The characteristics of the mucopolysaccharidoses are shown in Table 23–1. Disorders that result in

Table 23–1. The mucopolysaccharidoses.

Type	Lysosomal Enzyme or Biochemical Defect	Clinical Sample	Inheritance
Hurler, type IH	α-L-Iduronidase	WBC	AR
Scheie, type IS	α-L-Iduronidase	WBC	AR
Hunter, type II	Iduronosulfatase	S	XL
Sanfilippo A, type IIIA	Heparan-N-sulfamidase	WBC	AR
Sanfilippo B, type IIIB	α-N-Acetylglucosaminidase	S	AR
Sanfilippo C, type IIIC	Acetyl-CoA:α-glucosaminide N-acetyltransferase	WBC	AR
Sanfilippo D, type IIID	N-Acetylglucosamine-6-sulfatase	WBC	AR
Morquio A, type IVA	N-Acetylgalactosamine-6-sulfatase	SF	AR
Morquio B, type IVB	β-Galactosidase, specific for keratan sulfate	SF	AR
Maroteaux-Lamy, type VI	Aryl sulfatase B	WBC	AR
Sly, type VII	β-Glucuronidase	WBC	AR

AR = autosomal recessive, XL = X-linked; S = serum, SF = cultured skin fibroblasts, WBC = leukocytes.

heparan sulfate storage have progressive central nervous system involvement. Affected patients may have macrocephaly and develop communicating hydrocephalus. Frequently a period of normal development is followed by a plateau and then regression in skills. Dermatan sulfate storage is associated with progressive visceral and bone involvement. Affected patients may have hepatosplenomegaly, cardiomyopathy, or cardiac valvular involvement. Radiographs show a distinctive pattern of bony changes, termed **dysostosis multiplex.** The skull is elongated (dolicocephaly), the calvarium thickened, and the sella undercut or J-shaped (Figure 23–1). The lower thoracic and upper lumbar vertebral bodies have a "beaking" appearance; narrowing of their anterior surfaces results in a dorsal kyphosis or "gibbus" (Figure 23–2). The long bones become shortened and thickened with increased trabeculation. Chest radiographs show anterior thickening of the ribs (Figure 23–3). A Madelung deformity, with abnormal angulation of the distal humerus and ulna, may be present. Proximal metacarpals may develop a "baby-bottle" appearance (Figure 23–4). The pelvis may show flaring of the iliac bones, shallow acetabulae, and progressive coxa valga. Hypoplasia of the odontoid process and cervical spine instability may occur. In Morquio syndrome, the storage of keratan sulfate and chondroitin-6-sulfate is associated with a platyspondyly, or flattening of the vertebral bodies, which resembles that seen in the spondyloepiphyseal dysplasias (Figure 23–5).

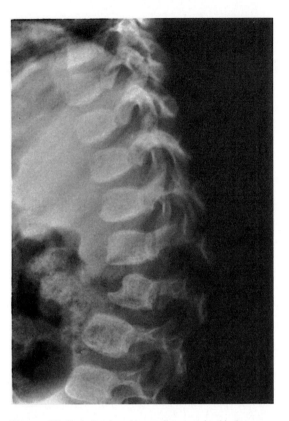

Figure 23–2. Lateral spine radiogram in Hurler syndrome. (Reproduced, with permission from Oski FA et al (editors), *Principles and Practice of Pediatrics,* 2nd ed, JB Lippincott, 1994.)

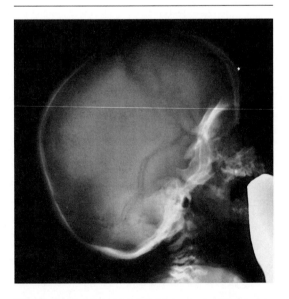

Figure 23–1. Lateral skull radiogram in Hurler syndrome. (Reproduced, with permission from Oski FA et al (editors), *Principles and Practice of Pediatrics,* 2nd ed, JB Lippincott, 1994.)

Hurler Syndrome (MPS Type IH): Hurler syndrome (MPS type IH), the prototype for this group of disorders, results from deficient activity of α-L–iduronidase. The disorder is inherited as an autosomal recessive trait and has an incidence of at least one in 100,000 births. There is storage of both heparan sulfate and dermatan sulfate. Affected patients are normal at birth; over the first year of life they develop corneal clouding, coarse facial features, and hepatosplenomegaly. Flattening of the midfacial area, widening of the nasal bridge, and gingival hyperplasia with thickening of the alveolar ridge is noted. Many patients have noisy breathing as infants and later develop upper airway obstruction that may result in sleep apnea or cor pulmonale. A dorsal kyphosis, or gibbus formation, develops in the thoracic and lumbar spine areas. Although they are large as infants, linear growth slows and minimal gain in height occurs after age 2–3 years. The skull enlarges; communicating hydrocephalus may become symptomatic. Decreased range of motion of joints gradually develops and results in a "jockey stance" and stiff hands and fingers (Figure 23–6). Some patients may also develop carpal tunnel syndrome or hearing

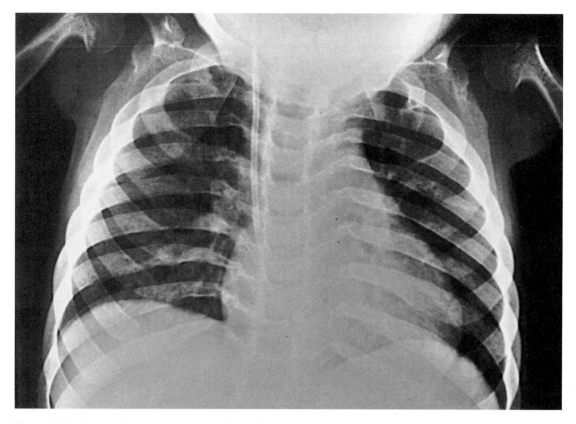

Figure 23–3. Chest radiogram in Hurler syndrome. (Reproduced, with permission from Oski FA et al (editors), *Principles and Practice of Pediatrics,* 2nd ed, JB Lippincott, 1994.)

impairments. Umbilical and inguinal hernias are common. Cardiac involvement, in the form of valvular disease or cardiomyopathy, often develops between 2 and 5 years of age. After 1 year of age, psychomotor development slows and then regresses. Although ambulatory as young infants, they become progressively debilitated and usually do not live past 10 years of age. Deaths most often result from cardiopulmonary or central nervous system involvement. There is no specific treatment except for symptomatic and supportive care. Bone marrow transplantation may be considered for young infants with Hurler syndrome, prior to major central nervous system or cardiac involvement.

Scheie Syndrome (MPS Type IS): Scheie syndrome (MPS type IS), is a milder, allelic form of Hurler syndrome that presents after 5 years of age. Although they also have deficient activity of α-L-iduronidase, affected patients do not have psychomotor impairment. Their life span may be normal. Aortic valvular lesions, carpal tunnel syndrome, glaucoma, retinal degeneration, and deafness often occur.

Hurler-Scheie Syndrome (MPS Type IH/IS): Patients with Hurler-Scheie syndrome (MPS type

IH/IS) have clinical features that are of intermediate severity compared to those noted with Hurler and Scheie syndromes. Some patients are compound heterozygotes for both Hurler and Scheie syndromes, whereas others have been found to have separate, distinct allelic mutations at the α-L-iduronidase locus. Clinical symptoms are apparent by 2 years of age; survival has been reported into young adult life.

Hunter Syndrome (MPS Type II): Hunter syndrome (MPS type II), is inherited as an X-linked trait and associated with both heparan sulfate and dermatan sulfate storage. The disorder results from deficient activity of iduronosulfatase. Severe (type A) and mild (type B) forms of the disorder exist. The clinical manifestations of the severe form of Hunter syndrome are similar to those of Hurler syndrome, except that the onset is later (between ages one and 2 years), there is a slower progression of the disease, and corneal clouding does not develop (Figure 23–7). Infiltrative ivory papules may be noted on the upper back and lateral upper arms and thighs. Significant behavioral problems and hearing impairment may occur. Hunter patients usually become debilitated during adolescence and do not live past the mid 20's. The mild form of Hunter syndrome, like the Scheie

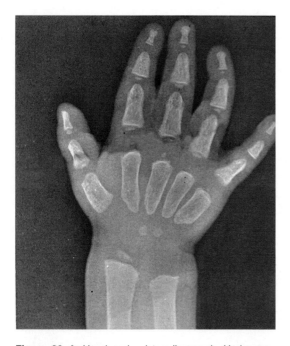

Figure 23–4. Hand and wrist radiogram in Hurler syndrome. (Reproduced, with permission from Oski FA et al (editors), *Principles and Practice of Pediatrics,* 2nd ed, JB Lippincott, 1994.)

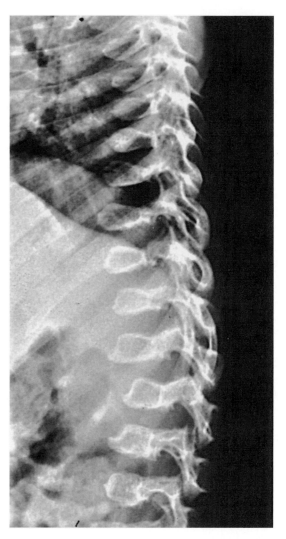

Figure 23–5. Lateral spine radiogram in Morquio syndrome. (Reproduced, with permission from Oski FA et al (editors), *Principles and Practice of Pediatrics,* 2nd ed, JB Lippincott, 1994.)

syndrome, is not associated with pyschomotor retardation. Type B patients may have a normal or near-normal life span. Female patients with Hunter syndrome may have X-chromosomal defects, eg, Turner syndrome, or have an autosomal recessive form of the disorder. Carrier detection is currently available only for families that have informative RFLP's at the iduronosulfatase locus.

Sanfilippo Syndrome (MPS Type III): Sanfilippo syndrome (MPS type III) is an autosomal recessive disorder that may result from one of four different enzymatic deficiencies which are clinically indistinguishable. The disorder may be as common as Hurler syndrome. Type A results from deficient activity of heparan-N-sulfatase (sulfamidase), type B from α-N-acetylglucosaminidase deficiency, type C from acetyl-CoA:α-glucosaminide N-acetyltransferase deficiency, and type D from N-acetylglucosamine-6-sulfatase deficiency. There is storage of heparan sulfate and progressive central nervous system degeneration. Most patients present between ages 2 and 5 years of age with behavioral problems and psychomotor delays. Many patients are hyperactive; seizure disorders are common. Some patients may have mild coarsening of facial features, hepatosplenomegaly, and dysostosis multiplex. They usually do not have short stature or corneal clouding. Patients with Sanfilippo syndrome usually become debilitated during late childhood and die during late adolescence (Figure 23–8).

Morquio Syndrome (MPS Type IV): Morquio syndrome (MPS type IV) is an autosomal recessive disorder associated with keratan sulfate storage alone or in combination with chondroitin-6-sulfate storage. Two clinically similar forms of the disorder exist. Type A results from deficient activity of N-acetyl-galactosamine-6-sulfate sulfatase (galactose-6-sulfatase) and type B is from deficient activity of a β-galactosidase, which is specific for keratan sulfate. Affected patients have short stature, bony dysplasia with flaring of the lower rib cage, and joint enlargement and laxity. Although the clinical onset is at about 1 year of age, most patients are not diagnosed until later during childhood. Corneal clouding and hepatosplenomegaly may be present but are usually

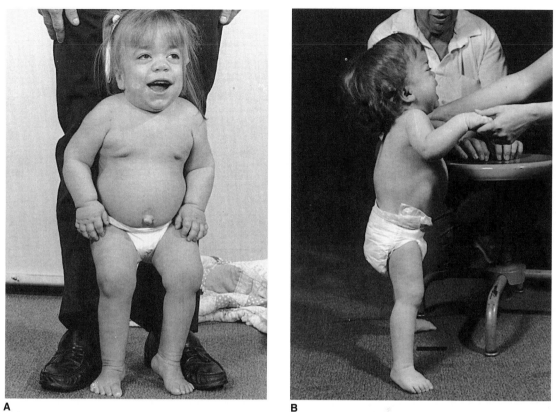

Figure 23–6. Hurler syndrome **(A)** age 37 months **(B)** age 27 months. Note the coarse facial features, dolicomacrocephaly, and dorsal kyphosis (gibbus). (Reproduced, with permission from Oski FA et al (editors), *Principles and Practice of Pediatrics,* 2nd ed, JB Lippincott, 1994.)

mild. Hearing impairment is common; cardiac valvular involvement may develop. Enamel hypoplasia may be noted in type A patients. Instability of the upper cervical spine usually requires posterior spinal fusion. Survival to adulthood is common. A milder form of the Morquio syndrome is also known.

Maroteaux-Lamy Syndrome (MPS Type VI): Maroteaux-Lamy syndrome (MPS type VI), also an autosomal recessive disease, is associated with deficient activity of aryl sulfatase B (N-acetylgalactosamine-4-sulfatase). Storage of dermatan sulfatase results in marked visceral and bony changes. The central nervous system is usually not involved until late in the course of the disease. Mild, intermediate, and severe forms of the disorder exist as noted with the Hurler, Scheie, and Hurler-Scheie phenotypes. The clinical features of the severe form resemble those in Hurler syndrome, except that psychomotor retardation does not occur. Corneal clouding is present; cardiac involvement and carpal tunnel syndrome are common. Death occurs in early adolescence (Figure 23–9). The mild form of the disorder may present with short stature, corneal clouding, and cardiac valvular involvement in young adults. Bone marrow

transplantation may be considered for young infants with Maroteaux-Lamy syndrome, prior to major cardiac involvement.

β-Glucuronidase Deficiency (MPS Type VII): β-Glucuronidase deficiency (MPS type VII), or Sly syndrome, is inherited as an autosomal recessive trait and characterized by the storage of heparan sulfate, keratan sulfate, chondroitin-4-sulfate, and chondroitin-6-sulfate. The disorder has clinical features that resemble the Hurler syndrome phenotype, but vary widely in onset and severity. Patients may present as early as the neonatal period with hydrops fetalis, or later during childhood without psychomotor retardation.

SPHINGOLIPIDOSES

Glycosphingolipids are macromolecules comprised of a ceramide (N-acylsphingosine) core, to which an oligosaccharide chain of neutral carbohydrates is attached. The carbohydrates may be sulfated (sulfatides); sialic acid residues may also be attached to the neutral carbohydrates (gangliosides). As with

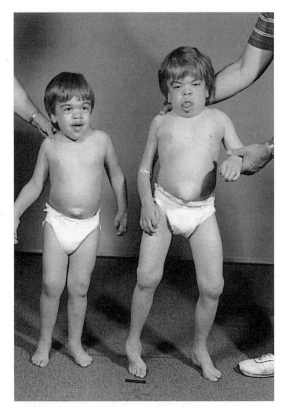

Figure 23–7. Hunter syndrome, brothers ages 5 and 15 years. (Reproduced, with permission from Oski FA et al (editors), *Principles and Practice of Pediatrics,* 2nd ed, JB Lippincott, 1994.)

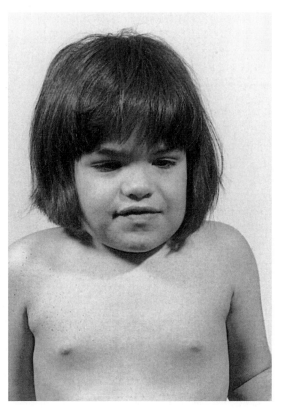

Figure 23–8. Sanfilippo syndrome, age 6 years. (Reproduced, with permission from Oski FA et al (editors), *Principles and Practice of Pediatrics,* 2nd ed, JB Lippincott, 1994.)

the MPSs, a series of lysosomal acid hydrolases are responsible for degradation of the compounds. Deficient activity of a specific hydrolase will result in intralysosomal storage of partially-degraded compounds, usually glycosphingolipids, gangliosides, or sphingomyelin. The disorders are confirmed by demonstration of deficient activity of their associated lysosomal acid hydrolase. Carrier detection and prenatal diagnosis are available, but only in a limited number of laboratories. Table 23–2 gives the characteristics of the sphingolipidoses.

GM$_1$ Gangliosidoses

GM$_1$ gangliosidoses are a group of autosomal recessive disorders associated with deficient activity of acid β-galactosidase. The subtypes vary widely in clinical manifestation. All result from progressive storage of macromolecules that contain β-galactoside residues, eg, GM$_1$ gangliosides, glycoproteins, oligosaccharides, and keratan sulfate-like MPSs.

Generalized Gangliosidosis (Type I): Generalized gangliosidosis (type I), which results from complete lack of β-galactosidase activity, presents shortly after birth with a rapidly progressive Hurler-like phenotype; death usually occurs by 2 years of age. Corneal clouding is usually not present. Significant cardiac involvement and peripheral edema may develop. One-half of patients have cherry-red spots in the macular area. Bone marrow and visceral organs show foamy histiocytes. Vacuolation of peripheral lymphocytes may be seen. Dysostosis multiplex is noted on radiographs (Figure 23–10).

Juvenile GM$_1$ Gangliosidosis (Type 2): Juvenile GM$_1$ gangliosidosis (type 2) is a milder form with less severe symptoms of MPS-like storage. Patients present with ataxia between one and two years of age, followed by progressive central nervous system involvement. Seizures and blindness commonly develop; death usually occurs between 3 and 10 years of age.

Adult GM$_1$ Gangliosidosis (Type 3): Adult GM$_1$ gangliosidosis (type 3) usually has its onset during adolescence with dysarthria, gait disturbances, and a progressive dystonia. If they occur, the features of MPS-like storage are mild. Most patients survive to their early adult years.

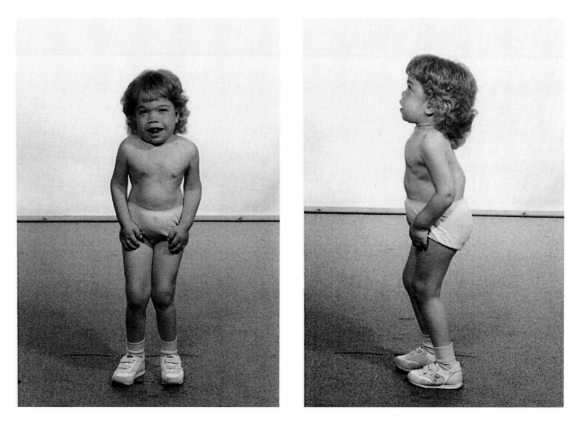

Figure 23–9. Maroteaux-Lamy syndrome, severe form, age 10 years. (Reproduced, with permission from Oski FA et al (editors), *Principles and Practice of Pediatrics,* 2nd ed, JB Lippincott, 1994.)

GM$_2$ Gangliosidoses

The GM$_2$ gangliosidoses are autosomal recessive disorders associated with cerebral degeneration and the storage of GM$_2$ ganglioside and related glycosphingolipids. There is deficient activity of the β-hexosaminidases or a sphingolipid activator protein. Isoenzymes of β-hexosaminidase are composed of varying combinations of two subunits, α and β. The gene for the α subunit is located on chromosome 15 and the gene for the β subunit is on chromosome 5. Two major isoenzymes, hexosaminidase A (hex A) and B (hex B), comprise the majority of total hexosaminidase activity. The isoenzyme hex A contains both α subunits and β subunits, whereas hex B has only β subunits. Mutations at the α subunit locus result in hex A deficiency and Tay-Sachs disease. Mutations at the β subunit locus result in total β-hexosaminidase deficiency and Sandhoff disease. Other forms of the disorder may be associated with lack of the GM$_2$ activator protein, which is needed for stabilization of the substrate-enzyme complex.

Tay-Sachs Disease, or GM$_2$ Gangliosidosis Type I:

Tay-Sachs disease, or GM$_2$ gangliosidosis type I, is most common in persons of Eastern European Jewish ancestry in whom the carrier rate is 1 in 27. The carrier rate among persons of other backgrounds is approximately 1 in 200. Affected children are normal at birth. Between 6 and 12 months of age they have the onset of hypotonia and psychomotor delay, that is followed by a rapidly progressive central nervous system degeneration with spasticity, seizures, and loss of vision. Death usually occurs by age 3 to 4 years. A cherry red spot in the macular area, which represents the storage of white GM$_2$ ganglioside surrounding and enhancing a normal red macular area, may be seen as early as 3 months of age. The disorder is associated with deficient activity of the A isoenzyme of β-hexosaminidase. Total β-hexosaminidase activity is usually normal. Education and carrier detection programs for Tay-Sachs disease have existed since the 1970s. At-risk couples, prior to the birth of an affected child, have been identified and offered genetic counseling and prenatal diagnosis. The incidence of Tay-Sachs disease has correspondingly decreased in Jewish communities since the carrier detection programs began. Couples, where at least one is of Eastern European Jewish ancestry, should be offered carrier testing for Tay-Sachs disease, preferably prior to conception. Testing in women after conception is more difficult because the placenta produces β-hexosaminidase, which inter-

Table 23–2. The sphingolipidoses.

Type	Lysosomal Enzyme or Biochemical Defect	Clinical Sample	Inheritance
GM₁ gangliosidosis	β-Galactosidase	WBC	AR
Tay-Sachs disease	β-Hexosaminidase, A isoenzyme	S, WBC	AR
Sandhoff disease	β-Hexosaminidase, total	S, WBC	AR
Fabry disease	α-Galactosidase	WBC	XL
Schindler disease	α-N-acetylgalactosaminidase	WBC	AR
Lactosylceramidosis	Neutral β-galactosidase	SF	AR
Gaucher disease	β-Glucosidase	WBC	AR
Farber disease	Ceramidase	WBC	AR
Niemann-Pick, type I	Sphingomyelinase	WBC	AR
Niemann-Pick, type IIS	Defect in cholesterol esterification	SF	AR
Krabbe disease	β-Galactosidase, specific for galactosylceramide	WBC	AR
Metachromatic leukodystrophy	Aryl sulfatase A	WBC	AR
Multiple sulfatase deficiency	Aryl sulfatases A, B, & C; heparan sulfamidase, iduronosulfatase, and other sulfatases	WBC	AR

AR = autosomal recessive, XL = X-linked; S = serum, SF = cultured skin fibroblasts, WBC = leukocytes.

feres with the interpretation of results from standard serum carrier testing. Leukocyte testing in pregnant women gives a more accurate indication of their carrier status, but is more costly and labor intensive. Delaying testing until after conception also may not allow enough time for completion of the carrier testing prior to the time that prenatal diagnosis would be performed.

Sandhoff Disease, or GM₂ Gangliosidosis Type 2: Sandhoff disease, or GM₂ gangliosidosis type 2, is associated with complete deficiency of β-hexosaminidase. Clinical manifestations are often indistinguishable from Tay-Sachs disease; hepatosplenomegaly, however, may also develop. The disorder may occur in a person of any background.

Juvenile Forms: Juvenile forms of both Tay-Sachs disease and Sandhoff disease are known which present with ataxia or developmental regression between 2 and 6 years of age. Cherry-red spots are not always present, but optic atrophy or retinitis pigmentosa may occur. Progressive loss of speech, athetosis, spasticity, and seizures lead to death between ages 5 and 15 years.

Adult Forms: Patients with adult forms of Tay-Sachs disease present before age 16 years with atypical spinocerebellar degeneration or psychoses.

Affected patients of all types have been found to have normal β-hexosaminidase activity when tested with artificial substrates, which is the common means for testing. Some of these patients will demonstrate deficient activity of β-hexosaminidase when natural substrates are used; other patients have a deficiency of a sphingolipid activator protein. Occasionally otherwise normal persons are found to have deficient activity of β-hexosaminidase. Such persons are usually

compound heterozygotes who have one mutant gene for the classic disorder and another which does not allow measurement of β-hexosaminidase activity with artificial substrates.

GM₃ Gangliosidosis

GM₃ gangliosidosis is a rare disorder associated with deficient activity of uridine diphosphate-N-acetylgalactosaminyl transferase. Affected patients have a rapidly progressing hypotonia, hyporeflexia, psychomotor retardation, and failure to thrive.

Fabry Disease

Fabry disease, or α-galactosyl–lactosyl ceramidosis, is an X-linked disorder associated with deficient activity of α-galactosidase, previously called α-galactosidase A. Storage of glycosphingolipids occurs in the eyes, kidneys, skeletal, and cardiac muscle, central and autonomic nervous system, and the vascular endothelium and smooth muscle. Most affected boys present by 10 years of age with acroparesthesia. There is an almost constant burning type of pain in the hands and feet. In addition, painful crises, lasting minutes to days, may involve the extremities or abdomen. Characteristic angiokeratoma corporis diffusum appear in the bathing suit area between the umbilicus and knees and occasionally on the conjunctiva or mucosal surfaces. Angiokeratomas are flat or slightly raised, dark red to blue-black, small macules that usually appear in clusters. Sweating may be decreased. Storage in the eye leads to a characteristic whorl-like corneal dystrophy and spoke-like or propeller-like cataracts. As the disease progresses, hypertension and proteinuria are noted, followed by renal failure that may occur as early as

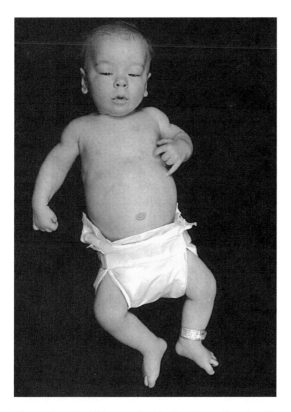

Figure 23–10. GM$_1$ gangliosidosis. (Reproduced, with permission from Oski FA et al (editors), *Principles and Practice of Pediatrics,* 2nd ed, JB Lippincott, 1994.)

age 30 or 40 years and require renal dialysis or transplantation. Cardiomyopathies, myocardial infarctions, and cardiac conduction defects may also occur. Aneurysms, vascular occlusions, or hemorrhages of the central nervous system may result from vascular endothelial involvement. Supportive and symptomatic treatment are available; enzyme replacement therapy is being developed. Symptomatic carrier females for Fabry disease may have a milder form of the disorder.

Schindler Disease

Schindler disease is a rare, autosomal recessive disease that results from deficient activity of α-N-acetylgalactosaminidase, previously termed α-galactosidase B. Affected patients have progressive psychomotor retardation, myoclonic seizures, and optic atrophy.

Lactosyl Ceramidosis

Lactosyl ceramidosis is a rare, autosomal disease associated with deficient activity of neutral β-galactosidase that cleaves the terminal β-galactosyl residues from lactosylceramide. Storage of lactosylceramide occurs in the viscera, brain, connective tissues, and reticuloendothelial system. Psychomotor delay and hypotonia are followed by progressive central nervous system degeneration, ataxia, optic atrophy, lymphadenopathy, hepatosplenomegaly, and death during childhood.

Gaucher Disease

Gaucher disease, the most common of the lysosomal storage disorders, is an autosomal recessive disorder that results from deficient activity of β-glucosidase and the subsequent storage of glucocerebroside in the reticuloendothelial system. There are three major forms of the disorder.

Type 1 (Adult, Non-neuronopathic): Type 1, the adult, non-neuronopathic form, is the most common and occurs in 1 in 6000 to 10,000 persons. It is most frequently diagnosed in persons of Eastern European Jewish ancestry but is panethnic. Type I Gaucher disease may present with splenomegaly and pancytopenia from hypersplenism at any age. Hepatomegaly also occurs and is associated with mildly elevated liver function tests, and occasionally progressive hepatic disease or cirrhosis. Storage of glucocerebroside in the bone marrow also affects hematologic parameters, interferes with growth and mineralization of the bones, and results in painful bone crises and infarcts, avascular necrosis of the femoral and humeral heads, and pathologic fractures. Skeletal radiographs and radioimaging are helpful in determining the degree of clinical involvement. The distal femur may show erosion and thinning of the cortex with an Erlenmeyer flask-type deformity. With advanced disease, cachexia and a yellow-brown discoloration of the skin from glucocerebroside disposition are noted. Although the central nervous system is usually not involved, an oculomotor apraxia may occur. Large, lipid-laden, fusiform histiocytes with dense eccentric nuclei, termed "wrinkled tissue paper" or "crumpled silk" cells, are noted in bone marrow preparations. Affected symptomatic type 1 Gaucher patients should be considered for enzyme replacement therapy using macrophage-targeted modified glucocerebrosidase. Although extremely expensive, enzyme replacement therapy poses considerably less risks than bone marrow transplantation, which is currently the only other alternative therapy.

Type 2 (Acute Neuronopathic or Infantile): Type 2 Gaucher disease, the acute neuronopathic or infantile form, is a rare condition characterized by progressive hepatosplenomegaly and central nervous system deterioration in early infancy. Most children die by 2 years of age.

Type 3 Gaucher Disease (Subacute Neuronopathic or Juvenile): Type 3 Gaucher disease, the subacute neuronopathic or juvenile form, often presents like type 1 with hepatosplenomegaly during childhood, but patients then develop a slowly progressive central nervous system deterioration after age 8 years. Many patients live to be young adults.

Atypical Cases: Atypical cases of Gaucher disease may result from deficiency of a sphingolipid activator protein for β-glucosidase.

Mutations in the gene for Gaucher disease correspond to the clinical presentation and type of the disease. In patients who have the conset of their disease during childhood, molecular genetic testing may be helpful in distinguishing type 3 from type 1.

Farber Disease

Farber disease, or ceramidosis, is a rare autosomal recessive disorder associated with deficient activity of ceramidase and the storage of ceramide and other gangliosides in the skin, lymph nodes, viscera, and brain. Connective tissue granulomas also form in response to the storage in the conjunctiva, pharynx, and upper respiratory tract. Patients affected with **type 1,** or the "classic," most common, form of the disorder, present between 2 weeks and 4 months of age with a hoarse cry, swollen painful joints, periarticular nodules, and pulmonary infiltration. With progression of the disease, skin nodules may develop over pressure points and in the periorbital and perioral regions. Valvular cardiac lesions, hepatosplenomegaly, and generalized lymphadenopathy also occur. Psychomotor regression, seizures, hypotonia, hyporeflexia, and failure to thrive precede death, which usually occurs within a few years after the onset of the disorder. Other very rare forms of the disorder differ in the age of onset, clinical severity, and degree of visceral involvement. Therapy is mainly supportive.

Niemann-Pick Disease

The heterogeneous group of autosomal recessive disorders known as Niemann-Pick disease are associated with storage of sphingomyelin, GM_2 and GM_3 gangliosides, cholesterol, bis(monoacylglyceryl) phosphate, and other glycosphingolipids in the reticuloendothelial system, viscera, and brain. The two major types of the disorder, types I and II, are further subdivided into acute (A), subacute (S), and chronic (C) forms according to the age of onset and severity. Type I forms are associated with deficient activity of sphinogomyelinase and the storage of sphingomyelin and cholesterol. Type II forms vary in the material stored, which may include sphingomyelin, cholesterol, glycolipid or bis(monoacylglyceryl)phosphate. Type IIS results from defects in cholesterol esterification. The basic defects in the other forms of type II are unknown. Affected patients with all forms of the disorder have lipid-filled "foam cells" in the bone marrow, liver, spleen, adrenals, brain, lymph nodes, and lungs. "Sea-blue histiocytes" may also be shown with Romanovsky staining. Accurate carrier and prenatal testing are presently only available for types IA and IS.

Type IA: The most common and severe form of this group of disorders, type IA Niemann-Pick disease, occurs most often in children of Eastern European Jewish ancestry. Affected children develop massive hepatosplenomegaly during the first year of life. Corneal opacities with a brownish discoloration of the anterior lens capsule, yellow-brown discoloration of the skin, lymphadenopathy, pulmonary infiltration, and failure to thrive also occur. Cherry-red macular spots are present in one-half of affected patients. Rapidly progressing central nervous system deterioration leads to death usually between 2 and 5 years of age.

Type IIA: Niemann-Pick disease resembles type IA, but the course of the disease is somewhat slower. Patients with type IIA may also have a neonatal, hepatitis-like presentation.

Type IS: Type IS Niemann-Pick disease, thought to be a milder allelic variant of type IA, presents with hepatosplenomegaly, pulmonary infiltration, and lymphadenopathy in childhood. Affected patients also have varying degrees of abnormalities in nerve conduction velocity, involvement of the central nervous system, and macular findings. Many patients live to adulthood.

Type IIS: Type IIS Niemann-Pick disease is associated with hepatosplenomegaly with cholestasis, lymphadenopathy, seizures, and central nervous system involvement. Most patients present between 2 and 7 years of age; they usually do not live past late childhood or adolescence. Some patients with type IIS, who have defects in cholesterol esterification, may benefit from lowered cholesterol intakes and medications that inhibit hydroxymethylglutaryl–CoA reductase.

Types IC and IIC: Types IC and IIC Niemann-Pick disease are adult forms associated with late onset hepatosplenomegaly and neurologic involvement.

Krabbe Disease

Krabbe disease, also known as globoid cell leukodystrophy, is an autosomal recessive disorder that is most common in persons of Scandinavian ancestry. Deficient activity of the β-galactosidase specific for removing the terminal β-galactosyl residues from galactosylceramide results in storage of galactosylceramide (galactocerebroside) in the central and peripheral nervous system. "Globoid cells" are large, distended, multinucleated, modified macrophages found in clusters in the perivascular areas of the white matter. There are infantile, late infantile, juvenile, and adult forms of the disorder.

Infantile Form: Patients with the infantile form of Krabbe disease present before 6 months of age with increased motor tone, irritability, hypersensitivity to external stimuli, episodic hypothermia, optic atrophy, and developmental regression. Seizures, peripheral neuropathies, and loss of vision and hearing develop. Cherry-red macular spots may be present. Cerebrospinal fluid protein levels are markedly elevated and nerve conduction velocities are decreased. Neuroimaging shows severe brain atrophy with demyelination and gliosis. The disorder is rapidly progressive with death usually occurring prior to 2 years of age.

Other Forms: The **late infantile form** of Krabbe's disease usually has its onset between 6 months and 3 years of age. The onset of the **juvenile form** occurs between 3 and 10 years of age and patients with the **adult form** present between 10 and 35 years of age. Affected patients have psychomotor regression, optic atrophy, spastic quadriparesis with pyramidal signs, acute polyneuropathy, spinocerebellar degeneration, and ataxia.

Metachromatic Leukodystrophy

Metachromatic leukodystrophy, or sulfatide lipidosis, results from deficient activity of aryl sulfatase A (galactosyl–3-sulfate-ceramide sulfatase, cerebroside sulfatase). Storage of galactosyl sulfatide (cerebroside sulfatide) occurs in the white matter of the central nervous system and in the peripheral nervous system. Galactosyl sulfatide and sulfated galactoglycerolipids also accumulate in the kidney, gallbladder, and other visceral organs. Demyelination, gliosis, spongy degeneration, and atrophy of the brain develops. The disorder was named for the metachromatic staining noted with acetic acid-cresyl violet stain prior to our understanding of the biochemistry involved. The disorder is inherited as an autosomal recessive trait and has three clinical forms which vary in age of onset.

Late-infantile Form: Patients with the late-infantile form of metachromatic leukodystrophy present between 1 and 2 years of age with psychomotor delay, ataxia, gait disturbances, weakness, or peripheral neuropathy. Progressive nervous system deterioration is associated with psychomotor regression, hypotonia, hyporeflexia, optic atrophy, seizures, and bulbar and pseudobulbar palsies. The macular areas may show a gray discoloration. Cerebrospinal fluid protein levels are elevated and nerve conduction velocities slowed. Neuroimaging shows atrophy of the white matter. Death usually occurs between 2 and 4 years after the onset of the disease.

Juvenile Form: Patients with the juvenile form of metachromatic leukodystrophy usually present between 5 and 7 years of age, although sometimes as late as age 20. Presenting symptoms include changes in personality or school performance, gait disturbances, ataxia, speech problems, or incontinence. The progression of the disease is slower than that noted with the late-infantile form; patients often live for 4 to 6 years after the onset of their disease.

Adult Form: The adult form has its onset after puberty with clinical features that resemble those of the juvenile form, but a slower course. Patients with the adult form may survive for 5 to 10 years or longer after the onset of their disease.

Some patients with the juvenile and adult forms of metachromatic leukodystrophy have normal levels of activity of aryl sulfatase A; their disease results from **deficiency of a cerebroside sulfatase activator protein** (sphingolipid activator protein 1). Healthy adults have been found to have reduced levels of activity of aryl sulfatase A when tested with artificial substrates, but normal levels of activity when natural radiolabeled substrates are used. This **pseudodeficiency** is not uncommon and can be problematic if present in a family with an affected child who wish prenatal testing.

Multiple Sulfatase Deficiency

Multiple sulfatase deficiency, or Austin disease, is a rare autosomal recessive disorder that results from impaired production, impaired activation, or increased degradation of multiple lysosomal and nonlysosomal sulfatases. Affected patients have decreased levels of activity of the lysosomal hydrolases aryl sulfatase A, aryl sulfatase B, iduronosulfatase, heparan sulfamidase, N-acetylglucosamine-6-sulfate sulfatase, and N-acetylgalactosamine-6-sulfate sulfatase. The disorders associated with these enzyme deficiencies include metachromatic leukodystrophy, Maroteaux-Lamy syndrome, Hunter syndrome, Sanfilippo syndrome A and D, and Morquio syndrome A, respectively. Affected patients also have deficient activity of aryl sulfatase C, a cytosolic steroid sulfatase, which results in X-linked ichthyosis, corneal opacities, and elevated blood cholesterol sulfate levels in affected males. Affected patients with multiple sulfatase deficiency have clinical manifestations that are a combination of those features seen with late-infantile metachromatic leukodystrophy, the mucopolysaccharidoses, and steroid sulfatase deficiency. The disorder usually presents by age 2 years with psychomotor delay or regression, coarse facial features, hepatosplenomegaly, weakness, deafness, and ichthyosis. Dysostosis multiplex is present on radiographs; urinary dermatan sulfate and heparan sulfate may be elevated. The course of the disease is similar to that for the late-infantile form of metachromatic leukodystrophy; most patients do not live past 10 years of age. A more severe form of the disorder with presentation at birth has been reported.

Other Types of Leukodystrophies

Other types of leukodystrophies, or disorders affecting the white matter, must be included in the differential diagnosis of the sphinogolipidoses that present with leukodystrophy.

Canavan Disease: Canavan disease, or spongy degeneration of the brain, an autosomal recessive disorder most common in children of Eastern European Jewish ancestry, is associated with deficient activity of aspartoacylase. Levels of N-acetylaspartic acid are elevated in the blood and urine. Affected patients present in early infancy with optic atrophy, macrocephaly, hyperreflexia, and rigidity. Progressive neurological deterioration results in death prior to 5 years of age.

Alexander disease, which is thought to result from astrocyte dysfunction, and Pelizaeus-Merzbacher disease, which appears to be related to mutations in the proteolipid protein gene on the X-chromosome, are nonlysosomal leukodystrophies. Adrenoleukodystrophy is discussed with the disorders of peroxisomal metabolism.

GLYCOPROTEINOSES (OLIGOSACCHARIDOSES)

Glycoproteinoses are rare autosomal recessive disorders that result from deficient activity of lysosomal acid hydrolases that remove carbohydrate residues from the oligosaccharide chains of glycoproteins. Because oligosaccharide linkages also are present in sphingolipids and mucopolysaccharides, more than one type of partially degraded compounds may accumulate in the individual disorders. Many of the clinical features of this group of diseases resemble those seen in the mucopolysaccharidoses, sphingolipidoses, and mucolipidoses. Increased urinary excretion of abnormal oligosaccharides and vacuolation of peripheral lymphocytes are noted. Carrier testing and prenatal diagnosis are available. Table 23–3 lists characteristics of the glycoproteinoses.

Fucosidosis
Fucosidosis, most common in persons of Italian or Spanish-American background, results from deficient activity of α-fucosidase which leads to the storage of fucose-containing sphingolipids, glycoproteins, and oligosaccharides.

Type I: Patients with the more severe form of fucosidosis, type I, present between 3 and 18 months of age with short stature, coarse facial features, macroglossia, hepatosplenomegaly, cardiac involvement, seizures, and psychomotor retardation. Dysostosis multiplex is present on radiographs. Sweat chloride levels may be elevated. Most children die before 10 years of age.

Type II: Patients with type II fucosidosis present between 1 and 2 years of age. Type II has a slower course; affected patients may survive to young adulthood. This form of the disorder does not usually have abnormal sweat chloride levels or hepatosplenomegaly, but angiokeratomas, as seen in Fabry disease, may occur.

Mannosidosis (α-Mannosidase Deficiency)
Mannosidosis is associated with deficient activity of α-mannosidase, which results in the storage of mannose-containing glycoproteins.

Type I: Patients with type I mannosidosis present between 3 and 12 months of age with coarse facial features, hepatosplenomegaly, psychomotor retardation, posterior spoke-like cataracts, corneal opacities, frequent infections, hearing loss, and hypotonia. Mild dysostosis multiplex is present on radiographs. Most affected patients do not live past 10 years of age.

Type II: Type II mannosidosis presents between age 1 and 4 years and has a slower course than type I. Patients may survive to young adulthood.

β-Mannosidase Deficiency
Deficient activity of β-mannosidase is associated with the onset of psychomotor retardation during childhood. Affected patients do not have abnormal facies or hepatosplenomegaly. Angiokeratomas are present. Combined deficiencies of β-mannosidase and heparan sulfamidase have been reported in one patient who had clinical features similar to those seen with Sanfilippo syndrome.

Table 23–3. Glycoproteinoses (oligosaccharidoses).

Type	Lysosomal Enzyme or Biochemical Defect	Clinical Sample	Inheritance
Fucosidosis	α-Fucosidase	WBC	AR
Mannosidosis	α-Mannosidase	WBC	AR
β-Mannosidase deficiency	β-Mannosidase	WBC	AR
β-Mannosidase deficiency variant	Combined deficient activities of both β-mannosidase and heparan sulfamidase	WBC	AR
Sialidosis	α-Neuraminidase	SF	AR
Sialolipidosis	? α-Neuraminidase specific for GM₃ and GD₂	SF	AR
Galactosialidosis	Protective protein that complexes with both α-neuraminidase and β-galactosidase	SF	AR
Aspartylglucosaminuria	Aspartylglucosaminidase	WBC	AR

AR = autosomal recessive, SF = cultured skin fibroblasts, WBC = leukocytes.

α-Neuraminidase Deficiency (Sialidoses)

The sialidoses, previously classified as type I mucolipidosis, are now known to be associated with deficient activity of the α-neuraminidase that cleaves the terminal α-N-acetyl–neuraminic acid (sialic acid) residues from glycoproteins and oligosaccharides.

Type I Sialidosis: Type I sialidosis, also known as the cherry-red-spot-myoclonus syndrome, has its onset between 8 and 25 years of age. The disorder is most common in persons of Italian background. Affected patients have progressive visual impairment with cherry-red macular spots and, occasionally, punctate lenticular opacities. Generalized, often debilitating, myoclonus develops. Acroparesthesia, delayed nerve conduction velocity, hyperreflexia, ataxia, nystagmus, and major motor seizures may occur. Most patients do not live past young adult life.

Type II Sialidosis: Type II sialidosis, also known as the dysmorphic form, varies in its onset and severity. Affected patients have a Hurler-like phenotype in addition to features of type I sialidosis. Type II sialidosis may present as a severe congenital form in the neonatal period, with a life span of a few months, or as a stillborn with hydrops fetalis. Patients with the infantile form present between birth and 12 months of age with hepatosplenomegaly and renal involvement. Those with the juvenile form present between ages 2 and 20 years with a milder phenotype; this form of the disorder is most common in Japan.

Sialolipidosis: Patients with sialolipidosis present within the first 2 months of life with hypotonia and progressive neurological dysfunction. Corneal clouding is present; other Hurler-like features are not seen. Most patients die during childhood; some may live to be young adults. This disorder was previously classified as mucolipidosis type IV. Lysosomal inclusions are found in tissues throughout the body; an abnormal ganglioside content may be noted in cultured skin fibroblasts from affected patients. The basic defect, which is unknown, may be associated with deficient activity of an α-neuraminidase specific for GM_3 and GD_2 gangliosides.

Galactosialidosis: Galactosialidosis results from lack of a protective protein that forms a complex with both α-neuraminidase and β-galactosidase. Affected patients have clinical features similar to those of type II sialidosis.

Aspartylglucosaminuria

Aspartylglucosaminuria is an autosomal recessive disorder, most common in persons from Finland, that results from deficient activity of aspartylglucosaminidase. Patients present between 1 and 5 years of age with gradual coarsening of facial features, sagging skin, and psychomotor deterioration. Lenticular opacities, acne, and photosensitivity are common. Joint laxity, macroglossia, short stature, hypotonia, and spasticity have occasionally been noted. Radio-

graphs show mild dysostosis multiplex. Most patients live well into their adult years.

DISORDERS OF LYSOSOMAL ENZYME TRANSPORT (MUCOLIPIDOSES)

The mucolipidoses, autosomal recessive disorders associated with deficient activity of multiple acid hydrolases, have clinical features of both the mucopolysaccharidoses and sphingolipidoses. Prior to our current understanding of the biochemistry involved, four types of the disorder existed. Types I and IV, now known to be associated with deficient activity of α-neuraminidase, are presently classified with the glycoproteinoses. Types II and III, which still retain the name mucolipidoses, are associated with faulty synthesis of the mannose-6-phosphate recognition marker needed for transport of the acid hydrolases into lysosomes. During post-translational processing, mannose-rich oligosaccharide side chains are attached to the lysosomal acid hydrolases. N-acetylglucosamine-1-phosphotransferase acts to attach N-acetylglucosamine-1-phosphate groups to the 6-hydroxyl position of the mannose residues. The N-acetylglucosamine is then removed by the action of a phosphodiesterase to expose mannosyl–6-phosphate, which is the signal for Golgi receptor sites that transport the hydrolases to their intralysosomal location. If the mannosyl–6-phosphate marker is not present, the hydrolases leave the cell and become elevated in extracellular fluids. Most patients with mucolipidoses types II and III have deficient activity of N-acetylglucosamine-1-phosphotransferase. Others have been found to have defective recognition function or reduced activity of phosphodiesterase. In affected patients, the activity of the lysosomal hydrolases in extracellular fluids, eg, plasma and serum, is markedly increased (often to 10–20 times normal), whereas the activity of the hydrolases in cells, eg, cultured skin fibroblasts, is markedly reduced. The specific activities when measured in leukocytes may be normal or decreased. In affected patients, the activities of aryl sulfatase A, β-galactosidase, β-hexosaminidase, and α-L–iduronidase may be measured in this manner to show the defect. The activities of acid phosphatase and β-glucosidase are not affected. Deficient activity of the phosphotransferase may also be shown in cultured skin fibroblasts from affected patients. Prenatal diagnosis is available for the mucolipidoses, but carrier detection is not accurate. Table 23–4 lists characteristics of the mucolipidoses.

Mucolipidosis Type II

Mucolipidosis type II presents shortly after birth with clinical features similar to those seen with Hurler syndrome and GM_1 gangliosidosis. Severe dysostosis is present from birth; gingival hypertrophy is prominent. Most affected patients die prior to 5

Table 23–4. Other lysosomal disorders.

Type	Lysosomal Enzyme or Biochemical Defect	Clinical Sample	Inheritance
Lysosomal enzyme transport defects			
Mucolipidosis type II	Activity of multiple enzymes elevated in S or P and reduced in WBC or SF	S or P and WBC or SF	AR
Mucolipidosis type III			AR
Lysosomal membrane transport defects			
Infantile free sialic acid storage	Free sialic acid	WBC	AR
Salla disease	Free sialic acid	WBC	AR
Cystinosis	Free cystine	WBC	AR
Other lysosomal disorders			
Pompe disease	α-1,4-Glucosidase	WBC, SF	AR
Wolman disease	Acid lipase	WBC	AR
Cholesteryl ester storage disease	Acid lipase	WBC	AR

AR = autosomal recessive, P = plasma, S = serum, SF = cultured skin fibroblasts, WBC = leukocytes.

years of age (Figure 23–11). The disorder is also known as "I"-cell disease because of the numerous, dense inclusions that are noted with phase-contrast microscopy in cultured skin fibroblasts from patients.

Mucolipidosis Type III

Mucolipidosis type III, or pseudo-Hurler polydystrophy, is a milder variant that presents between 4 and 5 years of age with mild psychomotor delay, joint stiffness, and clinical features similar to those seen with the intermediate form of Maroteaux-Lamy syndrome (MPS type VI). Affected patients may live to be young adults. Carpal tunnel syndrome and cardiac valvular involvement are common; atlantoaxial subluxation may occur.

LYSOSOMAL MEMBRANE TRANSPORT DEFECTS

Carrier-mediated transport systems are needed for the transport of small molecules from the lysosomal space into the cytosol. Defective transport of sialic acid and cystine results in lysosomal accumulation of these molecules, and the disorders known as free sialic acid storage disease and cystinosis, respectively (Table 23–4.)

Free Sialic Acid Storage Disorders

The free sialic acid storage disorders are associated with increased lysosomal levels of free sialic acid, or N-acetylneuraminic acid.

Infantile Free Sialic Acid Storage Disease: In the more severe infantile free sialic acid storage disease, generalized storage of sialic acid occurs. Af-

fected patients present within the first 2 months of life with coarse facies, hepatosplenomegaly, psychomotor retardation, hypopigmentation, anemia, ascites, and diarrhea. Dysostosis multiplex may be present on radiographs. Most affected patients do not live past the first few years of life.

Salla Disease: The milder form of the disorder, Salla disease, is most common in persons from Finland. Affected patients present between 3 and 12 months of age with coarse facies, hypotonia, ataxia, and psychomotor retardation. A slowly progressive central nervous system involvement with dysarthria, dystonia, and seizures occurs; many patients live into adult life.

Intermediate forms of the disorder have also been reported. All forms of the disorder are inherited as autosomal recessive traits. Elevated levels of sialic acid may be shown in leukocytes and cultured skin fibroblasts.

Cystinosis

Cystinosis is an autosomal recessive disorder characterized by the lysosomal accumulation of free cystine. Patients with the **infantile nephropathic type,** the most common form, present between 3 and 18 months of age with renal Fanconi syndrome, poor linear growth, fair complexion and light hair, hypohidrosis, and hypothyroidism. These patients have cystine deposition in the corneas, which may be evident with slit-lamp examination. Photosensitivity and a peripheral pigmentary retinopathy may also occur. Cystine crystals may also be noted in renal interstitial tissues, bone marrow, lymph nodes, and conjunctiva by electron microscopy. Untreated, the disorder leads to renal failure by age 10 years. Patients who un-

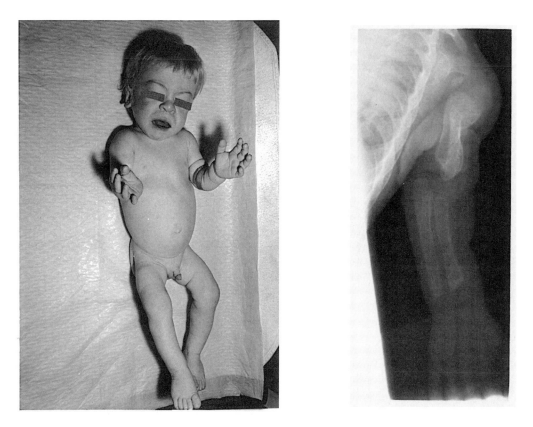

Figure 23–11. (A). Mucolipidosis II, I-cell disease. **(B)** Radiogram in Mucolipidosis II. Note the severe dysostosis multiplex and the "bone within bone" appearance. (Reproduced, with permission from Oski FA et al (editors), *Principles and Practice of Pediatrics,* 2nd ed, JB Lippincott, 1994.)

dergo renal transplantation have continued cystine deposition in extrarenal tissues and develop loss of vision, corneal erosion, diabetes mellitus, and neurological involvement as teenagers or adults. Treatment with cysteamine in enteral and eye drop forms may slow the progression of the disorder. **Intermediate, adolescent, and adult forms** of the disorder are also known. Elevated cystine levels may be shown in leukocytes or cultured skin fibroblasts.

OTHER DISORDERS OF LYSOSOMES

Pompe Disease

Pompe disease, or glycogenosis type II, is an autosomal recessive disorder associated with deficient activity of lysosomal acid α-1,4-glucosidase (acid maltase) and the lysosomal accumulation of glycogen in most tissues throughout the body. Patients with the **infantile form,** also known as generalized glycogenosis, present shortly after birth with a rapidly progressing generalized myopathy and hypertrophic cardiomyopathy. Hepatomegaly and macroglossia may be present. Biochemical abnormalities, eg, hypoglycemia, that are associated with cytosolic defects

in glycogen metabolism, do not occur. Most affected infants do not live past 1 year of age. Patients with **juvenile and adult forms** of Pompe disease usually present with myopathies at later ages; cardiac involvement is variable (Table 23–4).

Lysosomal Acid Lipase Deficiency

Deficient activity of lysosomal acid lipase results in the lysosomal accumulation of cholesteryl esters and triglycerides.

Wolman Disease: In the more severe form of the disorder, Wolman disease, affected infants present in the first few weeks of life with vomiting, diarrhea, steatorrhea, abdominal distention, hepatosplenomegaly, and calcification of the adrenal glands. Progressive lysosomal storage occurs throughout the body; there is severe failure to thrive. Most affected patients do not live past 6 months of age. Peripheral lymphocytes may be vacuolated; bone marrow examination may show foam cells and "sea-blue histiocytes." Plasma cholesterol and triglyceride levels are usually normal. Liver function tests are abnormal; portal fibrosis may occur.

Cholesteryl Ester Storage Disease: The milder form of the disorder, cholesteryl ester storage disease, is characterized by hepatomegaly that may not appear until adult life. Some affected patients also have splenomegaly, hepatic fibrosis, micronodular cirrhosis, esophageal varices, and intestinal involve-

ment. Adrenal calcification does not occur. Plasma cholesterol is elevated; atherosclerosis may develop (Table 23–4).

REFERENCES AND SUGGESTED READING FOR SECTION III: INBORN ERRORS OF METABOLISM

Berry GT et al: Branched-chain amino acid-free parenteral nutrition in the treatment of acute metabolic decompensation in patients with maple syrup urine disease. New Eng J Med 1991;**324**:175.

Bremer HF, Duran M, Kamerling JP, Przrembel H, Wadman SK. *Disturbances of Amino Acid Metabolism: Clinical Chemistry and Diagnosis.* Urban and Schwarzenberg, 1981.

Breningstall GN. Approach to diagnosis of oxidative metabolism disorders. Pediatric Neurology 1993;**9**:81.

Brown GK. Pyruvate dehydrogenase E1α deficiency. J Inher Metab Dis 1992;**15**:625.

Brown FR, Voight R, Singh A, Singh I. Perxoisomal disorders. Neurodevelopmental and biochemical aspects. Amer J Dis Child 1993;**147**:627.

Burton BK. Inborn errors of metabolism: the clinical diagnosis in early infancy. Pediatrics 1987;**70**:359.

Chelly J, Monaco AP. Cloning the Wilson disease gene. Nature Genetics 1993;**5**:317.

Clarke, LA. Mitochondrial disorders in pediatrics: clinical, biochemical, and genetic implications. Pediatric Clinics of North America 1992; **39**:319.

Desnick RJ (editor). *Treatment of Genetic Diseases.* Churchill Livingstone, 1991.

DeVivo DC. The expanding clinical spectrum of mitochondrial diseases. Brain and Development 1993 **15**:1.

DeVivo DC, DiMauro S. Mitochondrial diseases. Pages 1335–1356 in: *Pediatric Neurology,* 2nd ed, Swaiman KF (editor) Mosby, 1994.

Edwards CQ, Kushner JP. Screening for hemochromatosis. New Eng J Med 1993;**328**:1616.

Emery AEH, Rimoin DL (editors). *Principles and practice of medical genetics.* Churchill Livingstone, 1990.

Geet CV, Jaeken J. A unique pattern of coagulation abnormalities in carbohydrate-deficient glycoprotein syndrome. Pediatric Research 1993 **33**:540.

Hagberg BA, Blennow G, Kristiansson B, Stibler H. Carbohydrate-deficient glycoprotein syndromes: peculiar groups of new disorders. Pedatric Neurology 1993;**9**:255.

Hale, DE, Bennett MJ. (1992) Fatty acid oxidation disorders: a new class of metabolic diseases. J Pediatr 1993; **121**:1.

Holton JB (editor). *The inherited metabolic diseases.* Churchill Livingstone, 1987.

Hommes FA (editor). *Techniques in Diagnostic Human Biochemical Genetics.* Wiley-Liss, 1991.

Lindstedt S et al. Treatment of hereditary tyrosinaemia type

I by inhibition of 4-hydroxyphenylpyruvate dioxygenase. Lancet 1992;**340**:813–817.

Moser HW. Peroxisomal diseases. *Advances in Human Genetics* 1993;**21**:1.

Nyhan WL, Sakati ND. *Diagnostic Recognition of Genetic Disease.* Lea and Febiger, 1987.

Parini R et al. Nasogastric drip feeding as the only treatment of neonatal maple syrup urine disease. Pediatr 1993;**92**:280.

Peinemann F, Danner DJ. Maple syrup urine disease 1954 to 1993. J Inher Metab Dis 1994;**17**:3.

Robinson BH. Lacticacidemia. *Advances in Human Genetics* 1989;**18**:151.

Schaub J, VanHoof F, Vis HL. Inborn errors of metabolism. Vol 24, *Nestle Nutrition Workshop Series.* Raven Press, 1991.

Scriver CR, Beaudet AL, Sly WS, Valle D (editors). *The Metabolic Basis of Inherited Disease,* 6th ed, McGraw-Hill, 1989.

Seashore MR: Neonatal screening for inborn errors of metabolism: Update. Seminars in Perinatology 1990; **14**:431.

Seashore MR, Rinaldo P. Metabolic disease of the neonate and young infant. Seminars in Perinatology 1993;**17**:318.

Shapira E, Blitzer MG, Miller JB, Affrick DK. *Biochemical Genetics: A Laboratory Manual.* Oxford University Press, 1989.

Shoffner JM, Wallace DC. Oxidative phosphorylation diseases. Advances in Human Genetics 1990;**19**:267.

Tint GS et al. Defective cholesterol biosynthesis associated with the Smith-Lemli-Opitz syndrome. New Eng J Med 1994;**330**:107.

Tulinius MH et al. Mitochondrial encephalomyopathies in childhood. I. Biochemical and morphologic investigations. J Pediatr 1991;**119**:242.

Tulinius MH, et al. Mitochondrial encephalomyopathies in childhood II. Clinical manifestations and syndromes. J Pediatr **119**:251.

Waber L. Inborn errors of metabolism. Pediatric Annals 1990;**19**: 105.

Wappner RS. Biochemical diagnosis of genetic diseases. Pediatric Annals 1993;**22**:282.

Wappner RS, Brandt IK. Inborn errors of metabolism. In: Principles and Practice of Pediatrics, 2nd ed, Oski FA et al (editors), JB Lippincott, 1994.

Ward JC. Inborn errors of metabolism of acute onset in infancy. Pediatr Rev 1990;**11**:205.

SECTION IV.
Other Clinical Issues in Genetics & Primary Care

Special Senses & Skin

24

This chapter will review some well-characterized single gene disorders in which the principal manifestations are confined to the special senses or to the skin. Typically, such syndromes are a consideration if the patient demonstrates features in addition to the findings in the special senses or the skin. Table 24–1 lists some inherited disorders of vision.

INHERITED DISEASES OF VISION

Retinal Disease

Retinitis Pigmentosa (RP): Retinitis pigmentosa (RP) is a feature of a variety of syndromes and contiguous gene deletions. As a single gene disorder, RP affects about 1 in 4000 people in the United States and thus represents a common cause of blindness. Night blindness is prominent at the onset of RP; ultimately affected individuals lose central vision. Considerable clinical heterogeneity both within and between families makes diagnosis and prognosis a challenge. The physical findings, which include abnormal retinal vessels and pigmentary changes in the retina, and the electroretinogram, which is usually abnormal, do not always distinguish among the three Mendelian patterns of inheritance that RP manifests. Molecular analysis is beginning to clarify the mutations responsible for RP and to provide an effective tool for diagnosis and genetic counseling (Table 24–2).

Mutations in three different genes are associated with RP. These genes encode proteins that are important for vision: rhodopsin, peripherin-RDS, and a cyclic GMP-dependent cation channel protein in rod cells. Rhodopsin, a transmembrane photoreceptor protein that functions in the rod cell, undergoes a change in conformation in response to light, thus activating another protein, transducin, which converts the light energy to a signal sent to the brain. Peripherin-RDS is a protein that is not light-sensitive. It is essential for the stability of the photoreceptor outer segment discs. cGMP-dependent cation channel protein in rod cells is also important for visual function. Mutations and deletions in rhodopsin and mutations in peripherin-RDS may account for as many as one-third of autosomal dominant cases of RP.

The molecular analyses are beginning to establish genotype-phenotype correlations between the mutations and the RP phenotype and to clarify mode of inheritance in some families. Evidence is accumulating that one form of RP is not monogenic but results when the individual is a double heterozygote for mutations at two different loci, ROM1 (the gene for another photoreceptor protein) and peripherin-RDS.

Macular Disease

The inherited forms of macular disease usually have their onset in childhood. Mutations in peripherin/RDS have been described.

Table 24–1. Some inherited disorders of vision.

Disorder	Inheritance	Map Location
Macular degeneration (early onset) (MIM 153700)	AD	11q13
Stickler syndrome (arthro-ophthalmopathy) (MIM 108300)	AD	Not mapped
Hereditary corneal dystrophy (MIM 122000)	AD	Not mapped
X-linked micro-ophthalmia (Lenz syndrome)	XL	Not mapped
Retinal cone degeneration (MIM 180020)	AD	6q25–q26

Table 24–2. Inherited retinitis pigmentosa (RP).

Disorder	Inheritance	Map Location	Gene Defect
RP1 (MIM 180100)	AD	8p11–q21	Not mapped
RP2 (MIM 312600)	XL	Xp11.3	Not mapped
RP3 (MIM 312610)	XL	Xp21.1	Not mapped
RP4 (MIM 180380)	AD	3q21–q24	Rhodopsin
RP5 (MIM 180102)	AD	Not mapped	Not mapped
RP6 (MIM 312612)	XL	Xp21.3–p21.2	Not mapped
RP7 (MIM 179605)	AD	6p21.1–cen	Peripherin, photoreceptor
RP8 (MIM 180103)	AD	Not mapped	Not mapped
AD RP (MIM 180073)	AD	17	Phosphodiesterase, cyclic GMP
AD RP (MIM 180072)	AD	4p16.3	Retinal rod photoreceptor cGMP phosphodiesterase, β-subunit
AD RP (MIM 180071)	AD	5q31.2–q34	Retinal rod photoreceptor cGMP phosphodiesterase, α-subunit

Autosomal Dominant Stationary Night Blindness: Both autosomal dominant (MIM 163500) and X-linked recessive (MIM 310500) stationary night blindness exist. These disorders are associated with early onset night blindness that does not progress. Rod dysfunction is the basis of the disorder. Myopia may also be a clinical feature, particularly in the X-linked form. The genetic defects are not known. The X-linked form maps to Xp11.3.

Usher Syndrome: Usher syndrome is characterized by autosomal recessive retinitis pigmentosa associated with deafness. At least three different loci are known (Table 24–3).

Familial Exudative Vitreoretinopathy (MIM 133780): The clinical characteristics of familial exudative vitreoretinopathy include abnormal retinal vascularization, vitreous exudates, and retinal detachment that ultimately lead to blindness. Both autosomal dominant (MIM 133780) and X-linked recessive (MIM 305390) inheritance are recognized. The genes have not been mapped and the molecular abnormalities are unknown.

Retinoschisis: Progressive abnormalities of the retina and retinal vasculature lead to blindness in retinoschisis. X-linked inheritance has been established, and linkage markers at Xq22.1–p22.2 may be useful for diagnosis and genetic counseling. The molecular pathology is not known.

Table 24–3. Inherited forms Usher syndrome.

Autosomal Recessive Usher Syndrome	Map Location
Usher syndrome-1A (MIM 276900)	14q32
Usher syndrome-1B (MIM 276903)	11q13.5
Usher syndrome-2 (MIM 276901)	1q32

Ocular Albinism: Isolated ocular albinism is associated with retinal depigmentation, foveal hypoplasia, and translucent irises. At least two X-linked forms are known, OA1 and OA2. Both map to the short arm of the X-chromosome.

Color Blindness: Color-blindness is an X-linked trait that affects 8% of Caucasian males; this abnormality in color vision results from mutations in the genes for red, green, and blue photopigment proteins. The genes for these proteins have been cloned. They exist in a tandem array on the X-chromosome long arm. Relatively frequent crossovers between these genes result in gene rearrangements, some of which lead to genetic variation in color perception. Deletions in the red and green pigment genes are also associated with abnormal color vision.

Anterior Chamber

Rieger Eye Malformation: Rieger eye malformation comprises iris hypoplasia, posterior embryotoxon, and glaucoma. This syndrome is often associated with abnormal teeth and midfacial hypoplasia; other malformations such as empty pituitary sella may also occur. The condition is inherited in an autosomal dominant fashion in some families. Considerable genetic heterogeneity exists, and one form is linked to markers on 4q. Deletions in 4q23–q26 are also associated with the Rieger malformation.

Cataract: X-linked congenital cataract is linked to markers at Xp21.1–p22.3. The clinical phenotype of this disorder also includes microphthalmia and microcornea. Autosomal dominant and autosomal recessive inheritance of cataracts occur.

Aniridia: Autosomal dominant aniridia is distinct from aniridia associated with Wilms tumor and with deletions and mutations on chromosome 11. The features of this rare condition include absence of the iris, a high incidence of glaucoma, and cataracts. The

Table 24–4. Examples of syndromic deafness and their genetic map locations.

Syndrome	Map Location
Usher syndrome (Types 1A, 1B, 2)	11q13.5, 1q32, 14q32
Waardenburg syndrome	2q35–q37
Alport syndrome	Xq21–q22
Albinism-deafness	Xq26.3–q27
Norrie syndrome	Xp11.3–p11.4

Table 24–5. Inherited non-syndromic deafness.

Disorder	Inheritance
Congenital sensorineural deafness	XLR, AR, AD
Early-onset sensorineural deafness	XLR
Progressive mixed deafness with gusher	XLR (Xq13–q21.1)
Progressive high-tone neural deafness	AD
Progressive low-tone deafness	AD

preservation of visual acuity distinguishes the several different variants of this disorder.

Inherited Diseases of Hearing

There are more than 200 kinds of inherited deafness. Many of these are part of recognized syndromes that involve other systems as well. These will not be reviewed here, but a few are listed in Table 24–4. Whenever the physician identifies hearing loss, a careful search for other clinical findings such as diabetes, congenital heart disease, and gonadal dysgenesis will help to identify a syndrome with associated deafness. The evaluation should include, besides the careful hearing evaluation, assessment of vision, examination for craniofacial anomalies and other dysmorphic features, assessment of neurologic and intellectual function, and consideration of inborn errors of metabolism associated with deafness. All modes of inheritance have been established for deafness. Known loci for autosomal dominant non-syndromic deafness are on 1p, 5, and 13q; loci for X-linked non-syndromic deafness exist on Xq12 and Xq21.1. Possible sites of gene action include inner ear development, cochlear structure, and eighth nerve structure. Table 24–5 lists some known non-syndromic inherited forms of deafness.

Inherited Disorders of Smell

Kallmann Syndrome (MIM 308700): Kallmann syndrome is an X-linked disorder characterized by hypogonadotropic hypogonadism and anosmia. Hemizygous males express the full phenotype, while heterozygous females may demonstrate only anosmia.

The gene maps to Xp22.3; the protein is probably a cell adhesion molecule.

Skin

Albinism: Albinism is a condition characterized by little or no biosynthesis of melanin. Affected persons have depigmented skin and hair. The retina is also affected; this results in poor visual acuity, sensitivity to light, and nystagmus. There are several distinct genetic forms of albinism. Table 24–6 lists the different forms along with their location on the genome map and the recognized genetic defects. In the tyrosinase-negative form, mutations in the gene for tyrosinase result in loss of activity of tyrosinase and thus in lack of biosynthesis of melanin.

Vitiligo: Vitiligo is characterized by localized loss of pigment in the skin. Skin is normally pigmented early in life and over time loses this pigmentation. The disorder displays familial aggregation but not Mendelian inheritance patterns. Mutations at multiple loci may explain this observation.

Ectodermal Dysplasia: Anhidrotic ectodermal dysplasia (MIM 305100) is an X-linked disorder characterized by the presence of abnormal sweat glands, conical teeth, and decreased or fragile hair (Table 24–7). Affected children may develop hyperthermia because of the inability to sweat. The gene maps to Xq12–q13.1. The phenotype is fully expressed in males; female gene carriers usually have partial expression with minimal findings or no clear phenotypic abnormalities.

Table 24–6. Oculo-cutaneous albinism.

Disorder	Map Location	Defect
Oculocutaneous albinism IA (tyrosinase-negative) (MIM 203100)	11q14–q21	Tyrosinase
Oculocutaneous albinism II (tyrosinase-positive) (MIM 203200)	15q11.2–q12	PED (protein may be tyrosine transporter)

Table 24–7. Inherited skin disorders.

Disorder	Molecular Abnormality	Inheritance	Map Location
X-linked icthyosis	Steroid sulfatase deficiency	XLR	X
Anhydrotic ectodermal dysplasia (MIM 305100)	Unknown	XLR	Xq12–q13.1
Focal dermal hypoplasia (lethal in males) (MIM 305600)	Unknown	XLD	Xp22.31
Cutis laxa	Abnormal collagen and elastin fibers	XLR, AD, AR	X, autosomal locations unknown

REFERENCES AND SUGGESTED READING

Arnos KS: Hereditary hearing loss. N Engl J Med 1994; **331**:469.

Beighton P et al: Hearing impairment and pigmentary disturbance. Ann NY Acad Sci 1991;**630**:152.

Blethen SL, Taysi K: Autosomal dominant aniridia in association with craniopharyngioma. Am J Dis Child 1981;**7**:575.

Couke P et al: Linkage of autosomal dominant hearing loss to the short arm of chromosome 1 in two families. N Engl J Med 1994;**331**:425.

Drummond-Borg M, Deeb SS, Motulsky AG: Molecular patterns of X chromosome-linked color vision genes among 134 men of European ancestry. Proc Soc Natl Acad Sci USA 1989;**86**:983.

Dryja TP et al: Mutations within the rhodopsin gene in patients with autosomal dominant retinitis pigmentosa. N Engl J Med 1990;**323**:1302.

Gal A et al: Heterozygous missense mutation in the rod cGMP phosphodiesterase β-subunit gene in autosomal dominant stationary night blindness. Nature Genetics 1994;**7**:376.

Gilgenkrantz S et al: Hypohidrotic ectodermal dysplasia. Hum Genet 1989;**81**:120.

Gorski JL: Father-to-daughter transmission of focal dermal hypoplasia associated with nonrandom X-inactivation. Am J Med Genet 1991;**40**:332.

Humphries P, Kenna P, Farrar GJ: On the molecular genetics of retinitis pigmentosa. Science 1992;**256**:804.

Kajiwara K, Berson EL, Dryja TP: Digenic retinitis pigmentosa due to mutations at the unlinked peripherin/RDS and ROM1 loci. Science 1994;**264**:1604.

Kleinmann RE et al: Primary empty sella and Rieger's anomaly of the anterior chamber of the eye: A familial syndrome. N Engl J Med 1981;**304**:90.

Lee ST et al: Mutations of the P gene in oculocutaneous albinism, ocular albinism, and Prader-Willi syndrome plus albinism. N Engl J Med 1994;**330**:529.

Legius E et al: Genetic heterogeneity in Rieger eye malformation. J Med Genet 1994;**31**:340.

Nath SK, Majumder PP, Nordlund JJ: Genetic epidemiology of vitiligo: Multilocus recessivity cross-validated. Am J Hum Genet 1994;**55**:981.

Nathans J et al: Molecular genetics of human blue cone monochromacy. Science 1989;**245**:831.

Nathans J, Thomas D, Hogness DS: Molecular genetics of human color vision: the genes encoding blue, green, and red pigments. Science 1986;**232**:193.

Pearce WG, Kerr CB: Inherited variation in Rieger's malformation. Br J Ophthal 1965;**49**:530.

Reardon W: Genetic deafness. J Med Genet 1992;**29**:521.

Shapiro L, Weiss R: X-linked ichthyosis due to steroid-sulphatase deficiency. Lancet 1978;**i**:70.

Shapiro L et al: Enzymatic basis of typical X-linked ichthyosis. Lancet 1978;**i**:756.

Shastry BS: Recent developments in certain X-linked genetic eye disorders. Biochim Biophys Acta 1993;**1182**:119.

Shastry BS: Retinitis pigmentosa and related disorders: Phenotypes of rhodopsin and peripherin/RDS mutations. Am J Med Genet 1994;**52**:467.

Spillmann T: Genetic disease of hearing. Current Opinion in Neurology 1994;**7**:81.

Spritz RA et al: Detection of mutations in the tyrosinase gene in a patient with type IA oculocutaneous albinism. N Engl J Med 1990;**322**:1724.

Steele FR: Shedding light on inherited blindness: The genetics of retinitis pigmentosa: J NIH Research 1994; **6**:58.

Vollrath D, Nathans J, Davis RW: Tandem array of human visual pigment genes at Xq28. Science 1988;**240**:1669.

Wells J et al: Mutations in the human retinal degeneration slow (RDS) gene can cause either retinitis pigmentosa or macular dystrophy. Nature Genetics 1993;**3**:213.

Zonana J et al: Detection of de novo mutations and analysis of their origin in families with X linked hypohidrotic ectodermal dysplasia. J Med Genet 1994;**31**:287.

Congenital Malformations

25

Embryonic and Fetal Development

During embryonic and fetal life, cellular growth, migration, and differentiation result in a highly organized and sequential formation of complex structures and organ systems throughout the body. An **inductive interaction** of tissues leads to selective types of development at specified sites in the body. The means by which various tissues interact appears to be through "messengers" secreted by inducer cells or by direct physical contact of the inducer and responder cells or tissues. Normal differentiation requires that the specific inductive interaction, or hormonal influence, occur at a designated time in development. Inductive and responder cells and tissues must also be in their normal locations for proper development to occur.

The molecular and hormonal basis for induction and differentiation is complex and just starting to be understood. Much of the control of cellular differentiation appears to be at the level of mRNA processing, which controls gene expression at specific sites and times in developing tissues. Specific growth factors or signaling peptides [eg, transforming growth factor (TGF), nerve growth factor (NGF), fibroblast growth factor (FGF), insulin-like growth hormone (IGF), and platelet-derived growth factor (PDGF)], the hormones of the steroid-thyroxine-retinoic acid "super family," and corresponding binding proteins and nuclear receptors for the factors and hormones have been shown to influence fetal development. Isoforms of the compounds and receptors have differing actions during morphogenesis that are often tissue specific and may occur only in certain localized areas. For example, TGFα, an isoform of TGF, is an embryonic epidermal (epithelial) growth factor, whereas TGFβ is associated with the induction and differentiation of mesodermal cells. Various types of retinoic acid receptors (RARs) also differ in their function during development. RARβ appears to be involved with regulating programmed cell death (eg, loss of tissue between the digits for formation of the fingers) while, RARγ is associated with cartilage development. In addition, homeotic genes (composed of highly conserved common sequences of DNA known as "homeoboxes") and other related genes, eg, pax or "paired box" genes, transcribe proteins which regulate gene expression in specific areas, or fields, of the developing embryo.

The **first week** after fertilization is characterized by cell division and implantation. Approximately one-third to one-half of fertilized zygotes never implant. Of those that do implant, only 58% survive to the end of the second week. Major chromosomal abnormalities are found in approximately one-half of spontaneous early miscarriages.

The term **embryo** is used from the beginning of the second week to the end of the eighth week after fertilization. During this time there is formation of three primitive cell layers, consisting of the ectoderm, endoderm, and mesoderm, which differentiate by the end of the eighth week into the beginnings of all the major organ systems of the body. It is during this embryonic period of morphogenesis and organogenesis that most birth defects occur.

The term **fetus** is used from the ninth week of development to birth. During this fetal period there is continued growth and differentiation of tissues and organs. The brain, teeth, heart, abdominal wall, and external genitalia complete their development. Although major structural defects are less likely to occur during the fetal period, environmental factors such as mechanical forces, vascular disruptions, drugs, toxins, and infectious agents may disturb normal development.

Defects in morphogenesis may occur from lack of development of an organ or tissue (aplasia, hypoplasia), incomplete fusion or separation of structures (cleft palate), incomplete septation or canalization (duodenal atresia), persistence of early forms no longer needed (Meckel diverticulum), or improper migration or localization of cells, tissues, or organs (ectopic thyroid, undescended testes).

Table 25–1 lists examples of common major congenital anomalies and their corresponding defects in embryonic development. The most common major congenital anomalies are single, isolated defects that are associated with a multifactorial pattern of inheritance.

Congenital Malformations, Deformations, and Disruptions

Congenital malformations, deformations, and disruptions result from abnormal development of the embryo and fetus during early intrauterine life. Collectively they are responsible for up to 50% of hospi-

Table 25–1. Major congenital malformations and related defects in morphogenesis.[1]

System	Malformation	Defect in Morphogenesis	Time of Defect	Incidence	MIM Number
CNS	Anencephaly	Closure of anterior neural tube	26 days	1–2 per 1000	206500
	Meningomyelocele	Closure of posterior neural tube	28 days	1–2 per 1000	182940
	Holoprosencephaly	Development of prechordal mesoderm	23 days	1 in 16,000	157170, 236100
Face	Cleft lip	Closure of lip	36 days	1 in 1000	119530
	Cleft palate	Fusion of maxillary palatal shelves	10 weeks	1 in 2500	119540
Endocrine	Agenesis of thyroid	Development of thyroid gland	24 days	1 in 4000	218700
Heart	Ventricular septal defect	Closure of ventricular septum	6 weeks	1 in 800	None
	Patent ductus arteriosus	Closure of ductus arteriosus	9–10 months	1 in 1200	169100
	Transposition of great vessels	Directional development of the aorticopulmonary septum	34 days	1 in 3500	None
GI	TEF with esophageal atresia	Division of foregut into trachea and esophagus	30 days	1 in 3000	189960
	Malrotation of intestines	Rotation of intestine so that cecum lies to right	10 weeks	1 in 500	None
	Omphalocele	Return of midgut from yolk sac to abdomen	10 weeks	1 in 5000	164750, 310980
	Meckel diverticulum	Obliteration of vitelline duct	10 weeks	1 in 25–33	155140
	Diaphragmatic hernia	Closure of pleuroperitoneal canal	6 weeks	1 in 2000	222400
	Duodenal atresia	Recanalization of duodenum	8 weeks	1 in 10,000	223400
	Imperforate anus	Perforation of anal membrane	8 weeks	1 in 5000	207500
	Aganglionic megacolon	Migration of neural crest cells into wall of colon	5–7 weeks	1 in 5000	249200
	Biliary atresia	Canalization of bile ducts	After 5 weeks	1 in 20,000	210500
GU	Hypospadias	Fusion of urethral folds	12 weeks	1 in 300	146450, 241750
	Cryptorchidism	Descent of testicle into scrotum	7–9 months	1 in 33	219050
	Bicornuate uterus	Fusion of lower portion of Mullerian ducts	10 weeks	1 in 1000	192000
	Exstrophy of bladder	Migration of lower midline abdominal mesenchyme	30 days	1 in 30,000	None
	Bilateral renal agenesis	Development of metanephroi	5 weeks	1 in 3300	191830
Limbs	Radial aplasia	Genesis of radial bone	38 days	1 in 33,000	312190
	Syndactyly	Separation of digital rays	6 weeks	1 in 6000	185900–186300

[1] CNS = central nervous system, GI = gastrointestinal, GU = genitourinary, TEF = tracheoesophageal fistula. Adapted from Jones KL: *Smith's Recognizable Patterns of Human Malformation*, 4th ed, WB Saunders, 1988.

tal admissions, 10% of deaths during the perinatal period, and 40% of deaths within the first year of life. Congenital malformations, deformations, and disruptions result from various etiologies. Six to fifteen percent will be associated with chromosomal abnormalities (eg, Down syndrome), 2–10% will be due to single gene defects (eg, achondroplasia), 7–10% will be associated with environmental factors (eg, viral infections), 20–25% will be of multifactorial etiology, and the remaining 40–60% will be of unknown causes.

Malformations

Congenital malformations, by definition, are birth defects that result from single, localized abnormalities in morphogenesis or organogenesis, which are intrinsic to the embryo or fetus. **Major malformations** are defined as those which interfere with normal function and require medical attention. Major malformations occur in 3% of newborns. During the first 5 years of life an additional 2–3% of infants and children will be noted to have a major malformation which was not present or noted at birth. Approximately 0.7% of patients with major malformations will have multiple malformations. In contrast, **minor malformations** are not associated with serious health problems and are often only of cosmetic significance. Single minor malformations are noted in 14% of newborns, eg, ear tags or syndactyly of the second and third toes. The presence of two or more multiple minor malformations, however, should alert the clinician to the possibility of other major congenital malformations. Patterns of minor malformations may be important in establishing the diagnosis of a syndrome. They may also be helpful in establishing the time during gestation when an interference with development occurred. Table 25–2 list examples of common minor malformations.

Deformations

In contrast to malformations, which are intrinsic to the embryo or fetus, deformations and disruptions are usually associated with extrinsic factors which interfere with otherwise normal development. **Deformations** result from abnormal mechanical forces that change the form, shape, or position of a part of the body. Deformations are noted in 2% of newborns and most often occur as a result of intrauterine constraint or decreased fetal movement during the last trimester of gestation. They may be associated with decreased intrauterine size, oligohydramnios, or abnormal fetal positioning and presentation. Affected neonates may be noted to have compression and distortion of facial structures, abnormal positioning of the extremities and head, generalized or localized decreased joint mobility, joint dislocations, nerve palsies, torticollis, or craniostenosis. For example, compression of the fetal jaw on a shoulder may result in micrognathia.

Table 25–2. Examples of minor malformations.

Affected Area	Minor Malformations
Head	Flat or prominent occipital area Open metopic suture Absent or triple hair whorl at vertex
Ears	Bifid or notched ear lobe Cup-shaped ears Thickened or folded helix
Face	Prominent bridge or nose Long nasal septum Epicanthal folds Upward or downward slanting palpebral fissures Short palpebral fissures Short or long philtrum Relatively large or small mouth Relatively large or small jaw
Mouth	Bifid or long uvula Relatively large or small tongue
Limbs	Single transverse palmar crease Tapered fingers Overlapping fingers Syndactyly of second and third toes Increased space between toes Curving of fifth fingers Hypoplastic or hyperconvex nails
Skin	Dimples on sacrum or shoulders Skin tags Superficial hemangiomas Nevi
Other	Extra nipples Single umbilical artery Umbilical hernia Diastasis recti

Thoracic compression may result in pulmonary hypoplasia. Although usually extrinsic, deformations may also be related to intrinsic disorders of the fetus. Renal agenesis, eg, will also result in oligohydramnios because of the decreased contribution of fetal urine to the amniotic fluid volume during the last half of gestation. Infants with decreased fetal movement as a result of maternal or fetal neuromuscular disorders may have similar findings (fetal akinesia sequence, arthrogryposis, Pena-Shokier I phenotype). Because of the decreased movement of joints, these patients will also have absent flexion creases and webbing of the skin across the joints. Tables 25–3A–C list the causes of and findings associated with common deformations.

Disruptions

Disruptions are associated with extrinsic factors that result in the destruction of otherwise normally developed tissues or organs. Approximately 1 in 2000 neonates will have birth defects that are associated with **rupture of the amnion.** Rupture of the amnion during early pregnancy may result in the formation of amniotic bands or strands that can adhere

Table 25–3A. Classification and etiology of deformations.

Classification		Etiology

Intrauterine constraint	Extrinsic (external)	Small uterine cavity (1–2% women)
		    Multiple gestations (crowding)
		    Abnormal uterus (bicornate uterus)
		    Intrauterine fibroids or other masses
		Fetal positioning
		    Breech presentation (6% deliveries)
		    Transverse lie (1 in 300–600)
		    Face or brow presentation (1 in 500)
		Oligohydramnios
		    Rupture of amnion
		    Amniotic fluid leak
		    Maternal hypertension
		    Placental insufficiency
		    Monozygous twins with abnormal circulation pattern

	Intrinsic (embryo or fetus)	Oligohydramnios
		    Renal agenesis
		    Polycystic kidneys
		    Obstructive uropathy

Decreased fetal movement	Extrinsic	Maternal neuromuscular disease
		    Myasthenia Gravis
		    Myotonic dystrophy

	Intrinsic	Neuromuscular disease Fetal akinesia sequence Pena-Shokeir syndrome, type I

Table 25–3B. Deformations: birth defects that result from intrauterine constraint.

Affected System or Area	Clinical Findings
Extremities	Abnormal positioning of extremities: clubfoot (equinovarus deformity), metatarus adductus, dorsiflexion of feet (calcaneovalgus), tibial torsion
Joints	Joint dislocations: dislocated hips, knee (genu recurvatum), radial head
Nervous system	Nerve palsies (from compression of nerves): facial palsy, radial, posterior interosseous nerve (wrist drop), sciatic (foot drop, leg weakness)
Thorax	Thoracic compression: pulmonary hypoplasia, pectus carinatum or excavatum, scoliosis
Head and face	Orofacial compression: nasal compression, asymmetric ears, overfolded helices, micrognathia (compression of chin on shoulder), facial asymmetry Abnormal head positioning: torticollis, plagiocephaly (rhomboid shape), hyperextension of neck Cranium: craniostenosis, extreme molding
Genitalia	Compression of genitalia
Skin	Redundant skin (with oligohydramnios)
Vascular system	Vascular compromise with associated disruptions (See also Table 25–4.)

Table 25–3C. Deformations: birth defects that result from decreased fetal movement.

Affected System or Area	Clinical Findings (Fetal akinesia sequence; arthrogryposis)
Joints	Multiple congenital joint contractures: limited extension of head, abnormal positioning of hands and feet, camptodactyly of fingers (stiff, flexed), equinovarus foot deformity
Skin	Absent flexion creases and webbing of skin over joints; tight, thin skin
Orofacial	Micrognathia, depressed tip of nose, wide-spaced eyes, low-set ears
Lungs	Pulmonary hypoplasia
Skeleton	Thin, fragile bones
Other	Decreased motor mass Polyhydramnios (decreased fetal swallowing) Poor fetal growth Short umbilical cord

to the embryo or fetus. With fetal growth, the bands can tighten and compromise developing areas and lead to resorptive necrosis. The bands most often affect the limbs and the craniofacial and abdominal areas. Rupture of the amnion later during pregnancy results in oligohydramnios with associated fetal compression and deformation. Many severely affected fetuses are spontaneously aborted; others are stillborn or die early in the neonatal period. Careful examination of the placenta may reveal the bands and remnants of the amnion. Alternatively, disruptions may occur as a result of **vascular compromise.** Vascular disruptions may result from abnormal development of fetal blood vessels or circulation patterns, disturbances in placental circulation, or from maternal hypotension, vasoactive drugs, or agents (eg, cocaine). The decreased blood supply may involve almost any area of the developing embryo or fetus and results in an atresia, if it occurs early during gestation, or necrosis, if it occurs later in gestation. Patterns of malformations may

be seen with abnormal development or loss of circulation in certain embryonic vessels. For example, the hypoplasia of the pectoral muscles and distal limb defects seen with the Poland sequence can be related to decreased blood supply from the branches of the embryonic subclavian artery that supply a common area in the developing embryo destined to become these structures. Vascular anastomoses and discordant placental blood flow in **twins with a common placenta** predispose them to vascular disruptions. In approximately 1% of monozygous twins, intrauterine death of one twin may result in the release of thromboplastin or emboli to the surviving co-twin that can lead to ischemia in localized areas. Porencephaly, transverse limb reductions, gastroschisis, and intestinal atresias are common findings in monozygous twinning. Table 25–4 details the abnormalities associated with disruptions. Most disruptions occur as sporadic events that are not inherited. The prognosis is related to the severity of the defect that occurs.

Table 25–4. Disruptions and associated birth defects.

Disruption	Type	Associated Birth Defects
Rupture of the amnion (amniotic band syndrome)	Early	Craniofacial: anencephaly, encephalocele, meningocele, facial clefts and distortions, cleft lip, cleft palate (Robin sequence type), choanal atresia, ear malformations. Extremities: reduction limb defects, amputations, polydactyly, syndactyly, distal lymphedema, dislocated hips. Other: placental attachment to the head or abdomen, defects in the abdominal or thoracic wall, short umbilical cord, omphalocele.
	Late	Oligohydramnios. Compression type deformations.
Vascular disruptions	General	Cerebral and cerebellar infarction, microcephaly, hydranencephaly, porencephalic cysts, hemifacial microsomia, cleft lip or palate, pulmonary infarction, intestinal atresias (not duodenal), gastroschisis, liver infarction, renal infarction, limb amputations, transverse limb reductions defects, cutis aplasia.
	Embryonic aortic arches	Some cases of DiGeorge sequence. (See Table 25–5).
	Embryonic omphalomesenteric artery	Some cases of gastrochisis: small abdominal wall defect in umbilical area, herniated small intestine without a covering sac.
	Embryonic stapedial artery	Facio-auriculo-vertebral spectrum: abnormal development of 1st and 2nd branchial arches. Variable, usually unilateral, hypoplasia of lower facial bones and muscles, lateral cleft-like extension of corner of mouth, underdeveloped ear, deafness; abnormal cervical vertebrae. May have epibulbar dermoids, notch in upper eyelid, cleft lip and/or palate, congenital heart disease.
	Embryonic subclavian artery and branches	Poland sequence: unilateral absence of pectoralis muscle, syndactyly and short digits. Moebius sequence: 6th and 7th cranial nerve palsy. Klippel-Feil sequence: abnormal cervical vertebrae, short neck. (See also Table 25–5).
	Vitelline artery	"Vitelline artery steal." Sirenomelia sequence: abnormal caudal development. (See also Table 25–5).

Sequences, Associations, and Syndromes

Sequences, associations, and syndromes are categories of combinations of multiple malformations.

Sequences

Sequences are patterns of multiple birth defects that result from a single localized defect in morphogenesis. Although more than one birth defect is present, they may all be traced back to one basic defect and have a common etiology. The primary defect leads to secondary, and often tertiary defects in morphogenesis. Sequences may arise from malformations, deformations, or disruptions. One of the most commonly recognized sequences is meningomyelocele. The basic defect is the posterior neural tube failing to close. Secondary defects that occur with meningomyelocele include hydrocephalus (from altered cerebrospinal fluid flow and absorption), bladder and bowel incontinence and club feet (from denervation distal to the meningomyelocele), and spina bifida (from failure of the vertebral bodies to close over the defect). Sequences may also occur with deformations (eg, fetal akinesia sequence) or disruptions (eg, embryonic vessel abnormalities). Table 25–5 lists common sequences and the associated pattern of defects.

Associations

Associations are nonrandom combinations of malformations that occur more frequently than would be expected by chance alone, but are not considered of a high enough frequency to be considered a syndrome. Each affected patient will not have all the malformations that are associated. However, finding two or three of the constellation of malformations should lead to an evaluation for the other associated defects. Table 25–6 lists the clinical features of the CHARGE, MURCS, and VATER associations (Figure 25–1).

Syndromes

Multiple malformation syndromes are recognizable combinations or patterns of birth defects that cannot be explained on the basis of a single isolated defect. The combination of findings results from structural defects in more than one area or tissue in the developing embryo or fetus. Affected patients are more likely to resemble other patients with the same syndrome than they resemble their own siblings. Affected patients usually will not have all the findings of a syndrome, but they will have two or three key features which places them into a specific syndrome category. Syndromes are best categorized as to their major finding, eg, short stature, or combination of major findings, eg, facial and limb abnormalities. There are well over 1000 recognized syndromes; many are very rare. Over one-half of patients evaluated for multiple malformations will not have the characteristics of any known, recognized syndrome, association, or sequence. Table 25–7 lists the clinical findings of some of the more common malformation syndromes. The reader is referred to the recommended readings at the end of this chapter for extensive listings and catalogs of the syndromes. (See also Figures 25–2 through 25–9.)

Approximately 100 of the currently recognized syndromes have associated chromosomal abnormalities. Standard chromosomal analysis will detect large duplications, deletions, and abnormalities in the number of chromosomes, eg, Turner syndrome or Down syndrome. For others, specific DNA probes have been developed that can detect small molecular changes not usually noted with standard chromosomal analysis. Table 25–8 lists the chromosomal location of selected malformations and syndromes. Specific DNA probes are available for many of those listed. Deletions (del) of chromosomal regions result in structural and functional monosomies of multiple genes within the region, which independently contribute to the phenotype of the syndrome (contiguous gene syndromes). Duplications result in structural and functional trisomies of chromosomal regions.

Genomically Imprinted Genes

There are certain genes that are expressed only if they are of maternal origin and others that are expressed only if they are of paternal origin. Such genes, which are differently expressed depending on the parental origin, are "genomically imprinted." A normal complement of imprinted genes (one of each parental origin) must be functionally active for normal fetal development to occur. Deletion of a parental imprinted gene that is normally expressed results in no functional activity at the gene site. Genomic imprinting is known to occur in human chromosomal regions 15p11–13 (Prader-Willi and Angelman syndromes) and 11p15.5 (Beckwith or Beckwith-Wiedemann syndrome). Imprinting may also play a role in the development of some types of tumors (eg, Wilms) and Huntington disease.

Prader-Willi syndrome and Angelman syndrome are both associated with deletions in the 15q11–13 chromosomal region but have different clinical features (see Table 25–7). Prader-Willi syndrome results when the deletion occurs on a chromosome of paternal origin and is thought to result from functional deficiency of the SNRPN gene, or other genes, that are paternally expressed (maternally repressed) in the region. The SNRPN gene encodes for a small ribonucleoprotein-associated polypeptide SmN. In contrast, Angelman syndrome occurs only when the deletion is of maternal origin; deletion of a maternally expressed (paternally repressed) $GABA_A$ receptor gene appears to be associated. The cytogenetic and molecular findings in Beckwith syndrome are more complex. Although most cases of Beckwith syndrome are sporadic, some cases have been noted to occur with

Table 25–5. Examples of sequences and associated patterns of birth defects.

Sequence	MIM Number(s)	Primary Defect in Morphogenesis	Secondary Associated Malformations and Other Findings
Athyrotic hypothyroidism	218700	Failure of development of the thyroid gland	Immature bones of prenatal onset; large fontanels, immature facial bones. Myxedema with hoarse cry, full subcutaneous tissues, enlarged tongue and muscles. Delayed myelination, mental handicaps. Umbilical hernias. Dry skin, mottling, hypothermia. Constipation, prolonged jaundice, decreased activity. Usually sporadic; may be detected by newborn screening.
Cleft lip	119530	Failure of closure of lip	Cleft palate, defects in tooth development and incomplete growth of the alae nasi on the side of the cleft. Mild ocular hypertelorism. As an isolated finding, multifactorial or polygenic inheritance; more common in males than females.
Robin (Pierre Robin)	261800	Early hypoplasia of the mandibular area, which allows the tongue to be posteriorly located and impairs closure of the palatal shelves	Small mandible that has catch-up growth by one year of age. "U"-shaped cleft palate. Posterior placement of the tongue with airway obstruction. May be seen with trisomy 18, Stickler syndrome, deformations.
Frontonasal dysplasia (median facial cleft)	136760	Abnormal midline facial development	Ocular hypertelorism, "widow's peak" of midline hair. Broad nasal bridge, variable bifid nose, notched alae nasi. Median cleft lip. Midline deficit of frontal bone. Usually sporadic.
Septo-optic dysplasia	182230	Incomplete early morphogenesis of the anterior cephalic midline structures	Hypoplasia of optic chiasm, nerves, and discs. Visual defects, pendular nystagmus, field defects. Absence of septum pellucidum. Hypothalamic defects; varying degrees of panhypopituitarism. Usually sporadic; may occur with holoprosencephaly sequence.
Holoprosencephaly	157170 236100	Abnormal development of prechordal mesoderm	Missing or incomplete midfacial development: hypotelorism, lack of ethmoid bone, absent philtrum and nasal septum, single naris, proboscis, cleft lip, cleft palate. Incomplete cleavage and development of forebrain: anophthalmia, microophthalmia, cyclopia, iris colobomas, retinal defects, lack of optic nerves and olfactory lobes, single ventricle of the brain, absence of corpus callosum, fused thalami, incomplete development of anterior and posterior pituitary, microcephaly, severe mental retardation, apnea, seizures. Varies in severity and prognosis; may be seen with chromosomal defects (trisomy 13, 18p–, 13q–), Meckel-Gruber syndrome, and in diabetic progeny.
Anencephaly	206500	Failure of closure of the anterior neural tube	Incomplete development and subsequent degeneration of the brain. Incomplete development of the skull. Distorted facial features and ears. Occasionally cleft palate, abnormal cervical vertebrae, abnormal development of the anterior pituitary. May be associated with decreased maternal intake of folic acid, early rupture of the amnion with amniotic bands, maternal hyperthemia.
Meningomyelocele	182940	Failure of closure of the posterior neural tube	Spina bifida, defect in spinous process of vertebral bodies. Hydrocephalus. Neurological deficits caudal to the lesion, club foot, leg weakness, bladder and bowel incontinence. May be associated with decreased maternal intake of folic acid.

Table 25–5. *(Continued)*

Sequence	MIM Number(s)	Primary Defect in Morphogenesis	Secondary Associated Malformations and Other Findings
Exstrophy of bladder	None	Failure of mesoderm below umbilicus to invade cloacal membrane	Breakdown of cloacal membrane (midline abdominal wall below the umbilicus and anterior bladder wall) with exposure of the posterior bladder wall. Incomplete fusion of the genital tubercles, epispadias, inguinal hernias, separated pubic rami. May be part of the more extensive exstrophy of the cloaca sequence, with the additional involvement of urorectal septum (imperforate anus), and lumbosacral vertebral bodies (hydromyelia). More affected males than females.
Poland (subclavian artery supply disruption sequence, SASDS)	173800	Decreased blood supply from proximal embryonic subclavian artery to distal limb and pectoral areas	Unilateral absence or hypoplasia of pectoralis major muscles. Syndactyly and short digits. May also have asymmetric hypoplasia or aplasia of the areola or nipple, decreased subcutaneous tissues of the breast and pectoral areas, webbing of axilla, reduction defects in arm and forearm, rib defects, hemivertebrae, Sprengel anomaly of scapula, renal anomalies. May be seen with Moebius sequence. Usually sporadic; occasionally familial cases.
Moebius (congenital facial diplegia)	157900	Failure of development of the sixth and seventh cranial nerve nuclei. May result from decreased blood supply from branches of the embryonic subclavian artery	Bilateral 6th and 7th cranial nerve palsies. High nasal bridge, micrognathia, small mouth, expressionless face, ptosis. May involve other cranial nerves. May have other craniofacial and limb hypoplasias (Oromandibular-limb hypogenesis spectrum). Usually sporadic; occasionally autosomal dominant.
Klippel-Feil	148900	Abnormal early development of cervical vertebrae. May result from decreased blood supply from branches of the embryonic subclavian artery	Fused cervical vertebrae, hemivertebrae. Short, webbed neck, low hairline. Facial asymmetry. Torticollis, decreased movement of neck. Occasionally neurological defects from cord involvement, deafness, cleft palate; heart, renal, and other vertebral anomalies. Usually sporadic; may be autosomal dominant with variable expression. More affected females than males.
Sirenomelia	None	Alteration in early vascular development with blood returning to the placenta through a single vessel derived from the vitelline arteries. "Vitelline artery steal" of blood and nutrients from caudal structures of embryo and fetus	Single lower extremity with posterior alignment of the knees and feet. Absent sacrum; lumbosacral vertebral defects. Imperforate anus, absent rectum. Absent external and internal genitalia. Renal agenesis, absent bladder. Caudal regression sequence seen in diabetic progeny has similar findings but is of different etiology.
DiGeorge	188400	Abnormal differentiation of structures derived from the third and fourth pharyngeal pouches and the fourth branchial arch; may be related to abnormal development of the embryonic aortic arches	Hypoplasia or absence of parathyroids and thymus. Abnormal facies with hypertelorism, downward slanting eyes, short philtrum, anteverted nose, low-set ears with notched pinnae, micrognathia. Cardiac malformations of great vessels: aortic arch abnormalities, conotruncal defects, PDA, tetralogy of Fallot. Occasionally esophageal atresia, choanal atresia, imperforate anus, diaphragmatic hernia, hypothyroidism, nephrocalcinosis. Usually sporadic. Gene (DGCR) locus 22q11.21–q11.23; DNA probe available. Some cases autosomal recessive or autosomal dominant. May also be seen with chromosomal defects and maternal intake of alcohol, retinoic acid, or other vitamin A derivatives.

Table 25–6. Associations.

Association	MIM Number	Mnemonic	Major Birth Defects	Other Findings
CHARGE	214800	C	Colobomas, iris and retinal.	Micrognathia, cleft lip, cleft palate, facial palsy, DiGeorge sequence, renal anomalies, omphalocele, tracheoesophageal fistula, anal atresia, rib anomalies, ptosis, microcephaly, ocular hypertelorism. Some patients will have severe involvement and holoprosencephaly sequence. Etiology unknown; usually sporadic and not inherited.
		H	Heart defects; tetralogy of Fallot, PDA, double outlet right ventricle with atrioventricular canal, ventricular septal defect, atrial septal defect, right-sided aortic arch.	
		A	Choanal atresia	
		R	Retarded growth and development; postnatal growth deficiency, mental handicaps that vary from mild to severe-profound.	
		G	Genital anomalies, hypogonadism (males)	
		E	Ear anomalies, deafness	
MURCS	None	MU	Mullerian duct aplasia; absence of vagina, absent to hypoplastic uterus (Rokitansky sequence); primary amenorrhea, infertility.	Short stature, rib anomalies, upper limb defects, Sprengel scapular anomaly. Occasionally deafness, external ear defects, facial asymmetry, cleft lip and palate, micrognathia, gastrointestinal defects. Etiology unknown; usually sporadic and not inherited.
		R	Renal aplasia; renal agenesis and/or ectopy	
		CS	Cervicothoracic somite dysplasia; cervical and thoracic vertebral defects, occasionally Klippel-Feil sequence.	
VATER	192350	V	Vertebral anomalies; lower thoracic, lumbar and sacrococcygeal areas more common	Single umbilical artery, rib anomalies, defects of external genitalia, cardiac defects, lower limb anomalies, prenatal and postnatal growth deficiency, large fontanel. Only rarely will the patients have central nervous system involvement and psychomotor handicaps. Etiology unknown; usually sporadic and not inherited.
		A	Anal atresia with or without fistula	
		T	Tracheoesophageal fistula with esophageal atresia	
		E	Ear anomalies	
		R	Radial dysplasia that includes the thumb, or radial hypoplasia, preaxial polydactyly, syndactyly. Renal anomalies	

unbalanced duplications of the 11p15.5 chromosomal region of paternal origin. In other cases, balanced translocations or inversions of maternal origin are found.

Uniparental Disomy (UPD): Uniparental disomy (UPD) occurs when a set of one or more genes on both chromosomes are of the same parental origin. Normally one set is inherited from each parent. Uniparental disomy is uncommon, but may arise from correction of a trisomy early in pregnancy through loss of one of the three chromosomes. If the remaining chromosomes are both of the same parental origin, then genetic disorders associated with imprinting may occur. Prader-Willi syndrome (maternal UPD), Angelman syndrome (paternal UPD), and Beckwith syndrome have been reported to occur with uniparental disomy.

Uniparental Isodisomy: Correction of a monosomy, early in pregnancy, by duplication of the monosomic chromosome, also results in the set of genes being of the same parental origin; in this case the term uniparental isodisomy is used. Disorders as-

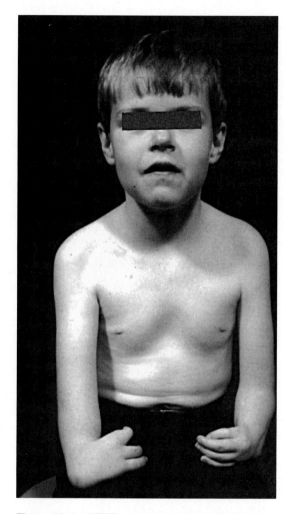

Figure 25–1. VATER association. Note distal limb defects with radial dysplasia. This boy also has vertebral anomalies, anal atresia, and normal intelligence. (Courtesy of David Weaver, M.D.)

sociated with imprinted genes may also occur with uniparental isodisomy. In addition, with uniparental isodisomy, if any of the duplicated genes are abnormal, autosomal recessive syndromes or biochemical genetic disorders may result.

Teratogens

Teratogens are environmental agents that produce congenital malformations or raise the incidence of congenital malformations in the general population. Teratogens may interfere with the growth and differentiation of tissues and organs and result in single or multiple malformations. They may also result in deformations or cause a disruption with resorptive necrosis of a normally developed structure. Table 25–9 illustrates the various times during gestation when major organ systems are susceptible to teratogens. If present

during the first two weeks after conception, teratogens may result in early loss of pregnancy. During the embryonic period of organogenesis, to the end of the eighth week after conception, teratogens may produce a spectrum of multiple birth defects. Later during the fetal period, from 9 weeks to term, teratogens are less likely to produce structural abnormalities, but they may interfere with the developing organ systems that have continued growth and differentiation during this time, eg, the brain, teeth, external genitalia, eyes, ears, and the palate.

In addition to being related to the time in gestation when the exposure occurs, the pattern and severity of the effects of teratogens may correspond to the dose and duration of the exposure and to the susceptibility of the fetus. Not every exposed fetus will be affected, and there is often a wide spectrum of effects when they do occur. Effects may differ, depending on whether there is just a one-time exposure or continued exposure throughout the pregnancy. The adverse fetal effect of a specific agent may occur only during a certain time, or "window," during gestation. For example, thalidomide has been shown to affect the developing limbs only if the mother took thalidomide between 20 and 40 days after conception. The extent of fetal effects may also be related to other modifying factors, eg, whether the fetus or mother is able to detoxify certain drugs and chemicals. For example, the level of activity of the enzyme epoxide hydrolase, involved with the metabolism of Dilantin, may determine whether the fetus will have fetal hydantoin (Dilantin) syndrome. If there is a lowered level of activity of epoxide hydrolase, then the fetus may be more susceptible to the effects of maternal Dilantin therapy. If there is a higher level of activity of epoxide hydrolase, then no fetal Dilantin effects may occur.

Some of the more common known teratogens, along with the associated birth defects and other clinical findings, are detailed in Tables 25–10A–D. There are four major categories of teratogens: infectious agents, drugs or pharmaceuticals, environmental chemicals and physical agents, and maternal disease. The listing is not inclusive of all known teratogens. Consultation with an expert in teratology should be considered prior to counseling for individual cases.

Congenital Infections

Congenital infections are well-known causes of birth defects and psychomotor handicaps. Congenital cytomegalovirus infection occurs in 1–3% of all pregnancies and congenital toxoplasmosis in 1 in 1000. Other less common congenital infections may occur with syphilis and rubella, varicella, parvovirus B19, and herpes simplex viruses. Even though immunization is available for rubella, as many as 25% of women in childbearing age may not have protective antibodies. The incidence of congenital rubella infections, as well as congenital syphilis infections, has

Table 25–7. Common malformation syndromes.[1]

Name	Major Clinical Features
I. Syndromes with short stature as a major clinical finding	
Aarskog syndrome (MIM 1000050) and Aarskog-Scott syndrome (Faciogenital dysplasia) (MIM 3054000)	Uncommon. Mild to moderate short stature, shawl scrotum, widow's peak; short, broad hands and feet (brachydactyly), mild syndactyly, transverse palmar creases; mild pectus excavatum. Facies: rounded, hypertelorism, broad nasal bridge, short anteverted nose, long philtrum, ptosis. Sex-influenced AD; or, X-linked semidominant; chromosomal location Xq13.
Bloom syndrome (MIM 210900)	Rare. Most common with Eastern European Jewish ancestry. Prenatal onset growth deficiency. Mild microcephaly, psychomotor handicap. Erythematous, sun-sensitive rashes on face and exposed areas. Malar hypoplasia, small mandible, narrow facies. Associated with chromosomal instability and increased chromatin exchange. Increased risk for neoplasia, leukemia. AR; gene location 15q26.1.
DeLange syndrome (Cornelia de Lange syndrome, Brachmann-deLange syndrome) (MIM 122470)	Incidence: 1 in 20,000. Short stature of prenatal onset. Psychomotor retardation, may be severe. Low-pitched cry in infancy. Microbrachycephaly. Bushy eyebrows which meet in midline (synophrys); hirsuitism. Characteristic facies with small, anteverted nose, thin lips with downward curving at angles of mouth, long philtrum. Limb defects; micromelia, phocomelia. Cardiac defects. Usually sporadic. Some patients with duplications of chromosomal region 3q25–29 have similar phenotype (Figure 25–2). (See also Chapter 8.)
Dubowitz syndrome (MIM 223370)	Rare. Prenatal and postnatal growth deficiency. Microcephaly; psychomotor delay. High-pitched, hoarse voice. Characteristic facies with high forehead, broad nasal bridge, telecanthus, short palpebral fissures, ptosis, blepharophimosis, epicanthal folds. Dysplastic ears; eczema-like skin disorder on face and in flexor creases; sparse hair and lateral eyebrows. AR.
Hallerman-Streiff (Oculomandibulodyscephaly with hypotrichosis syndrome) (MIM 234100)	Uncommon. Proportionate short stature; brachycephaly with frontal and parietal bossing. Microophthalmia, congenital cataracts. Hypotrichosis, cutaneous atrophy of scalp and nose, hypoplastic teeth. Characteristic facies with narrow, thin, small, pointed nose; small mouth and mandible; high arched palate. Varying psychomotor development. Sporadic, AR.
Noonan syndrome (MIM 163950)	Incidence: 1 in 1000–2500. Turner-like phenotype; occurs in both sexes. Prenatal onset short stature; psychomotor handicap. Low posterior hairline, short or webbed neck. Shield chest, pectus excavatum or carinatum; cubitus valgus. Males may have small penis, cryptorchidism. Facies: epicanthal folds, ptosis, hypertelorism, downward slanting palpebral fissures, myopia, keratoconus. Low-set or abnormal ears. Heart disease: pulmonary valvular or peripheral stenosis; other cardiac defects. Usually sporadic; some AD with variable expression (Figure 25–3). (See also Chapter 8.)
Opitz syndrome (G syndrome) (MIM 145410)	Rare. Moderate short stature. Mild to moderate mental handicap. Hypertelorism, widow's peak, posterior rotation of ears. Hypospadias, cryptorchidism, bifid scrotum. Hoarse voice and cry; esophageal motor dysfunction. May have cleft lip or palate and cardiac defects. AD with sex-limited expression for genital anomalies.
Robinow syndrome AD: (MIM 180700) AR: (MIM 268310)	Incidence: 1 in 500,000. Mild to moderate short stature. "Fetal face," macrocephaly, large anterior fontanels, prominent forehead, hypertelorism, triangular mouth, short anteverted nose, hyperplastic alveolar ridges. Genital hypoplasia in males and females. Short forearms. Hemivertebrae. AD or AR.
Rubenstein-Taybi syndrome (MIM 180849)	Incidence: 1 in 33,000. Short stature. Broad terminal phalanges, especially of thumbs and large toes, with medial deviation. Characteristic facies: beaked/straight nose, septum extends below alae nasi, downslanting palpebral fissures, epicanthal folds, hypoplastic maxilla. Microophthalmia, ptosis, low-set or malformed ears. Cryptorchidism. Cardiac and renal defects. Delayed bone age. Psychomotor delay, may be severe (Figure 25–4). Most cases sporadic; deletion 16p13.3, detected in 25% patients with DNA probe.
Russell-Silver syndrome (Silver syndrome) AR: (MIM 270050) XLR: (MIM 312780)	Common. Short stature of prenatal onset; delayed bone age. Hemiatrophy with asymmetry, especially of the limbs. Triangular facies with prominent forehead, down-turned corners of mouth. Cafe-au-lait spots, syndactyly, small incurved fifth finger. Precocious puberty, may have fasting hypoglycemia, occasional growth hormone deficiency. Excessive sweating. AD with incomplete penetrance, AR, or XLR.
Seckel syndrome (MIM 210600)	Uncommon. Severe microcephaly and short stature of prenatal onset. Psychomotor retardation. Large beaked nose, narrow face, relatively large eyes, low-set dysplastic ears, receding forehead, micrognathia. Dislocation of hips; hypoplastic proximal fibula and radius. Some patients have an increase in chromosomal breakage. AR.

Table 25–7. *(Continued)*

Name	Major Clinical Features
Williams syndrome (MIM 194050)	Incidence: 1 in 10,000–20,000. Mild to moderate short stature of prenatal onset. Mild microcephaly. Moderate psychomotor handicap. Friendly, loquacious personality, hoarse voice. "Elfin" facies with depressed nasal bridge, epicanthal folds, anteverted nose, short palpebral fissures, periorbital fullness, blue eyes, stellate pattern of iris, long philtrum, prominent lips. Small or missing teeth, enamel hypoplasia. Supravalvular aortic stenosis, and other cardiac defects. Bladder diverticula. Hypoplastic nails, brachydactyly. Hypercalcemia may occur in infants. Most sporadic. Associated with deletions in elastin gene located at 7p11.2; 92–95% of patients will be detected by DNA probe (Figure 25–5). (See also Chapter 8.)

II. Syndromes with overgrowth as a major clinical finding

Name	Major Clinical Features
Beckwith syndrome (Beckwith-Weidemann syndrome) (MIM 130650)	Incidence 1 in 20,000. EMG syndrome (exomphalos-macroglossia-gigantism). Large for gestational age at birth. Large muscle mass and accelerated osseous maturation. Characteristic facies with macroglossia, prominent eyes with relative infraorbital hypoplasia. Nevus flammeus on central forehead and eyelids. Large fontanels. Linear fissures on the lobes of ears anterior or posterior, and indentations or pits on the posterior rim of the helix. Large abdominal organs; hypoglycemia due to pancreatic hyperplasia. Omphalocele, umbilical hernia, diastasis recti. Hemihypertrophy, which may cross midline. Increased risk for the development of tumors (8%); Wilms, hepatoblastoma, neuroblastoma, gonadoblastoma. Usually sporadic. Gene locus at 11p15.5 is imprinted. Small number of cases associated with deletions/duplications; uniparental disomy noted in 25%. DNA probe available (Figure 25–6).
Sotos syndrome (MIM 117550)	Uncommon. Cerebral gigantism syndrome. Prenatal onset of large size, with relatively large head, hands, and feet. Advanced bone age. Prominent forehead, downward slanting palpebral fissures, hypertelorism, high narrow palate. Variable psychomotor delay, poor coordination. More common in males, usually sporadic.
Weaver syndrome (MIM 277590)	Rare. Accelerated growth and maturation of prenatal onset. Psychomotor delay, mild hypertonia. Facies: large bifrontal diameter, flat occiput, ocular hypertelorism, epicanthal folds, downslanting palpebral fissures, long philtrum, micrognathia, large ears. Broad thumbs, thin deep-set nails, decreased mobility to fingers, elbows, and knees. Relatively loose skin, inverted nipples, thin hair, umbilical hernia. Hoarse, low-pitched cry. Males more often affected than females. Sporadic.

III. Syndromes with early aging

Name	Major Clinical Features
Cockayne (MIM 216400–216411)	Rare. Growth deficiency, loss of adipose tissue, and senile changes that begin during infancy. Psychomotor handicap, peripheral neuropathy, deafness, unsteady gait, tremor. Small, thick skull. Retinal pigmentation, optic atrophy, cataracts. Photosensitive dermatitis. Hepatomegaly, cryptorchidism, hypertension, renal interstitial fibrosis. Defective DNA repair, no increase in incidence of neoplasia. AR.
Progeria (MIM 176670)	Rare. Hutchison-Gilford syndrome. Onset of senile changes between birth and 18 months. Alopecia, thin skin, hypoplastic nails, loss of adipose tissue, periarticular fibrosis, growth deficiency, atherosclerosis, osteoporosis. Facial hypoplasia, micrognathia. Average life span 14.2 years. Intelligence normal. Sporadic; possibly AD new mutation.
Werner syndrome (MIM 277700)	Rare. Diagnosis usually made between age 15 and 30 years. Short stature, loss of adipose tissue, patches of stiffened and calcified skin especially on face and lower legs. Premature aging; atherosclerosis with calcification, osteoporosis, diabetes, hypogonadism, cataracts, retinal degeneration. Appearance of advanced age by 30–40 years. Average age of death 47 years. Increased incidence of malignancy, especially sarcoma and meningioma. AR. Chromosomal breakage, deletions, translocations may occur.

IV. Syndromes with CNS malformations or mental handicap a major clinical finding

Name	Major Clinical Features
Angelman syndrome (MIM 105830)	Uncommon. Happy-puppet syndrome. Moderate-severe psychomotor handicap; seizures, ataxia. Hyperactive, frequent inappropriate laughter. Facies: large mouth, protruding tongue, prominent jaw, thin upper lip. Gene location 15q11–q13 imprinted; maternal deletion; less than 5% uniparental disomy. 85% confirmed by cytogenetics or DNA probe. Sporadic.
Bardet-Biedl (MIM 209900)	Uncommon. Polydactyly, postaxial; syndactyly. Psychomotor handicap. Obesity. Retinitis pigmentosa, loss of vision in late teenage or as young adult. Hypoplastic genitalia, hypogonadism. Gene location 16q21. AR.

Table 25–7. *(Continued)*

Name	Major Clinical Features
Lowe syndrome (MIM 309000)	Uncommon. Oculocerebrorenal syndrome. Congenital cataracts, glaucoma. Hypotonia, decreased or absent deep tendon reflexes, moderate to severe psychomotor handicap, behavioral problems. Postnatal growth deficiency. Fanconi-type renal tubular acidosis; renal failure as young adult. Facies: thin, deep set eyes. Gene location Xq26.1. XLR; female carriers may have lenticular opacities.
Meckel-Gruber syndrome (Meckel syndrome) (MIM 249000)	Rare. Prenatal growth deficiency, posterior or dorsal encephalocele, microcephaly, cerebral and cerebellar hypoplasia. Microophthalmia, cleft palate, micrognathia, ear anomalies, sloping forehead, short neck. Polydactyly. Dysplastic kidneys with cyst formation, hepatic cysts and fibrosis, incomplete development of external genitalia. Usually die within first weeks of life. AR.
Miller-Dieker syndrome (Lissencephaly syndrome) (MIM 247200)	Uncommon. Incomplete development of the brain, with a smooth surface and areas of pachygyria; hypoplastic or aplastic corpus callosum. Severe psychomotor handicap with hypotonia, seizures, microcephaly, bitemporal narrowing, high forehead. Vertical ridging of skin on forehead with crying. Small, anteverted nose, upward slanting palpebral fissures, micrognathia, low-set and/or posteriorly rotated ears. Usually die in first 3 months, or before 2 years of age. Gene location 17p13.3; 50% will have cytogenetic detection, over 90% detection with DNA probe. (See also Chapter 11.)
Prader-Willi syndrome (MIM 176270)	Incidence: 1 in 10,000–20,000. Hypotonia from birth, often requires tube feedings. Hyperphagia and obesity after 2–4 years of age. Compulsive, obsessive behaviors, especially toward foods. Mild to moderate psychomotor handicap. Characteristic facies with narrow bitemporal diameter, upward slanting palpebral fissures, almond-shaped eyes. Fair complexion. Hypogonadotropic hypogonadism in both sexes. Short stature, small hands and feet; may have growth hormone deficiency, responsive to replacement therapy. Usually sporadic. Gene location 15q11–q13 imprinted; paternal deletion; 20–25% uniparental disomy. 70% confirmed by cytogenetics or DNA probe (Figure 25–7).
Sjogren-Larsson (MIM 270150)	Rare. Short stature; ichthyosis; moderate to severe psychomotor handicap, especially in expressive language; spasticity, especially of legs. Occasionally pigmentary retinopathy, seizures, hypoplastic teeth; metaphyseal dysplasia with small irregular epiphyses. AR.

V. Syndromes with abnormalities in orofacial development

Name	Major Clinical Features
Mandibulofacial dysostosis (Treacher Collins syndrome) (MIM 136760)	Uncommon. Downward slanting palpebral fissures, malar and mandibular hypoplasia, coloboma of lower eyelid, partial or total absence of lower eyelashes, malformed ears and external ear canals, conductive deafness, cleft palate. AD, with wide variability in expression; 60% cases are new mutations.
Rieger syndrome (MIM 180500)	Uncommon. Iris dysplasia. Facies: broad nasal bridge, maxillary hypoplasia, thin upper lip, everted lower lip. Hypodontia. Hypospadias. Gene location 4q25–q27. AD with varying expression.
Stickler syndrome (Hereditary arthoophthalmodystrophy) (MIM 120140)	Incidence: 1 in 20,000. Hyperextensible joints with early onset degenerative joint disease. Mild skeletal epiphyseal dysplasia. Moderate-severe myopia with retinal detachment and/or cataracts. Flat facies with depressed nasal bridge and epicanthal folds. May have cleft palate with/without Robin sequence, deafness, dental anomalies. Hypotonia, marfanoid habitus. Defect: diminished amount of type II collagen in cartilage in some affected patients. AD, with variable expression.
Van der Woude syndrome (MIM 119300)	Incidence: 1 in 90,000. Lower lip pits. Hypodontia, missing teeth. Cleft lip, with or without cleft palate, cleft palate, cleft uvula. Gene location 1q32. AD, with approximately 80% penetrance.
Waardenberg syndrome, type I (MIM 193500)	Incidence: 1 in 30,000. Partial albinism, often as with white forelock; heterochromic iris; vitiligo. Deafness, bilateral, sensorineural. Broad, high nasal bridge with hypoplastic alae nasi. Median eyebrow flare. Lateral displacement of the inner canthi. Gene location 2q35. AD; some new mutations.

VI. Craniosynostoses (premature closure of cranial sutures)

Name	Major Clinical Features
Apert syndrome (Acrocephalosyndactyly, type I) (MIM 101200)	Incidence: 1 in 130,000. Premature closure of cranial sutures, especially of coronal suture. Shortened anteroposterior diameter of skull, flat face, shallow orbits, hypertelorism, downward slanting palpabral fissures, small nose, maxillary hypoplasia. Narrow palate, cleft palate, or bifid uvula. Variable syndactyly of digits, which can include total or partial fusion of all digits (mitten hands and feet). Distal thumb and large toe broad, fingers shortened. Syndactyly may be cutaneous or involve osseous structures. AD, many cases represent new mutations; advanced paternal age noted.
Carpenter syndrome (Acrocephalopolysyndactyly, type II) (MIM 201000)	Rare. Variable premature closure of the coronal, sagittal, and lambdoid sutures. Shallow supraorbital ridges. Lateral displacement of inner canthi. Short, curved digits, partial syndactyly, camptodactyly. Polydactyl feet. Hypogenitalism. AR.

Table 25–7. *(Continued)*

Name	Major Clinical Features
Crouzon syndrome (Craniofacial dysostosis) (MIM 123500)	Uncommon. Premature closure of coronal, lambdoid, and sagittal sutures. Shortened anteroposterior and widened lateral diameter of the skull. Shadow orbits, ocular proptosis, frontal bossing, hypertelorism. Hypoplastic maxilla. Conductive hearing loss. AD, variable expression, many cases represent new mutations.
Pfeiffer syndrome (Acrocephalosyndactyly, type V) (MIM 101600)	Rare. Premature closure of coronal and occasionally sagittal sutures. High forehead, hypertelorism, upward slanting palpebral fissures, small nose. Broad distal thumbs and great toes; partial syndactyly second-third toes, second-third-fourth fingers. AD, many cases represent new mutations.
Saethre-Chotzen syndrome (Acrocephalosyndactyly, type III) (MIM 101400)	Most common of the acrocephalosyndactyly syndromes. Variable premature closure of the coronal suture. Decreased anteroposterior diameter of the skull, high forehead, shallow orbits, ptosis, maxillary hypoplasia, narrow palate. Facial asymmetry. Large, late-closing fontanels. Small ears, prominent crus. Partial syndactyly second-third fingers, fourth-fifth toes. Broad great toes and thumbs; finger-like thumb. Short clavicles. Gene location 7p21. AD, wide variation in expression.
VII. Syndromes with abnormalities in facial and limb development	
Coffin-Lowry syndrome (MIM 303600)	Rare. Postnatal growth deficiency. Severe psychomotor handicap. Hypotonia. Facies: coarse appearance with downward slanting palpebral fissures, prominent eyebrows, maxillary hypoplasia, hypertelorism, short nose, prominent ears, hypodontia; thick, everted lower lip. Bifid, short, sternum, pectus carinatum. Hands large, with tapering digits. Gene location Xp22.2–p22.1. XLR.
Ectrodactyly-ectodermal dysplasia-clefting syndrome (EEC syndrome) (MIM 129900)	Rare. Variable features. Fair complexion, thin skin; thin, sparse hair; blue iris, photophobia, blepharophimosis, defects of lacrimal duct system. Missing teeth. Cleft lip and/or cleft palate. Malar and maxillary hypoplasia. Varying defects in the midportion of the hands and feet; syndactyly to ectrodactyly (missing digits). AD, variable expression and penetrance.
Larsen syndrome AD: (MIM 150250) AR: (MIM 245600)	Rare. Facies: flat, with depressed nasal bridge, hypertelorism. Dislocation of major joints. Long fingers, widened thumbs, short nails, short metacarpals. Talipes equinovalgus, equinovarus. AD, or AR.
Oculodentodigital syndrome (MIM 164200)	Rare. Small eyes, small corneas, short palpebral fissures. Small nose with hypoplastic alae nasi. Dental enamel hypoplasia. Small or missing middle phalanges of fingers or toes. Syndactyly of fourth-fifth fingers, third-fourth toes. Decreased mobility fifth fingers. Fine, dry, sparse, slow growing hair. Wide mandibular alveolar ridge. AD, variable expression.
Orofacial digital syndrome, type I (MIM 311200)	Incidence: 1 in 50,000. Webbing between the buccal mucous membrane and the alveolar ridge. Partial clefts in the lip, tongue, alveolar ridges. Anomalous teeth. Hypoplastic alae nasi cartilages. Asymmetric short digits, may have syndactyly, brachydactyly, polydactyly. 50% psychomotor delay. X-linked, lethal in utero in males.
Orofacial digital syndrome, type II (Mohr syndrome) (MIM 252100)	Rare. Mild short stature. Conductive hearing loss. Facies: lateral displacement of inner canthi; low nasal bridge, midline partial cleft of lip, cleft of tongue. Hypoplasia of maxillary zygomatic arch, body of mandible. Partial duplication of large toe and first metatarsal, cuneiform, and cuboid bones. Short hands, polydactyly. Intelligence usually normal. AR.
Trichorhinophalangeal (TRP) syndrome, type I AD: (MIM 190350) AR: (MIM 275500)	Rare. Facies: nose pear-shaped, hypoplastic nares, long prominent philtrum, narrow palate, micrognathia, large prominent ears. Hypodontia, caries. Sparse, thin hair with relative hypopigmentation. Thin nails. Short metacarpals and metatarsals; cone-shaped epiphysis second-fourth fingers and toes, asymmetric finger lengths, abnormal angulation of fingers. Gene location 8q24.12. AD or AR.
TRP, type II (Langer-Giedion syndrome) (MIM 150230)	Rare. Varying psychomotor handicap; microcephaly. Facies: large protruding ears, deep-set eyes, large bulbous nose with thick alae nasi, broad nasal bridge, simple elongated philtrum. Loose redundant skin in infancy, sparse scalp hair; multiple nevi. Epiphyses in hands cone-shaped, lack of modeling in metaphyseal regions; multiple exostoses of long tubular bones. Syndactyly, hypotonia, lax joints. Gene location 8q24.1–q24.3; 75% detected by cytogenetics, 90% by DNA probe.
VIII. Syndromes with abnormalities in limb development	
Holt-Oram syndrome (Cardiac-Limb syndrome) (MIM 142900)	Uncommon. Variable upper limb and shoulder girdle defects; hypoplasia, phocomelia, finger-like thumb; may be asymmetric. Cardiac defects: septal defects most common. AD, with variable expression. (See also Chapter 8.)
Thrombocytopenia-absent radius syndrome (TAR) (MIM 274000)	Rare. Thrombocytopenia with absent or hypoplastic megakaryocytes, leukemoid granulocytosis, eosinophilia, anemia. Absent or hypoplastic radius, usually bilateral. May have ulnar hypoplasia and other defects of the extremities. AR.

Table 25–7. *(Continued)*

Name	Major Clinical Features
IX. Bone dysplasias	
Achondrogenesis and hypochondrogenesis Type I: (MIM 200600) Type II: (MIM 200610) Type III: (MIM 200710) Type IV: (MIM 200720)	Rare. Severe chondrodysplasia and short-limbed bone dysplasia present at birth. Poorly ossified skeleton. Most die in utero or in perinatal period. Four types of the disorder. Type II results from decreased type II collagen. Defect in other types unknown. AR; some patients may represent AD new mutations. For this, and other bone dysplasias in this section, radiographs are usually diagnostic. Not all findings will be detailed in this table, however, and the reader is referred to the suggested readings.
Achondroplasia (MIM 100800)	Incidence: 1 in 26,000. Most common of the chondrodysplasias. Short-limbed bone dysplasia, present at birth. Large head, relatively small foramen magnum, short cranial base. Prominent forehead, flat nasal bridge, midfacial hypoplasia. Lumbar lordosis. Short hands. Fingers in "trident" or "Vulcan" position with second-third and fourth-fifth fingers held together. May develop hydrocephalus, spinal cord and/or root compression, sleep apnea. Gene locus 4p16.3. AD; 90% of cases represent new mutations (Figure 25–8).
Camptomelic dysplasia (Campomelic dysplasia) (MIM 211970)	Rare. Short-limbed bone dysplasia present at birth. Flat facial appearance. Large head, large brain with cellular disorganization; hydrocephalus. Bowed tibiae, short fibulae. Short, flat vertebral bodies. Hypoplastic scapulae. Small thorax. Tracheo-bronchiomalacia. Many die in the perinatal period from respiratory insufficiency. Gene locus 17q24.3–q25.1. AR.
Diastrophic dysplasia (Diastrophic nanism syndrome) (MIM 222600)	Uncommon. Short-limbed bone dysplasia present at birth. Short, thick tubular bones, scoliosis, incurving of feet (talipes equinovarus). Proximal placement of thumbs, small first metacarpals. Decreased mobility of joints; variable webbing across joints. Hypertrophied articular cartilage which presents as soft, cystic masses in the ears in early infancy. AR.
Hypochondroplasia (MIM 146000)	Uncommon. Mild features of achondroplasia. Less common than achondroplasia. Short stature, mild, short-limbed bone dysplasia. AD; some cases represent new mutations.
Metaphyseal chondrodysplasia, Schmid type (MIM 156500)	Rare. Mild to moderate short stature. Short tubular bones. Broad, irregular, splayed metaphyses. Tibial bowing, waddling gait, flared lower rib cage. AD, with variable expression.
Spondyloepiphyseal dysplasia (SED), congenita (MIM 120140)	Incidence: 1 in 100,000. Shortened-trunk bone dysplasia that is present at birth and involves the spine and epiphyses. Flat facies, malar hypoplasia, cleft palate, myopia, retinal detachments. Barrel chest, pectus carinatum. Defect: abnormal amount and mobility of α1 type II collagen chains. Gene locus 12q13.11–q13.2. AD.
Spondyloepiphyseal dysplasia (SED), tarda AD: (MIM 184100) AR: (MIM 271600) XLR: (MIM 313400)	Uncommon. Onset between 5 and 10 years of age. Short stature, flattened vertebral bodies with short spine, kyphosis, scoliosis; short neck, chest, and trunk. Epiphyseal irregularity; leads to osteoarthritis in hips, knees, and spine in affected adults. AD, AR, or XLR (most common) inheritance patterns.
Thanatophoric dysplasia (MIM 187600)	Incidence: 1 in 42,000. Severe, short-limbed bone dysplasia and chondrodysplasia, present at birth. Narrow thorax with short ribs. Most affected patients die shortly after birth from respiratory insufficiency. Usually sporadic.
X. Defects in collagen synthesis and structure	
Osteogenesis imperfecta (OI)	
OI type I: Autosomal dominant with blue sclera (MIM 120150)	Incidence: 1 in 15,000–20,000. Variable fractures, usually in early childhood, before puberty, or late in life. Normal teeth, near normal stature, little or no bone deformity. 50% mixed type hearing loss, onset in late adolescence. Mild joint hypermobility, mild increased bruising. Defect: decreased production of type I procollagen.
OI type II: Perinatal lethal AD: (MIM 166210) AR: (MIM 259400)	Incidence: 1 in 20,000–60,000. Severe bone involvement with undermineralized bones, absence of mineralization of skull, short extremities, small thoracic cavity, bowed legs at birth. Death from respiratory insufficiency, 60% during first day, 80% first month. Dark sclerae, beaked nose, Most patients represent AD new mutations; a few AR. Defect: mutations, rearrangements, deletions in genes for α1 and α2 polypeptides of type I collagen chains; mutations in C-terminal polypeptide of α1 type I procollagen.

Table 25–7. *(Continued)*

Name	Major Clinical Features
OI type III: Progressive deforming with normal sclera (MIM 259420)	Deformities at birth from in utero fractures. Undermineralized skeleton, thin ribs and long bones. Fractures at birth or by 1 year with deformity. Short adult height; kyphoscoliosis, respiratory insufficiency. Sclerae pale blue at birth, normal later. Dentogenesis imperfecta common; hearing loss common. Most patients represent AD new mutations; some AR. Defect: AD—point mutations in genes for α1 and α2 polypeptides of type I collagen chains. AR—mutation that prevents incorporation of α2 type I procollagen into molecules.
OI type IV: Autosomal dominant with normal sclera (MIM 166220)	At birth, some with fractures, some with femoral bowing. Short stature by age 2 years, mild to moderate bone deformity. Fractures occur prior to puberty, late in life. Dentogenesis imperfecta and hearing loss common. Normal or grayish sclera. One-third develop progressive scoliosis, pulmonary insufficiency. AD with intrafamilial variability. Defect: point mutations in genes for α1 and α2 type I collagen chains; deletions in α2 type I collagen chains.
Ehlers-Danlos syndrome (ED)	
ED type I. Gravis (MIM 130000)	Incidence: 1 in 20,000. Soft, velvety hyperextensible skin; joint hypermobility, easy bruising; tissue friability; thin, atrophic, cigarette paper scarring of skin; varicose veins. Prematurity. Life span normal. Diagnosis in childhood. Defect unknown. AD.
ED type II. A. Mitis (MIM 130010)	Uncommon. Similar to type I, less severe, prematurity not noted. Defect unknown. AD.
ED type II. B. Recessive (MIM 225320)	Rare. Similar to type I, aortic dilatation. Defect unknown. AR.
ED type III. Familial hypermobility (MIM 130020)	Common. Marked joint hypermobility, recurrent joint dislocations with degenerative joint disease. Skin soft but not hyperextensible. Mitral valve prolapse. Defect unknown. AD.
ED type IV. Vascular or ecchymotic (MIM 120180)	Incidence: 1 in 100,000–1,000,000. Thin, translucent skin with visible venous patterns. Hypermobility in small joints of hands and feet. Marked bruising. Tight, thin skin on face; thin nose. Varicose veins. Arterial rupture, anywhere, but most commonly small arteries in abdomen. Spontaneous rupture of colon, usually sigmoid. Rupture of pregnant uterus during last trimester. Keratoconus, peridontal disease. Diagnosis in late childhood or later. Death in 30s–40s from arterial rupture. Defect in type III procollagen structure, synthesis, or secretion. AD with 50% new mutations.
ED type V. X-linked (MIM 305200)	Rare. Similar to type II, with intramuscular hemorrhage. Defect unknown. XLR.
ED type VI. (MIM 225400)	Uncommon. Soft hyperextensible skin; joint hypermobility; severe kyphoscoliosis, marfanoid habitus. Recurrent intraocular bleeding, retinal hemorrhage, rupture of globe; loss of vision. Intraabdominal vascular rupture. Onset during childhood. Defect: decreased lysyl hydroxylase; abnormal posttranslational hydroxylation of type I and type III collagen. AR.
ED type VII. Arthrochalasis multiplex congenita (AMC); types A and B (MIM 130060)	Congenital dislocated hips. Marked joint hypermobility, recurrent joint dislocations. Mild-moderate short stature. Mild midfacial hypoplasia. Defect in conversion of type I procollagen to collagen. Types A and B: abnormal procollagen. AD.
ED type VII. AMC, type C (MIM 225410)	Similar to type VII: types A and B. Defect in conversion of type I procollagen to collagen: abnormal converting enzyme, procollagen N-protease. AR.
ED type VIII (MIM 130080)	Uncommon. Similar to type II. Bruising; soft hyperextensible skin; hypermobile joints; peridontal disease with loss of teeth. Defect unknown. AD.
ED type IX. Occipital horn syndrome (MIM 304150)	Uncommon. Abnormal copper metabolism with secondary lysyl oxidase deficiency. Defect in copper-transporting ATPase (Mc1); allelic to Menkes disease. Gene location: Xq13.3 XLR. (See also Section on Inborn Errors of Metabolism.)
ED type X (MIM 225310)	Similar to type II. Mild joint hypermobility and bruising. Defect in fibronectin. AR.

[1] AD = autosomal dominant; AR = autosomal recessive; CNS = central nervous system; XLR = X-linked recessive.

been rising in recent years. Not all maternal infections will be transmitted, but those that are transmitted often lead to widespread infection of the embryo and fetus. Infection early in pregnancy may cause fetal death and loss of the pregnancy. Infection of the developing central nervous system may result in cortical or cerebellar atrophy, microcephaly, intracranial calcifications, seizures, hypotonia or hypertonia, and varying degrees of psychomotor retardation. Infection of the developing eye may lead to congenital cataracts, glaucoma, chorioretinitis, microophthalmia, and visual impairment. Sensorineural deafness and intrauterine growth retardation (IUGR) also are common findings. Affected neonates often have a postnatal continuing systemic infection associated with hepatitis, hepatosplenomegaly, lymphadenopa-

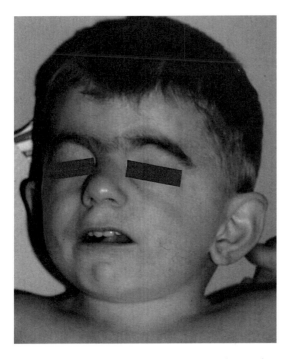

Figure 25–2. DeLange syndrome. Note eyebrows that meet in the midline (synophrys), thin lips that curve downward at the angles of the mouth, and small, anteverted nose.

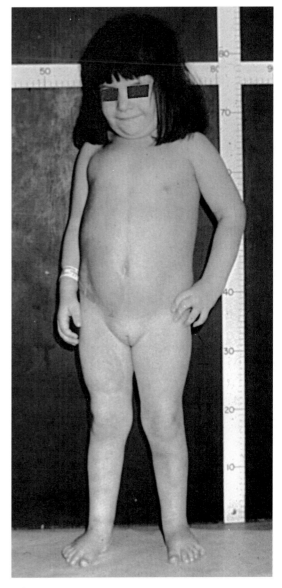

Figure 25–3. Noonan syndrome. Note short neck and broad "shield" chest. This girl also has peripheral pulmonic stenosis and a mild psychomotor handicap.

thy, hemolytic anemia, thrombocytopenia or purpura, and osteitis or osteochondritis. Postnatal viral cultures and serial IgG and IgM titers may confirm the suspected diagnosis.

Drugs and Pharmaceuticals

Prenatal exposure to drugs and pharmaceuticals may result in patterns of abnormalities which may be recurrently observed and considered a syndrome, as is seen with fetal hydantoin (Dilantin) or trimethadione exposures. Almost every anticonvulsant, except for perhaps phenobarbital and related compounds, has been shown to be teratogenic during pregnancy. For women of child-bearing age with seizure disorders, it is important that they receive appropriate counseling and guidance in regard to their medication, optimally prior to pregnancy. Discontinuance of anticonvulsant medications may result in the recurrence of maternal seizures, which, if generalized and associated with hypoxia, can also have adverse fetal effects. Birth defects have also been more recently associated with maternal use of lithium salts, retinoic acid (used for the treatment of cystic acne), and with angiotensin converting enzyme (ACE) inhibitors (commonly used for the treatment of hypertension). Theoretically, all drugs or pharmaceuticals should be considered as possible teratogens during pregnancy. The use of medications during pregnancy, whether prescribed or "over-the-counter," should be minimal and limited only to those needed to treat important maternal health conditions. The relative risks for the fetus and the mother should be considered when a significant maternal health condition is present which can only be treated with a drug with possible adverse fetal effects. After delivery, maternal medications, as well as some environmental chemicals, may be excreted in breast milk, which should also be consid-

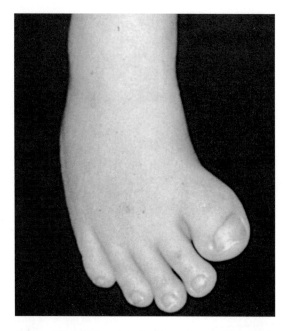

Figure 25–4. Rubenstein-Taybi syndrome. Photograph illustrates broad large toe and medial deviation of toes.

ered when formulating a treatment plan for the expectant mother.

Environmental Chemicals and Physical Agents

Environmental chemicals and physical agents may result in significant birth defects. Prenatal exposure to ethyl alcohol, which occurs in as many as one in 300 pregnancies, is considered the most common reason for psychomotor retardation in the Western world. Many of the major features of the fetal alcohol syndrome will occur with chronic maternal alcoholism during the entire pregnancy, while only minimal findings, usually disturbances in psychomotor development or behavior, may be noted in children who are less exposed, especially later in pregnancy. The use of "street" drugs or chemicals, eg, cocaine or toluene (glue sniffing), can also adversely affect the fetus and the neonate. Alcohol, street drugs, and an increased risk for congenital infection often occur together in the same pregnancy. Hypoxia, from smok-

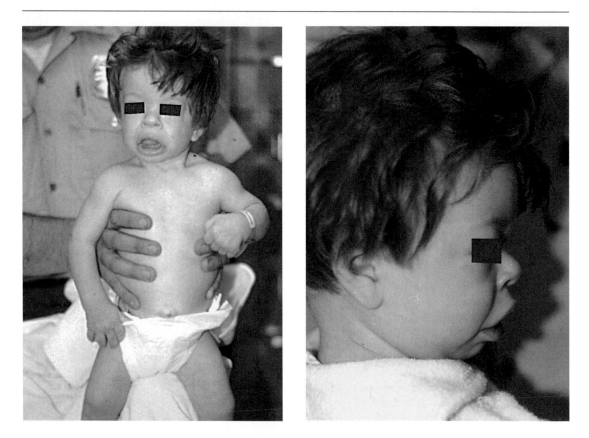

Figure 25–5. Williams syndrome. Note characteristic facial appearance. **(A)** Frontal view. **(B)** Profile. (Courtesy of David Weaver, M.D.)

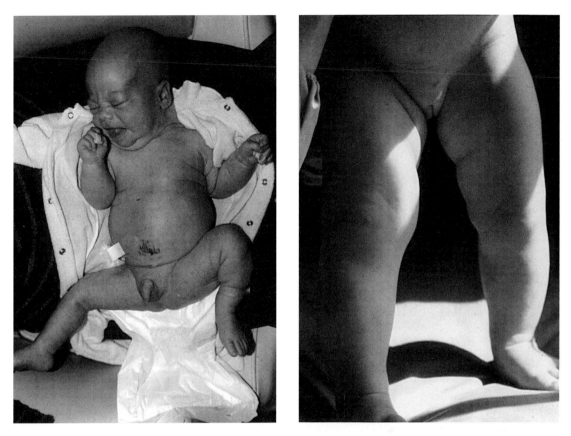

Figure 25–6. Beckwith syndrome. **(A)** Infant. Note repair of omphalocele and macroglossia. **(B)** Toddler. Note hemihypertrophy of leg. (Courtesy of David Weaver, M.D.)

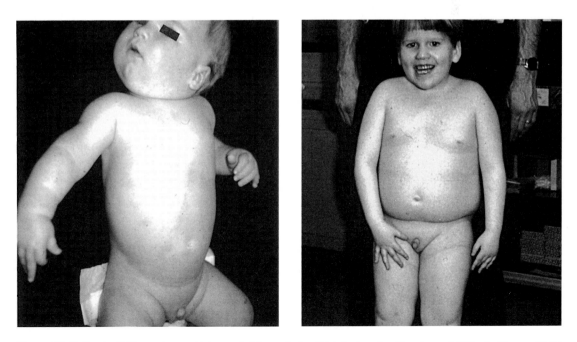

Figure 25–7. Prader-Willi syndrome. Note genital hypoplasia. **(A)** Infant male. (Courtesy of Wilfredo Torres, M.D.) **(B)** 4.5-year-old male.

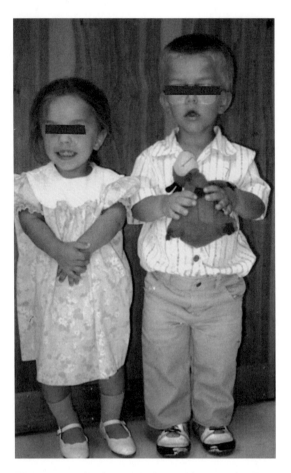

Figure 25–8. Brother and sister with achondroplasia. (Courtesy of Wilfredo Torres, M.D.)

ing, or maternal cardiovascular or pulmonary disease, may result in intrauterine growth retardation. Maternal hyperthermia and exposure to heavy metals or polyhalogenated biphenyls (PCB) have all been reported to have adverse fetal effects. Dietary iodine deficiency, excessive use of maternal inorganic iodides, or antithyroid medications given to the mother may result in fetal goiter and hypothyroidism. Nutritional folate deficiency has been associated with an increased incidence of neural tube defects. Maternal exposure to ionizing radiation from routine radiographic procedures does not usually carry an increased risk for abnormal structural development of the fetus. A total dose of over 10 rads, such as occurs with radiation therapy for malignancy, however, may have an adverse effect.

Maternal Disorders

Certain maternal disorders during gestation may adversely affect the fetus. The outcomes are usually related to the degree of control or severity of the maternal disease. Diabetes mellitus in the mother, especially if insulin-dependent, carries an increased risk for abnormalities in development of the brain, heart, and caudal region of the fetus (see also Chapter 12). Uncontrolled maternal phenylketonuria can be damaging to the developing central nervous system in utero and also lead to abnormalities in facial and cardiac fetal development. Certain maternal myopathies may result in decreased fetal movement and associ-

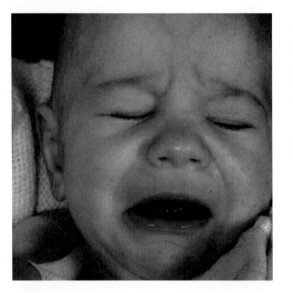
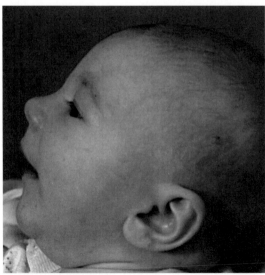

Figure 25–9. Maternal phenylketonuria (PKU) syndrome. Infant of a mother with PKU that was uncontrolled during the first 20 weeks of pregnancy. The infant also has severe, complex, congenital heart disease, hyperreflexia, and moderate psychomotor delay. Note mild facial dysmorphology and microcephaly. **(A)** Frontal view. **(B)** Profile.

Table 25–8. Chromosomal locations of selected malformations and syndromes.[1]

Malformation/Syndrome	Chromosomal Location	MIM Number
Aicardi syndrome	Xp22	304050
Achondroplasia	4p16.3*	100800
Angelman syndrome	15q11–13 (del)* (maternal)	234400
Anhidrotic ectodermal dysplasia	Xq12.2–13.1	305100
Aniridia-Wilms tumor	11p13 (del)*	194070
Bardet-Biedl syndrome	16q21	209900
Basal cell nevus syndrome	9q31	109400
Beckwith-Wiedemann syndrome	11p15.5*	130650
Bloom syndrome	15q26.1	210900
Cat eye syndrome	22q11.2	115470
Cleft palate, X-linked	Xq21.1–21.31	303400
Craniosynostosis, type I	7p21.3–p21.2	218450
Cri-du-chat syndrome	5p15.2 (del)*	123450
DiGeorge syndrome	22q11.2 (del)*	188400
Hirschsprung disease	10q11.2	249200
Hydrocephalus, aqueductal stenosis	Xq28	307000
Kallman syndrome	Xp23.3 (del)*	308700
Langer-Giedion syndrome	8q24.1 (del)*	150230
Lowe syndrome	Xq26.1	309000
Miller-Dieker syndrome	17p13.3 (del)*	247200
Nail-patella syndrome	9q34	161200
Polycystic kidney disease, type I	16p13.31	263200
Prader-Willi syndrome	15q11–q13 (del)* (paternal)	176270
Retinoblastoma	13q14 (del)*	180200
Rieger syndrome	4q25–q27	180500
Rubenstein-Taybi syndrome	16p13.3 (del)*	180849
Saethre-Chotzen syndrome	7q21	101400
Smith-Magenis syndrome	17p11.2 (del)*	182290
Velocardiofacial syndrome	22q11.2 (del)*	192430
Waardenburg syndrome, types I and III	2q35	193500
Williams syndrome	7q11.22 (del)*	194050
Wolf-Hirschhorn syndrome	4p16.3 (del)*	194190

[1] del = interstitial deletion; (paternal) or (maternal) indicate parental origin of deleted chromosomal region (see text); * = DNA probe available.

Table 25–9. Timetable of human development with times of increased susceptibility to teratogens.[1]

System	Cell Proliferation & Implantation _Early loss of pregnancy_	Embryonic Period _Major morphological abnormalities_						Fetal Period _Functional defects & minor morphological abnormalities_			
	Age in weeks after fertilization										
	0–2	3	4	5	6	7	8	9	16	20–36	38
CNS											
Eyes											
Ears											
Palate											
Teeth											
Heart											
Arms											
Legs											
Ext. gen.											

[1] CNS = central nervous system; Ext. gen. = external genitalia; darker shaded areas indicate highly sensitive time periods to teratogens; lighter shaded areas indicate less sensitive time periods to teratogens. Adapted from Moore KL: _The Developing Human,_ 4th ed., WB Saunders, 1988.

ated deformations and the fetal akinesis sequence (see also Chapter 11). Maternal systemic lupus erythematosus has resulted in loss of pregnancy and congenital heart block. Maternal endocrinopathies, eg, parathyroid and thyroid disorders, may result in the loss of pregnancy or changes in the corresponding fetal gland development and function.

The recurrence risks for the adverse effects of teratogens are related to repeated exposure of the fetus to such agents; continued public and professional education is needed to increase awareness of this problem.

Table 25–10A. Common teratogens: Congenital infections.[1]

Infection	Associated Birth Defects and Other Findings
Protozoa	
Congenital *Toxoplasmosis gondii*	Infection occurs in 0.1% of all pregnancies. 30–50% risk of transmission of maternal infection to fetus; increases with gestation: 25% first trimester, 54% 2nd trimester, 65% 3rd trimester. First trimester: early loss of pregnancy; 75% risk of severe manifestations. Risk of severe manifestations decreases during gestation; none if transmitted in third trimester. 10% of infected neonates symptomatic: microcephaly, hydrocephalus, diffuse intracranial calcification, seizures, psychomotor retardation, chorioretinitis, microphthalmia, cataracts, glaucoma, hepatomegaly, jaundice, anemia, thrombocytopenia, pneumonia, myocarditis, nephritis, rashes. Later onset symptoms: spasticity, blindness, deafness.
Spirochetes	
Congenital syphilis (*Treponema pallidum*)	Transmission of infection to fetus can occur at any time during gestation, but usually occurs after 4 months gestation. Of those infected, 50% infected are premature, stillborn, or die in perinatal period; 50% will have congenital syphilis. If infected late in pregnancy only 10% have congenital syphilis. Early congenital syphilis (findings during first 2 years of life): hydrops fetalis, large placenta, IUGR, hepatosplenomegaly, hepatitis, lymphadenopathy, jaundice, anemia, thrombocytopenia, leukemoid reactions, rhinitis, rashes, mucocutaneous lesions, condyloma lata, nephrosis, pneumonia, hydrocephalus, chorioretinitis, uveitis, optic atrophy, glaucoma. Late congenital syphilis: notched or peg-shaped teeth (Hutchinson), "mulberry" molars, osteitis and osteochrondritis, interstitial keratitis, deafness, frontal bossing, saddle nose, "saber" shins, synovial effusions (Clutton joints), deep linear facial scarring (rhagedes), psychomotor retardation, seizures, cranial nerve palsies.
Viruses	
Congenital cytomegalovirus (CMV)	30–40% of maternal infections transmitted to fetus. 1–3% of all neonates will be infected with CMV. 10–15% symptomatic at birth; of these, 20–30% neonatal mortality. General: IUGR. CNS: microcephaly, periventricular calcifications, hydrocephalus, seizures, severe-profound psychomotor retardation, deafness. Eye: chorioretinitis, optic atrophy, cataracts. Signs of systemic congenital viral infection in neonate as in rubella. Occasionally cardiac defects, biliary and esophageal atresias, omphalocele, cleft palate, hypospadias; unclear if related to CMV infection. 13–16% of those asymptomatic at birth will later have neurological impairments. Infected women may give birth to more than one infected child.
Congenital herpes simplex (HSV-1 and HSV-2)	10% maternal infections transmitted to fetus. Early loss of pregnancy, fetal death. Symptomatic neonates: microcephaly, intracranial calcification, hydranencephaly, chorioretinitis, psychomotor retardation, seizures, microphthalmia, PDA, scarring vesicular rash, hepatomegaly, hepatosplenomegaly, osteitis, adrenal failure, hypoplastic distal phalanges.
Congenital parvovirus B19 (Fifth disease)	33% or more of maternal infections transmitted to fetus and usually result in stillbirth, severe non-immune hydrops fetalis. With infection prior to 20 weeks, fetal death rate 3–9%. No structural anomalies noted.
Congenital rubella (German measles)	45–50% of maternal infections transmitted to fetus. Risk of transmission is 90% during first trimester, 25–30% in second trimester, and 53% in third trimester. Malformation risk highest if fetal infection occurs during first 8 weeks (26–61%), then declines with time during gestation. Psychomotor retardation may result from infection at any time during gestation. General: IUGR. CNS: microcephaly, sensorineural deafness, psychomotor retardation. Eye: cataracts, glaucoma, chorioretinitis, microphthalmia, strabismus. Cardiac defects: PDA, PPS, PS, ASD, VSD, tetralogy of Fallot. Congenital systemic viral illness in neonates associated with interstitial pneumonia, hepatosplenomegaly, hepatitis, lymphadenopathy, hemolytic anemia, thrombocytopenia, direct hyperbilirubinemia, myocarditis, nephritis, meningoencephalitis, osteitis (celery stalk appearance of long bones), rashes, "blueberry muffin" areas of dermal erythropoiesis. Late onset problems: diabetes mellitus, thyroid dysfunction.
Congenital varicella zoster (Chicken pox)	25% of maternal infections transmitted to fetus. Fetal varicella syndrome (FVS) occurs in up to 6.5% with fetal infection between 8 and 20 weeks. During second or third trimester: 0–1.1% adverse effects. Symptomatic neonates: 39% IUGR, 22% neonatal deaths. FVS: most common findings are hypoplasia and paresis of an extremity with scarring cicatricial (zigzag) skin lesions in a dermatome distribution and eye findings: microphthalmia, cataracts, chorioretinitis, optic atrophy, anisocoria. CNS: microcephaly, hydrocephaly, cortical atrophy, intracranial calcification, motor and sensory deficits, seizures, deafness, psychomotor retardation. Gastrointestinal and genitourinary anomalies have been reported.

[1] ASD = atrial septal defect; CNS = central nervous system; IUGR = intrauterine growth retardation; PDA = patent ductus arteriosus; PPS = peripheral pulmonic stenosis; PS = pulmonary valve stenosis; VSD = ventricular septal defect. Tables 25–10A through 25–10D do not include all known teratogens. It is recommended that a consultation be obtained with a person considered an expert in teratology prior to counseling in individual cases.

Table 25–10B. Common teratogens: Drugs and pharmaceuticals.[1]

Drug or Pharmaceutical	Associated Birth Defects and Other Findings
Angiotensin converting enzyme (ACE) inhibitors	
Enalapril, captopril, and others	Use during second and third trimester associated with hypoplasia of skull, renal failure, oligohydramnios deformation sequence. Prematurity, IUGR, and PDA reported but may or may not be associated. Neonatal hypotension may occur.
Antibiotics	
Streptomycin, and closely related aminoglycosides.	10–15% sensorineural hearing loss.
Tetracycline	Exposure after fourth month gestation: brown staining on deciduous teeth, increased caries, diminished growth of long bones. Permanent teeth may be affected if exposure later in pregnancy. Related to dose and duration of exposure.
Anticoagulants	
Coumadin (Warfarin)	Increased risk of early loss of pregnancy, stillbirth. One-third of exposed are affected. Exposure between 6 and 9 weeks: IUGR, psychomotor retardation, hypotonia, seizures, craniofacial abnormalities with severe nasal hypoplasia, choanal atresia; chondrodysplasia punctata (stippled epiphyses), hypoplastic nails, short fingers. Occasionally microcephaly, hydrocephalus, agenesis of the corpus callosum, optic atrophy, microphthalmia. Exposure in second and third trimester: IUGR, psychomotor retardation, seizures, optic atrophy.
Heparin	Use during pregnancy associated with 10–15% stillborn, 20% premature births.
Anticonvulsants	
Carbemazepine (Tegretol)	Phenotype similar to FHS. Prenatal and postnatal growth deficiency, psychomotor delay, microcephaly, narrow bifrontal diameter head, upward slanting palpebral fissures, epicanthal folds, short nose, long philtrum, cardiac defects, nail hypoplasia.
Diazepam (Valium)	First trimester exposure: may be at increased risk for cleft lip and/or palate.
Phenobarbital	Probably low risk. Very rarely features similar to FHS reported.
Phenylhydantoin (Dilantin)	10% with prenatal exposure will have fetal hydantoin syndrome (FHS). 33% of exposed will have some effect. Minimal effects: learning and behavioral difficulties. FHS: IUGR, postnatal growth deficiency, mild-moderate psychomotor retardation, large anterior fontanel, ridged metopic suture, midfacial hypoplasia with hypertelorism, depressed nasal bridge, short anteverted nose, bowed upper lip, cleft lip and/or cleft palate, hypoplasia of nails and distal digits, cardiac defects, ocular colobomas, hernias. Variable fetal susceptibility (see text). May have an increased risk for neuroblastoma or other tumors of neural tissue origin.
Primidone (Mysoline)	Probably low risk. Very rarely features similar to FHS reported.
Trimethadione (Tridione)	Early exposure: 25% early loss of pregnancy. 83% have at least one malformation. 33% die during first year of life. Fetal trimethadione syndrome (FTS): IUGR, postnatal growth deficiency, psychomotor retardation, delayed speech. Midfacial hypoplasia, short anteverted nose, flat nasal bridge, synophrys (eyebrows which meet in midline), upward slanting palpebral fissures and "V"-shaped eyebrows, strabismus, ptosis, cleft lip and/or cleft palate, cupped ears with overlapping helices, cardiac defects; abnormal kidneys and external genitalia.
Valproic acid (Depakene, Depakote)	29% Fetal valproate syndrome (FVS): IUGR, narrow bifrontal diameter head, high forehead, shallow orbits, epicanthal folds, telecanthus, flat nasal bridge, short anteverted nares, long thin philtrum, thin upper lip, small mouth, micrognathia, minor ear anomalies, cleft lip and/or palate, cardiac defects (VSD, coarctation of aorta, PDA, HLH), internal and external anomalies of genitalia, long fingers and toes, hyperconvex nails, defects in closure of neural tube (1–2%), psychomotor retardation.
Antithyroid medications	
Propylthiouracil, carbamizole, methimazole, [131]I	Hypothyroidism, psychomotor retardation. Limb and scalp defects noted with methimazole.
Chemotherapeutic	
Alkylating agents (chlorambucil, busulphan, cyclophosphamide)	10–35% exposed: early loss of pregnancy, IUGR, psychomotor retardation. Microphthalmia, cleft palate, genitourinary, and limb malformations.
Folic acid antagonists (aminopterin, methotrexate)	Early exposure: early loss of pregnancy. Later first trimester: IUGR, malformations of the skull, defects in ossification of skeleton, prominent eyes, ocular hypertelorism, hypoplastic supraorbital ridge, cleft lip and palate, malformed ears, micrognathia, limb and vertebral abnormalities, defects in closure of the neural tube, mild psychomotor retardation.

Table 25–10B. *(Continued)*

Drug or Pharmaceutical	Associated Birth Defects and Other Findings
Hormones	
Androgenic progestins (ethisterone, norethindrone)	High dose, 1–2% risk, if taken prior to 12 weeks after conception, for masculinization of female fetus; ambiguous genitalia in female. Progestins may have increased cardiovascular anomalies.
Androgens	Masculinization of female fetus if exposure prior to 12 weeks after conception.
Corticosteroids	1% risk for cleft palate or adrenal atrophy.
Diethylstilbesterol	Female offspring: cervical and vaginal anomalies (22–58%); 18–47% spontaneous abortions, infertility, fallopian tube abnormalities (18–47%), ectopic pregnancies (2.6–6.5%); preterm deliveries (10–30%); adenocarcinoma vagina (1.4–14 per 1000). Male offspring: conflicting reports of genitourinary malformations; possible increased risk for infertility and testicular malignancy.
Oral contraceptives, combined progestogens and estrogens	Conflicting reports of 2- to 4-fold increase in VATER association.
Inorganic iodides/iodine	
Dietary iodine deficiency	Endemic in certain areas. If occurs during the first one-half of gestation results in maternal and fetal goiter and hypothyroidism. Various degrees of psychomotor retardation, spastic diplegia, deafness, strabismus, nystagmus.
Dietary iodine excess (mucolytic agents, or as a thyroid-suppression medication)	Exposure after first trimester at risk for prenatal goiter, polyhydramnios (decreased fetal swallowing); neonatal massive thyromegaly with respiratory obstruction, feeding difficulties, transient hypothyroidism, occasionally hyperthyroidism.
Tranquilizers and psychotropics	
Lithium	First trimester exposure: 6 times risk of congenital heart disease, especially Ebstein anomaly of tricuspid valve; overall malformations 11%. Usually no effect on fetus after 45 days after conception.
Thalidomide	Effect only between 20 and 40 days after conception. Phocomelia (arms more affected than legs), polydactyly, syndactyly, facial capillary hemangiomas, hydrocephalus, eye and ear defects; esophageal or duodenal atresia, cardiac (tetralogy of Fallot), and renal anomalies. Usually normal psychomotor development.
Vitamins	
Folic acid	Decreased maternal intake of folic acid associated with an increased risk for defects in closure of the neural tube. Recommend at least 400 micrograms folic acid daily.
Retinoic acid: Etretinate (Tegison)	Similar defects to isotretinoin. Very long half-life; adverse fetal affects have been noted after 3 years discontinuance. Recommend not conceive until further information available.
Retinoic acid: Isotretinoin (Accutane)	Highest risk from 2–5 weeks after conception. Spontaneous abortions (40%). 25% with malformations. Features are similar to DiGeorge sequence and associated with abnormal migration of cranial neural crest cells. Craniofacial defects (81%): facial asymmetry, missing or small ears, abnormal middle ear, accessory parietal sutures, narrow sloping forehead, micrognathia, Robin sequence-type cleft palate, midfacial hypoplasia with flat nasal bridge, ocular hypertelorism. Cardiac defects (33%): conotruncal defects, VSD, aortic arch abnormalities. Abnormal thymus, immunodeficiency (33%). CNS (86%): microcephaly, hydrocephalus, posterior fossa cysts, cortical blindness, facial palsies, defects in closure of the neural tube, psychomotor retardation. Hypoplastic kidneys, hydroureter. Other defects reported. Recommend discontinue for at least 1 month before conceiving.
Vitamin A	With megadoses, over 15,000 units per day: sirenomelia and oculo-auriculo-vertebral sequences, genitourinary malformations. Recommend maximum of 8000 units per day during pregnancy.

[1] ASD = atrial septal defect; CNS = central nervous system; FHS = fetal hydantoin syndrome; HLH = hypoplastic left heart; IUGR = intrauterine growth retardation; PDA = patent ductus arteriosus; VSD = ventricular septal defect. Tables 25–10A through 25–10D do not include all known teratogens. It is recommended that a consultation be obtained with a person considered an expert in teratology prior to counseling in individual cases.

Table 25–10C. Common teratogens: Environmental chemicals and physical agents.[1]

Chemical or Physical Agent	Associated Birth Defects and Other Findings
Alcohol (ethyl alcohol)	Most common cause of mental retardation in Western world; 1 in 300–1 in 2000 live births. Wide range of dose-related effects from fetal alcohol syndrome (FAS) to only behavioral or learning difficulties. FAS: 30–50% or more of infants of mothers with chronic alcoholism. Early loss of pregnancy. Prenatal and postnatal growth deficiency, psychomotor retardation, poor coordination, attention deficit disorders with hyperactivity. Microcephaly, absence of corpus callosum; characteristic facies with midfacial hypoplasia, epicanthal folds, flat nasal bridge, short palpebral fissures, microphthalmia, unilateral ptosis, short upturned nose and indistinct philtrum, thin upper lip, malformed teeth. Joint contractures, abnormal palmar creases, congenital heart disease (ASD, VSD), scoliosis, renal anomalies. Disagreement on minimal amount of alcohol needed to produce a fetal effect. Recommend: abstain from use during pregnancy.
Cocaine	Exposure occurs in up to 10% of all pregnancies. Spontaneous abortions, prematurity, abruptio placenta. Exposure in first trimester: 15.7% vascular disruptions, with associated porencephaly, gastrointestinal, genitourinary, and limb reductions defects. Psychomotor retardation, behavioral difficulties. Often occurs with polydrug use. During first trimester, only occasional recreational use, usually not associated with increased risk of malformations.
Ionizing radiation	Malformations usually only noted with large doses used for treating malignancies, or doses over 10 rads. Early loss of pregnancy, microcephaly, eye anomalies, cataracts, spina bifida cystica, cleft palate, skeletal and visceral malformations, psychomotor retardation. Most diagnostic radioimaging studies do not affect the fetus directly or result in malformations; more likely there is a possible risk for DNA mutations in germ cells and increased risk (1.5 times general population risk) for leukemia.
Maternal hyperthermia	Temperature 38.9°C or more; usually over a 24-hour period or more with intercurrent illness; as minimal as 30–45 minutes in sauna or hot tub. Exposure between 4 and 14 weeks: IUGR, microcephaly, hypotonia, microphthalmia, midfacial hypoplasia, micrognathia, cleft lip and/or palate, malformed ears, Moebius sequence, neural tube defects, seizures, psychomotor retardation.
Methylmercury	Found in seed grains treated with methylated mercurial fungicides and in fish from contaminated waters. If exposed between 2 and 5 weeks after conception: severe microcephaly, spasticity, psychomotor retardation.
Polyhalogenated biphenyls (PCBs, PBBs)	Found in contaminated cooking oil. Cutaneous and mucosal hyperpigmentation (brown staining) of the skin, IUGR, exophthalmus, natal teeth, gum hypertrophy, nail dystrophy, acne, conjunctivitis.
Toluene (glue sniffing)	Features similar to FAS with prenatal and postnatal growth deficiency, microcephaly, psychomotor retardation, craniofacial defects, caudal regression sequence.
Tobacco (nicotine)	Dose-related IUGR, fetal loss, neonatal deaths, prematurity.

[1] ASD = atrial septal defect; FAS = fetal alcohol syndrome; IUGR = intrauterine growth retardation; VSD = ventricular septal defect. Tables 25–10A through 25–10D do not include all known teratogens. It is recommended that a consultation be obtained with a person considered an expert in teratology prior to counseling in individual cases.

Table 25–10D. Common teratogens: Maternal disorders.[1]

Maternal Disorder	Associated Birth Defects and Other Findings
Diabetes mellitus	Outcome varies with degree of control of maternal diabetes during pregnancy. Insulin-dependent diabetic at higher risk than non-insulin dependent or gestational diabetics. Increased risk of early loss of pregnancy. 8% risk for major malformations of heart (transposition of great vessels), anencephaly, spina bifida, hydrocephaly, holoprosencephaly, cleft lip and/or palate, renal anomalies, VATER association-like findings, caudal regression sequence similar to sirenomelia sequence, and hypoplasia-unusual facies syndrome. (See also Chapter 12.)
Hyperparathyroidism	Usually occurs with parathyroid adenomas. Increased risk for loss of pregnancy and stillbirth. Fetal and neonatal hypoparathyroidism, hypocalcemia, tetany.
Hyperthyroidism	Usually occurs with Graves disease. Increased risk for loss of pregnancy. If thyroid-stimulating globulins present, fetal and neonatal hyperthyroidism. Treatment with antithyroid medications can result in fetal hypothyroidism.
Hypoparathyoidism	Fetal and neonatal hyperparathyroidism; hypercalcemia, demineralized skeleton, fractures, bowing of long bones. Occasionally IUGR, pulmonary artery stenosis, VSD, hypotonia.
Hypothyroidism	Increased risk for loss of pregnancy. Because fetal thyroid development is independent of maternal thyroxine levels, fetal and neonatal thyroid development and function not affected.
Myopathies	Myotonia congenita and myasthenia gravis associated with fetal akinesis sequence. (See also Deformations and Chapter 11.)
Phenylketonuria	Outcome varies with degree of control of maternal phenylalanine (phe) levels during pregnancy. Uncontrolled (phe level over 20 mg/dl) throughout pregnancy: psychomotor retardation (92%), microcephaly (73%), congenital heart disease (12%), prenatal onset growth deficiency (40%), spontaneous early miscarriage (24%). Abnormal facies similar to FAS (Figure 25–9). (See also Section on Inborn Errors of Metabolism.)
Systemic lupus erythematosus	Early loss of pregnancy, congenital heart block.

[1] FAS = fetal alcohol syndrome; VSD = ventricular septal defect. Tables 25–10A through 25–10D do not include all known teratogens. It is recommended that a consultation be obtained with a preson considered an expert in teratology prior to counseling in individual cases.

REFERENCES AND SUGGESTED READING

Beighton P (editor): *McKusick's Heritable Disorders of Connective Tissue,* 5th ed. Mosby, 1993.

Buyse ML (editor): *Birth Defects Encyclopedia,* Center for Birth Defects Information Services, Inc., 1990.

Byers PH: Disorders of collagen biosynthesis and structure. Pages 4029–4077 in: *The Metabolic and Molecular Bases of Inherited Disease,* 7th edition. Scriver CR et al (editors). McGraw Hill, 1995.

Emery AEH, Rimoin DL (editors): *Principles and Practice of Medical Genetics,* 2nd edition. Churchill Livingstone, 1990.

Evans RM: The steroid and thyroid hormone receptor superfamily. Science 1988;**240:**889.

Gilbert SF: *Developmental Biology,* 3rd ed. Sinauer Associates, 1991.

Goodman RM, Gorlin RJ: *The Malformed Infant and Child: An Illustrated Guide.* Oxford University Press, 1983.

Graham JM: *Smith's Recognizable Patterns of Human Deformation,* 2nd ed. WB Saunders, 1988.

Hall JG (editor): Medical Genetics I. Ped Clin NA (Feb) 1992; **39:**1.

Hall JG (editor): Medical Genetics II. Ped Clin NA (April) 1992; **39:**199.

Hall JG, Froster-Iskenius NG, Allanson JE: *Handbook of Normal Physical Measurements.* Oxford Medical Publications, 1989.

Johnston MC: Understanding human embryonic development. Pages 31–63 in: *Human Malformations and Related Anomalies.* Stevenson RE, Hall JG, Goodman RM (editors). Oxford University Press, 1993.

Jones KL: *Smith's Recognizable Patterns of Human Malformations,* 4th ed. WB Saunders, 1988.

Kimmel CA, Buelke-Sam J (editors): *Developmental Toxicology,* 2nd ed. Raven Press, 1994.

Ledbetter DH, Ballabio A: Molecular cytogenetics of contiguous gene syndromes. Pages 811–839 in: *The Metabolic and Molecular Bases of Inherited Disease,* 7th ed. Scriver CR et al (editors). McGraw Hill, 1995.

McKusick VA: *Mendelian Inheritance in Man: catalogs of autosomal dominant, autosomal recessive, and X-linked phenotypes,* 11th ed. Johns Hopkins University Press, 1994.

Milton DA: Pattern formation during animal development. Science 1991;**252:**234.

Moore KL: *The Developing Human: Clinically Oriented Embryology,* 4th ed. WB Saunders, 1988.

Sapienza C, Hall JG: Genetic imprinting in human disease. Pages 437–458 in: *The Metabolic and Molecular Bases of Inherited Disease,* 7th ed. Scriver CR et al (editors). McGraw Hill, 1995.

Schardein JL: *Chemically Induced Birth Defects,* 2nd ed. Marcel Dekker, 1993.

Stevenson RE, Hall JG, Goodman RM (editors): *Human Malformations and Related Anomalies.* Vols 1 and 2. Oxford University Press, 1993.

Tabin CJ: Retinoids, homeoboxes, and growth factors: Toward molecular models for limb development. Cell 1991;**66:**199.

Wilkie AOM, Amberger JS, McKusick VA: A gene map of congenital malformations. J Med Genetics 1994;**31:** 507.

SECTION V.
Appendices

Prototype Pedigrees

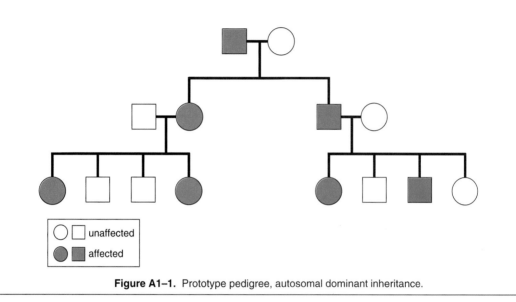

Figure A1–1. Prototype pedigree, autosomal dominant inheritance.

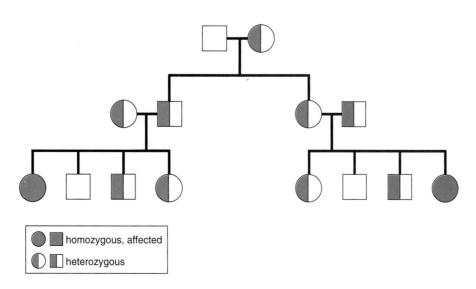

Figure A1–2. Prototype pedigree, autosomal recessive inheritance.

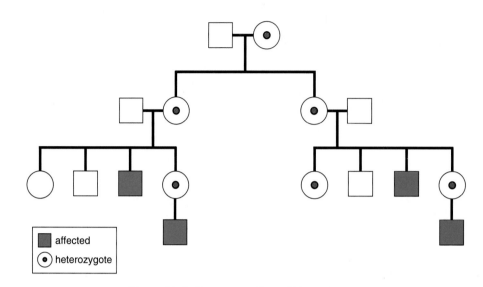

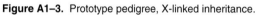

Figure A1–3. Prototype pedigree, X-linked inheritance.

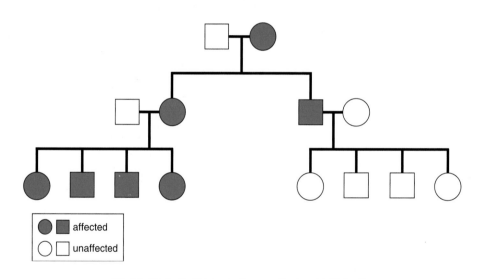

Figure A1–4. Prototype pedigree, mitochondrial inheritance.

MIM Numbers & Chromosomal Locations for the Inborn Errors of Metabolism

II

Display A2–1. Key to Appendix II abbreviations.

Abbreviation	Term
AR	Autosomal recessive
ATP	Adenosine triphosphate
cAMP	Cyclic adenosine monophosphate
CoA	Coenzyme A
ETF	Electron transfer flavoprotein
GTP	Guanosine triphosphate
MIM	Mendelian Inheritance in Man[1]
mtDNA	Mitochondrial DNA
NADH	Reduced form of nicotinamide-adenine dinucleotide

[1] From McKusick VA: *Mendelian Inheritance in Man: Catalogs of autosomal dominant, autosomal recessive, and X-linked phenotypes,* 11th ed. Johns Hopkins University Press, 1994, and OMIM (on-line version), 1995.

Table A2–1. Disorders of amino acids and organic acids.

Disorder(s) of	Name	MIM Number	Chromosomal Location
Phenylalanine and tyrosine metabolism			
	Phenylketonuria; phenylalanine hydroxylase deficiency	261600	12q22-q24.1
	Phenylketonuria; dihydropteridine reductase deficiency	261630	4p15.3
	Phenylketonuria; dihydrobiopterin synthetase deficiency	261640	11q22.3–q23.3
	Phenylketonuria; GTP cyclohydrolase I deficiency	233910	14q22.1–q22.2
	Tyrosinemia type I; fumarylacetoacetate hydrolase deficiency	276700	15q23-q25
	Tyrosinemia type II; tyrosine aminotransferase deficiency	276600	16q22.1-q22.3
	4-Hydroxyphenylpyruvic acid dioxygenase deficiency	276710	12q14–qter
	Alkaptonuria	203500	3q2
Methionine metabolism			
	Hypermethioninemia	250850	
	Homocystinuria; cystathionine synthase deficiency	236200	21q21-22.1
	Homocystinuria; 5,10-methylenetetrahydrofolate reductase deficiency	236250	1p36.3
	Homocystinuria; 5-methyltetrahydrofolate:homocystine methyltransferase deficiency	156570	1
	Sulfite oxidase deficiency	272300	
	Molybdenum cofactor deficiency	252150	
	Histidinemia	235800	12q22-q23
	Urocanic acidemia	276880	
	Formiminotransferase deficiency	229100	
Urea cycle			
	N-Acetylglutamate synthetase deficiency	237310	
	Carbamyl phosphate synthetase I deficiency	237300	2p
	Ornithine transcarbamylase deficiency	311250	Xp21.1
	Citrullinemia	215700	9q34
	Argininosuccinic aciduria	207900	7cen-q11.2
	Argininemia	207800	6q23
	Ornithine aminotransferase deficiency	258870	10q26
Glycine metabolism			
	Nonketotic hyperglycinemia	238300	9p13
Lysine metabolism			
	Familial hyperlysinemia	238700	
	Saccharopinuria	268700	
	Glutaric acidemia type I; glutaryl-CoA dehydrogenase deficiency	231670	19p13.2
Branched chain amino acids			
	Hypervalinemia	277100	
	Hyperleucine-isoleucinemia	238340	
	Maple syrup urine disease; decarboxylase $E_1\alpha$ subunit deficiency	248600	19q13.1-13.2
	Maple syrup urine disease; decarboxylase $E_1\beta$ subunit deficiency	248611	6p22-p21
	Maple syrup urine disease; dihydrolipoyl acyltransferase (E_2) deficiency	248610	1p31
	Maple syrup urine disease; lipoamide dehydrogenase (E_3) deficiency	246900	7q31-q32
	Isovaleric acidemia	243500	15q13-q15
	3-Methylcrotonyl-CoA carboxylase deficiency	210200	
	3-Methylglutaconic aciduria	250950	
	3-Hydroxy-3-methylglutaric acidemia	246450	1pter-p33

Table A2–1. *(Continued)*

Disorder(s) of	Name	MIM Number	Chromosomal Location
	Mevalonic aciduria	251170	12q24.1
	2-Methylacetoacetyl-CoA thiolase (β-ketothiolase) deficiency	203750	11q22.3–q23.1
	Propionic acidemia, type pccA	232000	13q32
	Propionic acidemia, type pccB	232050	3q21-q22
	Holocarboxylase synthetase deficiency	253270	21q22.1
	Biotinidase deficiency	253260	3p25
	Methylmalonic acidemia, mutase deficiency	251000	6p21.2-p12
	Defects in adenosylcobalamin formation, type cblA	251100	
	Defects in adenosylcobalamin formation, type cblB	251110	
	Combined methylmalonic acidemia and homocystinuria, type cblC	277400	
	Combined methylmalonic acidemia and homocystinuria, type cblD	277410	
	Combined methylmalonic acidemia and homocystinuria, type cblF	277380	
	Defects in methylcobalamin formation, type cblE	236270	
	Defects in methylcobalamin formation, type cblG	250940	
Proline and hydroxyproline metabolism			
	Hyperprolinemia type I	239500	
	Hyperprolinemia type II	239510	
	Hyperhydroxyprolinemia	237000	
	Iminoglycinuria	242600	
γ-Glutamyl cycle			
	5-Oxoprolinuria; glutathione synthetase deficiency	266130	
	Glutathione synthetase deficiency confined to erythrocytes	231900	
	γ-Glutamyl-cysteine synthetase deficiency	230450	
	γ-Glutamyl transpeptidase deficiency	231950	21q11.1-q11.2
	5-Oxoprolinase deficiency	260005	
Oxalate metabolism			
	Hyperoxaluria type I	259900	2q36-q37
	Hyperoxaluria type II	260000	16q13
Amino acid transport			
	Cystinuria	220100	2p
	Hartnup disease	234500	
	Lysinuria protein intolerance	222700	
	Hyperammonemia-hyperornithinemia-homocitrullinuria syndrome	238970	13q34

Table A2–2. Disorders of carbohydrate metabolism.

Disorder(s) of	Name	MIM Number	Chromosomal Location
Galactose metabolism			
	Galactosemia; galactose-1-phosphate uridyl transferase deficiency	230400	9p13
	Galactokinase deficiency	230200	17q21-q22
	Uridine diphosphate galactose-4-epimerase deficiency	230350	1pter-p32
Fructose metabolism			
	Fructose-1-phosphate aldolase B deficiency	229600	9q13-q32
	Fructose-1,6-diphosphatase deficiency	229700	
Glycogen storage disorders (GSD)			
	GSD type zero; glycogen synthetase deficiency	240600	
	GSD type Ia; glucose-6-phosphatase deficiency	232200	17
	GSD type Ib; glucose-6-phosphate transport defect	232220	
	GSD type Ic; inorganic phosphate transport defect	232240	
	GSD type II; lysosomal acid maltase deficiency	232300	17q23
	GSD type III; debrancher deficiency	232400	1p21
	GSD type IV; brancher deficiency	232500	3p12
	GSD type V; muscle phosphorylase deficiency	232600	11p13-qter
	GSD type VI; hepatic phosphorylase deficiency	232700	14
	GSD type VII; phosphofructokinase deficiency	232800	1cen-q32
	GSD type VIII; defect unknown	None	
	GSD type IXa; hepatic phosphorylase kinase deficiency, AR	172490	16q12-q13
	GSD type IXb; hepatic phosphorylase kinase deficiency, X-lined	306000	Xp22.2-p22.1
	GSD type IXc; hepatic and muscle phosphorylase kinase deficiency	261750	
	GSD type X; cAMP-dependent protein kinase deficiency ?	(172490)	
	GSD type XI; phosphoglucomutase ?	171900	1p31
Other disorders of carbohydrate metabolism			
	Glycerol kinase deficiency	307030	Xp21.3-p21.2

Table A2–3. Disorders of mitochondrial fatty acid oxidation.

Name	MIM Number	Chromosomal Location
Medium chain acyl-CoA dehydrogenase deficiency	201450	1p31
Long chain acyl-CoA dehydrogenase deficiency	201460	2q34-q35
Long chain 3-hydroxyl acyl-CoA dehydrogenase deficiency	143450	
Short chain acyl-CoA dehydrogenase deficiency	201470	12q22-qter
2,4-Dienoyl-CoA reductase deficiency	222745	
Carnitine plasma membrane transporter deficiency	212140	
Carnitine palmityl transferase I deficiency	255120	1p32
Carnitine palmityl transferase II deficiency	255110	
Glutaric acidemia type II; α-ETF subunit deficiency	231680	15q23-q25
Glutaric acidemia type II; β-ETF subunit deficiency	231680	19
Ethylmalonic-adipic acidemia	231680	15q23-q25

Table A2–4. Lactic acidosis and disorders of mitochondrial oxidative phosphorylation.

Disorder(s) of	Name	MIM Number	Chromosomal Location
Pyruvate metabolism			
	Pyruvate carboxylase deficiency	266150	11q
	Phosphoenolpyruvate carboxykinase deficiency	261650	
	Pyruvate dehydrogenase $E_1\alpha$ subunit deficiency	312170	Xp22.2-p22.1
	Pyruvate dehydrogenase $E_1\beta$ subunit deficiency	179060	3p13-q23
	Pyruvate dehydrogenase E_2 subunit deficiency	245348	
	Pyruvate dehydrogenase E_3 subunit deficiency	246900	7q31-q32
The Krebs Cycle			
	Fumarase deficiency	136850	1q42.1
Mitochondrial oxidative phosphorylation			
	Complex I of respiratory chain; NADH:ubiquinone oxidoreductase def.	252010	
	Complex I of respiratory chain; subunits ND1, ND2, ND3, ND4, ND5, ND6	516000–516006	mtDNA
	Complex II of respiratory chain; succinate:ubiquinone oxidoreductase def.	252011	
	Complex III of respiratory chain; ubiquinol:ferrocytochrome c oxidoreductase deficiency	124000	
	Complex III of respiratory chain; cytochrome b subunit	516020	mtDNA
	Complex IV of respiratory chain; cytochrome c oxidase deficiency	220110	
	Complex IV of respiratory chain; cytochrome c oxidase subunit I	516030	mtDNA
	Complex IV of respiratory chain; cytochrome c oxidase subunit II	516040	mtDNA
	Complex IV of respiratory chain; cytochrome c oxidase subunit III	516050	mtDNA
	Complex V of respiratory chain; ATP synthetase deficiency	164360	10
	Complex V of respiratory chain; ATP synthetase, subunit ATPase 6	516060	mtDNA
	Complex V of respiratory chain; ATP synthetase, subunit ATPase 8	516070	mtDNA
	Leigh syndrome	256000	
	Alpers syndrome	203700	
	Chronic progressive external ophthalmoplegia	258450	
	Luft syndrome	238800	
	Kearns-Sayre syndrome	530000	mtDNA
	Pearson syndrome	557000	mtDNA
	Leber hereditary optic neuropathy (LHON)	535000	mtDNA
	Neuropathy, ataxia, and neuropathy (NARP)	551500	mtDNA
	Mitochondrial encephalomyopathy with lactic acidosis and stroke-like episodes (MELAS)	540000	mtDNA
	Myoclonic epilepsy and ragged-red fibers (MERRF)	545000	mtDNA
	Diabetes mellitus and deafness	520000	mtDNA
	Myoneurogastrointestinal encephalopathy syndrome (MNGIE)	550900	mtDNA

Table A2–5. Disorders of peroxisomes.

Name	MIM Number	Chromosomal Location
Zellweger syndrome	214100	7q11.23
Neonatal adrenoleukodystrophy	202370	
Infantile Refsum disease	266510	
Hyperpipecolic acidemia	239400	
Rhizomelic chondrodysplasia punctata	215100	
Adrenoleukodystrophy	300100	Xq28
Pseudo-neonatal adrenoleukodystrophy	264470	
Pseudo-Zellweger syndrome	261510	3p23-p22
Hyperoxaluria type I	259900	2q36-q37
Acatalasemia	115500	11p13
Glutaryl-CoA oxidase deficiency	231690	

Table A2–6. Porphyrias.

Name	MIM Number	Chromosomal Location
Congenital erythropoietic porphyria	263700	10q25.2-q26.3
Erythropoietic protoporphyria	177000	18q21.3-q22
Hepatoerythropoietic porphyria	176100	1p34
Acute intermittent porphyria	176000	11q24.1-q24.2
Porphyria cutanea tarda	176100	1p34
Hereditary coproporphyria	121300	9
Variegate porphyria	176200	
δ-Aminolevulinic acid dehydratase deficiency	125270	9q34

Table A2–7. Disorders of purines and pyrimidines.

Name	MIM Number	Chromosomal Location
Gout, primary hyperuricemia	138900	
Lesch-Nyhan syndrome	308000	Xq26-27.2
Phosphoribosylpyrophosphate synthetase overactivity	311850	Xq22-q24
Adenylosuccinase deficiency	103050	22q13.1
Adenine phosphoribosyl transferase deficiency	102600	16q22.2-q22.3
Xanthine oxidase deficiency	278300	2
Myoadenylate deaminase deficiency	102770	1q21-p13
Hereditary orotic aciduria	258900	3q13
Dihydropyrimidine dehydrogenase deficiency	274270	1p22-q21

Table A2–8. Disorders of metal metabolism.

Name	MIM Number	Chromosomal Location
Wilson disease	277900	13q14.3
Menkes disease	309400	Xq13.3
Occipital horn syndrome	304150	Xq13.3
Acrodermatitis enteropathica	201100	
Familial (idiopathic) hemochromatosis	235200	6p21.3

Table A2–9. Disorders of bone metabolism.

Name	MIM Number	Chromosomal Location
Vitamin D dependency type I	264700	12q14
Vitamin D dependency type II	277420	
Familial hypophosphatemic rickets	307800	Xp22
Hypophosphatasia, infantile form	241500	1p36.1-p34
Hypophosphatasia, childhood form	241510	1p36.1-p34
Hypophosphatasia, adult form	146300	1p36.1-p34
Hyperphosphatasia with osteoectasia	239000	

Table A2–10. Other recently characterized inborn errors of metabolism.

Name	MIM Number	Chromosomal Location
Smith-Lemli-Opitz syndrome	270400	7q34-qter
Carbohydrate-deficient glycoprotein syndrome	212065	

Table A2–11. Lysosomal storage disorders.

Disorders of	Name	MIM Number	Chromosomal Location
Mucopolysaccharides (MPS)			
	Hurler syndrome; MPS type IH	252800	4p16.3
	Scheie syndrome; MPS type IS	252800	4p16.3
	Hurler-Scheie syndrome; MPS type IH/IS	252800	4p16.3
	Hunter syndrome; MPS type II	309900	Xq27-28
	Sanfilippo syndrome type A; MPS type IIIA	252900	
	Sanfilippo syndrome type B; MPS type IIIB	252920	
	Sanfilippo syndrome type C; MPS type IIIC	252930	
	Sanfilippo syndrome type D; MPS type IIID	252940	12q14
	Morquio syndrome type A; MPS type IVA	253000	16q24.3
	Morquio syndrome type B; MPS type IVB	253010	3pter-p21
	Maroteaux-Lamy syndrome; MPS type VI	253200	5q11-q13
	β-Glucuronidase deficiency; MPS type VII	253220	7q21.1-q22

Table A2–11. *(Continued)*

Disorders of	Name	MIM Number	Chromosomal Location
Sphingolipids			
	Generalized gangliosidosis; GM$_1$ Gangliosidosis, type 1	230500	3p21.33
	Juvenile GM$_1$ Gangliosidosis, type 2	230600	
	Adult GM$_1$ Gangliosidosis, type 3	230650	
	Tay-Sachs disease	272800	15q23-q24
	Sandhoff disease	268800	5q11
	GM$_2$ Gangliosidosis, sphingolipid activator protein deficiency	272750	5q32-q35
	GM$_3$ Gangliosidosis	305650	
	Fabry Disease	301500	Xq22.1
	Schindler disease	104170	22q11
	Lactosyl ceramidosis	245500	
	Gaucher disease, type 1	230800	1q21
	Gaucher disease, type 2	230900	1q21
	Gaucher disease, type 3	231000	q21
	Farber disease	228000	
	Niemann-Pick disease, sphingomyelinase deficiency, type I	257200	11p15.4-15.1
	Niemann-Pick disease, type II, cholesteryl esterification defect	257220	18q11-q12
	Niemann-Pick disease, type II, other	257250	
	Krabbe disease	245200	14q31
	Metachromatic leukodystrophy (MLD); arylsulfatase A deficiency	250100	22q13.31-qter
	MLD, cerebroside sulfatase activator protein deficiency	249900	10q21-q22
	Multiple sulfatase deficiency	272200	
	Canavan disease	271900	17pter-p13
Glycoproteins (Oligosaccharides)			
	Fucosidosis	230000	1p34
	Mannosidosis, α-mannosidase deficiency	248500	19p13.2-q12
	β-Mannosidase deficiency	248510	
	β-Neuraminidase deficiency	256550	6p21.3
	Sialolipidosis	252650	10pter-q23
	Galactosialidosis	256540	20q12-q13.1
	Aspartylglucosaminuria	208400	4q32-q33
Lysosomal enzyme transport			
	Mucolipidosis type II; I-cell disease	252500	4q21-q23
	Mucolipidosis type III, Pseudo-Hurler polydystrophy	252600	
Lysosomal membrane transport			
	Infantile free sialic acid storage disease	269920	
	Salla disease	269920	
	Cystinosis, early onset, infantile nephropathic type	219800	
	Cystinosis, late onset, juvenile or adolescent type	219900	
Other disorders of lysosomes			
	Pompe disease, acid maltase deficiency	232300	17q23
	Wolman disease	278000	10q23.2-q23.3
	Cholesteryl ester storage disease	278000	10q23.2-q23.3

Five Cases to Test Diagnostic Skills

III

CASE 1

A 28-year-old Man Diagnosed With Cancer of the Colon

Complete each set of questions.

Part I

A 28-year-old man is admitted to the surgery service and diagnosed with cancer of the colon. The surgeon asks the patient's consulting internist whether he should be concerned about a genetic cause for this cancer, and if he should obtain any corresponding special preparation of the cancer at operation the next day. As the internist, you ask yourself some questions in an effort to formulate an answer, and begin to formulate a plan.

1. List three kinds of genetic aberrations that can contribute to the cause of cancer.
2. Describe a method to look for each of these abnormalities and identify the tissues required.
3. For each kind of abnormality, describe a mechanism by which it leads to cancer.

Part II

As the consulting internist in Part I, you feel that a more detailed assessment of the patient would help you consider the genetic implications of this cancer. You decide to see the patient, take a more complete history, and perform a brief physical examination.

1. List four features of the history that might suggest that there are genetic factors operating in the cause of this cancer.
2. Other than the intestinal obstruction associated with this colon cancer, what features of the physical examination will help you rule genetic factors in or out? List as many as you can and tell what implications those findings have for the role of genes.

Part III

The patient tells you that his uncle also had cancer of the colon. The uncle was 40 years old at the time.

This uncle is his mother's brother. The patient does not know about his mother's history in this regard, because she refuses to discuss the topic with him.

1. Using whatever literature you find helpful, list at least two genetic conditions that you should consider in this patient given that history.
2. Draw a pedigree consistent with one of these conditions; tell how you would exclude it or confirm it. Indicate which members of the family are at risk for developing this disease. Discuss how you would use molecular genetic tools to answer these questions; using any literature of your choice, give three examples of molecular analyses for identification of persons at risk.

CASE 2

An Infant With Features Suggesting Down Syndrome

Complete each set of questions.

Part I

You are called to the nursery to see an infant whose features suggest Down syndrome (trisomy 21) when the infant is 4 days old. The infant is still in the hospital after birth because of gastrointestinal obstruction, which has been operated on. Upon taking the family history you determine that the mother is 36 years old, the father is 44 years old, and there are two siblings, a girl 3 years old and a boy 2 years old. You perform a karyotype on white blood cells from the baby.

1. Describe at least two karyotypes that would confirm the diagnosis of Down syndrome in this infant.
2. Does either of these karyotypes predict a difference in severity of the phenotype?
3. Where are the genes that account for the Down syndrome phenotype? What is known about the mechanisms by which these genes account for Down syndrome?

Part II

Having confirmed the diagnosis of Down syndrome, you begin to speak with the family about your finding in the chromosome study.

1. Write one paragraph explaining this diagnosis in terms that the non-physician/scientist family would understand.
2. List five critical pieces of information you wish to get across.

Part III

The family asks you whether there is a risk to them of having another child with Down syndrome and whether others in their family share this risk. They want to know if there are any more tests that you can do that will address this question.

1. What is the risk to them and other family members?
2. What information can you get from the karyotype to answer this question?
3. Are there other tests you can perform to address this risk?
4. List two tests you might perform and tell how either result would affect the answer to the family's question. Explain two mechanisms that increase the risk of having a child with trisomy 21.

CASE 3

A 27-year-old Woman With Muscle Weakness and Visual Disturbance

Complete each set of questions.

Part I

A 27-year-old woman is being evaluated for muscle weakness and a visual disturbance. Histologic examination of muscle tissue reveals mitochondria that are abnormal in shape and position. A disorder of mitochondrial function is suggested as a diagnosis.

1. Outline the major metabolic steps that take place in the mitochondria to support energy metabolism and summarize the overall importance of oxidative phosphorylation.
2. Discuss why some tissues are more affected by mutations that affect mitochondrial function than others.
3. Can mutations affecting mitochondrial oxidative phosphorylation explain muscle weakness and a visual disturbance?

Part II

This woman and her family raise the question of whether genetic factors play a role in the mitochondrial disorders being considered to explain her symptoms. She notes that her mother developed similar symptoms at about age 30 years.

1. List three patterns of inheritance that can be associated with genetic abnormalities in mitochondrial oxidative phosphorylation and tell what the molecular basis for each would be.
2. This woman has two brothers and a sister; she also has a daughter. Construct three pedigrees: one that would be consistent with each of the proposed patterns of inheritance for this family and list the kinds of mutations that would explain the inheritance.

Part III

You discover a molecular genetics laboratory that will examine muscle tissue from the woman described.

1. Using the literature, list at least four specific molecular genetic abnormalities for which you would ask the laboratory to look. Predict the inheritance pattern for each.
2. Draw a pedigree consistent with one of these abnormalities, indicating which members of the family are at risk for developing this disease, and what molecular abnormality you would find in muscle cells and in white blood cells of other affected individuals.
3. Write a short paragraph to give to the family explaining how this molecular abnormality relates to the disease and what the test results mean.

CASE 4

An Infant Girl With Syndactyly Involving the Fingers of Both Hands and One Foot

Complete each set of questions.

Part I

You are called to the nursery to see an infant girl with syndactyly involving the fingers of both hands, and one foot. On the left hand, the thumb is normal, three fingers are shortened and syndactylous, and one finger appears short with a narrowed ring of tissue around it. The right hand is similar, but only two fingers are syndactylous. The toes of the affected foot are syndactylous, shortened, and have no nails.

1. What other features of the physical examination would help you to categorize this group of abnormalities as genetic or non-genetic?
2. List four ways that defects in morphogenesis can occur.
3. Explain how genes can be involved in the control of morphogenesis.

Part II

You take a complete family history and note that the parents are both 27 years old, and this is their second child. Their other child is a girl who is two years old and is healthy. There are no known congenital malformations in the family, and the parents are healthy and unrelated. There were no exposures to known teratogens during the pregnancy.

1. How does the history affect your assessment of whether this is genetic or non-genetic?
2. What genetic mechanisms should still be considered?

Part III

The parents ask if there are any tests that can help you understand this group of abnormalities better.

1. What tests would be helpful? Tell how the results of these tests would influence your assessment.
2. Describe two scenarios: one in which you propose a genetic mechanism and one in which you propose a non-genetic mechanism.
3. For each scenario, tell what features of the examination, the history, and the test results lead you to your conclusion.

CASE 5

A 35-year-old Woman With Her Fourth Pregnancy

Complete each set of questions.

Part I

A woman comes to your obstetrical practice to confirm her suspected pregnancy and begin prenatal care. She is 35 years old and this is her fourth pregnancy. She has one living child and had three spontaneous miscarriages between her son and this pregnancy.

1. List three points you would discuss with her in reference to genetic risks.
2. List three questions you would ask her to identify any genetic risks she may carry. Tell how the answers would allow you to assess this risk.
3. Without knowing anything else about her history, are there any tests you would want her to be informed about that could assess her risk of having a child with a genetic condition or congenital malformations?

Part II

She tells you that her grandparents were Jewish.

1. How does this new information influence your estimation of genetic risks?
2. List two other questions you would be prompted to ask.
3. List three other ethnic backgrounds which would raise your estimate of the genetic risks to this pregnancy.
4. What test could you do to evaluate the risks?

Part III

The patient wants to know more about prenatal diagnosis to address genetic risks. You are concerned about how your patient is feeling about the information you have discussed. You are aware that cultural factors often influence the ways in which people look at pregnancy, risks for babies with abnormalities, and prenatal diagnosis.

1. What prenatal tests will you discuss with this woman?
2. Write a brief paragraph explaining the risks and benefits of the tests you are suggesting that she consider.
3. List three questions you might ask, to develop understanding of the cultural, family, and ethical issues that may be important in her decision to have or decline these tests.

ANSWERS

Case 1

Part I
1. Mutations in proto-oncogenes.
   Mutations in tumor suppressor genes.
   Chromosomal translocations that place genes related to growth under inappropriate genetic control.
   Chromosomal deletions.
   Amplification of genes that control cell growth and division.
2. Molecular techniques to identify mutations in proto-oncogenes or tumor suppressor genes.
   Karyotype with possible use of FISH to identify translocations.
3. Proto-oncogene mutations and tumor suppressor gene mutations lead to abnormal function of proteins that stimulate cell division, receptors that activate those proteins and are in turn activated by other signalling proteins, proteins that suppress cell division and growth, proteins that control programmed cell death, proteins that interact with DNA and control its replication or that turn specific genes off or on.

Part II
1. Family history of cancer.
   Congenital malformations.
   Multiple primary tumors.
   Early onset.
2. Evidence for the above.

Part III
1. Li-Fraumeni syndrome.
   Lynch family cancer syndrome.
   Mutations in BRCA1.
   Familial adenomatous polyposis of the colon (APC).

Gardner syndrome (also APC gene).

Turcot syndrome.

Hereditary non-polyposis colon cancer (HNPCC).

2. See prototype pedigrees in the appendix for all modes of inheritance.

Case 2

1. Standard trisomy 21.

Unbalanced translocation, eg, 14/21.

Mosaicism for trisomy 21.

2. Trisomy and unbalanced translocation have the same phenotype.

Phenotype is variable and unpredictable in mosaicism.

3. 21q22.1-q22.2, is the Down syndrome "critical region"; the genes in this region that are involved are not precisely known.

Part II

1. Read the counseling section in the chapter dealing with cytogenetics, construct such a paragraph and have a colleague read and critique it.

2. Many systems of the body can be affected in Down syndrome, including the central nervous, skeletal, cardiovascular, hematopoietic, systems and thyroid gland.

Ongoing medical care addressing these systems is crucial.

Developmental delay with mental retardation is always a part of the disorder.

Many children with Down syndrome are able to learn the tasks of daily living and grow in adults who can contribute to their communities.

Maternal age is a factor in occurrence; recurrence risk to a future pregnancy depends on maternal age and the presence or absence of a balanced translocation in the parent.

Risk to other family members is minimal unless there is a balanced translocation being inherited in the family.

Prenatal diagnosis is available.

Part III

1. See table in Chapter 7.

2. Information from the karyotype

A. Balanced translocation in infant

1. Karyotype both parents: If one of them carries a balanced translocation, other relatives of that parent may also carry it and this can be determined by performing a karyotype on them;

2. If neither parent carries this translocation, the risks to these other relatives are the same as the general population: age-related risks for the mother.

B. Standard trisomy in the infant

1. Risks to other relatives same as general population; there is no solid evidence for familial tendency to nondisjunction, al-

though there are a few families that suggest that possibility.

C. Mosaicism

1. No evidence for increased risk to relatives, although gonadal mosaicism cannot be excluded.

3. Maternal serum screening using the triple screen can be offered. Prenatal diagnosis can be offered to other family members contemplating pregnancy. While the risks of invasive procedures are low, they are probably higher than such relatives have for a chromosomal abnormality unless the age of the mother is more than 35 years.

4. A. Amniocentesis or chorionic villus sampling

B. Increased risks of trisomy 21 or other autosomal trisomies in a child.

C. Maternal age: Mechanism is non-disjunction in meiosis I or meiosis II, the incidence of which occurs as maternal age advances. The causes at the cellular level of non-disjunction are not known.

D. Translocation: Mechanism is abnormal segregation in meiosis because of inability of homologs to line up correctly. See Chapter 2 for diagram.

Case 3

Part I

1. See Chapter 16 on mitochondrial inheritance and mitochondrial disease for pathways that review how oxidative phosphorylation accomplishes electron transport and generates ATP.

2. Tissues with the highest number of mitochondria and the greatest need for energy are generally most affected. These include nervous system, skeletal muscle, cardiac muscle, eye muscles, and optic nerve.

3. The mutations disrupt energy metabolism in energy-requiring tissues such as skeletal muscle, optic nerve, and retina.

Part II

1. All these mutations affect energy metabolism by disrupting genes coding for subunits in the oxidative phosphorylation pathway.

A. Mitochondrial inheritance: Point mutations in genes on the mitochondrial chromosome.

B. Sporadic (not inherited): Deletions in genes on the mitochondrial chromosome.

C. Autosomal recessive: Mutations in nuclear genes coding for subunits in the oxidative phosphorylation pathway where homozygosity is necessary for expression.

D. Autosomal dominant: Mutations in nuclear genes coding for subunits in the oxidative phosphorylation pathway that are expressed when only one copy of the gene is mutant.

Table A3–1. Disorders of oxidative phosphorylation. Mutations in nuclear DNA (AR unless noted)[1]

Disorder	Complex subunits	Clinical phenotypes
1. Deficiency of Complex I (NADH:ubiquinone oxidoreductase	At least 35 polypeptides; 7 encoded by mtDNA	(1) Muscle weakness (2) Muscle weakness with brain disease and lactic acidosis (3) Central nervous system disease
2. Deficiency of Complex II (succinate: ubiquinone oxidoreductase	4 components, encoded only by nDNA	(1) Central nervous system disease (2) Muscle weakness
3. Deficiency of Complex III (ubiquinol: ferrocytochrome c oxidoreductase)	11 subunits; 1 encoded by mtDNA	(1) Muscle weakness (2) Disease of heart muscle (3) Muscle weakness with brain disease and lactic acidosis
4. Deficiency of Complex IV (cytochrome c oxidase)	13 Subunits; 3 encoded by mtDNA	(1) Muscle weakness (2) Muscle weakness with brain disease and lactic acidosis
5. Deficiency of Complex V (ATP synthase)	12–14 subunits; 2 encoded by mtDNA	(1) Muscle weakness (2) Muscle weakness with brain disease and lactic acidosis
6. Deficiency of coenzyme Q_{10} (CoQ_{10})		(1) Muscle weakness and seizures
7. Defects in intergenomic signaling		
A. Depletion of mtDNA		(1) Muscle weakness and lactic acidosis (2) Liver failure (3) Muscle weakness
B. Multiple mtDNA deletions		(1) AD form of CPEO[2]

[1] AD = autosomal dominant; CPEO = chronic progressive external ophthalmoplegia; Leigh syndrome = subacute necrotizing encephalomyopathy; MNGIE = mitochondrial neuropathy, gastrointestinal disorder, encephalopathy syndrome; mtDNA = mitochondrial DNA; nDNA = nuclear DNA. Modified from Seashore, MR and Wappner, R, Genetics in Primary Care and Clinical Specialities, Appleton&Lange, in press.
[2] CPEO = chronic progressive external ophthalmoplegia = eye muscle weakness.

Table A3–2. Disorders of oxidative phosphorylation. Mutations in mitochondrial DNA[3].

Disorder	Clinical Phenotypes	Inheritance Pattern
A. Large-scale rearrangements (deletions or duplications) of mtDNA	a. Kearns-Sayre syndrome[4] b. Variants of Kearns-Sayre syndrome c. Pearson syndrome (anemia)	Sporadic, not inherited Sporadic, not inherited Sporadic, not inherited
	d. Diabetes mellitus and deafness	Maternal inheritance
B. Point mutations of mtDNA		
1. Structural mtDNA genes	a. LHON;[6] optic nerve disorder b. NARP;[7] abnormal gait, pigmented degeneration of retina	Maternal inheritance Maternal inheritance
2. Synthetic mtDNA mutations [point mutations in mtDNA that affect transfer RNA tRNA)]	a. MELAS; lactic acidosis and stroke-like episodes b. MERRF; myoclonic epilepsy (seizures) and ragged-red (muscle) fibers c. MiMyCa; maternally inherited disorder with adult onset muscle and cardiac muscle disease d. Maternally inherited diabetes and deafness	Maternal inheritance Maternal inheritance Maternal inheritance Maternal inheritance

[3] Modified from Seashore, MR and Wappner, RS, Genetics in Primary Care and Clinical Specialites, Appleton & Lange.
[4] CPEO = chronic progressive external ophthalmoplegia = eye muscle weakness.
[5] CPEO = chronic progressive external ophthalmoplegia = eye muscle weakness.
[6] Leber hereditary optic neuropathy.
[7] neuropathy, ataxia, and retinitis pigmentosa.

2. See Appendix I for prototype pedigrees. Note the mutations listed in the tables.

Part III

1. See tables from Chapters 15 and 16 reproduced here.
2. Draw a pedigree based on the prototype pedigrees. For mitochondrial inheritance, point mutations would be seen in the tissues and the white blood cells of the affected person and the matrilineal relatives. For sporadic inheritance, only the affected person would have the deletion, and it would not be seen in the leukocytes. For the autosomal mutations, the mutations should be seen in tissues and white cells of affected persons and affected relatives. Various molecular techniques can be used depending on the specific mutations, including RFLP analysis, specific oligonucleotide analysis, and DNA sequencing.
3. Write such a paragraph based on the information in the chapters on mitochondrial inheritance and neuromuscular diseases. Have a colleague read and critique it.

Case 4

Part I

1. Genetic abnormalities may be more symmetrical, whereas deformations or abnormalities caused by amniotic bands are more likely to be asymmetrical. The presence of malformations in other systems such as skeletal, cardiac, and central nervous system suggests a general mechanism that may be genetic.
2. Lack of development of an organ or tissue (aplasia or agenesis).
   Incomplete fusion or separation of structures.
   Incomplete septation or canalization.
   Persistence of early forms no longer needed.
   Improper migration or localization of cells, tissues, or organs.
3. Mutations could affect:
   mRNA processing that is needed for site specific expression.
   Genes that code for growth factors or signalling peptides or their receptors.
   Genes that code for proteins involved in apoptosis (programmed cell death).
   Homeotic genes (homeobox) or pax genes (paired box).

Part II

1. Lack of family history for congenital malformations is evidence against genetic disorders but does not exclude them.
2. Recessive or X-linked disorders; new dominant mutations.

Part III

1. Physical exam for other abnormalities; radiographs for bony abnormalities underlying the syn-

dactyly. Abnormal findings might be evidence for a single gene syndrome associated with syndactyly.
2. Outline how you would discuss one of the mechanisms in Part II answer 2; have a colleague read and critique it.
3. New dominant mutation: Features consistent with known syndrome, no family history, radiographs showing abnormal metacarpals or fused bones.
   Recessive disorder: Features consistent with known syndrome, no family history, radiographs consistent.
   Deformation or amniotic bands: Distal abnormalities only, circumferential bands, no family history, no bony abnormalities on radiographs.

Case 5

Part I

1. Maternal age and risk of chromosome abnormalities.
   Three spontaneous abortions and risk of mother or father carrying balanced translocation.
   Risks that everyone carries, some of which can be addressed by maternal serum screening, such as neural tube defects.
2. Family history of congenital malformations, stillbirths, early infant deaths.
   Ethnic background with respect to specific genetic risks.
   Family history of specific genetic conditions by systems: CNS, blood, kidney, musculo-skeletal, hearing, vision, skin, cancer, cardiovascular, metabolic.
3. Maternal serum triple screen.
   Amniocentesis.
   CVS.

Part II

1. If Ashkenazi, risk of this mother being a carrier of the Tay-Sachs mutation is about 1/25; testing for the carrier state is available.
2. Askenazi?
   Any known Tay-Sachs carriers?
   Any known Gaucher disease, Canavan disease, other conditions known to be more common among those of Jewish ancestry?
3. Consider the following:

European and U.S. Caucasians	Cystic fibrosis, PKU
Ashkenazi Jews	Tay-Sachs disease, Gaucher disease (adult)
West Africans	Sickle cell anemia
Mediterranean peoples	β-Thalassemia, Sickle cell anemia
Asian peoples	α-thalassemia, Sickle cell anemia
French-Canadians	Tay-Sachs disease (not Askenazi mutation)

4. Appropriate screening tests for carrier status: Molecular tests for CF, PKU; enzyme analysis for TS, Gaucher disease; Hb electrophoresis, MCV for hemoglobinopathies.

Part III
1. Serum triple screening.
   Amniocentesis.
   CVS.
   Ultrasound.
2. Referring to chapter 7, write such a paragraph and have a colleague read and critique it.

3. How strong a role do religious beliefs and convictions play in your ideas about having children and raising a family?
   What are your beliefs about a family's choice as to whether to have a child who has a serious birth defect or disease that limits physical or intellectual function?
   Do you believe a woman ought to be able to choose to terminate a pregnancy when the child is affected with such a condition?
   How would your husband and family react to the birth of a child with such serious medical problems?

REFERENCES AND SUGGESTED READING

Seashore, MR. Clinical genetics, pages 249–263 in: *Medical Complications During Pregnancy,* 4th ed, Burrow GN, Ferris TF (editors) Saunders, 1995.

INDEX

LANGE
medical books

Available at your local health science bookstore
or by calling
Appleton & Lange toll free
1-800-423-1359 (in CT 203-406-4500).

A smart investment in your medical career

(more on reverse)

Clinical Cardiology, 6/e
Cheitlin, Sokolow, & McIlroy
1993, ISBN 0-8385-1093-0, A1093-2

Fluid & Electrolytes
Physiology & Pathophysiology
Cogan
1991, ISBN 0-8385-2546-6, A2546-8

Basic & Clinical Biostatistics, 2/e
Dawson-Saunders & Trapp
1994, ISBN 0-8385-0542-2, A0542-9

Basic Gynecology and Obstetrics
Gant & Cunningham
1993, ISBN 0-8385-9633-9, A9633-7

Review of General Psychiatry, 4/e
Goldman
1995, ISBN 0-8385-8421-7, A8421-8

Principles of Clinical Electrocardiography, 13/e
Goldschlager & Goldman
1990, ISBN 0-8385-7951-5, A7951-5

Basic & Clinical Endocrinology, 4/e
Greenspan & Baxter
1994, ISBN 0-8385-0560-0, A0560-1

Occupational Medicine
LaDou
1990, ISBN 0-8385-7207-3, A7207-2

Primary Care of Women
Lemcke, Pattison, Marshall, & Cowley
1995, ISBN 0-8385-9813-7, A9813-5

Clinical Anesthesiology, 2/e
Morgan & Mikhail
1996, ISBN 0-8385-1381-6, A1381-1

Dermatology
Orkin, Maibach, & Dahl
1991, ISBN 0-8385-1288-7, A1288-8

Rudolph's Fundamentals of Pediatrics
Rudolph & Kamei
1994, ISBN 0-8385-8233-8, A8233-7

Genetics in Clinical Medicine and Primary Care
Seashore
1995, ISBN 0-8385-3128-8, A3128-4

Smith's General Urology, 14/e
Tanagho & McAninch
1995, ISBN 0-8385-8612-0, A8612-2

Clinical Oncology
Weiss
1993, ISBN 0-8385-1325-5, A1325-8

General Ophthalmology, 14/e
Vaughan, Asbury, & Riordan-Eva
1995, ISBN 0-8385-3127-X, A3127-6

CURRENT Clinical References

CURRENT Critical Care Diagnosis & Treatment,
Bongard & Sue
1994, ISBN 0-8385-1443-X, A1443-9

CURRENT Diagnosis & Treatment in Cardiology
Crawford
1995, ISBN 0-8385-1444-8, A1444-7

CURRENT Diagnosis & Treatment in Vascular Surgery
Dean, Yao, & Brewster
1995, ISBN 0-8385-1351-4, A1351-4

CURRENT Obstetric & Gynecologic Diagnosis & Treatment, 8/e
DeCherney & Pernoll
1994, ISBN 0-8385-1447-2, A1447-0

CURRENT Diagnosis & Treatment in Gastroenterology
Grendell, McQuaid, & Friedman
1996, ISBN 0-8385-1448-0, A1448-8

CURRENT Pediatric Diagnosis & Treatment, 12/e
Hay, Groothuis, Hayward, & Levin
1995, ISBN 0-8385-1446-4, A1446-2

CURRENT Emergency Diagnosis & Treatment, 4/e
Saunders & Ho
1993, ISBN 0-8385-1347-6, A1347-2

CURRENT Diagnosis & Treatment in Orthopedics
Skinner
1995, ISBN 0-8385-1009-4, A1009-8

CURRENT Medical Diagnosis & Treatment 1996
Tierney, McPhee, & Papadakis
1996, ISBN 0-8385-1465-0, A1465-2

CURRENT Surgical Diagnosis & Treatment, 10/e
Way
1994, ISBN 0-8385-1439-1, A1439-7

LANGE Clinical Manuals

Dermatology
Diagnosis and Therapy
Bondi, Jegasothy, & Lazarus
1991, ISBN 0-8385-1274-7, A1274-8

Practical Oncology
Cameron
1994, ISBN 0-8385-1326-3, A1326-6

Office & Bedside Procedures
Chesnutt, Dewar, Locksley, & Tureen
1993, ISBN 0-8385-1095-7, A1095-7

Psychiatry
Diagnosis & Therapy 2/e
Flaherty, Davis, & Janicak
1993, ISBN 0-8385-1267-4, A1267-2

Neonatology
Management, Procedures, On-Call Problems, Diseases and Drugs, 3/e
Gomella
1994, ISBN 0-8385-1331-X, A1331-6

Practical Gynecology
Jacobs & Gast
1994, ISBN 0-8385-1336-0, A1336-5

Drug Therapy, 2/e
Katzung
1991, ISBN 0-8385-1312-3, A1312-6

Ambulatory Medicine
The Primary Care of Families
Mengel & Schwiebert
1993, ISBN 0-8385-1294-1, A1294-6

Poisoning & Drug Overdose, 2/e
Olson
1994, ISBN 0-8385-1108-2, A1108-8

Internal Medicine
Diagnosis and Therapy, 3/e
Stein
1993, ISBN 0-8385-1112-0, A1112-0

Surgery
Diagnosis & Therapy
Stillman
1989, ISBN 0-8385-1283-6, A1283-9

Medical Perioperative Management
Wolfsthal
1989, ISBN 0-8385-1298-4, A1298-7

LANGE Handbooks

Handbook of Gynecology & Obstetrics
Brown & Crombleholme
1993, ISBN 0-8385-3608-5, A3608-5

HIV/AIDS Primary Care Handbook
Carmichael, Carmichael, & Fischl
1995, ISBN 0-8385-3557-7, A3557-4

Pocket Guide to Diagnostic Tests
Detmer, McPhee, Nicoll, & Chou
1992, ISBN 0-8385-8020-3, A8020-8

Handbook of Poisoning
Prevention, Diagnosis & Treatment, 12/e
Dreisbach & Robertson
1987, ISBN 0-8385-3643-3, A3643-2

Handbook of Clinical Endocrinology, 2/e
Fitzgerald
1992, ISBN 0-8385-3615-8, A3615-0

Clinician's Pocket Reference, 7/e
Gomella
1993, ISBN 0-8385-1222-4, A1222-7

Surgery on Call, 2/e
Gomella & Lefor
1996, ISBN 0-8385-8746-1, A8746-8

Internal Medicine On Call
Haist & Robbins
1991, ISBN 0-8385-4052-X, A4052-5

Obstetrics & Gynecology On Call
Horowitz & Gomella
1993, ISBN 0-8385-7174-3, A7174-4

Pocket Guide to Commonly Prescribed Drugs
Levine
1993, ISBN 0-8385-8023-8, A8023-2

Handbook of Pediatrics, 17/e
Merenstein, Kaplan, & Rosenberg
1994, ISBN 0-8385-3657-3, A3657-2

 Appleton & Lange • P.O. Box 120041 • Stamford, CT • 06912-0041 • 1-800-423-1359